canine anatomy

The National Veterinary Medical Series for Independent Study

canine anatomy

Bonnie J. Smith, D.V.M., Ph.D.

Assistant Professor
Virginia-Maryland Regional College of Veterinary Medicine
Blacksburg, Virginia

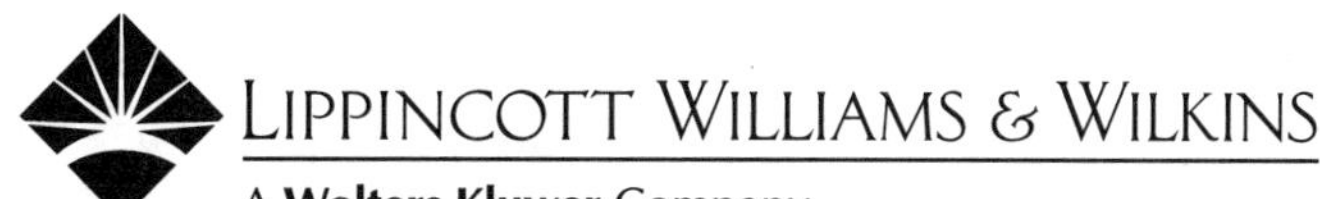

Lippincott Williams & Wilkins
A **Wolters Kluwer** Company
Philadelphia • Baltimore • New York • London
Buenos Aires • Hong Kong • Sydney • Tokyo

Acquisitions Editor: Elizabeth A. Nieginski
Editorial Director, Development: Julie Scardiglia
Senior Development Editor: Melanie Cann
Managing Editors: Marette D. Magargle-Smith, Karla M. Schroeder
Marketing Manager: Jennifer Conrad

9 8 7 6 5 4 3 2 1

Library of Congress Cataloging-in-Publication Data

Smith, Bonnie J.
Canine anatomy / Bonnie J. Smith
p. cm. — (The National veterinary medical series for independent study)
Includes index.
ISBN 0-683-30080-6
1. Dogs—Anatomy. I. Title. II. Series
SF767.D6S55 1999
636.7'0891—dc21 98-31094
CIP

Dedication

I offer this book to many folks:
My treasured daughters, Lanner and Kestrel
My dogs, especially Trell
My students, who have been many and hopefully will be many more,
and
My editor, who really made it happen

Contents

Preface

The objective of *NVMS Canine Anatomy* is to provide a quick review of the most salient points of canine gross anatomy for those in the veterinary medical field. The book is written in the characteristic "narrative outline" format of the National Veterinary Medical Series (NVMS), a format that simplifies the presentation of the material and maximizes the ease with which information on a particular topic can be found. The concise yet comprehensive coverage of information and the many study questions with complete explanations are two features that make the book useful for readers with many different needs—a freshman veterinary student who needs a concise review to accompany her course work, an upperclassman who needs a quick review of anatomy preparatory to performing a physical or radiographic examination or a surgical procedure, and a recent graduate who needs to prepare for the national board examinations would all find this book useful. The beautifully rendered illustrations by Caitlin Duckwall and the clinical correlations facilitate learning and help the reader draw parallels between basic science and clinical practice.

I have endeavored to discuss anatomy for the veterinarian's sake (rather than for the anatomist's sake), from the perspective of what among the vast scope of anatomical information is important to the general veterinarian. Although seeking to be generous in the information provided and to present a depth appropriate to a veterinarian's (rather than to a veterinary technician's) education, I have made an effort to avoid superfluous levels of detail. The focus is on basic anatomical description of the major body systems, as well as features of relevance to clinical medicine.

This text can be used in two ways: either to *review* material after studying it in-depth in lecture and laboratory, or to *preview* material before undertaking an in-depth study. In either case, however, the reader must remember that this book is meant to supplement and enhance traditional textbooks and atlases of canine anatomy, not to replace them.

My hope is that several types of readers will find this text useful, and that the book will help to bring the fascinating and truly relevant subject of canine anatomy "alive" for the reader.

Bonnie J. Smith

PART I

OVERVIEW

Chapter 1

Approach to Anatomic Study and Anatomic Terminology

I. APPROACHES TO GROSS (MACROSCOPIC) ANATOMY

A. Systematic (systemic) anatomy. In this approach, the study of anatomy is organized according to body systems. All aspects of the systems are studied, progressing from one body region to the next:

1. Integument
2. Skeletal and muscular systems
3. Nervous system
4. Circulatory system (including lymphatics)
5. Respiratory system
6. Digestive system
7. Urinary system
8. Genital system
9. Endocrine system

B. Regional (topographic) anatomy. This approach considers all systems within a given region, whether that region contains all of a particular body system or not. Organs and structures are considered in relation to each other.

1. Head and neck
2. Back
3. Thoracic limb
4. Pelvic limb
5. Thorax
6. Abdomen
7. Pelvis and perineum

C. Functional anatomy focuses on the relation of structure and function to each other. For example, muscles crossing the cranial surface of the elbow joint are flexors of the joint, whereas those crossing the caudal surface are extensors.

D. Applied anatomy is concerned with the practical application of knowledge about anatomy to the assessment of the health and condition of a patient, and to the diagnosis and/or treatment of clinical conditions. For example, a ready site to take the pulse of a dog is the femoral artery within the femoral triangle.

E. Clinical anatomy deals with how structure and function relate to clinical signs and entities observed in the practice of medicine. For example, avulsion of the roots of the brachial plexus produces, in addition to signs referable to motor and sensory damage to the affected limb, a drooping eyelid and miotic pupil in the ipsilateral eye because the sympathetic nerves to the eye also travel through the region of the brachial plexus.

II. ANATOMIC TERMINOLOGY

A. Anatomic nomenclature. Although anatomic nomenclature may at first seem obscure, the naming of structures typically follows one of several patterns. Knowledge of these patterns often not only simplifies learning the terminology, but also facilitates retention, because the names are often descriptive of certain aspects of the structure.

1. **Practical names.** Anatomic structures are commonly named according to the qualities listed below. Combining these descriptors leads to even more descriptive names for many structures (e.g., lateral digital extensor muscle, a name that describes the position as well as the function of the muscle).
   a. **Function** (e.g., adductor muscle of the thigh, levator palpebrae muscle)
   b. **Position relative to other similar structures** (e.g., superficial inguinal ring, ventral conchae)
   c. **Location** (e.g., infraorbital foramen, subscapularis muscle)
   d. **Appearance or form** (e.g., greater curvature of the stomach, triangular ligament of the liver)
2. **Eponymous names** relate the structure to a person, usually the person who first described the structure (e.g., canal of Schlemm, foramen of Monro). Because eponyms are useless from a practical standpoint, the *Nomina Anatomica Veterinaria* discourages their use. However, because many eponyms are firmly entrenched in clinical use, some of the more common ones are sometimes used in this text.
3. **Other names.** Some structures bear names that have little practical application to the structure (e.g., radial nerve, sympathetic nervous system).

B. **Anatomic position and planes.** In the **anatomic position,** the dog (or any other quadruped) stands erect on all four limbs, facing left, with the tail slightly raised (Figure 1–1). An **anatomic plane** is any surface, real or imaginary, along which any two points can be connected by a straight line (see Figure 1–1).

1. The **median plane** divides the head, body, or any limb longitudinally into equal right and left halves. For any structure, there is only a single median plane. The terms "me-

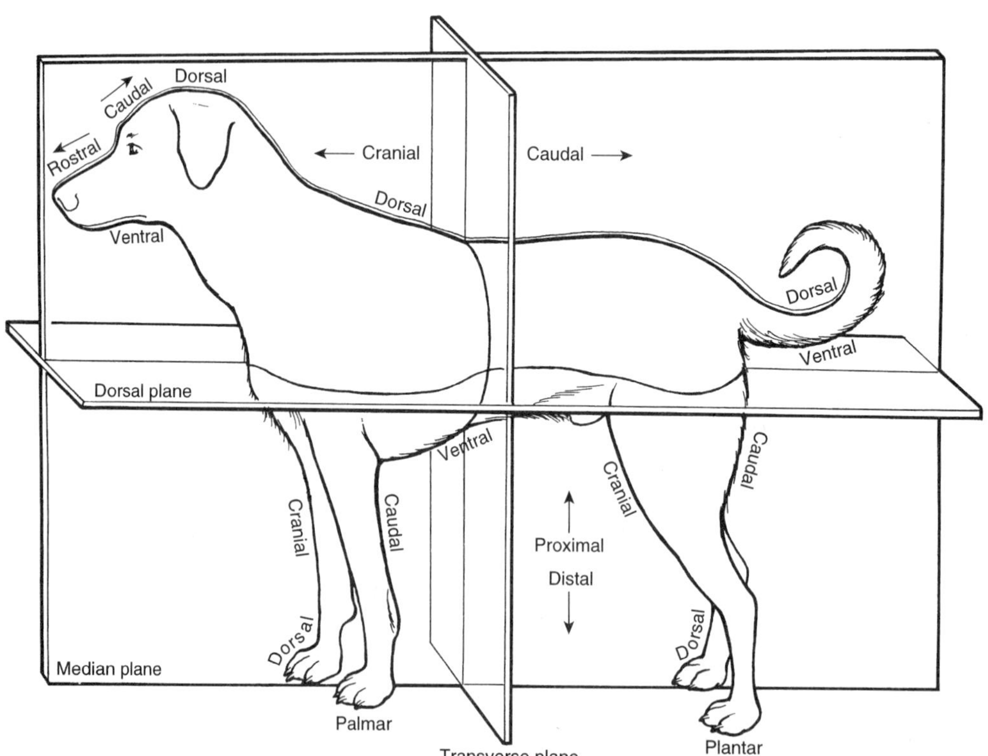

FIGURE 1–1. Anatomic position, anatomic planes, and anatomic directional terms.

dian" and "medial" are not synonymous—"median" refers to a specific anatomic plane, whereas "medial" is a directional term (Table 1–1).

2. A **sagittal (paramedian) plane** passes through the right or left side of the body parallel to the median plane. For any structure, there is potentially an infinite number of sagittal planes.
3. A **transverse plane** passes through the head, body, limb, or organ at right angles to the structure's long axis. The transverse plane is the one that divides the body or limbs into the informal "cross-sections" referred to in relation to procedures such as computer-assisted tomography (CAT).
4. A **dorsal plane** runs at right angles to both the median and transverse planes (horizontally, in the standing dog), dividing the body into dorsal and ventral portions.
5. A **coronal plane** is essentially the same as a transverse plane when the dog is positioned in the anatomic position. Therefore, the term is infrequently used in the study of veterinary anatomy.

C. **Anatomic directional terms** are generally arranged in pairs of opposites (see Table 1–1). The construction of these adjectives is such that the information they convey remains the same, regardless of the position of the animal's body. For example, regardless of the posture of the dog, the skin of the abdomen is always "superficial" to the liver. However, with the dog in dorsal recumbency, the abdominal skin can be said to be "over" the liver, whereas with the dog standing, the abdominal skin is "under" the liver.

D. **Terms describing anatomic movements** describe motions of joints, not of body regions. Thus, while it is correct to say that the triceps brachii extends the elbow, it is incorrect to say that this muscle extends the arm.

1. **Flexion, extension,** and **hyperextension**
   a. **Flexion** decreases the angle of a joint, as when the elbow or finger is bent.
   b. **Extension** increases the angle of a joint, as when the elbow or finger is straightened.
   c. **Hyperextension (dorsiflexion)** extends a joint beyond a linear or straight configuration, so that the angle of the joint is extended beyond 180 degrees. For example, the human carpus is hyperextended when the wrist is bent so that the dorsal surface of the hand bends back toward the arm. Note that some joints of the dog are normally held in a hyperextended position (e.g., the joints of the metacarpophalangeal, metatarsophalangeal, and distal interphalangeal joints when the limbs are weight-bearing).

2. **Adduction** and **abduction**
   a. **Adduction** moves a body part toward the median plane, as when a limb is tucked under the body.
   b. **Abduction** moves a body part away from the median plane, as when a limb is pulled to the side.

3. **Protraction** and **retraction**
   a. **Protraction** moves a structure cranially or rostrally, or moves it away from the central body, as when the tongue is projected from the mouth.
   b. **Retraction** moves a structure back toward the body, as when the tongue is replaced in the mouth.

4. **Elevation** and **depression**
   a. **Elevation** moves a structure dorsally, as when the shoulder is shrugged or the eyelid is opened.
   b. **Depression** moves a structure ventrally, as when the eyelid is closed.

5. **Supination** and **pronation**
   a. **Supination** rotates the thoracic limb so that the palmar/caudal surface faces medially, as when the dog turns the weight-bearing surface of its paw "upward" to remove a burr between the pads.
   b. **Pronation** rotates the thoracic limb so that the palmar/caudal surface faces medially, laterally, or caudally, as when the dog turns the supinated paw "downward" in order to stand.

TABLE 1–1. Directional Terms in the Study of Anatomy

Term	Definition
Superficial	Closer to the external body surface
Deep	Closer to the center of the body, away from the surface
Dorsal	
Exclusive of the limbs	Nearer the back (vertebral column) and the corresponding surfaces of the head, neck, and tail
On the limbs	The "front" or upper surface of each limb distal from the carpus or tarsus
Ventral	Nearer the belly or lowermost surface of any body surface, except the limbs
Medial	Toward or relatively near the median plane
Lateral	Away or relatively far from the median plane
Cranial	
Exclusive of the limbs/head	Toward the head
On the limbs	The forward surface of each limb as far distally as the carpus or tarsus
Caudal	
Exclusive of the limbs	Away from the head, toward the tail
On the limbs	The rear surface of each limb as far distally as the carpus or tarsus
Proximal	
Exclusive of the limbs	Nearer the main mass or origin of a structure
On the limbs	Nearer to the body; the attached end
Distal	
Exclusive of the limbs	Away from the main mass or origin of a structure
On the limbs	Farther from the body; the free end
Inner	Toward the center of a body cavity, organ, or structure
Outer	Away from the center of a body cavity, organ, or structure
Anterior	In veterinary medicine, this term is restricted to describing some structures of the head, particularly the eye (meaning closer to the cornea or the rostral part of the head)
Posterior	In veterinary medicine, this term is restricted to describing some structures of the head, particularly the eye (meaning closer to the optic nerve or the caudal part of the head)
Rostral	Toward the nose (used to describe structures on the head)
Caudal	Away from the nose, toward the occiput (used to describe structures on the head)
Dorsal	The surface of either paw from the carpus or tarsus on distally that lies opposite the surface bearing the pads; in other words, the forward-facing or upper surface
Palmar	The surface of the forepaw from the carpus or tarsus on distally that bears the carpal, metacarpal, and digital pads

continued

TABLE 1–1. Directional Terms in the Study of Anatomy

Term	Definition
Plantar	The surface of the hindpaw from the tarsus on distally that bears the metatarsal and digital pads
Axial	Used in reference to the digits to mean toward the functional axis of the limb*
Abaxial	Used in reference to the digits, to mean away from the functional axis of the limb*

*The functional axis of the limb passes between the third and fourth digits.

6. **Inversion** and **eversion**
   a. **Inversion** rotates the pelvic limb so that the plantar/caudal surface faces medially (similar to supination).
   b. **Eversion** rotates the pelvic limb so that the plantar/caudal surface faces laterally or caudally (similar to pronation).
7. **Rotation** describes an essentially circular movement of a part (rather than a joint) around its long axis, as when the head of the humerus rotates in the glenoid cavity of the scapula. The direction of the rotation is described by the direction of movement of the cranial or lateral surface of the part being moved; thus, when the femur rotates medially, the cranial surface moves medially.
8. **Circumduction** describes a combined movement, involving both flexion/extension and abduction/adduction. The resulting movement essentially describes a circle.

Chapter 2

The Common Integument and Mammary Glands

I. COMMON INTEGUMENT

A. Introduction

1. **Definition.** The term "common integument" refers to the **skin,** along with its **associated hair, glands, pads,** and **claws.**
2. **Functions.** The integument is the largest organ and serves multiple functions essential to life.
   a. **Protection.** The integument, which covers the entire external surface of the body and blends with the mucous membranes at the body's several natural openings, protects underlying structures.
      (1) The integument protects underlying structures from **abrasive, thermal,** or **chemical injury.** Specialized, thickened regions of the skin are present in certain areas (e.g., the pads, the skin of the nose) to provide additional protection against physical trauma.
      (2) The integument offers protection against **invasion by microorganisms.**
      (3) The integument, which is nearly impermeable to water, presents a **water barrier** that protects against desiccation (offering protection against fluid and electrolyte imbalances) and overhydration.
   b. **Provision of sensory information.** Most of the skin's surface is generously supplied with numerous types of general sensory afferent endings (e.g., temperature, pressure, touch, pain).
   c. **Secretion**
      (1) The mammary glands (see II) are actually modified sweat glands.
      (2) The skin also produces various substances related to its own function, as well as pheromones.
   d. **Synthesis.** Vitamin D synthesis takes place in the skin.
   e. **Thermoregulation**
      (1) **Prevention of excessive heat loss.** The shunting of blood away from the skin's surface can minimize heat loss.
      (2) **Dissipation of excessive body heat.** In dogs, the role of the skin in dissipation of excessive body heat is minimal; most dissipation of excessive body heat in dogs occurs via pronounced panting. Sweat glands are present in canine skin, but are quite few in number as compared with the number in other species.

B. Skin

1. **Layers**
   a. The **epidermis,** the superficial layer of the skin, consists of multiple layers of cells that are constantly renewed. Cells are produced in the deepest layers of the epidermis and are pushed to the surface by the multiplying cells beneath. As the cells move to the surface, they undergo degenerative changes, eventually die, and are sloughed when they reach the surface. In this manner, the skin is continuously provided with new layers of cells at the external surface to replace those lost to wear. The epidermis is avascular.
   b. The **dermis,** the deep layer of the skin, consists of a dense feltwork of collagen fibers that is generously supplied with vessels and nerves. The dermis is also invaded by numerous epidermal ingrowths, including hair follicles and sweat, sebaceous, and other glands. The dermis and epidermis are interdigitated. In addition to creating a secure attachment between the two layers, this interdigitation provides a vast surface area for the diffusion of oxygen, nutrients, and waste materials. In this manner, the avascular epidermis receives nutrients and oxygen, and dispenses with waste.

c. The **superficial fascia** is **not part of the skin;** rather, it **underlies the skin** and serves to bind the skin to the muscles beneath. In addition, it provides a pathway for vessels and nerves to reach the skin. The superficial fascia is subdivided into:
   (1) The **superficial layer of the superficial fascia,** which is fatty and relatively loose
   (2) The **deep layer of the superficial fascia,** which is membranous and stronger

2. **Muscles.** There are essentially two types of muscle in the skin: those contained within the skin and those associated with, but actually lying beneath, the skin.
   a. The **arrector pili muscles** are contained within the skin and are associated directly with hair follicles. These muscles erect the hairs against the cold and in behavioristic displays.
   b. The **cutaneous muscles** are anchored in the dermis and closely affixed to the superficial fascia. Contraction of these muscles causes movement of the skin, or of structures associated with the skin (e.g., the whiskers on the muzzle). Prominent cutaneous muscles include the **sphincter colli,** the **platysma,** and the **cutaneous trunci.**

3. **Vascularization.** Blood is supplied to the skin via **cutaneous arteries** that pass between or through the muscles en route to the skin. These arteries and their accompanying veins run parallel to the skin surface. The blood supply to the skin is divided into three plexuses:
   a. The **subdermal plexus** is the deepest and is formed from the termination of cutaneous arteries. This plexus represents the major blood supply to the skin.
   b. The **cutaneous plexus** is intermediate in position, and forms a network around the hair follicles and glands. Branches leave the cutaneous plexus and proceed superficially to form the most superficial plexus.
   c. The **subpapillary plexus** is the most superficial plexus, lying just deep to the epidermis and serving as a source of nutrients and oxygen for this avascular layer. The subpapillary plexus also serves as the "sink" for waste products produced by the epidermal layer.

Canine Clinical Correlation

The parallel course of the cutaneous arteries forms the basis for the success of skin grafting techniques. Because of significant differences between the arterial pattern in human beings versus dogs, human skin grafting techniques cannot be directly extrapolated to dogs.

4. **Innervation.** Both autonomic and sensory components supply the skin.
   a. The **autonomic innervation** controls blood vessel caliber, skin gland activity, and piloerection.
   b. The **sensory innervation** is provided via larger nerve trunks that enter the dermis and then divide into smaller branches that accompany the blood vessels en route to the dermal and epidermal tissues. The pattern of skin innervation generally follows a segmental pattern, in which a given spinal nerve typically supplies a specific skin region (i.e., a **dermatome**).
      (1) Dermatomes are generally readily recognizable as slightly overlapping sequential segments of the skin on the trunk.
      (2) Dermatomes of the limbs and head are often less readily discernible.

Canine Clinical Correlation

Because a dermatome reliably represents the field of distribution of a spinal nerve, testing of a skin region for an intact sensory response can be used to test integrity of spinal nerve function: if a sensory deficit is found in a given dermatome, the conclusion can be reliably drawn that the spinal nerve supplying that area has sustained some impairment.

C. **Hair** is a uniquely mammalian feature; in fact, it is one of the defining characteristics of the taxonomic Class Mammalia. Most members of the Class, including dogs, possess a haircoat that covers nearly the entire body surface. There are three major types of hair:

1. **Guard hairs** form the outermost layer of hair that covers most of the skin surface.
   - **a.** These hairs are regularly arranged in broad tracts that follow the contour of the body and give the dog's coat its smooth appearance. Guard hairs are generally thick, long, and (relative to the undercoat) stiff.
   - **b.** The arrangement of the guard hairs effectively promotes runoff of rain or other moisture. Unless a dog is submerged in water for a considerable period or the contour of the haircoat is disturbed while the dog is wet, the guard hairs are surprisingly effective in preventing the water from penetrating to the skin, thereby preventing chilling.
2. **Wool hairs** form the innermost layer of hair over most of the skin surface.
   - **a.** Wool hairs are thinner, more undulating, and softer than guard hairs, and they are also generally shorter and more numerous than the guard hairs of the outer coat.
   - **b.** This is the hair layer that provides most of the direct insulation and warming effect for the dog.
     - **(1)** The insulating effect of the wool hairs is reflected by the fact that this layer of hair is often thickest in the winter, and then is shed or thinned out in the warmer months.
     - **(2)** Breeds possessed of a thick outer coat and an abundant undercoat, such as huskies, can tolerate subfreezing weather for prolonged periods of time (provided they can escape the wind), whereas breeds with a short outer coat and essentially no undercoat, such as Doberman pinschers, can become chilled in surprisingly mild weather and have very poor tolerance for cold temperatures.
3. **Tactile hairs** (e.g., "whiskers") are specialized hairs that have been adapted to provide sensory information from the environment. The base of the tactile hair resides in a blood-filled sinus that greatly amplifies the motion of the hair and increases its sensitivity, allowing tactile hairs to detect even the slightest touch.
   - **a.** Tactile hairs are notably thicker than any other hair on the body, and usually protrude outward beyond the surrounding haircoat.
   - **b.** Tactile hairs are mostly concentrated on the head, and thus are associated with the other sensory specializations of this region (i.e., vision, hearing, taste).

D. **Pads.** In dogs, four **digital pads** are accompanied by a **carpal pad** and a **metacarpal pad** on the forepaw and a **metatarsal pad** on the hindpaw (Figure 2–1). It is of interest to note that the metacarpal pad, though entirely non-weightbearing, is essentially of the same structure and thickness as those pads that do continually contact the ground. The pads consist of a hairless epidermal pad supported by a digital cushion.

1. The **epidermal pad** is extremely thickened and cornified (and usually heavily pigmented). It possesses numerous conical papillae that provide traction as the dog walks.
2. The **digital cushion** consists of typical dermis and a markedly thickened subcutis containing abundant reticular, collagenous, and elastic fibers interspersed with adipose tissue. The eccrine sweat glands are contained within the adipose tissue of the footpad.

E. **Claws.** The claw is an epidermal structure, formed from a modification of the superficial layers of the epidermis. The claw is often deeply pigmented.

1. The claw consists of a **sole** (the most distal portion), two laterally compressed **walls** (which form the axial and abaxial surfaces of the claw), and a **central dorsal ridge** that is thicker than the walls. The **claw fold** is a fold of skin at the proximal border of the claw that is continuous with the horn (i.e., the outermost layer) of the claw.
2. The proximal, or coronary, border of the claw rests under the unguicular ridge of the distal phalanx. The periosteum of the distal phalanx is continuous with the dermis of the claw, and these two tissues occupy the space between the bone of the distal phalanx and the epidermal tissues of the claw itself.

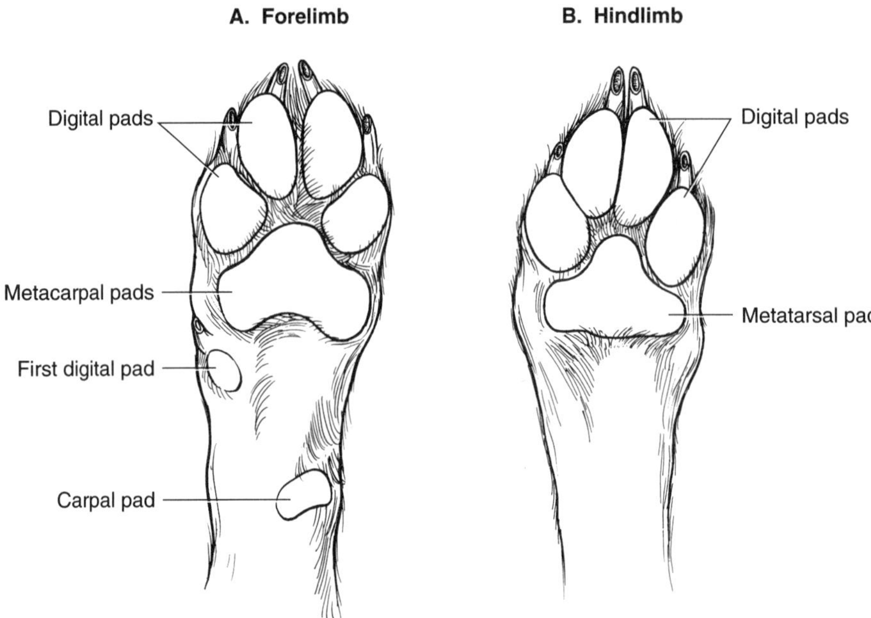

FIGURE 2–1. Footpads on the forelimb and the hindlimb of the dog. Note that there is no tarsal equivalent to the carpal pad.

Canine Clinical Correlation

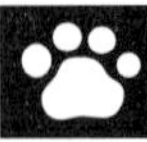

The profuse bleeding that can occur when a toenail is clipped too short originates in the well-vascularized dermal tissues between the claw and the bone of the distal phalanx.

F. Glands

1. **Sebaceous glands** are present in the skin and are associated with hair follicles. The ducts of the sebaceous glands open at the base of the hair follicles. Sebaceous glands are best developed along the dorsum, and are largest at the mucocutaneous junctions of the lips, vulva, and eyelids. The **tarsal glands of the eyelids** are modified sebaceous glands.
2. **Sweat glands**
   a. **Eccrine sweat glands** are present in the footpads. The ducts of these glands open directly onto the surface of the footpads. The function of these sweat glands relates to **territorial marking,** as much if not more than to thermoregulation.
   b. **Apocrine sweat glands** are present in the skin. The ducts of the apocrine sweat glands open into the hair follicles superficial to the ducts of the sebaceous glands.
3. **Circumanal glands** (Figure 2–2). Numerous circumanal glands are located in the skin directly surrounding the entire circumference of the anus. These glands open directly onto the skin's surface and must not be confused with the glands of the anal sacs.
4. **Anal sac glands** are sebaceous in nature, and lie within the walls of the paired, spherical anal sacs. Therefore, the ducts of these glands open into the anal sacs, rather than directly onto the surface of the skin (see Figure 2–2).
5. **Tail area glands** are sebaceous glands located in a diamond-shaped area on the dorsal aspect of the tail approximately at the level of Cd 7–9. Hairs in this region are larger than surrounding hairs. The modified skin in this region is believed to function in individual recognition and identification.

II. MAMMARY GLANDS.

MAMMARY GLANDS. The mammary gland is another uniquely mammalian feature and, in fact, is the characteristic for which the taxonomic Class Mammalia is actually named. In females, the development of the mammary glands exceeds that of the males, even in nonparous bitches, and is maximal in bitches that bear and nurse puppies.

A. Location and number. The mammary glands are located in bilateral lines on each side of the ventral midline.

1. The teats are often staggered in their arrangement, which facilitates access of the puppies to their food source.
2. Larger breeds typically have four to six glands on each side of the midline, whereas smaller breeds most typically have four glands on each side. When five pairs are present, the glands are identified according to their location as **cranial thoracic, caudal thoracic, cranial abdominal, caudal abdominal,** and **inguinal.**

B. Structure. Mammary glands are modified sweat glands. Each mammary gland is comprised of a separate collection of epithelial glandular tissue, the associated papilla (teat), connective tissue, and the covering skin.

1. The **glandular tissue** proliferates extensively during pregnancy and lactation. When lactation ceases, the mammary tissue involutes remarkably so that relatively little is left. En-

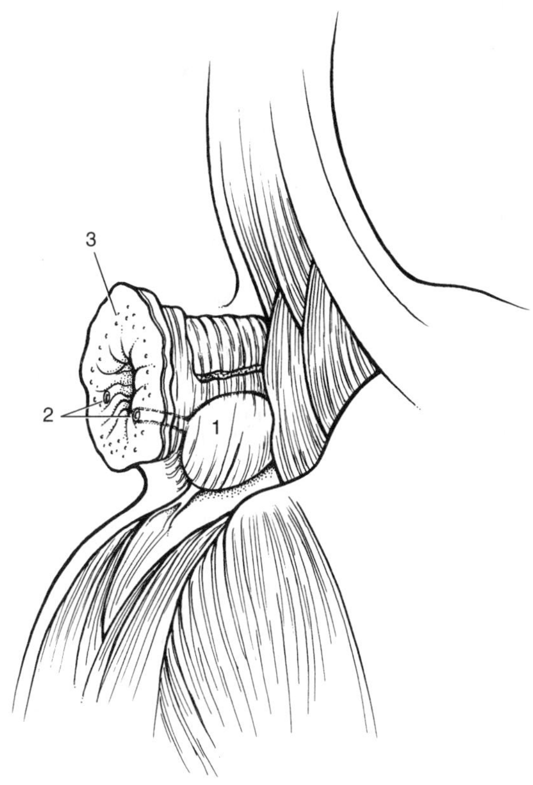

FIGURE 2–2. The anal sacs (*1*) and circumanal glands (*2*) of the dog. The circumanal glands are located in the skin surrounding the circumference of the anus and open directly onto the skin's surface. The walls of the anal sacs contain numerous microscopic glands (the glands of the anal sac, not shown). These glands produce a secretion that functions in individual recognition and territorial marking. The orifices of the glands of the anal sac open directly into the anal sac. The anal sacs open into the anal canal, and then onto the skin surface via a single duct (*3*). (Modified with permission from Dyce KM, Sack WO, Wensing CJG: *Textbook of Veterinary Anatomy.* Philadelphia, WB Saunders, 1987, p 366.)

suing pregnancies, however, result in a proliferation of tissues similar to that of the previous lactation.

2. Within each mammary gland, subdivisions of glandular tissue are separate both anatomically and functionally from each other. **Duct systems** within each subdivision coalesce into progressively larger passageways leading to the teat. The smallest passages deep within the gland lead to the **gland sinus** (located within the gland), to the **teat sinus** (located within the body of the teat), to the **teat canal** (located in the distal end of the teat), which opens onto the teat surface at the **teat orifice.** Because multiple ducts remain separate from each other, multiple teat orifices are present on the end of each teat, resulting in a sieve-like pattern of pinhole-sized openings that is usually visible to the naked eye in a bitch who has nursed a litter.

C. **Vascularization.** The mammary glands are extremely vascular, owing to the necessity of passing 400 liters of blood through the mammary gland to produce a single liter of milk! The arterial vessels anastomose freely with each other, forming an extensive plexus around the various glands. The veins also anastomose in a similar manner, resulting in a vast venous plexus that parallels the arterial one.

1. **Arterial supply**
   a. The **thoracic mammae** receive arterial supply primarily from the **internal thoracic artery;** the **internal intercostal** and **lateral thoracic arteries** may also contribute.
   b. The **abdominal** and **inguinal mammae** receive arterial supply from the **cranial** and **caudal superficial epigastric arteries.**
2. **Venous drainage.** The venous drainage of the mammae follows the arterial supply, with the **cranial** and **caudal superficial epigastric veins** draining the majority of blood from the glands.
3. **Lymphatic drainage.** The following description is a general one, and considerable variation may be encountered clinically.
   a. **Thoracic mammae.** Lymph from the cranial and caudal thoracic mammae drains to the **axillary lymph node.**
   b. **Cranial abdominal mamma.** Lymph drainage from the cranial abdominal mamma is somewhat inconsistent. Typically this gland also drains to the **axillary lymph node,** but also often joins the drainage of the caudal abdominal mamma to the **superficial inguinal lymph node.**
   c. **Caudal abdominal mamma.** Lymph from the caudal abdominal mamma drains caudally, either into the lymphatic mesh surrounding the inguinal mammary gland, or directly into the **superficial inguinal lymph node.**
   d. **Inguinal mamma.** Lymph from the inguinal mamma drains into the **superficial inguinal lymph node.**

Canine Clinical Correlation

The occasional communication of the mammary lymphatic network, both cranially and caudally, as well as from right to left, becomes important in considering the metastasis of mammary adenocarcinoma. If communication among lymphatic networks occurs, one cancerous gland may potentially metastasize to any of the others. Similarly, drainage of the mammary glands to the ipsilateral superficial inguinal lymph nodes can result in metastasis of the disease elsewhere in the body.

D. **Innervation.** Nerves are distributed throughout the mammary glands, to the glandular parenchyma, vessels, smooth muscle of the teat, and the skin of the gland and teat.

a. **Sensory innervation**
   (1) **Thoracic mammary glands.** Sensory innervation is provided via the ventral cutaneous nerves.
   (2) **Abdominal** and **inguinal mammae.** These mammae are innervated via the ventral superficial branches of the first three lumbar nerves.

b. **Sympathetic innervation** parallels the vascularization of the mammae.

Chapter 3

The Skeletomuscular System

I. INTRODUCTION. The combination of body organs and tissues that serves the function of supporting and moving the body has been considered in differing ways.

A. As separate "skeletal" and "muscular" systems. Possibly as a result of the distinct physical characteristics of bone and muscle, these two systems are sometimes considered entirely independently of each other. Indeed, bone is a physically hard and enduring substance, has no intrinsic mobility in life, and persists in recognizable form long after the soft tissues have decomposed following death. Muscle, in contrast, is a soft tissue without durable form, capable of active movement during life (thereby conferring motion to the organism), that decomposes rapidly after death.

B. As the "locomotory" system. This terminology has the advantage of considering the skeletal muscles and bones as a functioning unit. However, this particular identifying term leaves much to be desired in being descriptive of the system.

C. As the "skeletomuscular" or "musculoskeletal" system. These terms seem to combine the best of the two previous ones, in considering skeletal muscles and bones as a single unit functionally (because neither is capable of significant action alone) while nonetheless recognizing that this single functional unit is composed of two very different morphological types of organs (hard bone and soft muscle). In considering which of these two terms to employ, this author's preference is to use the former, because consideration of this system is best undertaken once the bones are understood.

II. SKELETON (Figure 3–1). Functions of the skeleton include **support, protection, leverage,** a **repository** for minerals, **fat storage,** and **hematopoiesis.**

A. Bone is the major component of the skeleton. The dynamic nature of bone is somewhat belied by its strength, durability, and lack of mobility, but the fact that it is a **well-vascularized, vital tissue** capable of responding to its environment and also subject to various types of metabolic as well as traumatic injury must always be kept in mind.

1. **Histology.** Bone consists of a **living, cellular part (osteoblasts** and **osteocytes)** surrounded by a **matrix** synthesized by the osteoblasts and osteocytes. The matrix has an organic and an inorganic portion. Both of these portions are under control of the osteoblasts and osteocytes, and can be modified according to the physical or physiologic demands of the body.
2. **Classification of bones.** Bones can be classified according to:
   a. **Location** (see Figure 3–1)
      (1) The **axial skeleton** includes the skull, vertebral column, ribs, and sternum (i.e., the bones that comprise the central axis of the body).
      (2) The **appendicular skeleton** includes the bones of the limbs.
   b. **Shape** (Figure 3–2)
      (1) **Long bones** are found in the limbs, where they provide an attachment site for limb muscles and levers for movement. They have identifiable structural regions:
         (a) The **metaphyses** are the morphologically specialized proximal and distal ends of the bones.
         (b) The **diaphysis** is the **shaft** of the bone (i.e., the elongate central portion that comprises the longest part of the bone).
         (c) The **epiphyses** are the regions between the metaphyses and the central region of the bone. In a growing animal, the epiphyses are separated from the meta-

FIGURE 3–1. Skeleton of the dog. Note that the os penis is nearly hidden by the thigh in this view.

physes and the diaphysis by cartilaginous **epiphyseal growth plates,** which are active sites of endochondral bone formation and bone elongation. After growth is complete, the epiphyseal plates ossify or "close," and the three regions of the long bones blend smoothly together.

Canine Clinical Correlation

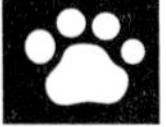

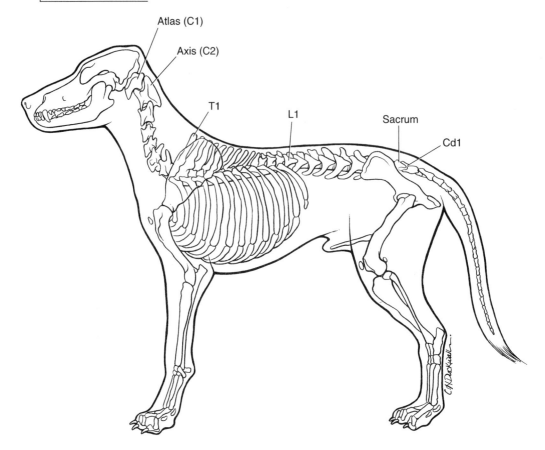

Growth of bone is accomplished at the epiphyseal plates of long bones, as well as at **ossification centers.** Ossification centers are often present in seemingly irregularly placed regions of developing bones, such as the anconeal process of the ulna. A general familiarity with the ossification centers of bones as well as the approximate ages at which they close is helpful in distinguishing these normally radiolucent areas from fracture sites in young animals.

(2) Short bones are found only in the carpus and tarsus. These bones are highly irregular in shape and size but, in general, are relatively small.

(3) Flat (squamous) bones are found in most regions of the skull and in the ribs. These bones generally serve a **protective** or **reinforcing** function.

(4) Irregular bones include the bones of the vertebral column, the bones of the pelvis, and the bones of the skull that are not flat.

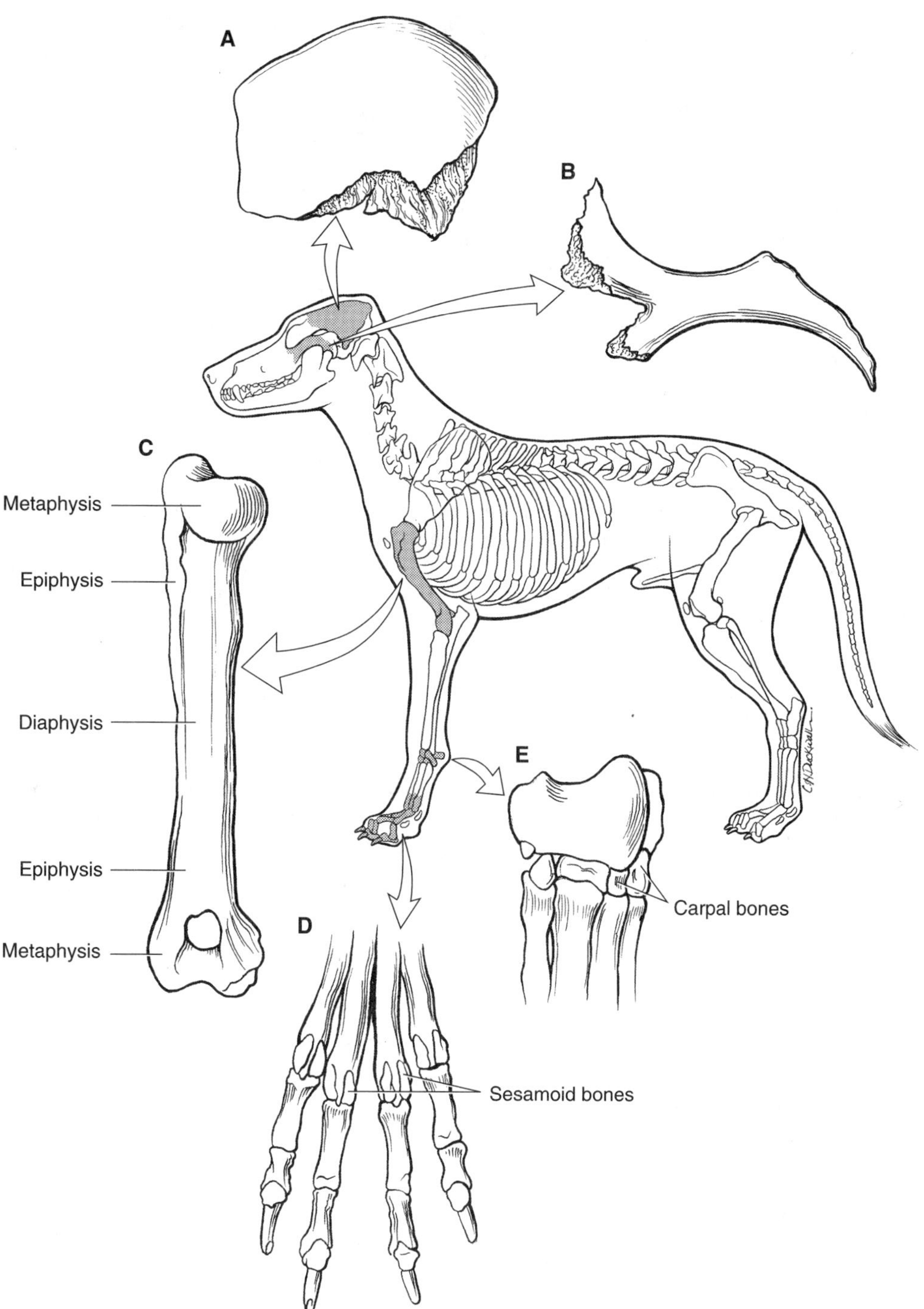

FIGURE 3–2. Various shapes of bones. (*A*) The left parietal bone of the skull is an example of a flat bone. Flat bones, which are usually gently curved or sculpted, are irregular in form when compared with each other as a group; therefore, they do not possess regularly identifiable group characteristics like the long bones do. (*B*) Irregular bones, such as the zygomatic bone, usually possess prominent, irregular, outward-jutting processes that provide attachment sites for skeletal muscles or articulation sites for other bones. (*C*) Long bones (e.g., the humerus), found in the limbs, are enlarged at their proximal and distal ends, where they are covered by hyaline cartilage and specialized in contour for the formation of joints with other bones. (*D*) Palmar view of the sesamoid bones of the distal interphalangeal joint, shown in articulation with adjacent bones. Sesamoid bones are so named because of their resemblance to sesame seeds. (*E*) Seven short bones are found in the carpus as well as in the tarsus.

(5) **Sesamoid bones** are located in tendons (or, less commonly, in ligaments) near freely mobile joints. These bones can be smaller than 1 mm in diameter [e.g., the sesamoid bones of the dorsal surface of the distal interphalangeal (DIP) joints], or fairly large [e.g., the patella (the largest sesamoid bone of the body)]. Sesamoid bones function in reducing friction and wear of tendons.

B. **Cartilage** comprises a relatively small part of the skeleton. Somewhat like bone, cartilage is also composed of cells surrounded by an intercellular matrix. However, one of the fundamental differences of bone and cartilage is that cartilage is **avascular;** thus, cartilage responds poorly to injury and does not heal well. Three types of cartilage are found within the skeleton:

1. **Hyaline cartilage** lines the surface of synovial joints and is characterized by a matrix possessing abundant natural lubricants. Hyaline cartilage also forms the cartilaginous portion of the ribs, comprises most of the laryngeal cartilages, and serves as the anlage for long bone development. Thus, hyaline cartilage is the most commonly found form of cartilage in the skeleton.
2. **Fibrocartilage** is particularly durable and resilient, possessing a matrix comprised of extensive bundles of collagenous fibers. Fibrocartilage is more restricted in its distribution than hyaline cartilage; it is found in most symphyses (pelvic, intervertebral) and in the menisci of the stifle and temporomandibular joints.
3. **Elastic cartilage** possesses a matrix containing large amounts of elastic fibers. The resulting cartilage has a great deal of flexibility, but nonetheless considerable strength. Elastic cartilage forms the skeleton of the pinna, the external nose, and the epiglottis.

Canine Clinical Correlation

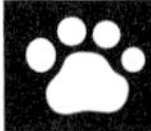

The avascular nature of cartilage significantly reduces its healing capacity. Hence, injury to cartilage is usually more serious than injury to bone, because the vascular nature of bone promotes rapid and secure healing. In a healthy animal, bone that has healed following an injury is essentially identical in strength to its condition prior to trauma. However, torn cartilage will not heal. Cartilage fragments or trailing, partially detached cartilage within a joint induce further damage, and must be removed surgically. The joint is then typically permanently compromised in its strength and function.

C. **Articulations (joints)** are formed where one bone contacts another. Bones at joints are held together by any one or a combination of fibrous, elastic, or cartilaginous tissue.

1. **Classification.** Articulations vary in their function and, therefore, their mobility.
   a. **Fibrous joints (synarthroses)** are capable of **minimal to no movement.** The main goal of synarthroses is to hold the bones together. Several subtypes of fibrous joints may be identified:
      (1) **Sutures,** such as those found among the flat bones of the cranium
      (2) **Syndesmoses,** in which a considerable amount of connective tissue intervenes between the two bones in question (e.g., the tibiofibular joint, the attachment of the hyoid apparatus to the skull)
      (3) **Gomphoses,** the specialized joints that hold the teeth in their alveoli
   b. **Cartilaginous joints (amphiarthroses)** permit only **limited motion,** mainly stretching or compression.
      (1) **Hyaline cartilage joints** are mainly characteristic of growing bone and are lost as the animal matures.
      (2) **Fibrocartilaginous joints** are features of the mature skeleton. They are found in the pelvic symphysis, mandibular symphysis, and between the sternebrae and vertebral bodies. These joints occasionally ossify with advanced age.
   c. **Synovial joints (diarthroses, "true joints")** permit a **relatively wide range of motion.** The

range of motion at a joint may be in a single plane (e.g., such as occurs at the elbow), or in multiple directions (e.g., such as occurs at the hip). Motions that can take place at joints, depending on the form of the joint, include flexion, extension, hyperflexion (dorsiflexion), abduction, adduction, rotation, and circumduction (see Chapter 1 II D).

(1) Components. Synovial joints (Figure 3–3) consist of:

(a) Two bones, the ends of which are covered by **hyaline cartilage**

Canine Clinical Correlation

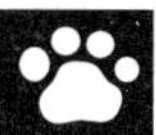

Osteochondritis dissecans is a commonly occurring disease in which a dissecting or abrading injury to articular cartilage produces pain and lameness. Surgical intervention is required. The most common site for this lesion in dogs is the shoulder, but the elbow, tarsocrural joint (hock), stifle, and femoral head may also be affected.

(b) A **joint cavity** that lies between the two apposing bones

(c) A **joint capsule** that entirely surrounds the joint cavity, extending both proximal and distal to it

(i) The **outer, fibrous layer** is a protective, strengthening structure.

(ii) The **inner, synovial layer** secretes the viscous and slick synovial fluid,

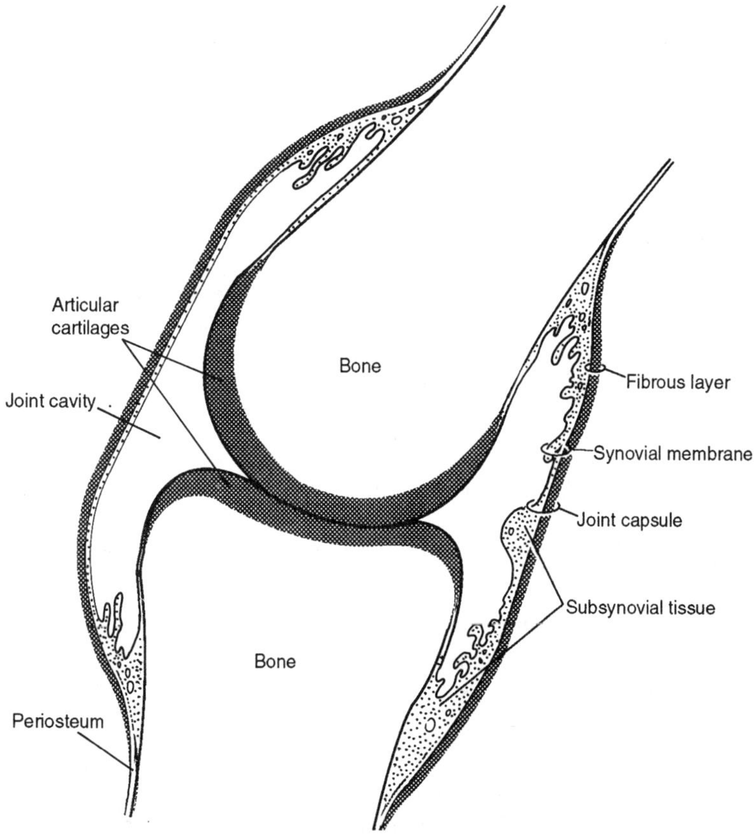

FIGURE 3–3. A typical synovial joint. (Reprinted with permission from Dellmann H-D, Carithers JR: *NVMS Cytology and Microscopic Anatomy*. Baltimore, Williams & Wilkins, 1996, p 114.)

which provides lubrication for the joint's movement. Additionally, the synovial fluid provides a route for the diffusion of oxygen and nutrients to, and the removal of waste products from, the joint's cartilage.

(d) Other components. Some synovial joints (e.g., the stifle joint) possess modifications related to the form or function of the joint (e.g., fat pads, intraarticular ligaments).

(2) Types. Synovial joints can be classified according to the amount of mobility afforded by the joint. There are seven subcategories of synovial joints; the most familiar subtypes are **ball-and-socket** and **ginglymus (hinge)** joints.

D. **Ligaments** are collections of dense regular connective tissue of varying thickness and size that cross the joints and hold them together. They are actually implanted in the bones proximal and distal to the joint.

1. In most cases, the ligaments are distinct enough to be readily identified as thick collagenous bands passing in a proximal to distal direction along the joint.
2. In some instances, ligaments are poorly distinguished from the joint capsule surrounding the joint. In such cases, the entire joint capsule is sometimes considered as a sort of a diffuse ligament. The joint capsule may be annularly thickened on the cranial/dorsal and caudal/palmar/plantar surfaces to form an **extensor** or **flexor retinaculum,** which serves to bind the tendons to the bone and prevent them from bowing.

Canine Clinical Correlation

Like cartilage, ligaments are avascular in nature; therefore, injury to ligaments is in some ways more serious than injury to bone. Ligaments that are partially detached from the bone are unable to form attachments to the bone that are as secure as the original; therefore, sprained and torn ligaments are unable to optimally support the joint and are more prone to subsequent injury than an intact ligament.

III. SKELETAL MUSCLE.

Shortening of the skeletal muscles acts to produce a change in position of one or both of the bones to which the muscles attach. Muscle groups are typically arranged in sets to allow opposing actions on a joint (e.g., the hypaxial and epaxial muscles on opposite sides of the vertebral column).

A. Structure

1. Histology

a. Myocytes (fibers). Skeletal muscles are composed of a legion of individual muscle cells.

b. Connective tissue surrounds individual cells, larger groups of cells (to form **fascicles),** and the entire muscle.

c. Deep fascia. The deep fascia is intimately bound to the muscle surface. It cannot be stripped from the muscle.

(1) Three layers of the deep fascia are defined:

(a) An **outer investing fascia** lies over the superficial surface of the body musculature (i.e., it "lines" the body musculature from the superficial side).

(b) The **inner investing fascia** lies on the deep surface of the musculature of the body wall (i.e., it "lines" the body musculature from the deep side).

(c) Intermediate investing fasciae arise as septa from the outer investing fascia and pass among and around individual muscles and neurovascular bundles.

(2) Functions. The deep fascia is particularly well-developed among the muscles of the limbs, and often provides direct attachment for muscle fibers as either supplementary anchorage, or as a separate aponeurotic site of origin or insertion.

(3) **Fascial planes.** Distinct fascial planes separating muscles are present among the muscles of the trunk, neck, and head, as well as on the limbs.

Canine Clinical Correlation

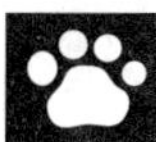

Infection can spread along, but will seldom cross, the various fascial planes of the body. Since the advent of powerful antimicrobials, the importance of knowing the disposition of these fascial planes has decreased somewhat; however, familiarity with their positioning can still be useful, in that opening the fascial planes at their most ventral sites can facilitate drainage of fluids or pus.

2. **Attachment to bone.** The connective tissue investing the muscle converges at each end of the muscle to form the attachments anchoring the muscle to the bone. The traction of skeletal muscles on bone induces a remodeling response, producing an elevation at the site of attachment. Thus, recognizable crests, tubercles, and trochanters become permanent features of the bone.
   a. **Types of attachments**
      (1) **Tendons** are distinct bundles of collagenous fibers.
      (2) **Aponeuroses** are broad, flat sheets of connective tissue.
   b. **Sites of attachment.** Skeletal muscles attach proximally and distally to different bones, always cross at least one joint, and may extend considerable distances and cross multiple joints.
      (1) The **proximal attachment (origin)** is the attachment of the muscle closest to the body.
      (2) The **distal attachment (insertion)** is the attachment of the muscle farthest from the body.
3. **Regions.** Many limb muscles are subdivided into recognizable regions.
   a. **Head.** The head is the region of the muscle arising from a given area (e.g., the long head of the triceps muscle). The various heads of a muscle may arise from divergent bones, but will converge to the same tendon (e.g., the radial, ulnar, and humeral heads of the deep digital flexor muscle).
   b. **Belly.** The belly is the expanded midportion of the muscle. Some individual skeletal muscles may have multiple bellies. In contrast to the head of a muscle, various bellies of a muscle share a similar origin as well as the same tendon of insertion (e.g., the several bellies of the humeral head of the deep digital flexor muscle).

B. **Types of skeletal muscle.** Skeletal muscles take various gross forms (Figure 3–4), depending on the orientation and abundance of the fibers within the muscle.

1. **Fusiform muscles** are elliptical with rounded cross-sections. The muscle fibers are parallel to the long axis of the muscle.
2. **Flat muscles** (e.g., the styloglossus or splenius muscles) are strap-like or sheet-like in form.
3. **Pennate muscles.** The muscle fibers lie at an angle to the long axis of the muscle.
   a. **Unipennate muscles** (e.g., the abductor pollicis longus muscle) attach at an angle along only one side of a tendon.
   b. **Bipennate muscles** (e.g., the gastrocnemius muscle) attach at an angle along both sides of a tendon.
   c. **Multipennate muscles** (e.g., the deltoideus muscle) attach to a tendon from multiple angles.
4. **Sphincter muscles** (e.g., the precapillary sphincters, the sphincter of the urinary bladder) are circular in form and serve to close a structure when contracted.

C. **Accessory structures**

1. **Sesamoid bones** [see II A 2 b (5)] develop within tendons at sites of excessive wear to protect the associated tendon from injury.

2. **Bursae** are connective tissue sacs lined by synovial tissue that typically develop between a bony prominence and a tendon, muscle, or ligament. Bursae reduce friction of the associated structure over the bone.
3. **Synovial tendon sheaths** are double-layered sacs similar in form to a greatly elongated bursa. Tendon sheaths also facilitate movement and reduce friction.

D. Vascularization. Muscles are highly vascular organs, owing to their high metabolic rate.

1. **Arteries** provide branches to nearby muscles in a remarkably constant pattern, though variations do exist. Anastomosis of arteries within the muscle is common.
2. **Veins** generally parallel the arteries and take the same names.
3. **Lymphatic vessels** accompany the arteries.

E. Innervation

1. **Motor nerves** accompany the arterial supply into the muscles. Skeletal muscles of a given action group are typically innervated by the same nerve (e.g., the radial nerve innervates the elbow extensors).
2. **Sensory nerves** of various types (e.g., spindles, stretch receptors, paciniform corpuscles) send input away from the muscles along the same pathway as the motor nerves.

Chapter 4

The Nervous System

I. INTRODUCTION. The nervous system is a system that is widely diverse structurally, but nonetheless functions as an exquisitely integrated whole, permitting the animal to receive information from its environment, as well as its own body, and to appropriately respond.

A. Functional components include the:

1. **Sensory component,** which receives input from the environment as well as from the animal's own body
2. **Somatic motor component,** which effects messages sent from the brain to the voluntary (skeletal) muscles
3. **Visceral motor component,** which effects messages sent from the brain to the smooth muscles of the various internal organ systems and structures of the skin

B. Basic structural unit. The **neuron** (nerve cell) is the structural unit of the nervous system. Neurons are immensely diverse in their exact form, size, and location; however, all neurons have dendrites, a cell body, an axon, and telodendria.

1. The **dendrites** are **afferent (sensory, "incoming") processes** specialized to receive information from the internal or external environment and send that information to the central portion of the neuron.
2. The **cell body** is the enlarged portion of the neuron; it contains most of the cytoplasm and organelles.
3. The **axon** is a **single efferent (motor, "outgoing")* process** that conveys information from a neuron to other neurons or effector organs (e.g., muscles, glands).
4. The **telodendria** (*telo,* "end") are the **terminal processes of the axon;** they are specialized for sending information to other neurons or effectors.

C. Conceptual divisions. Division of the nervous system into separate regions is artificial, but nonetheless necessary to approaching the study of this complex organ system. The nervous system can be considered on the basis of **structure** and on the basis of **function.**

1. **Structural division**
   a. **Central nervous system (CNS)**
      (1) **Components** include the **brain** and **spinal cord.** The CNS is the part of the nervous system that is **encased in bone.**
      (2) **Functions** of the CNS include:
         (a) **Reception** of all sensory information
         (b) **Integration** of sensory information
         (c) **Initiation** and **coordination** of motor activity
   b. **Peripheral nervous system (PNS)**
      (1) **Components.** The PNS includes the **cranial** and **spinal nerves,** which extend to and from the periphery and the CNS.
      (2) **Functions.** The PNS **conveys information:**
         (a) **To the CNS,** from sensory receptors sensing both the internal and external environments
         (b) **From the CNS,** in the form of motor commands to the muscles and glands of the body

---

*Remember: "**e**fferent" equals "**e**xiting."

2. **Functional division**
   a. **Somatic nervous system**
      (1) The **afferent component** carries and processes **sensory input** (both conscious and unconscious) from the **internal and external environments.**
      (2) The **efferent component** is involved with **motor control of voluntary muscle.**
   b. **Visceral nervous system**
      (1) The **afferent component** carries and processes **sensory input from the visceral organs.**
      (2) The **efferent component** [the **autonomic nervous system (ANS)**] is **motor** only, and is composed of those parts of the CNS and PNS that affect smooth muscle, cardiac muscle, and the glands of the viscera and skin. The efferent visceral nervous system is composed of the **sympathetic** and **parasympathetic systems.**
         (a) **Sympathetic division.** The sympathetic division is often referred to as the **"fight or flight" system.** Sympathetic activity decreases vegetative activities (e.g., digestion of food, renal filtration of blood), diverting blood flow and energy to sensory organs and large skeletal muscle masses to maximize sensory input and prepare the animal to defend itself or flee. The sympathetic division is also sometimes referred to as the **thoracolumbar system,** because its neuronal cell bodies are located in the lateral horn of the thoracolumbar regions of the spinal cord, or the **adrenergic system,** because of the release of epinephrine associated with activation of this system.
         (b) **Parasympathetic division.** This division is frequently described as the **"vegetative"** or **"autopilot" system,** because parasympathetic activity returns the body to an unexcited state, suitable for maintaining status quo. The sympathetic division is also sometimes referred to as the **craniosacral system,** because its neuronal cell bodies are located in the brain stem or the sacral region of the spinal cord, or the **cholinergic system,** because of its use of acetylcholine as its exclusive transmitter.

II. STRUCTURAL CLASSIFICATION

A. CNS

1. **Brain.** The brain is the **central receiving, integrating,** and **controlling portion of the CNS.**
   a. **Histology**
      (1) The **grey matter** of the brain is composed of the neurons' cell bodies and their supporting structures.
      (2) The **white matter** is composed of axons collected into neural pathways.
   b. **Gross anatomy**
      (1) **Brain.** The brain consists of the **cerebral hemispheres** (involved with sensory function, memory, integration, thought, and consciousness), the **cerebellum** (a center of coordination), and the **brain stem** (involved with visceral reflexes).
      (2) **Supportive and protective structures** include the **cranial vault of the skull** and three layers of **meninges** (Figure 4–1). From superficial to deep, these meninges are the dura mater, the arachnoid, and the pia mater.
         (a) The **dura mater** ("tough mother") is a thick and fibrous membrane consisting of an **outer layer** (the periosteum of the skull) and an **inner layer,** sometimes referred to as the "true" dura.
            (i) The **epidural space** is a potential space between the inner and outer dural layers. The **meningeal arteries** and **venous sinuses of the brain** lie between the two layers of the dura.
            (ii) The **subdural space** is a potential space just deep to the inner dura, between the dura and the arachnoid (the next meningeal layer).
         (b) The **arachnoid** is a thin, membranous layer deep to the dura. The arachnoid is connected to the next meningeal layer by a thin lacework of trabeculae. (The spiderweb-like appearance gave rise to its name, which means "spiderlike.")

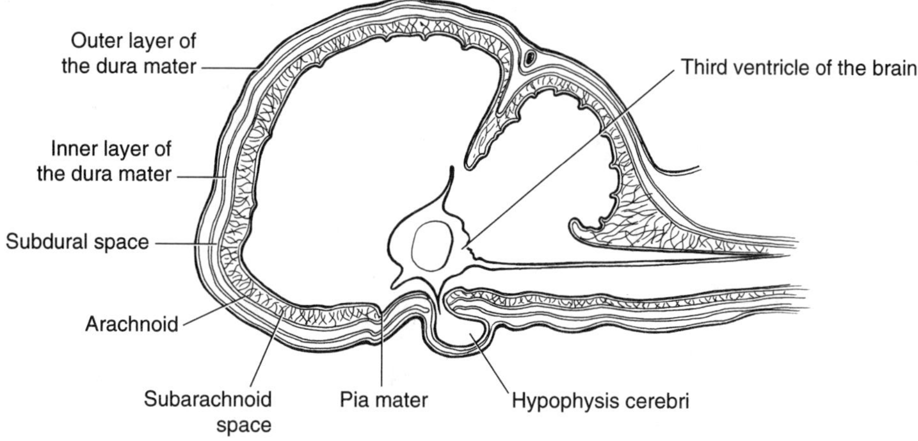

FIGURE 4–1. Schematized lateral view of the meninges of the brain. The subarachnoid space (*cross-hatched area*) is where the cerebrospinal fluid is located.

(i) The arachnoid layer provides a passage for and supports the relatively large distributing **cortical arteries.**

(ii) The **subarachnoid space** lies deep to the arachnoid layer, and contains the **cerebrospinal fluid.**

(c) The **pia mater** ("tender mother") is a delicate membrane that is intimately attached to the surface of the brain, closely following the contours of the sulci. The pia mater conducts the small blood vessels that directly supply the brain and brain stem.

2. **Spinal cord.** The spinal cord relays **sensory information to the brain,** relays **motor commands from the brain,** and plays a part in numerous **reflex arcs.**
   a. The spinal cord is **shorter than the vertebral canal** (Figure 4–2).
      (1) The discrepancy between the lengths of the vertebral column and the spinal cord develops because the spinal cord grows little after birth, but the vertebral column grows considerably.
      (2) The gradual elongation of the vertebral column as the animal grows draws out the length of the lumbar and sacral spinal nerve roots. This collection of elongate nerve roots is vaguely reminiscent of a horse's tail, hence the anatomic term **cauda equina.**
   b. The spinal cord is of **uneven diameter** in its course through the vertebral canal (Figure 4–3).
      (1) The **cervical intumescence** is an enlargement associated with the increase in neurons innervating the thoracic limbs, extending from spinal cord segments C6–T1.
      (2) The **lumbar intumescence** is an enlargement associated with the increase in neurons innervating the pelvic limbs, extending from spinal cord segments L5–S1.
      (3) The **conus medullaris,** the gradually narrowing region of the cord caudal to the lumbar intumescence, terminates at approximately the level of vertebrae L6–L7. The conus medullaris is comprised of spinal cord segments S2 through Cd5.
      (4) The **filum terminale** is a band of glial and ependymal cells, containing no nervous elements, extending from the distal end of the conus medullaris and terminating at approximately the level of the fifth caudal vertebra (Cd5).
   c. The surface of the spinal cord is marked by **dorsal** and **ventral median fissures** that divide the cord into symmetric right and left halves (Figure 4–4).
      (1) **Grey matter.** On cross-section, the spinal cord contains a butterfly-shaped inner region composed of neuronal cell bodies.

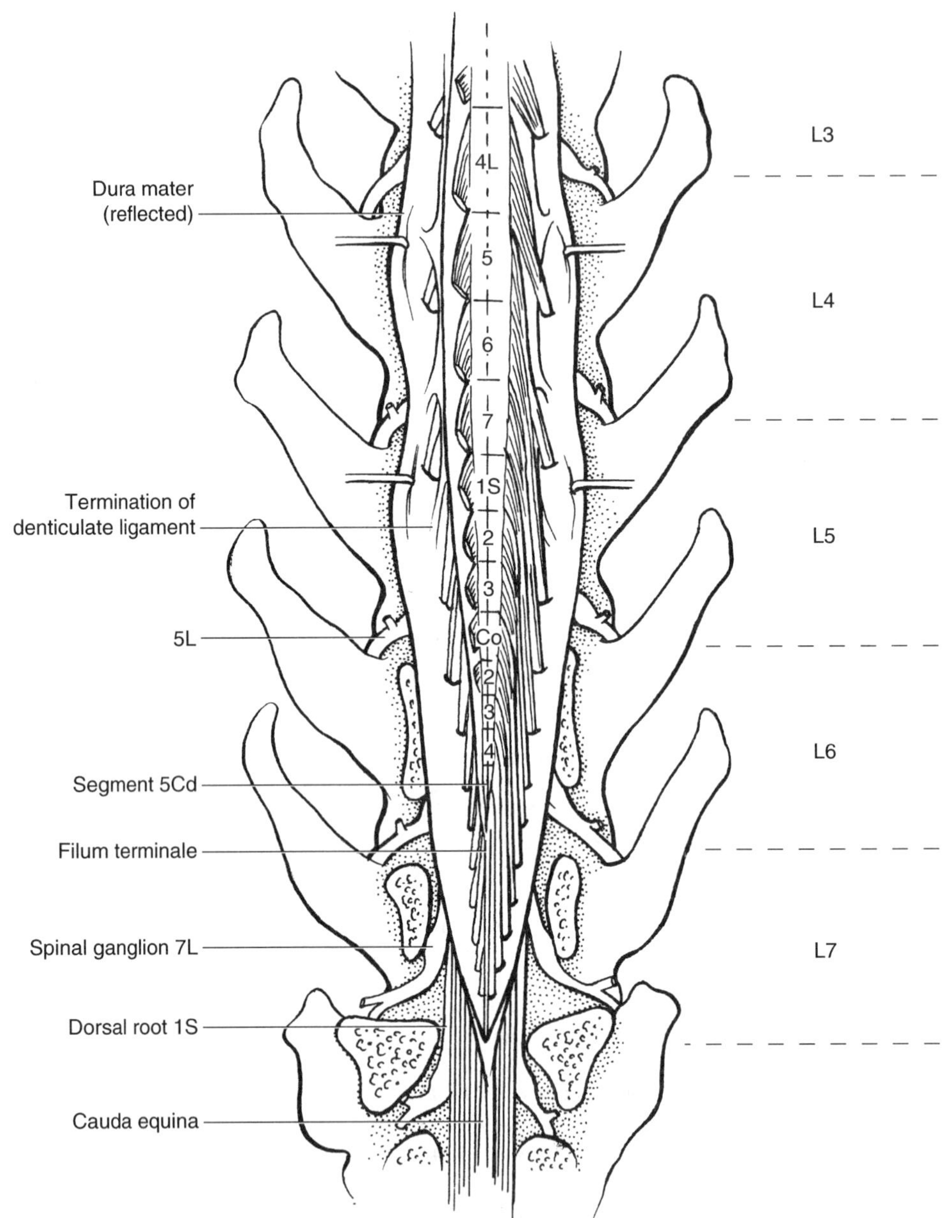

FIGURE 4–2. The termination of the spinal cord within the vertebral canal. The S3 segment of the spinal cord terminates at approximately the level of vertebrae L5–L6. (The cord tends toward the greater of those lengths in smaller dogs.) Note the elongation of the terminal spinal nerve roots as they travel to their exit points. (Modified with permission from Fletcher TS, Kitchell RL: Anatomic studies on the spinal cord segments of the dog. *Am J Vet Res* 27: 1759–1767, 1966.)

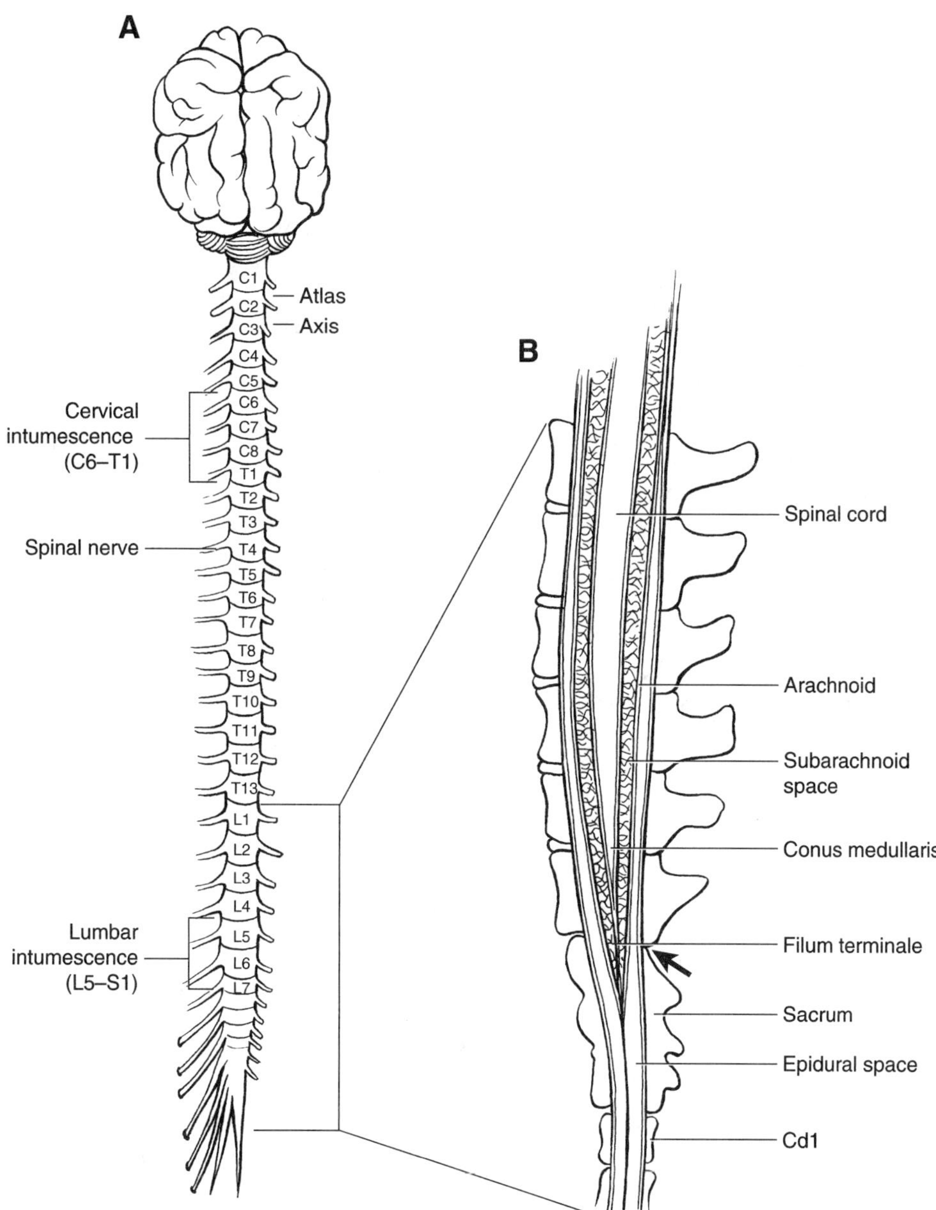

FIGURE 4–3. (*A*) The central nervous system (CNS) removed from the skull and vertebral column. (*B*) Median section of the caudal vertebral canal, spinal cord, and associated structures. Note that the lumbosacral junction (indicated by the *bold arrow*) is the preferred site for inserting the needle when performing a spinal tap.

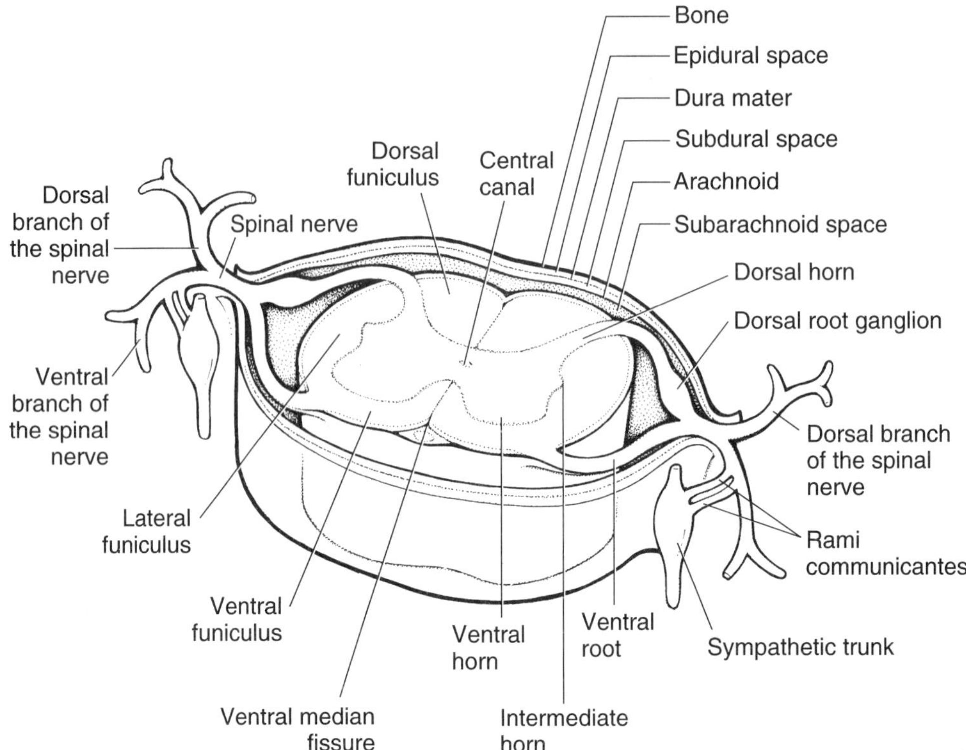

FIGURE 4–4. Cross-section of the spinal cord. The spinal nerve, which contains both sensory (dorsal) and motor (ventral) components, is a mixed spinal nerve.

(a) At the center of the grey matter lies the **central canal,** a longitudinal cavity containing cerebrospinal fluid.

(b) The upper wings of the "butterfly" are the **dorsal horns,** and the lower wings are the **ventral horns.** The **dorsal roots** continue from the dorsal horn to the periphery of the cord. Similarly, the **ventral roots** continue from the ventral horn to the cord's periphery.

(c) In the thoracolumbar region of the spinal cord, an additional enlargement of grey matter is present, referred to as the **intermediate horn.** This region contains the cell bodies of the sympathetic nervous system.

(2) **White matter.** The grey matter is surrounded by white matter, composed of myelinated axons. The white matter is divided into regions by the fissures and the horns of the grey matter.

(a) The **dorsal funiculus** lies between the dorsal median fissure and the dorsal roots.

(b) The **lateral funiculus** lies between the dorsal and ventral roots.

(c) The **ventral funiculus** lies between the ventral roots and the ventral median fissure.

d. The **spinal meninges** are essentially the same as those of the brain; in fact, they are contiguous with the brain meninges.

(1) The **spinal dura mater** differs from that of the brain in that the outer layer does not fuse with the periosteum of the surrounding bone.

(a) **Epidural** and **subdural spaces** are present, as with the brain dura mater. The epidural space contains venous plexuses and fat.

(b) The **spinal dura mater filament** is an extension of the dura mater that surrounds the filum terminale.

(2) The **spinal arachnoid** is similar to that of the brain. Like the subarachnoid space

of the brain, the subarachnoid space of the spinal cord contains cerebrospinal fluid.

(a) The **cerebellomedullary cistern (cisterna magna)** is a dilatation of the subarachnoid space in the atlantooccipital region (i.e., at the cranial end of the spinal column).

(b) The **lumbar cistern** at the **lumbosacral junction** is the extension of the subarachnoid space caudally beyond the S3 segment of the spinal cord.

Canine Clinical Correlation

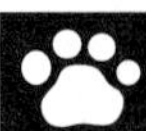

Spinal taps, used to obtain cerebrospinal fluid for analysis, can be performed at the cerebellomedullary cistern or at the lumbosacral junction. The **cerebellomedullary cistern** is accessible to needle puncture because of the incontinuity of the bony laminae in this area; however, because of the presence of the spinal cord within this space, iatrogenic injury to the cord is a risk. At the **lumbosacral junction,** the needle enters the region of the cauda equina (see Figure 4–3B). Here, the nerve roots are elongated and relatively mobile, so they tend to move out of the needle's path, reducing the chance of iatrogenic injury.

(3) The **pia mater** is also similar to that of the brain, and conducts the blood supply to the spinal cord. **Denticulate ligaments** are bilateral thickenings of the pia mater positioned along its lateral margins that attach to the dura mater. The denticulate ligaments effectively suspend the spinal cord within the fluid-filled subarachnoid space; thus, the surface of the spinal cord is surrounded on all sides by cerebrospinal fluid.

Canine Clinical Correlation

The spaces defined by the meninges provide the means of inducing two types of regional anesthesia. **Epidural anesthesia** is accomplished by introducing anesthetic material into the epidural space. This form of anesthesia is slower in onset and longer in duration, owing to the separation of the anesthetic from the spinal cord by the deep layer of the dura mater as well as the other two meningeal layers (see Figure 4–4). **Spinal anesthesia** is accomplished by introducing the anesthetic into the subarachnoid space. This form of anesthesia is quicker in onset (and also more likely to cause side effects) than epidural anesthesia because only the pia mater separates the subarachnoid space from the spinal cord.

3. **Cerebrospinal fluid** is the nutritive and protective fluid of the CNS. It fills the internal chambers of both the brain (the ventricles) and the spinal cord (the central canal), as well as the subarachnoid space surrounding both the brain and spinal cord.
   a. **Production.** Cerebrospinal fluid is continually produced by ultrafiltration of the blood at the **choroid plexuses,** capillary tufts that extend into the ventricular cavities. Cerebrospinal fluid normally flows freely from its production sites in the ventricles of the brain caudally to a point near the junction of the brain and the spinal cord. Here, the cerebrospinal fluid either:
      (1) Flows caudally through the **central canal of the spinal cord**
      (2) Enters the **lateral apertures,** via which it gains access to the **subarachnoid spaces** of the brain and spinal cord
   b. **Resorption.** Because cerebrospinal fluid is continually produced, it must also be resorbed to prevent abnormal accumulation of fluid and associated pathologic CNS changes. There are **two major routes of cerebrospinal fluid return** to the systemic circulation.

(1) **Through the arachnoid villi.** The arachnoid villi are protrusions of the arachnoid membrane (not capillary tufts) that extend into the dural venous sinuses. The walls of the villi are extremely thin, being composed only of a layer of endothelial cells and an associated thin layer of fibroblasts.

(a) When the venous pressure exceeds the cerebrospinal fluid pressure, the villi are passively collapsed. Cerebrospinal fluid remains within the subarachnoid space, and the collapsed villi act as valves, preventing blood from entering the cerebrospinal fluid.

(b) When cerebrospinal fluid pressure exceeds venous pressure, the villi expand, and cerebrospinal fluid passes across the membrane until equilibrium is reached.

(2) **Across the meningeal sheaths of the cranial and spinal nerve roots.** After crossing the meningeal sheaths of the cranial and spinal nerve roots, the transudated cerebrospinal fluid enters the lymphatics associated with the nerves.

B. PNS

1. **Spinal nerve roots** emerge from the spinal cord segments in bilaterally symmetrical pairs, one per segment (see Figure 4–4).

a. The **dorsal nerve roots** are formed from **afferent (sensory) fibers** that originate in the body and travel to the spinal cord. The **dorsolateral sulcus** is a groove present where the dorsal roots enter the spinal cord.

(1) The cell bodies of these neurons are located in the **dorsal root ganglion,** which lies in the intervertebral foramen (see Figure 4–4).

(2) Some of the sensory fibers of the dorsal root ganglion innervate specific segmental regions of skin referred to as **dermatomes,** which are most readily recognizable over the skin of the neck and trunk. Dermatomes overlap in a fashion that results in any given skin locus receiving innervation from three spinal nerves, reducing the likelihood of sensory deprivation in a given region following injury.

Canine Clinical Correlation

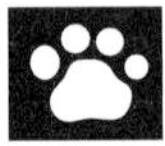

Because the innervation of dermatomes is constant, testing for sensory deficit in dermatomes can be used as a means of mapping peripheral nerve, nerve root, or spinal cord injury.

b. The **ventral nerve roots** are formed from **efferent (motor) fibers** that originate in the brain and travel to the body via the spinal cord.

(1) The cell bodies of these neurons lie in the **ventral horn** of the spinal cord (see Figure 4–4). The axons from these cells may innervate skeletal muscle, or synapse with neurons in peripheral ganglia that in turn innervate smooth muscle or glands.

(2) The region of musculature innervated by a single spinal nerve is referred to as a **myotome.** As is the case with the skin and dermatomes, muscles are also innervated by multiple nerves, reducing the chance of complete muscle denervation following injury to a single spinal nerve.

2. **Spinal nerves** are **formed by the junction of a dorsal and ventral nerve root** (see Figure 4–4). This junction physically takes place near the intervertebral foramen. Because the resulting nerve contains both sensory and motor components, the nerve is sometimes referred to as a **mixed spinal nerve.**

a. **Number and location.** Spinal nerves in the dog usually number **36 pairs,** one for each spinal cord segment plus one additional cervical spinal nerve. The first cervical nerve exits the CNS between the skull and vertebra C1. The remaining spinal nerves all exit the CNS through the intervertebral foramen just caudal to the vertebra of the same number.

b. **Branches.** The course of the mixed spinal nerve is rather short, because that nerve quickly divides into specific branches.

(1) The **meningeal branch** is the first branch of the spinal nerve, providing sensory innervation to the meninges.

(2) The **dorsal primary branch** passes dorsally to innervate the skin and muscles of the back (i.e., the **epaxial musculature).** The dorsal branches typically divide into **medial** (motor to epaxial musculature) and **lateral** (skin sensory) **branches.**

(3) The **ventral primary branch** passes ventrally to supply **all hypaxial structures,** including the limbs. Ventral branches also divide into **lateral** and **medial branches,** with the lateral branch being sensory to the skin.

(a) Certain of the ventral branches take on specific names, such as the **intercostal nerves** (T1–T12), the **costoabdominal nerve** (T13), the **cranial** and **iliohypogastric nerves** (L1 and L2, respectively), and the **ilioinguinal nerve** (L3).

(b) In the regions of the limbs, the ventral branches communicate to form the **brachial** and **lumbosacral plexuses,** associated with the thoracic and pelvic limbs, respectively.

(4) The **communicating branch (ramus communicans)** is unique. It carries motor and sensory fibers related only to **visceral structures** (i.e., smooth muscle and glands). The *Nomina Anatomica Veterinaria* no longer distinguishes grossly between white and grey rami communicantes.

III. FUNCTIONAL CLASSIFICATION

A. Terminology.

Terminology. Four adjectives are combined in various ways to describe the functional components of the nervous system.

1. **"General"** refers to **nonspecialized sensations** such as touch, temperature, proprioception, and pain (i.e., things essentially related to forms of touch).
2. **"Special"** refers to the **specialized senses** of vision, hearing, smell, and taste, as well as balance.
3. **"Somatic"** refers to the **external body surface** of the head, body wall, and extremities.
4. **"Visceral"** refers to the **viscera (organs).**

B. Somatic nervous system

1. **Somatic afferent nerves carry sensory information** from general free nerve endings as well as from specialized receptors **to the CNS.**

a. **Classification.** Afferent nerves can be classified according to the type of information conveyed.

(1) **General somatic afferent nerves** carry information regarding the forms of touch (e.g., light touch, pressure, temperature, pain) from the external body surface to the CNS.

(2) **Special somatic afferent nerves** carry information regarding vision, hearing, and balance.

b. **Pathway.** The afferent pathway involves one peripheral neuron and at least one central neuron.

(1) **Peripheral neuron.** The receptor of the neuron (either a free nerve ending or an ending making contact with a specialized receptor) receives the input and passes it to the cell body lying in the dorsal root ganglion. The impulse passes through the cell body and into the axon, entering the spinal cord through the dorsal root. The axon can either:

(a) Terminate and synapse in the spinal cord grey matter on the central neuron

(b) Pass cranially in a white matter funiculus of the spinal cord to reach a portion of the grey matter of the brain stem

(2) **Central neuron.** The central neuron is located in the grey matter of either the spinal cord or brain stem. After synapsing with the peripheral neuron, the central neuron sends information to neurons in higher brain centers.

2. **Somatic efferent nerves** function mainly in **regulating muscular activities necessary for voluntary movement and posture maintenance.**
   a. **Classification**
      (1) **General somatic efferent nerves** supply the voluntary muscles of the head, neck, body wall, and limbs.
      (2) **Special somatic efferent nerves** supply the voluntary muscles of the head and neck that arise from the embryonic branchial arches (rather than from the myotomes).
   b. **Pathway**
      (1) The efferent pathway involves two neurons, one in the CNS [an upper motor neuron (UMN)] and one in the PNS [a lower motor neuron (LMN)].
         (a) **UMN.** The cell bodies of these neurons are located in the cortical and brain stem nuclei. The axon of the UMN descends through the brain and, depending on the length of the axon, the spinal cord to terminate on a lower motor neuron (LMN). The location of the LMN cell body depends on the source of the original UMN.
         (b) **LMN.** The cell body of the associated UMN lies in the grey matter of the brain stem, for cranial nerves, or the ventral horn of the spinal cord, for spinal nerves. The axon of the LMN courses through either a cranial nerve or a spinal nerve to terminate on voluntary skeletal muscle fibers.
      (2) **Reflex arcs** are relatively shorter circuits passing from the periphery to the spinal cord and back out again. Reflex arcs are self-contained among the sensor, the spinal cord, and the effector, and require no input from higher centers (though a reflex can be modified by conscious action of higher centers). Many reflex arcs are protective (e.g., the withdrawal reflex) or regulatory (e.g., the stretch reflex).
         (a) **Simple reflex arcs** consist of a single sensory and a single motor neuron that synapse in the spinal cord.
         (b) **Complex reflex arcs** consist of more than two neurons, including one or more association neurons (interneurons) within the substance of the spinal cord.

Canine Clinical Correlation

When performing a neurologic examination, it must be remembered that because spinal reflexes require no higher input in order to complete an associated movement, withdrawal of a limb in response to a pinch does not necessarily imply that the dog felt the pinch, because pain perception is a function of higher brain centers.

C. Visceral nervous system

1. **Visceral efferent nerves** compose the **ANS,** which is **strictly motor in nature** and affects body systems over which minimal or no conscious or voluntary control can be exerted (e.g., digestive system, vasodilatory responses).
   a. **Pathway.** Three neurons, two peripheral and one central, form this pathway.
      (1) **UMN.** Cell bodies of the UMN lie in the grey matter of the autonomic centers of the brain. Axons from the UMN descend from the brain via tracts through the brain stem or spinal cord.
      (2) **Preganglionic neuron.** The cell bodies of the preganglionic neurons lie in either the brain or sacral spinal cord (parasympathetic nerves) or in the lateral horn of the spinal cord (sympathetic nerves). The preganglionic neuron sends its myelinated axon out to the PNS via either a cranial or spinal nerve. The preganglionic neuron terminates by forming a synapse with a postganglionic neuron in a ganglion (i.e., a collection of neuronal cell bodies outside of the CNS).
      (3) **Postganglionic neuron. The postganglionic neuron is unique to the ANS.** The cell body of the postganglionic neuron lies in an autonomic ganglion. The postganglionic neuron sends its unmyelinated axon peripherally to synapse on endings associated with smooth or cardiac muscle, or with glands.

b. Sympathetic ANS. The sympathetic division of the ANS is characterized by ganglia that are relatively close to the preganglionic cell bodies, and target organs that are relatively far from the postganglionic cell bodies. Thus, in general, the sympathetic division may be characterized by **short preganglionic** and **long postganglionic fibers.** The topography of the sympathetic ANS is described in detail in IV B; a brief overview is given here.

(1) Sympathetic preganglionic fibers originate in the lateral horn of the spinal cord. From here, preganglionic axons pass sequentially through the **ventral branches of the spinal nerves,** the **rami communicantes,** and the **sympathetic chain,** a bilaterally symmetrical series of ganglia located on each side of the vertebral column (usually one at each intervertebral foramen).

(a) These ganglia are referred to as **paravertebral ganglia** by virtue of their position. The paravertebral ganglia of a given side are interconnected by a narrow line of nerve fibers, giving rise to the outdated but nonetheless descriptive term, "string of pearls" (Figure 4–5).

(b) Within the sympathetic chain, the preganglionic axon has **three possible fates:**

(i) It may synapse immediately within the paravertebral ganglion at the same level where it will exit.

(ii) It may pass through the paravertebral ganglion at the level of origin without synapsing, and ascend or descend to synapse in a paravertebral ganglion of a different level.

(iii) It may pass through the chain without synapsing at all, to form a **splanchnic nerve** that synapses with a **prevertebral ganglion.** Prevertebral ganglia lie on the surface of the large vessels ventral to the vertebrae. Fibers leaving the prevertebral ganglia form a network of nerve fibers (i.e., a **plexus)** around the adjacent vessels. Fibers leave these plexuses and pass outward to their target organs along with the arteries.

(c) The preganglionic sympathetic neuron is said to be **cholinergic,** because the neurotransmitter released by the cell is **acetylcholine.** Sympathetic tone increases the cardiac and respiratory rates, and decreases gastrointestinal and secretory rates.

(2) Sympathetic postganglionic fibers originate from cells in the **paravertebral** or **prevertebral ganglia.** The **cells of the adrenal medulla** are actually specialized postganglionic sympathetic neurons, derived from the neural crest cells of the embryo. The postganglionic sympathetic neuron is described as **adrenergic,** because **norepinephrine** is usually released as the neurotransmitter.

(a) Sympathetic postganglionic fibers that pass back to a **spinal nerve** along a second ramus communicans deliver sympathetic innervation to sweat glands or to smooth muscle in vessel walls or arrector pili muscles.

(b) Sympathetic postganglionic fibers that pass to **perivascular plexuses** and **splanchnic nerves** deliver sympathetic innervation to visceral structures of the head, neck, thorax, abdomen, and pelvis. Sympathetic innervation to the **pelvic viscera** is carried from the abdomen into the pelvis by the paired **hypogastric nerves,** which carry the fibers to the **pelvic plexus.**

c. Parasympathetic ANS (see Figure 4–5)

(1) The parasympathetic division is described as **cholinergic,** because **acetylcholine** is released as the neurotransmitter by both the pre- and postganglionic neurons. Parasympathetic tone decreases the cardiac and respiratory rates, and increases gastrointestinal and secretory rates.

(2) The parasympathetic division is characterized by ganglia that are relatively far from the preganglionic cell bodies, and target organs that are relatively close to the postganglionic cell bodies. Thus, in general, the parasympathetic division may be characterized by **long preganglionic** and **short postganglionic fibers.** The topography of the parasympathetic ANS is described in detail in IV C; a brief overview is given here.

(3) Parasympathetic preganglionic fibers

(a) The **cranial parasympathetic preganglionic fibers** leave the brain along with the **oculomotor nerve (cranial nerve III),** the **facial nerve (cranial nerve VII),**

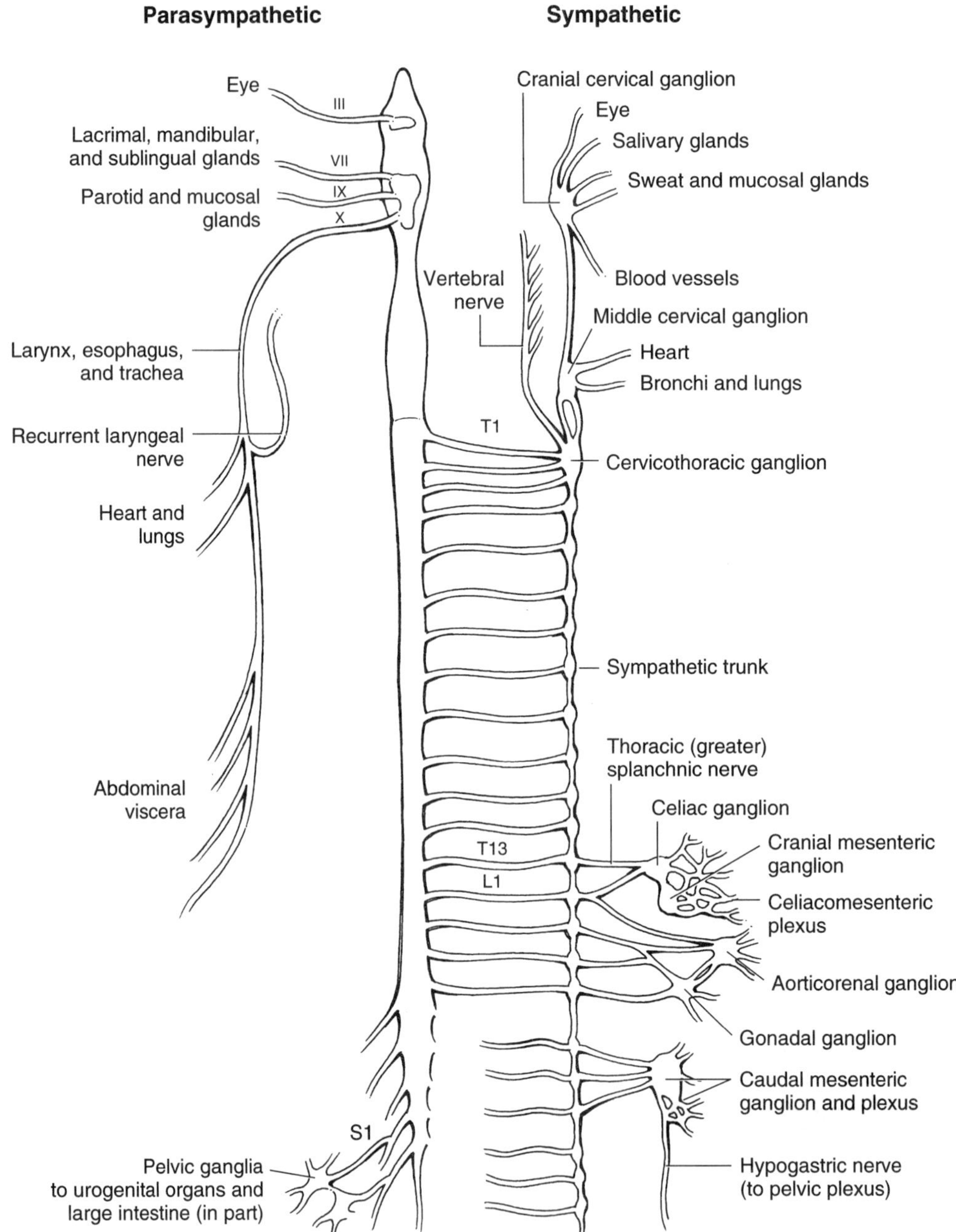

FIGURE 4–5. The autonomic nervous system (ANS). Note the craniosacral location of the cell bodies in the parasympathetic division, and the thoracolumbar location of the cell bodies in the sympathetic division. In the sympathetic ANS, the synapse between pre- and postganglionic fibers takes place in a physical position relatively close to the origin of the first neuron [rather than on or near the target organ], giving the sympathetic nervous system the characteristic of having short preganglionic fibers and long postganglionic fibers. Conversely, in the parasympathetic ANS, the parasympathetic fibers enter into small ganglia and synapse on or near the surface of their target organs; therefore, the preganglionic fibers are very long and the postganglionic fibers are short in the parasympathetic ANS.

the **glossopharyngeal nerve (cranial nerve IX),** and the **vagus nerve (cranial nerve X).**

(i) These fibers supply parasympathetic innervation to the viscera and other smooth muscles of the head, neck, thorax, and most of the abdomen.

(ii) The vagus nerve innervates the thoracic and the abdominal viscera as far caudally as the left colic flexure. The origin of the Latin name—*vagus,* "wanderer"—becomes apparent when considering the nerve's range of distribution.

(b) The **sacral parasympathetic preganglionic fibers** leave the sacral spinal cord and form the **pelvic nerve.** The pelvic nerve carries preganglionic parasympathetic fibers to the **pelvic plexus.** Autonomic fibers synapse in small ganglia in the plexus, and then leave the plexus to distribute to target organs of the lower abdominal and pelvic viscera along routes established by arteries.

d. The parasympathetic and sympathetic divisions of the ANS are compared in Table 4–1.

2. Visceral afferent nerves carry **sensory information from visceral organs** or **certain specialized sense organs to the CNS.**

a. Classification

(1) General visceral afferent nerves carry sensory information from the visceral organs (e.g., stretch of the gut tube by gas accumulation). The afferent fibers of the viscera must not be thought of as typical of those of the remainder of the body in terms of the type of sensory information to which they are sensitive. Rather than being sensitive to a wide variety of stimuli (e.g., light touch, motion, temperature), most visceral afferent fibers are **sensitive mainly to the sensation of stretch,** which is usually perceived as pain.

(2) Special visceral afferent nerves carry smell and taste.

b. Pathway. Visceral afferent pathways pass in a retrograde fashion (i.e., toward the CNS) along pathways established by the ANS (usually those of the sympathetic division). Therefore, though not part of that system, discussion of the visceral afferent nerves most conveniently follows discussion of the autonomic system because much of the terminology is the same.

(1) In the **cervical region,** visceral afferent fibers pass along cervical splanchnic nerves, toward the sympathetic chain, and through the rami communicantes, thereby gaining access to the spinal nerves and finally the spinal cord.

(2) In the **thoracoabdominal region,** visceral afferent fibers pass up the splanchnic nerves, into the sympathetic chain, and through the rami communicantes to a spinal nerve and finally, the spinal cord.

(3) In the **pelvic region,** two routes are present.

(a) Cranial pelvic viscera. The afferent neurons pass through the sympathetic pathways to the lumbar splanchnic nerves, then to the sympathetic chain and

TABLE 4–1. Summary Comparison of the Sympathetic and Parasympathetic Divisions of the Autonomic Nervous System

	Location of Preganglionic Cell Bodies	Length of Preganglionic Axon	Length of Postganglionic Axon	General Action	Neurotransmitter
Sympathetic	Thoracolumbar spinal cord	Short	Long	Accelerates	Acetylcholine (preganglionic) Norepinephrine (postganglionic)
Parasympathetic	Craniosacral spinal cord	Long	Short	Calms	Acetylcholine

through the rami communicantes to the spinal nerve, and finally, into the spinal cord.

(b) Caudal pelvic viscera. Afferent neurons follow the pelvic nerve (a parasympathetic path) to the midsacral regions of the spinal cord.

IV. AUTONOMIC NERVOUS SYSTEM (ANS) TOPOGRAPHY (See Figure 4–5)

A. Key concepts.
Key concepts. The location and course of the sympathetic and parasympathetic components of the ANS may be confusing and may, at times, even appear frankly irrational. Imperative to understanding the topography of the ANS is the immediate awareness of two facts which, though simple, are key to grasping the organization of the ANS organization. The apparent "wanderings" of various parts of autonomic nerves is attributable to the following two facts:

1. **Essentially all organs must receive dual innervation from both sympathetic and parasympathetic sources.** (When considering this fact, it must be kept in mind that the term "organs" includes the visceral organs as well as other structures, such as arterioles, sweat glands, and salivary glands.)
2. **The cell bodies of the sympathetic and parasympathetic neurons are severely restricted in their distribution.**
   a. The cell bodies of **sympathetic neurons** are located only in the **thoracolumbar spinal cord** (usually T1–L4 or L5), within the intermediate horn.
   b. The cell bodies of **parasympathetic neurons** are located only in the **brainstem and sacral spinal cord.**

B. Sympathetic ANS
Sympathetic ANS (see Figure 4–5). The topography of the sympathetic ANS is best understood by beginning at the cell bodies and following the fibers cranially and caudally, rather than beginning at the cranial extremity and passing to the caudal one. Though this approach "starts in the middle" and works to both ends, it actually follows the true path of the fibers within the system.

1. **Cell bodies** of the sympathetic ANS are located in the **thoracolumbar spinal cord.**
2. **Preganglionic fibers.** The sympathetic neurons send their axons out of the spinal cord through the ventral root, and the fibers travel with the spinal nerve for a very short distance.
   a. The sympathetic axons **part company with the spinal nerve** via a **white ramus communicans.** Because these fibers have just come from the spinal cord and have not yet synapsed anywhere, they are referred to as "preganglionic."
   b. The preganglionic fibers pass through this communicating branch, and enter the **sympathetic trunk.** Recall that the sympathetic trunk is the paired chain of pre- and postganglionic sympathetic and visceral afferent fibers positioned on the ventrolateral surfaces of the thoracolumbar vertebral bodies; a series of regularly-arranged **paravertebral ganglia** of the sympathetic chain is typically located at the site of junction with each entering white ramus communicans.
3. **Postganglionic fibers.** After entering the sympathetic trunk, the axons take one of various alternative paths [see III C 1 b (1) (b)], synapsing with one of the ganglia at some level, and emerge again from the sympathetic chain through a grey ramus communicans.
   a. The **cervicothoracic (stellate) ganglion** is a large ganglion formed, as the name suggests, from the fusion of the most caudal cervical ganglion with the most cranial (one or two) thoracic ganglia. The sympathetic trunk is split just ventral to the cervicothoracic ganglion by the passage of the subclavian artery. The **ansa subclavia** is the term given to the side of the loop passing ventral to the artery.
   b. The **middle cervical ganglion** is a variably-developed ganglion that is usually located near the cervicothoracic ganglion. The **cervical sympathetic trunk** extends cranially from the middle cervical ganglion, carrying sympathetic fibers up to the head. It travels in intimate contact with the vagus nerve, within the carotid sheath directly on the surface of the common carotid artery.

4. **Target organs.** After passing through a ganglion, the postganglionic fibers travel to their target organs to provide sympathetic innervation. The directness of this route varies according to the region supplied. Obviously, structures near the thoracolumbar area receive their sympathetic innervation via a fairly direct route, while those structures in more remote areas (e.g., the head, neck, pelvis) receive sympathetic innervation via a more complicated route.
   a. **Skin and body wall of the thoracolumbar region.** The skin and body wall of the thoracic and lumbar regions receive the most direct sympathetic input. The postganglionic fibers simply travel directly with the spinal nerves to these areas.
   b. **Thoracic viscera.** Sympathetic innervation of the thoracic viscera is also fairly direct. The postganglionic fibers leave the large ganglia of the cranial thorax (i.e., the cervicothoracic and middle cervical ganglia) and course along the surfaces of the regional arteries (thus following an already-established path and also gaining physical support) to their target organs.
   c. **Neck.** The neck receives sympathetic input via the **vertebral nerve,** a large nerve that leaves the cervicothoracic ganglion to travel cranially through the transverse foramina of the cervical vertebrae. Postganglionic fibers simply leave the vertebral nerve at each intervertebral foramen to travel with the spinal nerve, much as in the thoracolumbar area.
   d. **Head.** The head receives sympathetic input from fibers that arrive at the **cranial cervical ganglion,** having traveled up the cervical sympathetic trunk in intimate association with the vagus nerve (the two together are referred to as the **vagosympathetic trunk**).
      (1) Many postganglionic fibers leave this ganglion and travel directly along the surfaces of the arteries supplying the head.
      (2) Other postganglionic fibers join cranial nerves IX, X, XI, and XII to distribute along with them.
   e. **Abdominal viscera** receive sympathetic innervation via the **splanchnic nerves,** which depart from the late thoracic and early abdominal region of the sympathetic trunk and carry preganglionic sympathetic fibers into the abdomen. These fibers then synapse in various ganglia and distribute their postganglionic fibers to the abdominal viscera along the surfaces of the regional arteries.
      (1) The **major** and **minor splanchnic nerves** carry fibers to the large ganglia associated with the digestive viscera (i.e., the celiacomesenteric and cranial mesenteric ganglia) and distribute to the digestive organs of the abdomen.
      (2) The **lumbar splanchnic nerves** carry fibers to the cranial mesenteric, gonadal, and aorticorenal ganglia and their associated nerve plexuses.
   f. **Pelvic viscera** receive their sympathetic innervation through the **hypogastric nerves,** which depart from the caudal mesenteric ganglion and carry postganglionic sympathetic nerves into the pelvic region to enter the **pelvic plexus.** From the pelvic plexus, the postganglionic fibers again follow the common pattern of distributing to target organs by traveling along the surfaces of regional arteries.

C. **Parasympathetic ANS.** The topography of the parasympathetic nervous system is somewhat simpler than that of the sympathetic component. **Cell bodies** of the parasympathetic ANS are located in the **brain stem** and **sacral spinal cord** (see Figure 4–5).

1. **Neurons originating in the brain stem.** Parasympathetic neurons with cell bodies located in the brain stem send their preganglionic fibers out together with the fibers of one of four cranial nerves [i.e., the oculomotor (III), facial (VII), glossopharyngeal (IX), or vagus (X) nerve].*

*It must be noted that the parasympathetic fibers are only one component of these cranial nerves—other types of fibers, including general motor and sensory fibers, compose a large part of each nerve under discussion here.

a. **Head.** The head receives parasympathetic innervation from fibers traveling with cranial nerves III, VII, and IX.
   (1) **Oculomotor nerve (cranial nerve III).** Parasympathetic fibers traveling with **cranial nerve III** supply the **eye.** These fibers pass first to the **ciliary ganglion.** The postganglionic fibers supply muscles controlling the curvature of the lens (ciliary muscles) and the pupillary sphincter.
   (2) **Facial nerve (cranial nerve VII).** There are two parasympathetic components to **cranial nerve VII.** These components supply the:
      (a) **Lacrimal glands.** The first parasympathetic component of cranial nerve VII initially passes to the **pterygopalatine ganglion.** After leaving the pterygopalatine ganglion, postganglionic parasympathetic fibers provide innervation to the lacrimal gland and to glands and smooth muscle of the nasal and oral cavities. Confusion sometimes arises when it is mentioned that some of these postganglionic fibers travel with branches of cranial nerve V, the trigeminal nerve. However, it must be noted that these fibers do so only after having originated with cranial nerve VII and passed through the pterygopalatine ganglion. Thus, cranial nerve V has nothing to do with the origin of the nerve fibers.
      (b) **Sublingual salivary glands.** The second parasympathetic component of cranial nerve VII passes initially to the **mandibular ganglion.** Parasympathetic postganglionic fibers then innervate the mandibular and sublingual salivary glands.
   (3) **Glossopharyngeal nerve (cranial nerve IX).** Parasympathetic fibers traveling with **cranial nerve IX** supply the **parotid** and **zygomatic salivary glands.** The parasympathetic component of cranial nerve IX passes first to the **otic ganglion.** After leaving the otic ganglion, parasympathetic postganglionic fibers travel to the parotid and zygomatic salivary glands.

b. **Viscera of the neck, thorax,** and **most of the abdomen** receive parasympathetic innervation from fibers traveling with the **vagus nerve (cranial nerve X).** Parasympathetic fibers traveling with the vagus nerve first pass to and through, without synapsing, the **proximal vagal ganglion** (a sensory ganglion dealing with the ear but not parasympathetic function). They then pass to and through, again without synapsing, the **distal vagal ganglion,** positioned just outside the skull (another sensory ganglion, dealing with visceral sensory innervation but not parasympathetic function). Distal to the distal vagal ganglion, the vagus nerve joins company with the cervical sympathetic trunk, with the two structures often bound in a common epineurium. Here, the two nerves appear to be a single structure and are referred to together as the **vagosympathetic trunk.** The vagosympathetic trunk has two components, one directing sympathetic input cranially to the head, and the other conducting parasympathetic input caudally to the body cavities.
   (1) **Neck.** The **recurrent laryngeal nerves** depart from each vagus approximately at the level of the middle cervical ganglia. These nerves dispatch parasympathetic input to the **heart (cardiac nerves),** before ascending the neck *en route* to the larynx. From this point caudally, the vagus nerve is composed entirely of parasympathetic fibers.
   (2) **Thorax.** The vagus continues caudally dorsal to the hilus of the lung, and detaches several large **bronchial branches** as it passes. The right and left vagus nerves undergo a branching and rejoining to form dorsal and ventral **vagal trunks.** Branches of the vagal trunks supply branches to the esophagus as they pass the diaphragm and enter the abdomen.
   (3) **Abdomen.** Other branches of the dorsal and ventral vagal trunks provide parasympathetic innervation to the various digestive abdominal viscera from the stomach through the intestines as far caudally as the left colic flexure. These fibers pass through the prevertebral ganglia, enter the plexuses surrounding the ganglia, and pass on by following the arterial supply.

2. **Neurons originating in the sacral spinal cord.** The **pelvic viscera** (i.e., digestive, urinary, and reproductive organs) receive parasympathetic innervation from cell bodies located within the sacral spinal cord.

a. **Preganglionic fibers** leave the sacral spinal cord with the spinal nerves, and then separate from them shortly after exiting the intervertebral foramina (similar to the initial course of the thoracolumbar segments of the sympathetic nerves). The parasympathetic fibers then coalesce to form the **pelvic nerve,** which enters the **pelvic plexus** on the lateral rectal wall.

b. **Postganglionic fibers.** Parasympathetic fibers synapse in small ganglia within the pelvic plexus, and postganglionic fibers join with the sympathetic input that has arrived through the hypogastric nerve to be distributed along the course of the regional arteries. Note that the field of distribution of parasympathetic fibers from the pelvic plexus ascends into the abdomen to supply the field of the colon not reached by the vagus nerve (which stopped at the left colic flexure).

Chapter 5

The Circulatory System

I. INTRODUCTION

A. Function. The circulatory system moves blood through the body, distributing it to organs, tissues and cells, and then returns the blood and associated extravasated fluid to the central vascular compartments.

B. Components. The circulatory system is composed of the:

1. **Heart,** the muscular pump that moves blood through the vascular tree
2. **Arteries,** vessels that carry blood away from the heart, and toward the capillary beds
3. **Capillaries,** vessels through which blood moves very slowly, and across which diffusion of gases, nutrients, and metabolic waste products occurs
4. **Veins,** vessels that carry blood toward the heart, and generally away from the capillary beds
5. **Lymphatic vessels,** vessels that originate in tissue spaces and return excessive tissue fluid to the central circulation

C. Adult versus fetal circulation

1. **Adult circulation**
   a. **Circulatory cycle.** In adults, the systemic and pulmonary circulations are entirely separate (Figure 5–1).
      (1) **Systemic circulation.** This portion of the circulatory cycle passes blood to the capillary beds of the body via the arteries, and returns that blood to the heart.
      (2) **Pulmonary circulation.** This portion of the circulatory cycle passes the deoxygenated blood to the lungs for oxygenation, and returns that blood to the heart for rerouting through the body.
   b. **Circulation pattern.** The normal adult circulation pattern is of course a circle, and choosing a beginning point is somewhat arbitrary. However, for the sake of discussion: blood moves from the **left atrium,** to the **left ventricle,** to the **systemic arteries,** to the **capillary beds of the body,** to the **systemic veins,** to the **right atrium,** to the **right ventricle,** to the **pulmonary arteries** (which are carrying deoxygenated blood), to the **capillary beds of the lungs,** to the **pulmonary veins** (which are carrying oxygenated blood), to the **left atrium,** to renew the cycle.
2. **Fetal circulation.** The fetal circulation pattern (Figure 5–2) is notably modified because two features necessary for fetal life are incompatible with life in the adult.
   a. **Umbilical arteries** and **vein.** The umbilical arteries and vein conduct blood to and from the placenta.
      (1) The paired **umbilical arteries** carry **deoxygenated, waste-laden blood** from the caudal region of the aorta, past the cranial surface of the urinary bladder, and through the umbilicus to the placenta.
         (a) In some adult animals, portions of the umbilical arteries between the aorta and the bladder persist; in this case, the arteries are still identified in the adult as the umbilical arteries, and they terminate on the urinary bladder as the cranial vesical arteries.
         (b) The rest of the umbilical arteries fibrose and are recognized as the round ligaments of the bladder.
      (2) The unpaired **umbilical vein** carries **oxygenated, nutrient-laden blood** from the placenta to the fetus, entering at the umbilicus and passing to the liver.
   b. **Shunts.** Because gas exchange and nutrient transfer take place in the placenta, blood flow through the fetal lungs and liver is of minimal importance.

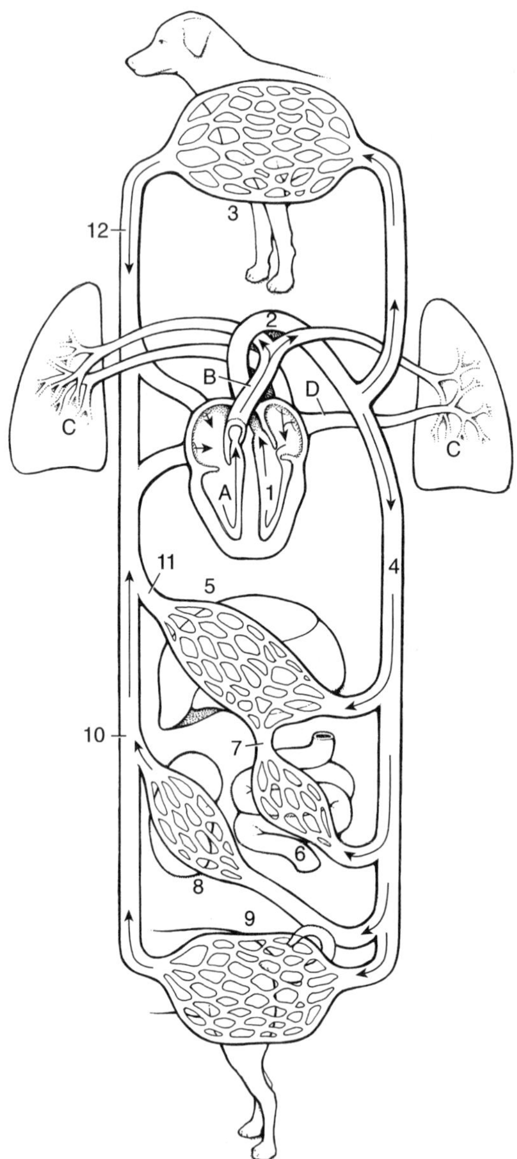

FIGURE 5–1. Schematic drawing of the systemic and pulmonary circulation. Structures of the systemic circulation are identified with numbers: (*1*) Left ventricle, (*2*) aorta, (*3*) capillary bed of the head, neck, and forelimb, (*4*) abdominal aorta, (*5*) liver, (*6*) capillary bed of the intestines, (*7*) portal vein, (*8*) capillary bed of the kidneys, (*9*) capillary bed of the caudal part of the body, (*10*) caudal vena cava, (*11*) hepatic veins, (*12*) cranial vena cava. Structures of the pulmonary circulation are identified with letters: (*A*) right ventricle, (*B*) pulmonary trunk, (*C*) capillary bed of the lungs, (*D*) pulmonary vein.

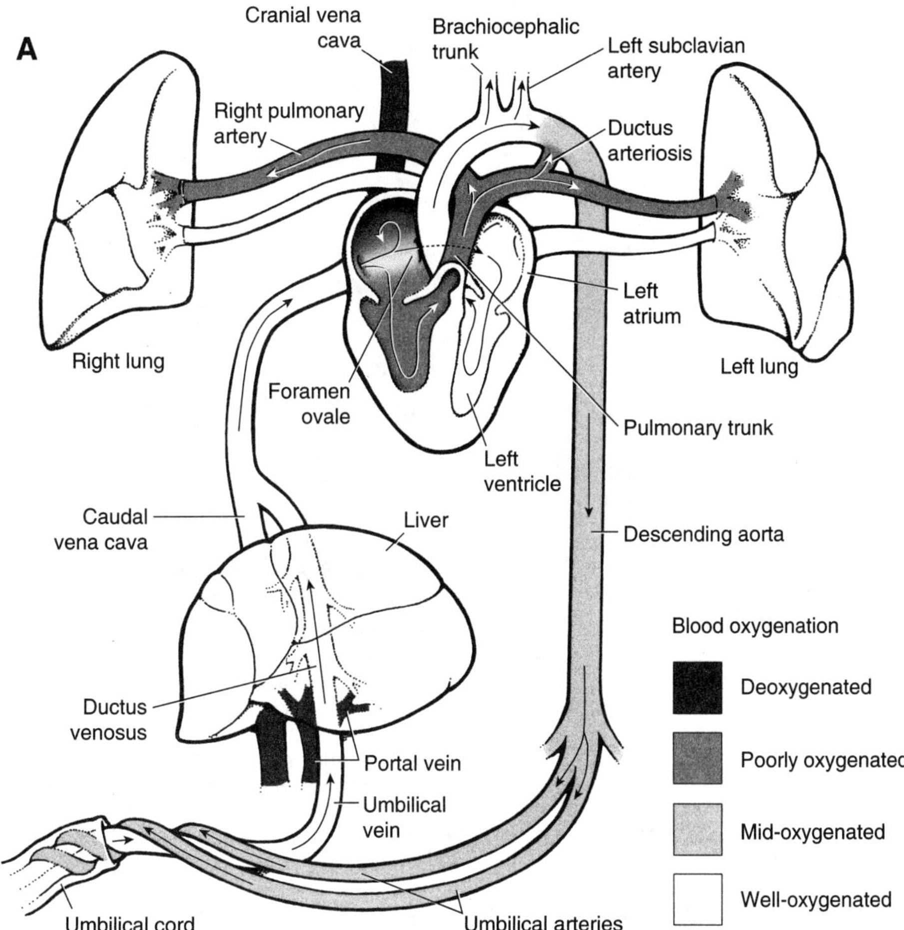

FIGURE 5–2. Comparison of the fetal and adult circulations. (*A*) The fetal circulation. *Arrows* indicate the direction of the blood flow. Note where the oxygenated blood (*white*) mixes with the deoxygenated blood (*black*): in the liver, in the caudal vena cava, in the right atrium, and at the entrance of the ductus arteriosus into the descending aorta. (*continued*)

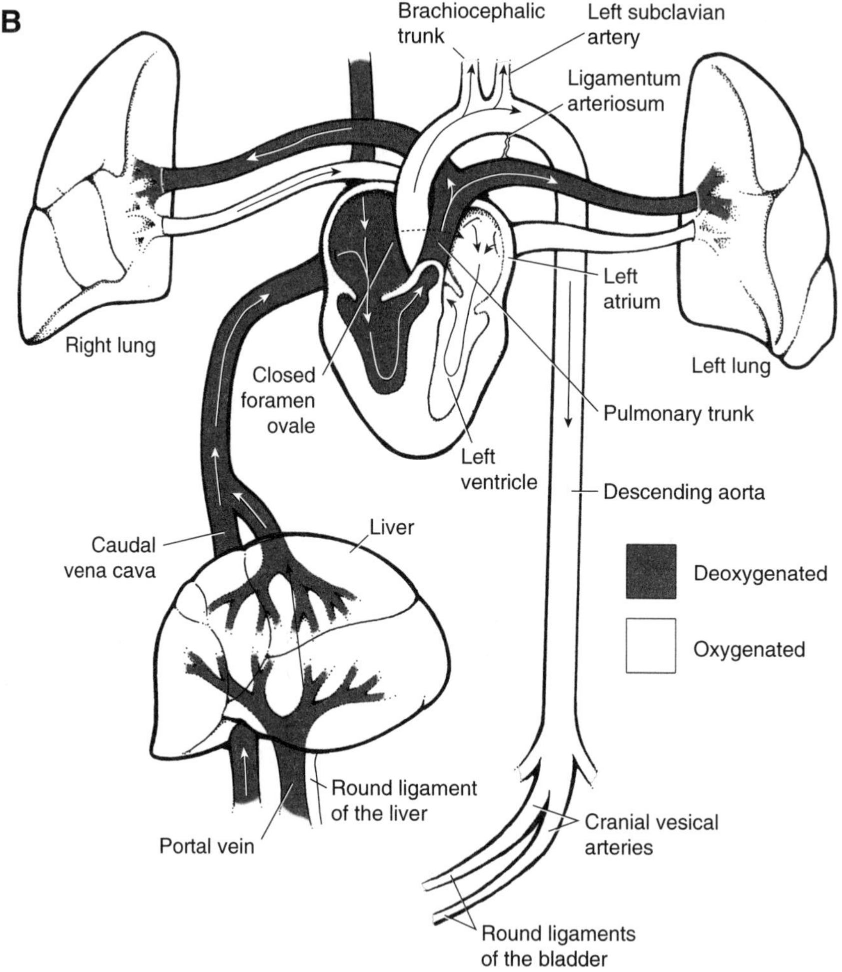

FIGURE 5–2—*continued* (*B*) The adult circulation. The adult remnant of the umbilical vein is the ligament teres hepatis (round ligament of the liver). The adult remnant of the foramen ovale is the fossa ovalis, a depression in the right side of the interatrial septum. The adult remnant of the ductus arteriosus is the ligamentum arteriosum, a ligamentous attachment between the aorta and the pulmonary artery. *Arrows* indicate the direction of blood flow. Oxygenated blood is *black;* deoxygenated blood is *white.*

(1) Pulmonary shunts

(a) The **foramen ovale** is an opening between the two atria, through which blood passes from the right atrium directly into the left atrium, thereby skirting the right ventricle and the lungs.

(b) The **ductus arteriosus** is a direct vascular connection between the pulmonary artery and the aorta. A small amount of blood exits the right ventricle; the ductus arteriosus diverts most of this blood from the pulmonary circulation to the systemic circulation.

(2) Hepatic shunt. The **ductus venosus** is a venous shunt within the liver that carries most of the nutrient-laden and oxygenized blood directly to the caudal vena cava. Because the mother's liver metabolizes food, those nutrients are ready for use by the fetus and therefore have no need to pass through the fetal hepatic parenchyma.

Canine Clinical Correlation

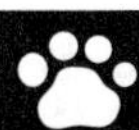

Persistence of various of the features of the fetal circulation are commonly seen in clinical practice, with clinical signs related to alterations in the abnormal blood flow. **Patent foramen ovale** and **persistent ductus arteriosus** occur fairly commonly, with signs referable to inadequate oxygenation of the blood. **Portacaval shunts** (persistence of the ductus venosus) are relatively less common, but when observed, are characterized by signs referable to nitrogen intolerance (e.g., seizures) following meals. Direct entrance of the nutrient-laden blood into the systemic circulation is responsible for the clinical signs.

II. THE HEART

A. Function

1. **Systemic pump.** The **left side of the heart** (i.e., the left atrium and ventricle) is associated exclusively with receiving oxygenated blood from the lungs, and sending it outward to the capillary beds of the body (Figure 5–3).

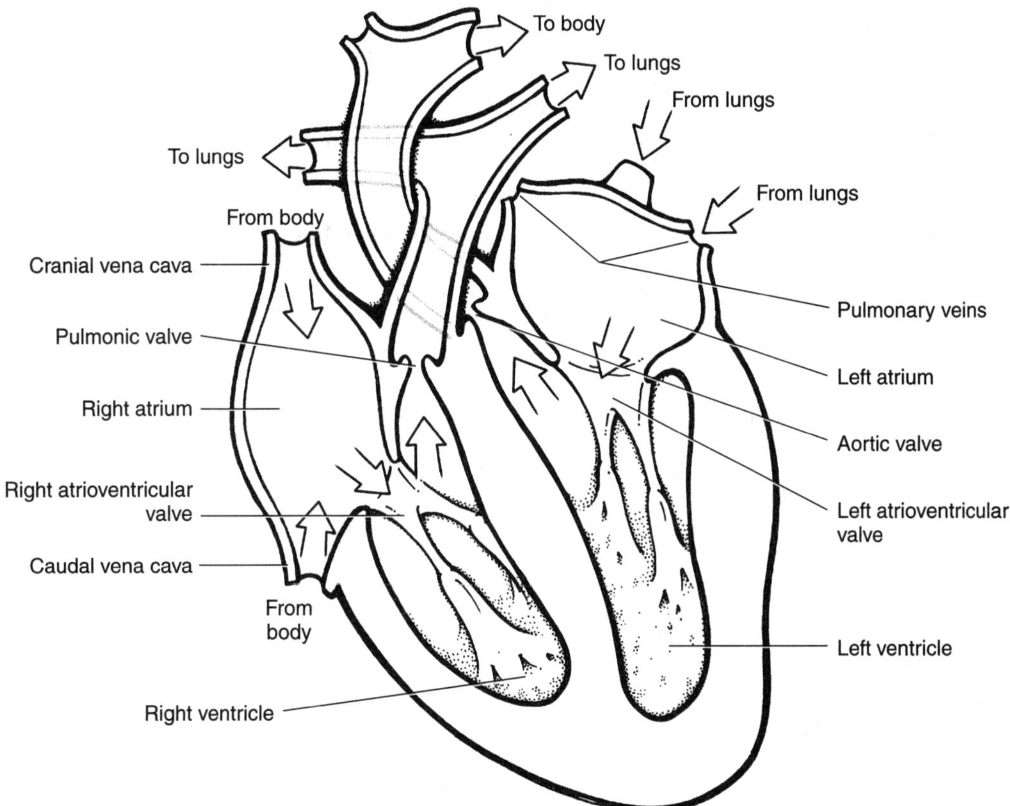

FIGURE 5–3. Flow of blood through the heart.

a. Blood passes to and through the body's capillary beds by the direct action of the heart.
b. Because blood forms a single fluid column, blood is "pushed" back to the heart through the systemic veins by the forward driving force of the blood in the arteries.

2. **Pulmonary pump.** The **right side of the heart** (i.e., the right atrium and ventricle) is associated exclusively with receiving deoxygenated blood from the body, and sending it outward to the capillary beds of the lungs (see Figure 5–3). Like the systemic pump, direct action of the heart is responsible for the passage of blood to and through the capillary beds of the lungs, and the forward driving force of the blood in the arteries returns the blood to the heart via the pulmonary veins.

B. **Vascularization. Coronary arteries** directly supply the myocardium with blood. The coronary arteries are the first branches of the aorta, arising immediately distal to the aortic valve leaflets. Thus, the heart receives highly oxygenated arterial blood before any other organ, even the brain!

C. **Innervation** of the heart is both intrinsic and extrinsic.

1. **Intrinsic.** The **sinuatrial** and **atrioventricular nodes** excite the cardiac muscle, causing it to contract. These nervous tissues are intrinsically rhythmic; the sinuatrial node essentially controls the atrioventricular node.
2. **Extrinsic.** The **autonomic nervous system (ANS)** regulates the heart's inherent rhythmicity, thereby either increasing or decreasing the heart rate.

III. THE ARTERIAL TREE.

The arteries of the body are classified according to size and mural structure, which are both related to function of the artery. The arterial walls are composed of elastic tissue, muscular tissue, or both, with the elastic tissue component being greater in arteries that carry blood at the highest pressure.

A. **Conducting arteries** (e.g., the aorta) are the **largest arteries** of the body. They are located relatively **close to the heart,** and thus **carry blood under high pressure. Elastic tissue** is the predominant component of the walls of conducting arteries.

1. The elastic tissue allows **expansion of the wall during systole** and **rebound of the wall in diastole.** Elastic rebound serves to continue the propulsion of blood through the vascular tree while the heart is in diastole. This pulsation decreases progressively as the arteries decrease in size (and is completely lost at the level of the capillary bed).

Canine Clinical Correlation

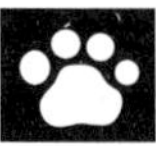

The elastic expansion and rebound of the larger arteries produces a pulse that can be monitored clinically as a measure of heart rate.

2. In the largest of the conducting arteries, the elastic tissue is sufficient in amount to color the entire artery pale yellow or white.

B. **Distributing arteries.** Most of the named arteries in the body are distributing arteries, which arise from conducting arteries or other distributing arteries in a series of branches that become progressively smaller. As the pressure continues to decrease in each successive branching, the walls of the distributing arteries tend to possess more muscle tissue and less elastic tissue.

1. **Distribution.** Distributing arteries are **mostly paired** (i.e., present on the right and left of

the body), with notable exceptions including the three major arteries to the abdominal viscera (i.e., the celiac, cranial mesenteric, and caudal mesenteric arteries).

2. **Characteristics of arterial channels.** The main arterial channels have certain characteristics in common, regardless of their location in a limb or body cavity. They tend to:
   a. Be greatly flexible but only slightly to moderately extensible
   b. Pass on the medial surface (which is relatively more protected than the lateral surface) of limbs
   c. Pass along the flexor rather than extensor surfaces of joints (thereby minimizing stretch)
   d. Not pass directly through muscle (thereby avoiding significant compression during flexion of the muscle)
3. **Anastomoses** between certain distributing arteries **permit collateral circulation** to a given area, as well as allowing equalization of pressure should one of the associated arteries become temporarily compressed (e.g., by muscular contraction or movement of a joint). However, such collateral channels are rarely able to compensate for acute and complete compromise of the other partner in the anastomosis.
4. **End arteries** are those that **supply a given region of an organ or tissue without the benefit of potential anastomoses.** Occlusion of an end artery unavoidably produces ischemia of the affected tissue, which can progress to an infarct (tissue death of the affected area).

C. **Arterioles,** which are not given specific names, are present at the termination of the smallest arteries. Arterioles are only slightly larger than capillaries. Spirally-arranged muscle fibers in their walls and precapillary sphincters located just at the junction of the arteriole and the capillary bed allow the arterioles to **regulate blood flow** to the capillary bed. The muscle fibers in the walls of the arterioles are innervated by nerves of the ANS.

IV. CAPILLARY BEDS

A. **Structure.** Capillary beds are networks of capillaries that extend between an arteriole and a venule (i.e., the smallest component of the venous system).

1. **Capillaries** are **barely larger than the diameter of an erythrocyte** in all species; in the dog, they are approximately 7 μm in diameter. The **capillary walls** are formed by **a single layer of endothelial cells supported by a thin basal lamina.**
2. **Sinusoids,** specialized forms of capillary beds, have **wider lumens** than typical capillaries and are commonly **fenestrated,** permitting ready exchange of colloidal substances across their beds. Sinusoids often contain **phagocytic cells** and are found in the bone marrow, spleen, and liver.
3. **Arteriovenous anastomoses** are direct connections between arterioles and venules that allow blood to circumvent the capillary beds. Arteriovenous anastomoses possess a thick muscular wall that when open, causes blood to bypass the capillary bed, and when closed, causes blood to enter the capillary bed. They are widely distributed throughout the body, and are usually found in organs with intermittent function (e.g., the gut, where they close during digestion to allow blood to flow into the gut's capillary beds).

B. **Function.** The capillary beds are where the **transfer of respiratory gases** (i.e., carbon dioxide and oxygen), **uptake of nutrients,** and **removal of metabolic wastes** occurs. The exchange of gases and other materials is facilitated by the **slow rate of blood flow** through the capillaries (0.5 mm/sec, as compared with 0.5 m/sec in the aorta) and the **extremely thin diffusion barrier** created by the endothelial cell walls of the capillary.

1. **Gas exchange** is caused by differences in concentration (i.e., the partial pressure) of the respiratory gases in various locations.
   a. **In the lungs,** carbon dioxide moves from the blood into the alveoli, while oxygen uptake occurs in the opposite direction.
   b. **In the peripheral tissues,** carbon dioxide moves from the tissues into the blood, while oxygen moves into the tissues.

2. **Movement of nutrients** and **metabolic waste products** is actually achieved by a mechanism of **fluid exchange.** The driving force for this exchange is differences in osmotic pressure.
   a. On the **arterial side** of the capillary bed, the blood pressure is greater than the tissue osmotic pressure, and an ultrafiltrate of nutrient-laden plasma passes out of the capillary bed to bathe the tissues. This loss of fluid from the capillary bed establishes the mechanism for fluid return at the venous side of the capillary bed by increasing the osmotic pressure of the blood within the bed—the osmotic pressure is increased by the removal of fluid, which leaves "solids" behind, while at the same time lowering the osmotic pressure of the tissues by "diluting" the materials there.
   b. On the **venous side** of the capillary bed, the blood pressure is less than the tissue osmotic pressure, and fluids from the tissue that are high in metabolic waste products move into the capillary.

Canine Clinical Correlation

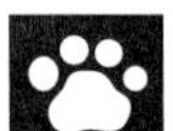

Edema results from the accumulation of fluid in tissue spaces when the normal uptake of fluid from capillary beds is compromised. Normal uptake of fluid from the capillary beds can be compromised as a result of disequilibrium of the oncotic pressures (e.g., as a result of venous stasis), or from increased capillary permeability (e.g., as a result of inflammation). **Bruising (hematoma)** develops when the integrity of the capillary bed is compromised by trauma, and erythrocytes leak into the tissues, die, and degrade.

C. **Distribution.** Capillary bed density is directly related to the metabolic demands of the tissue in question: the density is higher in active tissues (e.g., muscle) and lower in less active tissues (e.g., cartilage).

V. THE VENOUS SYSTEM.

The veins of the body, like the arteries, are classified according to size and mural structure.

A. **Terminology.** When considering the relation of named veins to each other, the tendency is to regard them similarly to arteries, thinking of the smaller veins as "branches" of the larger ones. However, it must be remembered that the direction of blood flow in veins is opposite to that in arteries; therefore, smaller veins do not actually branch off larger ones, but rather flow into them. Thus, correct terminology describes the deep brachial vein as a **"tributary,"** rather than a "branch," of the brachial vein.

B. **Structure**

1. The **venous walls are less robust than the arterial walls,** because blood is received by the venous side of the circulatory system at a low pressure, after having passed through the capillary beds. Thus, the strong "push" of the heart is diminished and the blood is moved through the veins almost secondarily by the force of the heart moving blood into the capillary bed from the opposite side. The larger veins possess some smooth muscle in their walls.
2. Veins tend to be **larger in diameter and less regular in lumenal shape** than their companion arteries.
3. Veins are **considerably compressible** by external forces (e.g., muscle contraction), a feature that assists significantly in venous return. Veins of the limbs and of mobile viscera possess **valves** that prevent backflow of blood.

C. **Distribution.** In general, the venous pattern is more variable than the branching of the arteries. However, several generalizations can be made:

1. **Most distributing arteries are accompanied by veins of the same name** (e.g., brachial artery, brachial vein). This is true in the limbs, on the body wall, and in the body cavities. Occasionally, one of these veins may be doubled, particularly in the limbs.
2. **Departures from close parallels with the arterial pattern are seen in several regions,** including the great vessels of the heart, liver, lungs, and brain.
3. **Two general sets of veins develop on the limbs and body wall:**
   a. A **deeper set** paralleling the arteries of the region
   b. A **superficial set** having essentially no direct relation to the deeper arteries and veins (e.g., the cephalic and lateral saphenous veins)

D. **Portal systems** are formed when a vein conducts blood from one capillary bed to another or to a sinusoidal bed, rather than from a capillary bed to a venule and then to the heart. Examples of portal systems include those associated with the liver and the hypophysis; there are few portal systems within the body.

VI. THE LYMPHATIC SYSTEM

(Figure 5–4). The lymphatic system is similar in form and function to the venous system.

A. **Function.** The lymphatic system serves as an adjunct to the venous system for returning tissue fluid to the circulatory system.

1. **Lymph** is fluid taken up by the lymphatic system from the tissue spaces. This fluid is part of the fluid transudated from the capillary bed that was not retrieved by the venous system. Like blood, lymph has **fluid** and **cellular components.** The cellular components include occasional erythrocytes and white blood cells, as well as numerous lymphocytes.

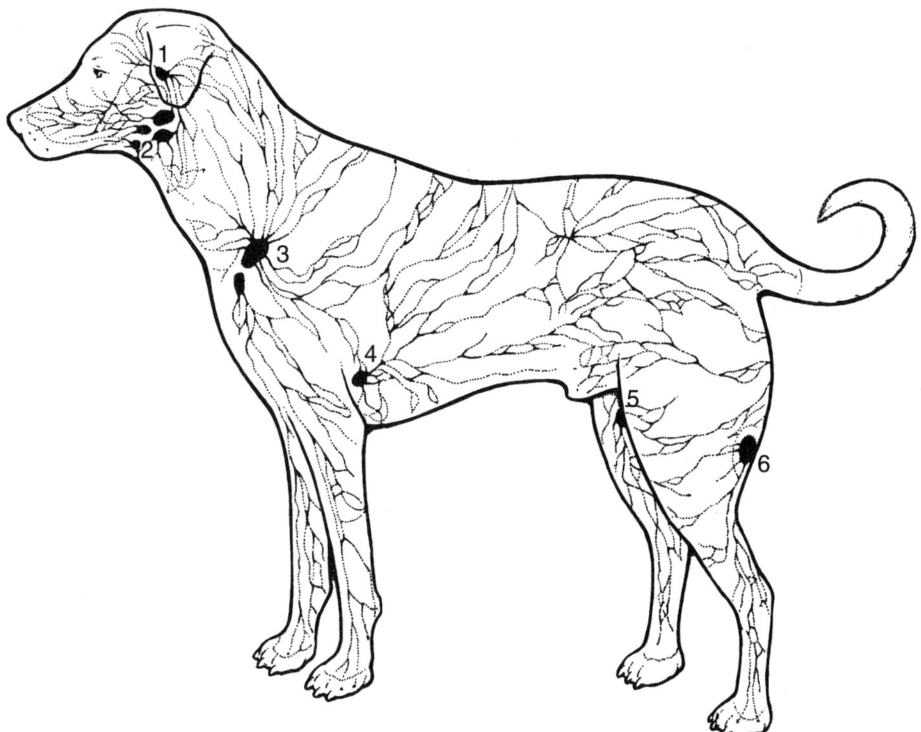

FIGURE 5–4. Superficial lymph drainage of the dog. (*1*) Parotid node, (*2*) mandibular nodes, (*3*) superficial cervical nodes, (*4*) accessory axillary nodes, (*5*) femoral node, (*6*) popliteal node.

2. **Chyle** is fluid within the lymphatic system that contains droplets of fat acquired in the gut via the **lacteal,** a lymphatic vessel positioned centrally within each villus.
3. **Proteins** continually enter the lymphatic system from the tissue spaces, and are filtered through lymph nodes as a part of the immune function of those organs.

B. Distribution. Though a basic pattern of the lymphatic system can be described, the details of its exact design are highly variable from one individual to the next.

C. Components

1. **Lymph capillaries** are simple endothelial tubes that are both larger and more irregular in diameter than the adjacent blood capillaries. The lymph capillaries begin blindly within the tissue spaces and are particularly numerous in the mucous membranes, serous surfaces, and the cutaneous dermis. They are entirely lacking in the central nervous system (CNS), globe of the eye, bone marrow, splenic parenchyma, and superficial fascia.
2. **Lymph vessels** form from the coalescing of lymphatic capillaries. They tend to roughly follow the venous pattern of a given area and are more numerous than the veins they tend to accompany. They possess more numerous valves than veins of similar size. The larger lymph vessels possess small amounts of smooth muscle and elastic fibers in their walls. **Lymph flow** is mainly passive (though contractile or pulsatile regions of some larger lymphatic channels have been described). Features assisting lymph flow include:
   a. Contraction of limb or body wall musculature
   b. Alternating pressure in the thoracic cavity produced by respiratory movements
   c. Massage of the lymph vessels by pulsation of adjacent arteries
   d. Valves
3. **Lymph nodes** are located at intervals along the lymphatic vessels. They are generally positioned within fatty tissue near the flexor sides of joints, in angles formed by the larger blood vessels, in the mediastinum, and in the mesentery.
   a. Lymph nodes are composed of an external capsule and an internal scaffold that supports lymphatic cells. Lymph enters the lymph nodes via **afferent lymph vessels,** passes through the cellular interior of the node, exits the node through **efferent lymph vessels,** and rejoins the general lymphatic circulation.
   b. **Functions.** Lymph nodes serve two essential functions:
      (1) They filter the blood, removing and processing antigenic materials.
      (2) They serve as a source of immune cells (lymphocytes).
4. **Lymph ducts** form from the convergence of lymphatic vessels.
   a. The **lumbar duct** receives drainage from the pelvic limbs. It passes cranially along the sublumbar musculature and enters the **cisterna chyli,** an erratically-shaped dilatation of the lymphatic channels that looks like a sac positioned roughly between the diaphragmatic crura.
   b. The **common lymphatic duct** drains the digestive viscera, and also enters the cisterna chyli.
   c. The **thoracic duct** continues cranially from the cisterna chyli, passes between the diaphragmatic crura, and ascends along the right dorsal border of the aorta. Typically, it terminates at the junction of the left external jugular vein and the cranial vena cava. In many cases, the thoracic duct bifurcates or even trifurcates near its termination, thus ending as a plexus rather than a single vessel. The thoracic duct thus forms the main channel for lymphatic return from the body: it receives lymph from the pelvic limbs, pelvis, abdomen, and left side of the thorax.

Canine Clinical Correlation

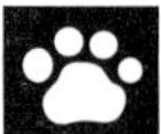

Rupture of the thoracic duct can occur following blunt trauma to the chest, as in a dog that has been hit by a car. **Chylothorax** may result from accumulation of chyle in either the thoracic or pleural cavities. Thoracocentesis yielding a fluid high in lymphocytes is diagnostic.

d. The **right lymph duct** drains the right side of the thorax and thoracic limb, terminating variably in the veins near the base of the heart.
e. The **tracheal ducts** course in the carotid sheath, and drain the head and neck. The left tracheal duct usually joins the thoracic duct, and the right tracheal duct usually ends near the right brachiocephalic vein.

D. **Lymphaticovenous communications** have been demonstrated among some of the larger lymphatic channels and adjacent veins, but normally carry minimal to no lymph.

Canine Clinical Correlation

Lymphatic channels provide the **main route of metastasis for various forms of carcinoma,** notably mammary and prostate adenocarcinomas. Owing to direct lymphaticovenous communications, as well as to the normal return of lymph or chyle to the central circulation, malignant cells can gain entry to the systemic circulation, allowing them to be widely disseminated throughout the body. Thus, surgical treatment of cancer commonly involves removal of lymph nodes and sometimes larger lymph channels as well.

Chapter 6

The Endocrine System

I. INTRODUCTION

A. Function. The endocrine system is composed of numerous ductless glands that produce hormones, which are released directly into the blood, lymph, or tissue fluid. Hormones released into tissue fluid affect the immediately adjacent tissues or organs, whereas hormones released into blood or lymph affect tissues or organs far removed from the gland. Though each of the endocrine glands has its own distinctive function, the action of the system as a whole **serves to integrate the activity of other body systems throughout the life of the individual.** Actions of the various hormones include:

1. Supplementing the nervous system response to internal and external stimuli
2. Influencing routine, daily functions (e.g., control of metabolism and homeostasis, immune system functioning)
3. Playing a role in more time-specific functions (e.g., growth in young animals, sexual differentiation in adolescent animals, normal aging)

B. The endocrine system as a "system." The variations among the glands that comprise the "endocrine system" has led some authors to refer to this group of organs as the "endocrine glands," rather than the "endocrine system." However, despite the differences, the similarities in structure and, particularly, in function, present a cogent argument for considering this group as a functional (if not morphological) system.

1. **Unique characteristics of the endocrine system**
   a. Its **component parts are separate anatomically** (i.e., they are not bound physically into a continuous whole).
   b. Unlike other more "conventional" organ systems, the various endocrine organs **have diverse embryologic origins.**
   c. The **substances produced by the components of the endocrine system are distinct structurally and functionally from each other.**
2. **Similarities among components of the endocrine system** include:
   a. An **absence of secretory ducts**
   b. Many epithelioid parenchymal cells, and **relatively little stroma**
   c. A **well-vascularized parenchyma**
   d. Intimate association with the adjacent **blood vessels, lymphatics,** or **tissue fluid**
   e. Hormone production

C. Classification of endocrine organs

1. **Primary endocrine organs** secrete hormones as their sole function. Primary endocrine organs include the:
   a. **Hypophysis cerebri (pituitary gland)**
   b. **Epiphysis cerebri (pineal gland)**
   c. **Thyroid gland**
   d. **Parathyroid glands**
   e. **Adrenal glands**
2. **Major endocrine organs** have a significant endocrine function in addition to serving in other capacities. Major endocrine organs include the:
   a. **Ovaries**
   b. **Testes**
   c. **Pancreas**
   d. **Placenta**

3. **Minor endocrine organs** have a relatively small (and usually local) endocrine function, which they perform in addition to some other, more major, function. Minor endocrine organs include the **kidneys** and **gastrointestinal mucosa.**

II. PRIMARY ENDOCRINE GLANDS

A. Hypophysis cerebri (pituitary gland, "hypophysis"). The term "hypophysis cerebri" is a positional description of the gland (Greek, *hypo* = beneath, *physis* = growth; *cerebri* = cerebrum—i.e., ventral to the main bulk of the brain). The term "pituitary" stems from the erroneous interpretation of the hypophysis cerebri as the source of nasal exudate (*pituita*).

1. **Appearance.** The hypophysis is a dark, round to elliptical body depending from the ventral midline of the diencephalon. The size of the hypophysis varies considerably among breeds as well as among individuals of the same breed.
2. **Location.** The hypophysis lies within a bony recess at the base of the skull.
3. **Components**
   a. The hypophysis appears grossly to be a single structure, but actually has two portions, each having a separate embryologic origin:
      (1) The **neurohypophysis** develops from the hypothalamus as a ventrally directed evagination of the neural ectoderm. The neurohypophysis retains its original connection to the hypothalamus as the stalk that suspends it from the brain. The interior of this stalk contains a cavity that is continuous with the third ventricle.
      (2) The **adenohypophysis** develops from the oral cavity as a dorsally directed invagination of oral ectoderm.
   b. A third portion of the gland, the **pars intermedia,** lies immediately adjacent to the neurohypophysis and is separated from the adenohypophysis by a cleft within the gland. This portion also develops from the invaginated oral ectoderm.
4. **Function.** The hypophysis is sometimes called the **"master gland,"** because it secretes hormones that control the other endocrine organs. The pituitary gland produces:
   a. **Somatotropic (growth) hormone**
   b. **Follicle-stimulating hormone**
   c. **Luteinizing hormone**
   d. **Prolactin**
   e. **Oxytocin**
   f. **Thyroid-stimulating hormone**
   g. **Adrenocorticotrophic hormone**
   h. **Melanophore-stimulating hormone**
   i. **Vasopressin**

B. Epiphysis cerebri (pineal gland, "epiphysis"). As with "hypophysis cerebri," the term "epiphysis cerebri" describes the position of the gland (Greek, *physis* = growth; *epi* = upon; *cerebri* = cerebrum). The term "pineal" stems from the fact that the pineal gland in humans is similar in appearance to a pine cone.

1. **Appearance and location.** The epiphysis is a small, dark outgrowth of the dorsal aspect of the brain, lying just cranial to the rostral colliculi. In the intact brain, it is not visible from the external surface. The epiphysis is a solid cellular structure and often contains multiple foci of calcification referred to colloquially as "brain sand."
2. **Function.** The function of the epiphysis has been a subject of long debate. It is known that the epiphysis produces **melatonin** and functions as a **biological clock,** regulating both diurnal and seasonal variation in gonadal activity.

C. Thyroid gland

1. **Appearance.** The thyroid gland of the dog is present as two separate lobes, most usually lacking any connection across the midline. The lobes of the thyroid gland are elongated symmetrical ovals, and are generally dark red in color.

2. **Location.** The thyroid gland lies on the ventrolateral surface of the trachea immediately caudal to the larynx, extending roughly across the level of the first five to eight cartilage rings. In this position, the gland may be palpable, particularly if enlarged.
3. **Components.** Two types of endocrine cells are present within the thyroid gland:
   a. Follicular cells, which represent the majority of the secretory cells in the gland
   b. Parafollicular cells (C cells), which are far fewer in number
4. **Function**
   a. **Thyroid hormone** is produced by the **follicular cells.** The hormone is stored within the gland and released as needed. Thyroid hormone exerts significant control over many body systems, because it controls many of the body's metabolic processes.
   b. **Calcitonin** is produced by the **parafollicular cells;** it stimulates the skeleton to take up calcium, thus lowering levels of calcium in the blood.

D. Parathyroid glands

1. **Appearance and location.** The parathyroid glands are among the smallest of the endocrine glands. In the dog, the parathyroid glands are generally present as four, tiny, separate glands that lie near, on, or embedded in the substance of the thyroid gland. Their exact positioning is variable.
   a. The **external parathyroid glands** are the more cranial pair of glands. They often lie within the fascia near the thyroid, rather than within the substance of the thyroid gland itself (hence the name). On close inspection, the external parathyroid glands may be visible as small, well-circumscribed pale ovals in the craniodorsolateral area of each thyroid gland.
   b. The **internal parathyroid glands** are the more caudal pair of glands. They lie deep to the thyroid capsule, and are occasionally embedded within the thyroid parenchyma on its medial surface. This pair of glands is not visible from the surface.
2. **Function.** The parathyroid glands produce **parathormone,** which is essential for the normal metabolism of calcium. Parathormone affects calcium metabolism in several ways:
   a. It promotes calcium absorption from the gut.
   b. It mobilizes calcium from the skeleton.
   c. It induces excretion of calcium in the urine.

Canine Clinical Correlation

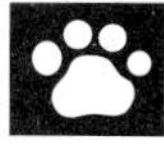

The close physical proximity of the thyroid and parathyroid glands raises an important point when considering thyroid surgery. Great care must be taken not to damage the parathyroid glands, because their function, which is necessary for life, is different from that of the thyroid glands.

E. Adrenal glands

1. **Appearance.** The adrenal glands are paired organs that are flat, elongated, and roughly rectangular; they are often asymmetrical in size and form.
2. **Location.** The adrenal glands lie retroperitoneally on the ventral surface of the sublumbar musculature, between the craniomedial border of the kidney and either the aorta (for the left gland) or the caudal vena cava (for the right gland). The adrenal glands lie "sandwiched" between two companion vessels, the common trunk of the caudal phrenic and cranial abdominal artery and vein (see Chapter 47, Figure 47–1). Identifying this vein, which passes ventral to the gland, is commonly the most ready way to find the gland. The artery passes dorsal to the gland.
3. **Components.** The adrenal gland is composed of two distinctly different tissues (structurally as well as functionally).

a. The **adrenal cortex** is derived from **mesenchymal cells** of the coelomic mesoderm. It produces **steroid hormones** (which are fatty substances); as a result, it is pale.
b. The **adrenal medulla** is derived from **neural ectodermal cells** that invade the developing cortex. The adrenal medulla is quite dark in comparison with the cortex.

4. **Function**
   a. The **adrenal cortex** produces **mineralocorticoids** and **glucocorticoids,** which are essential for life. These hormones **regulate mineral balance through the kidney** and also affect **carbohydrate metabolism.**
   b. The **adrenal medulla** produces **epinephrine** and **norepinephrine,** hormones that play a role in dealing with mental or physical stress. These hormones affect the sympathetic nervous system, and as a result, the adrenal medulla is often thought of as a "sympathetic ganglion."

III. OTHER ENDOCRINE TISSUES.

The other endocrine tissues are smaller groups of cells within other, nonendocrine organs of the body. Thus, these endocrine tissues are not visible grossly, and will be mentioned only briefly here.

A. Endocrine tissue of the pancreas. The endocrine pancreas consists of a myriad of **pancreatic islets** intercalated randomly among the exocrine part of the organ. The endocrine pancreas secretes **insulin,** which functions in the regulation of blood sugar levels.

B. Endocrine tissue of the ovary. The **corpus luteum** develops from the remainder of the follicle following ovulation and is an active source of **progesterone.** In pregnant bitches, the corpus luteum provides levels of progesterone sufficient to maintain the pregnancy until the placenta assumes adequate progesterone production.

C. Endocrine tissues of the placenta. During the last two trimesters of pregnancy, endocrine cells within the placenta produce **progesterone** in quantities sufficient to maintain the pregnancy to term.

D. Endocrine tissues of the testis. The **interstitial cells** are the source of male androgens, including **testosterone.**

E. Endocrine tissues of the kidney. The **juxtaglomerular cells** of the kidney are structurally and functionally modified smooth muscle cells of the afferent and efferent arterioles that contain secretory granules. In species other than the dog, these granules have been demonstrated to contain **renin,** which plays a role in increasing the blood pressure. Although it has not been proven, it is assumed that the granules of the juxtaglomerular cells in dogs contain renin as well.

F. Enteroendocrine cells are individual cells with an endocrine function that are scattered throughout the mucosa of the digestive and respiratory tracts. Secretion of various hormones have been controversially ascribed to these cells, and at present, no consensus has been reached.

Canine Clinical Correlation

Various disorders of the endocrine system occur frequently in dogs. Among the more common disorders are **diabetes mellitus, diabetes insipidus, hyper-** and **hypoadrenocorticism, hyperthyroidism, interstitial cell tumors** (in males), and **hypophyseal adenoma.**

STUDY QUESTIONS

DIRECTIONS: Each of the numbered items or incomplete statements in this section is followed by answers or by completions of the statement. Select the ONE numbered answer or completion that is BEST in each case.

1. In the normal anatomic position, the dog:

(1) lies in lateral recumbency with the head facing left.
(2) lies in ventral recumbency with the limbs extended parallel to the vertebral column.
(3) lies in dorsal recumbency with the limbs extended parallel to the vertebral column.
(4) stands on all four feet with the head facing left and the tail slightly raised.
(5) sits facing left with the tail outstretched.

2. The anatomic plane that divides the body into equal right and left halves is the:

(1) dorsal plane.
(2) medial plane.
(3) transverse plane.
(4) coronal plane.
(5) median plane.

3. Which one of the following adjectives is used by anatomists to describe a structure located near the external surface of the body?

(1) "Apical"
(2) "Above"
(3) "Superficial"
(4) "Upper"
(5) "Top"

4. In a dog that has sustained a spinal nerve injury, identification of the sensory deficit on the body surface can be used to identify which spinal nerves have sustained injury. How can this be explained?

(1) The skin is segmentally innervated by spinal nerves
(2) Each spinal nerve innervates a specific, nonoverlapping region of skin
(3) Sclerotomes are detectable on the skin's surface
(4) The parallel course of the cutaneous arteries and nerves allows for clinical identification of spinal nerve deficits

5. Which one of the following statements concerning the various glands of the skin in dogs is correct?

(1) Sweat glands are most numerous in the pads of the feet, where most of the dog's body heat is dissipated.
(2) Circumanal glands lie within paired sacs on each side of the anus.
(3) Sebaceous glands are present within the skin and are associated with hair follicles.
(4) Glands of the tail area surround the base of the tail over the dorsum of the back and caudal surfaces of the thighs.

6. Which one of the following is an example of a fibrous joint?

(1) Pelvic symphysis
(2) Mandibular symphysis
(3) Temporomandibular joint
(4) Intercarpal joints
(5) Sagittal suture of the skull

7. Which one of the following statements regarding afferent nerves is true?

(1) Afferent nerves of the visceral nervous system convey sensory information from the internal and external environments to reflex centers in the spinal cord.
(2) Afferent nerves of the visceral nervous system convey motor commands from the brain to effector organs.
(3) Afferent nerves of the somatic nervous system carry sensory information from the visceral organs to the brain.
(4) Afferent nerves of the somatic nervous system carry motor commands from the brain to the visceral organs.
(5) The cell bodies of the afferent nerves of the somatic nervous system are located in the dorsal root ganglia of the spinal cord.

8. Which one of the following statements concerning the meninges of the brain and spinal cord is true?

(1) The meninges consist of three layers, which from superficial to deep are the dura mater, arachnoid membrane, and pia mater
(2) The superficial-to-deep sequence of the meninges on the brain is inverse to that of the spinal cord.
(3) The cerebrospinal fluid (CSF) is contained in the subdural space of both the brain and spinal cord.
(4) The arachnoid membrane is the finest, most delicate layer, reminiscent of a spiderweb, that immediately surrounds the surface of the brain and spinal cord.

9. Which one of the following statements regarding the spinal cord is true?

(1) It contains nerve cell bodies within its white matter and axonal processes within its grey matter.
(2) It possesses neurons associated with the parasympathetic nervous system in the region of the intermediate horn.
(3) It extends the length of the vertebral canal.
(4) It receives sensory neurons through the dorsal horn.

10. Which one of the following statements regarding cerebrospinal fluid (CSF) is true?

(1) CSF is produced by the arachnoid villi.
(2) CSF fills the ventricles and sinuses of the brain and the central canal of the spinal cord.
(3) CSF is produced in times of stress to maintain the proper pH of the brain tissue.
(4) CSF cushions the brain and spinal cord.
(5) CSF is best obtained via a spinal tap in the midthoracic region.

11. Which one of the following statements regarding the hypophysis cerebri is true?

(1) It is the pineal gland.
(2) It is classified as a major endocrine organ.
(3) It produces substances that control the function of other endocrine organs.
(4) One portion is derived embryologically from neuroectoderm and the other is derived from mesoderm.

12. Which statement concerning the thyroid and parathyroid glands is true?

(1) The thyroid gland produces two separate substances with two separate effects.
(2) The parathyroid glands are simply small groups of cells intercalated diffusely with those of the thyroid gland.
(3) The thyroid and parathyroid glands share the same excretory ducts.
(4) The thyroid glands are bilaterally symmetrical glands that lie on each side of the esophagus.
(5) The thyroid gland is directly under the influence of estrogen or testosterone, and becomes functional after puberty.

DIRECTIONS: Each of the numbered items or incomplete statements in this section is negatively phrased, as indicated by a capitalized word such as NOT, LEAST, or EXCEPT. Select the ONE numbered answer or completion that is BEST in each case.

13. Which one of the following structures is NOT derived from the epidermis?

(1) Hair
(2) Footpads
(3) Claws
(4) Cutaneous arteries
(5) Cutaneous glands

14. Which one of the following statements regarding the spinal nerves is INCORRECT?

(1) Dorsal branches of spinal nerves innervate epaxial structures (e.g., muscle, skin).
(2) The dorsal roots of several branches intermingle to form the brachial and lumbosacral plexuses.
(3) Spinal nerves carry fibers from the autonomic nervous system (ANS).
(4) Neurons associated with spinal reflexes pass through spinal nerves.

15. All of the following statements regarding veins are true EXCEPT:

(1) They only carry deoxygenated blood.
(2) Their walls contain smooth muscle.
(3) They are usually larger in diameter and thinner-walled than arteries.
(4) A deep set of veins parallels the arteries and a superficial set travels alone.
(5) Skeletal muscle contraction assists the veins in returning blood to the central circulation.

ANSWERS AND EXPLANATIONS

1. The answer is 4 [Chapter 1 II B; Figure 1–1]. In the normal anatomic position, the dog stands on all four feet with the head facing left and the tail slightly raised.

2. The answer is 5 [Chapter 1 B 1]. The median, not the medial, plane divides the body into equal right and left halves. The terms "median" and "medial" are not interchangeable. The dorsal plane runs at right angles to both the median and transverse planes (horizontally, in the standing dog), dividing the body into dorsal and ventral portions. Transverse planes pass through the head, body, limb, or organ at right angles to the structure's long axis. A coronal plane is essentially the same as a transverse plane when the dog is positioned in the anatomic position.

3. The answer is 3 [Chapter 1 II C; Table 1–1]. "Superficial" is a term that retains its meaning regardless of the posture of the animal, whereas "apical," "above," "upper," and "top" can have different meanings depending on how the animal is positioned.

4. The answer is 1 [Chapter 2 I B 4 b]. The surface of the skin is supplied segmentally by spinal nerves in an overlapping pattern, creating dermatomes. Sclerotomes are embryonic precursors of vertebral bodies. The course of the cutaneous vessels and nerves in the skin is unrelated to the ability to identify spinal nerve lesions by clinically assessing sensory deficits.

5. The answer is 3 [Chapter 2 I F]. Sebaceous glands are present within the skin and are associated with hair follicles. Although sweat glands are most numerous in the pads of the feet, dogs dissipate most of their body heat by panting. Circumanal glands open directly onto the skin surrounding the anus. The glands of the tail area are present on the dorsal surface of the tail.

6. The answer is 5 [Chapter 3 II C 1 a]. The sagittal suture of the skull is a fibrous joint. Fibrous joints (synarthroses) are capable of minimal to no movement and mainly function to hold bones together. The pelvic and mandibular symphyses are cartilaginous joints. The temporomandibular and intercarpal joints are synovial joints.

7. The answer is 5 [Chapter 4 III A 2 b (1)]. The cell bodies of the afferent nerves in the somatic nervous system are located in the dorsal root ganglia of the spinal cord. Afferent nerves are sensory nerves, carrying information toward the brain. In the somatic nervous system, afferent nerves refer information from the skin surface as well as some from deeper structures. Afferents of the visceral nervous system carry information only from internal structures, and to the brain rather than to the spinal cord.

8. The answer is 1 [Chapter 4 II A 1 b]. The meninges are, from superficial to deep, the dura mater, the arachnoid, and the pia mater, and the sequence is the same for both the brain and spinal cord. Cerebrospinal fluid (CSF) is contained within the subarachnoid space, and the pia mater is the layer that is in closest proximity to the surface of the brain and spinal cord.

9. The answer is 4 [Chapter 4 II B 1 a]. The sensory (afferent) fibers that originate in the body enter the spinal cord through the dorsal horn. The grey matter of the spinal cord is composed of nerve cell bodies, and the white matter is composed of myelinated axons. The intermediate horn contains the cell bodies of the sympathetic nervous system. The spinal cord is shorter than the canal.

10. The answer is 4 [Chapter 4 II A 3]. Cerebrospinal fluid (CSF), the nutritive and protective fluid of the central nervous system (CNS), is produced continually by the choroid plexuses and resorbed by the arachnoid villi. The sinuses of the brain are venous sinuses, and are filled with venous blood. Spinal taps are most safely performed in the lumbosacral region of the dog, where nerve roots, rather than spinal cord tissue, is located.

11. The answer is 3 [Chapter 6 II A 4]. The hypophysis cerebri is the pituitary gland. This gland is a primary endocrine organ because its only function is to produce hormones. Major endocrine organs have a significant endocrine function, but they also serve in other capacities. The two parts of the hypophysis, the neurohypophysis and the adenohypophysis, are derived from neural ectoderm and oral ectoderm, respectively.

12. The answer is 1 [Chapter 6 II C–D]. The thyroid gland is a bilaterally-symmetrical gland that lies on each side of the trachea at the level of the larynx. It produces thyroid hormone, which affects numerous organs of the body, and calcitonin, which is involved in calcium metabolism. The thyroid gland is under the control of the pituitary gland, and functions throughout life. Neither the parathyroid glands nor the thyroid gland secrete their products via ducts. The parathyroid glands lie near, on, or in the substance of the thyroid gland; they are not small groups of cells intercalated with those of the thyroid gland.

13. The answer is 4 [Chapter 2 I]. The cutaneous arteries are not derived from the epidermis; in fact, the epidermis is avascular. Hair, footpads, claws, and the cutaneous glands develop from invasion of the dermis by epidermal outgrowths.

14. The answer is 2 [Chapter 4 II B 2 b (3) (b)]. The ventral branches of the spinal nerves, not the dorsal branches, mingle to form the brachial and lumbosacral plexuses. The dorsal branches of spinal nerves innervate epaxial structures (e.g., the muscles and skin). Spinal nerves carry fibers from the autonomic nervous system (ANS) as well as the peripheral nervous system. The neurons associated with spinal reflexes also pass through spinal nerves.

15. The answer is 1 [Chapter 5 I C 1 b, 2 a (2); V]. The pulmonary veins of the adult and the umbilical vein of the fetus carry oxygenated blood. Veins are defined according to direction of blood flow in them (i.e., toward the heart) rather than by the characteristics of the blood they contain. The larger veins contain some smooth muscle in their walls. The veins are usually larger in diameter and thinner-walled than their companion arteries. There is a superficial and a deep set of veins. Skeletal muscle contraction plays an important role in venous return.

PART II

HEAD

Chapter 7

Introduction to the Head

I. FACTORS CONTRIBUTING TO THE COMPLEX NATURE OF THE HEAD

A. Multiple roles

1. **Receipt of sensory input.** Specialized structures related to all five of the body's senses are present on the head. Because the head is the first portion of the animal's body to enter a new area, it is plainly advantageous from an adaptive point of view for all of the specialized structures delivering sensory input from the environment to be represented in the head.
   a. The head is the sole site where organs or tissues related to the special senses of **sight, smell, hearing,** and **taste** are found.
   b. Even for the more general sense of touch, specialized structures in the form of **vibrissae (tactile hairs)** are present. Vibrissae permit amplification of the touch sense so that even minimal stimulation is perceived by the brain.
2. **Protection of the brain.** The brain is contained within the cranial vault of the skull.
   a. The brain itself is a subject of immense intricacy, and adds exponentially to consideration of the complex nature of the head.
   b. Study of head structure is further complicated by the necessity for multiple openings in the skull to allow cranial nerves to exit the skull, as well as to allow the egress and ingress of blood vessels.
3. **Alimentation.** The teeth, the tongue, and the muscles of mastication are also among the many structures of the head.
4. **Facial expression.** The muscles of facial expression are located in the head. Facial expression is an acutely important part of communication among animals of the same, as well as different, species (i.e., intra- and interspecific communication); in fact, this function is as important in the life of the animal as more routine functions performed by the same muscles, such as closing the eyes and lips.

B. Complicated embryologic development. Embryologic development of the head is complicated and elaborate as a result of the multiple structures that are located in this area.

C. Small area. The head is a relatively small structure. "Packaging" of the brain, as well as structures related to special sensing, general sensing, alimentation, and facial expression, into such a small area further complicates what would be a complex situation even if these structures were dispersed over an area twice the size of the head!

II. HEAD MORPHOLOGY.

Over the centuries, humans have selectively bred dogs to induce variations in features of the canine body, including the morphology of the head. Although these features are often far from adaptive for the dog, the selection has nonetheless been highly effective in producing three distinct forms of the canine head: **mesaticephalic, dolichocephalic,** and **brachycephalic** (Figure 7–1).

A. Morphologic forms. Most of the variability among the three canine head forms is expressed in the facial region of the skull. Though the cranial vault obviously varies to some degree among these forms, cranial modifications are far less extreme than those of the facial region.

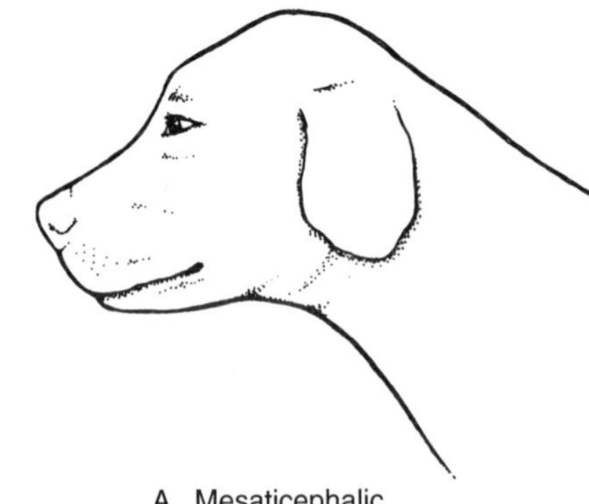

A. Mesaticephalic

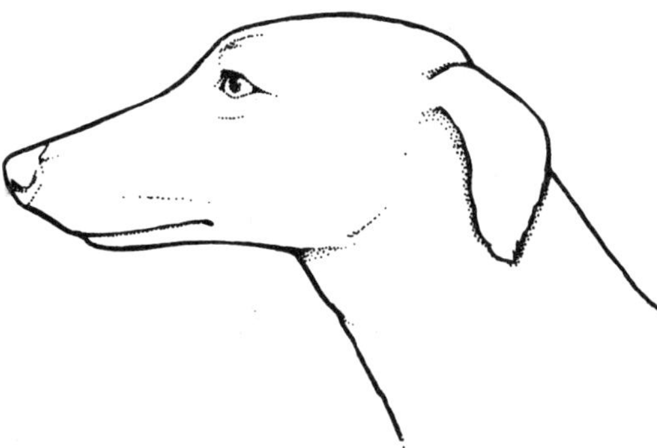

B. Dolichocephalic

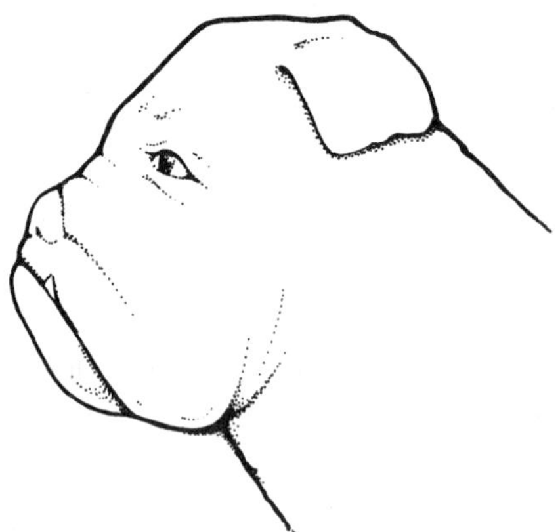

C. Brachycephalic

Figure 7–1. Canine head morphology.

1. **Mesaticephalic**
   a. **Appearance.** The mesaticephalic head is the least changed from the ancestral form. Proportions of the head are in concert with each other, and the overall form of the head forms a harmonious whole.
      (1) The **facial** and **cranial regions** are usually of nearly the same length and width.
         (a) The cranium is wide and usually roughly square-shaped.
         (b) The junction of the facial and cranial regions is characterized by a notable elevation from the level of the face to the higher level of the cranium. This point is called the **stop.**
      (2) The **eyes** are moderately widely spaced, and fit well within their orbits.
      (3) The **upper** and **lower jaws** are of the same length, and the dental arcades meet evenly along their full extent.
   b. **Breeds.** Many of the working and sporting breeds (e.g., beagles, Alaskan malamutes, huskies, the various breeds of pointers and terriers, Labrador retrievers) have mesaticephalic heads, related to the maximal brain space afforded by the cranial vault of the mesaticephalic form. Selection in relatively recent years has led some ancestrally working breeds with a sound mesaticephalic head form, such as collies, German shepherds, and Doberman pinschers, to approach—and in some cases, convincingly attain—the dolichocephalic form. The associated loss of intelligence, particularly in breeds that historically had been selected for that intelligence related to their working capabilities (e.g., collies), seems particularly lamentable.
2. **Dolichocephalic**
   a. **Appearance.** Generally, the dolichocephalic form departs from the mesaticephalic form by being longer and more narrow.
      (1) The **facial** and **cranial regions** are usually of nearly the same length and width. The cranium is narrow and low. Because the cranial region is not as high as in mesaticephalic breeds, the stop is less pronounced.
      (2) The **eyes** are smaller and more closely spaced than in mesaticephalic breeds, but they still fit well within their orbits, and may even be recessed into the orbit to some degree.
      (3) The **lower jaw** is sometimes notably shorter than the upper jaw, a condition referred to as **brachygnathism** (*brachy* = short; *gnatha* = jaw). Still, most of the time, the upper and lower dental arcades meet fairly evenly.
   b. **Breeds** with this head form include greyhounds, Afghan hounds, and salukis.
   c. **Clinical conditions** related strictly to the dolichocephalic form of the head are not marked, but in the opinion of many observers, extreme forms of the dolichocephalic skull are associated with a loss of intelligence owing to a decrease in brain size.
3. **Brachycephalic**
   a. **Appearance.** The brachycephalic form departs from the generalized mesaticephalic form in that it is shorter and wider.
      (1) The **facial region** is considerably shorter than the **cranial region.** The cranium is sometimes high and rounded; as a result of the height of the cranium, the stop is usually very pronounced.
      (2) The **eyes** are large and often widely spaced. They usually protrude considerably from their orbits.
      (3) The **lower jaw** is usually longer than the upper jaw, a condition referred to as **prognathism**.
   b. **Breeds** with this head form include English bulldogs, Boston terriers, Pekingese, and Chihuahuas.
   c. **Clinical conditions** related strictly to the brachycephalic form of the head are numerous and typically include:
      (1) Complications related to malocclusion
      (2) Difficulties in nasal breathing
      (3) Open-mouth breathing and swallowing difficulties resulting from elongation of the soft palate
      (4) Ocular problems

(5) Dermatologic problems associated with prominent skin folds, which develop as a result of shortening of the nasal and maxillary areas

(6) Difficulties for bitches in parturition stemming from the particularly large and round heads of the puppies

B. Though a given breed may be classified as belonging to one of these categories, gradations among the degree of expression of these classifying features exist among the breeds as well as among individuals within a given breed. Thus, some individuals of a breed characterized as dolichocephalic may have features that approach those of a mesaticephalic breed, and vice versa. However, selection for the brachycephalic form has typically been so efficacious that individuals with this head form seldom deviate far from the classic depiction.

Chapter 8

Skeleton of the Head and Dentition

I. INTRODUCTION. The complete skeleton of the head consists of the skull, the hyoid apparatus, and the cartilages of the external ear and nose (Figure 8–1). In its final form, the skeleton of the head is composed of 46 separate bones (some of these bones are formed via fusion of separate bones during development). Knowledge of the names and locations of many of these bones is clinically important in order to describe lesions of the skull or associated organs. Memorization of the bones of the skeleton of the head becomes much less daunting when one realizes that many of the bones are paired, which reduces the number of separate names from 46 to 27. Furthermore, if one concedes that not all of the bones are of profound clinical importance, 9 more names can be eliminated from the list, reducing the number of names that must be memorized to 18. (In the lists in sections I A 2 and I B, the bones that are in boldface type are the most clinically important bones of the head.)

A. Skull. Of the 46 bones of the mature skeleton of the head, **37** of these bones (including the mandible) belong to the skull.

1. **Definition.** Authors of textbooks generally adopt one of two definitions of what bones comprise the skull.
   - **a.** In a broad sense, the skull is defined as the **fused bones** and the **inner ear bones,** together with the **mandible.** The approach taken in this text is to adopt this broader view.
   - **b.** In a narrow sense, the skull is defined as the fused bones of the head without mobile joints (i.e., exclusive of the mandible), together with the inner ear bones.
2. **Regions and bones of the skull**
   - **a.** The **cranium** is that part of the skull exclusive of the mandible. Note that this differs from the common colloquial use of this term, which is often used to designate only that part of the skull that houses the brain.
     - **(1)** The **facial region (visceral region, viscerocranium)** of the cranium is the rostral part of the skull that projects forward from the braincase. This region houses or supports the eyes, nose, tongue, and other structures of the face; hence the term "viscerocranium." The bones of the viscerocranium are as follows:
       - **(a) Paired bones** include the:
         - (i) **Incisive**
         - (ii) **Nasal**
         - (iii) **Maxilla**
         - (iv) **Zygomatic**
         - (v) **Palatine**
         - (vi) **Lacrimal**
         - (vii) **Pterygoid**
         - (viii) **Ventral concha**
         - (ix) Dorsal concha
       - **(b) Unpaired bones** include the vomer.
     - **(2)** The **neural region (neurocranium, braincase)** is the caudal part of the skull that provides a complete bony housing for the brain. The bones of the neurocranium are as follows:
       - **(a) Paired bones** include the:
         - (i) **Parietal**
         - (ii) **Frontal**
         - (iii) **Temporal**

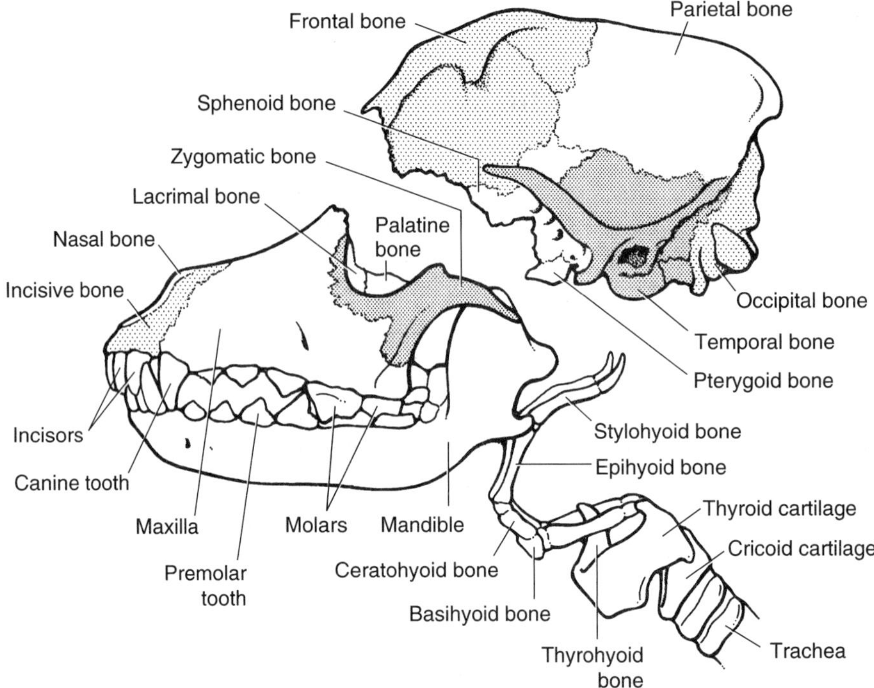

Figure 8–1. The bony skeleton of the head, lateral view.

(b) Unpaired bones include the:

(i) Occipital (forms from fusion of paired supra-, basi-, and exoccipital bones)

(ii) Basisphenoid

(iii) Presphenoid

(iv) Ethmoid

(v) Interparietal

b. The **mandible ("lower jaw")** is the portion of the skull that carries the ventral arcade of teeth and articulates by a synovial joint with the ventral cranial region. The mandible is considered to be a single bone composed of similar halves.

c. The **bones of the inner ear** comprise a minute but essential portion of the skull. These bones are paired and include the:

(1) Malleus

(2) Incus

(3) Stapes

3. Morphology of the skull. Although the description of the skull given in this chapter generally applies to all breeds, the spectrum of morphologic skull forms that exists among various breeds of dogs obviously affects the proportions or development of the various skull bones. **The general description given here is based on the mesaticephalic head form.**

a. Dolichocephalic skulls adhere fairly closely to this description, though the elements are elongated in a rostrocaudal direction and compressed to some degree in the dorsoventral dimension.

b. Brachycephalic skulls deviate markedly from this description, **most notably in the facial region** as visible from all aspects.

4. Functions of the skull

a. Protection. One of the more obvious functions of the skull is to protect the brain.

Aside from the foramen magnum (by which the spinal cord exits the skull), the cranial cavity opens to the exterior only at multiple smaller holes (i.e., foramina) where veins exit the skull, arteries enter, and nerves enter or leave (Table 8–1).

b. **Housing.** The skull houses the organs of special sense (i.e., vision, hearing, equilibrium, smell, and taste).

c. **Provision of attachment sites.** The skull provides attachment sites for the teeth, the tongue, the larynx, and numerous muscles.

d. **Prehension of food.** The hinge between the mandible and the rest of the skull allows the animal to open and close its mouth, enabling it to take food into the body.

B. Hyoid bones. The **hyoid apparatus** (see Chapter 12 V) suspends the tongue and larynx from the skull in the intermandibular space. The bones of the hyoid apparatus are as follows:

1. **Paired bones** include the:
   a. **Stylohyoid**
   b. Ceratohyoid
   c. Epihyoid
   d. Thyrohyoid

2. **Unpaired bones** include the **basihyoid.**

C. Cartilages of the external ear and nose are also considered part of the skeleton of the head.

II. SKULL

A. Lateral surface of the skull (excluding the mandible). The lateral aspect of the skull is divided into rostral and caudal areas by the position of the orbit. These correspond largely to the facial and neural regions, respectively (Figure 8–2).

1. **Rostral to the orbital region (the viscerocranium).** The wall of the lateral facial surface is relatively smooth, bowing slightly laterally from the midline.

   a. **Maxilla.** The region of the lateral facial wall of the skull that is rostral to the orbital region is formed mainly by the maxilla.

      (1) The maxilla carries the **upper arcade of teeth exclusive of the incisors** (i.e., the canine teeth and all of the premolars and molars). The alveolar juga (tooth sockets) of the molars produce recognizable elevations along the maxilla's ventral margin.

      (2) Approximately halfway along the length of the lateral facial region, the **infraorbital foramen** presents as a large ovoid foramen situated with its long axis oriented dorsoventrally. Note that this position is not directly below the orbit, as the name would imply—the name is taken from the position of the infraorbital foramen in the human skull, in which the foramen indeed lies below the orbit. The infraorbital foramen provides passage for the infraorbital artery, vein, and nerve.

   b. **Incisive bone.** The most cranial extremity of the skull's lateral surface is formed by the incisive bone, which borders the nasal opening and carries the incisor teeth.

   c. **Zygomatic arch.** The zygomatic arch, a heavy arch of bone projecting laterally from the skull, is a prominent feature of the lateral view of the skull. The arch forms a bridge between the facial and neurocranial regions.

      (1) The zygomatic arch is formed from the articulation of the separate **zygomatic bone** cranially with the **zygomatic process of the maxillary bone** and caudally with the **zygomatic process of the temporal bone.**

      (2) The caudoventral region of the zygomatic arch provides the site for articulation of the mandible with the remainder of the skull at the **mandibular fossa.**

2. The **orbital region** includes the **orbit** and the **pterygopalatine fossa.**

   a. The **orbit** is a funnel-shaped region that houses the eye (i.e., the globe and its adnexa). In addition, the ventromedial region of the orbit provides passage for various nervous and vascular structures.

TABLE 8–1. Major Foramina, Fissures, and Canals of the Skull

Foramina, Fissure, or Canal	Transmitted Structures
Externally visible	
Mental foramina	Branches of the inferior alveolar a, v, n
Mandibular foramen	Branches of the inferior alveolar a, v, n
Mandibular canal	Inferior alveolar a, v, and n between the mandibular foramen and the mental foramina
Palatine fissure	Anastomoses between the palatine and the infraorbital and nasal aa and vv
Major palatine foramen	Major palatine a, v, n
Minor palatine foramina	Branches of the major palatine artery
Caudal palatine foramen	Major palatine, a, v, n
Sphenopalatine foramen	Sphenopalatine a, v Caudal nasal n
Infraorbital foramen	Infraorbital a, v, n
Maxillary foramen	Maxillary a, v, n
Infraorbital canal	Maxillary/infraorbital a, v, n between the maxillary and infraorbital foramina
Optic canal	Optic n (CN II) External opthalmic artery External opthalmic vein
Orbital fissure	Oculomotor n (CN III) Trochlear n (CN IV) Ophthalmic division of trigeminal n (CN V_1) Abducens n (CN VI) Dorsal external opthalmic vein
Rostral alar foramen	Maxillary a, v Maxillary division of trigeminal n (CN V_2)
Caudal alar foramen	Maxillary a, v
Alar canal	Maxillary a, v throughout length Maxillary division of trigeminal n (CN V_2) through rostral portion
Round foramen	Maxillary division of trigeminal n (CN V_2) *en route* to alar canal
Oval foramen	Mandibular division of trigeminal n (CN V_3) Emissary vein from cranial cavity
Musculotubal canal	Auditory tube
Foramen lacerum	A loop of the internal carotid a
Stylomastoid foramen	Facial n (CN VII)
Tympanooccipital fissure	Glossopharyngeal n (CN IX) Vagus n (CN X) Spinal accessory n (CN XI) Sympathetic nn Small vv

continued

TABLE 8–1. Major Foramina, Fissures, and Canals of the Skull

Foramina, Fissure, or Canal	Transmitted Structures
Retroarticular foramen	Temporomandibular articular v
Hypoglossal canal	Hypoglossal n (CN XII)
Foramen magnum	Spinal cord
	Basilar a
	Venous plexus
	Spinal part of spinal accessory n (CN XI)
Internally visible	
Round foramen	Maxillary division of trigeminal n (CN V_2)
	Emissary vein from the cavernous sinus
Carotid canal	Internal carotid a
Internal acoustic meatus	Facial n (CN VII)
	Vestibulocochlear n (CN VIII)
Jugular foramen	Glossopharyngeal n (CN IX)
	Vagus n (CN X)
	Spinal accessory n (CN XI)
	Sigmoid sinus
Foramen magnum	Spinal cord
	Basilar a
	Venous plexus
	Spinal part of spinal accessory n (CN XI)

Organized according to physical proximity on the skull.

a = artery; aa = arteries; CN = cranial nerve; n = nerve; nn = nerves; v = vein; vv = veins.

(1) **Orbital aperture.** The rostral orbital aperture tends to be nearly round in brachycephalic breeds, oval in dolichocephalic breeds, and somewhere in between these two forms in mesaticephalic breeds.

(2) **Orbital borders**

(a) The rostral and medial orbital borders are formed from the zygomatic process of the maxilla, as well as the lacrimal and frontal bones. The zygomatic process of the frontal bone demarcates the dorsocaudal edge of the bony orbital border.

(b) The lateral orbital border is formed by the zygomatic arch. The frontal process of the zygomatic bone demarcates the ventrocaudal edge of the bony orbital border.

(c) The canine bony orbit is incomplete; the two processes forming its dorso- and ventrocaudal borders do not meet. In the intact state, this gap between the zygomatic process of the frontal bone and the frontal process of the zygomatic bone is closed by the **orbital ligament.**

b. The **pterygopalatine fossa** is contiguous with the orbit, and only poorly demarcated from it. In the prepared skull, the two areas are continuous. However, in the intact state, the periorbita separates the two. In the intact state, the pterygopalatine fossa is largely filled by the substance of the pterygoid muscles.

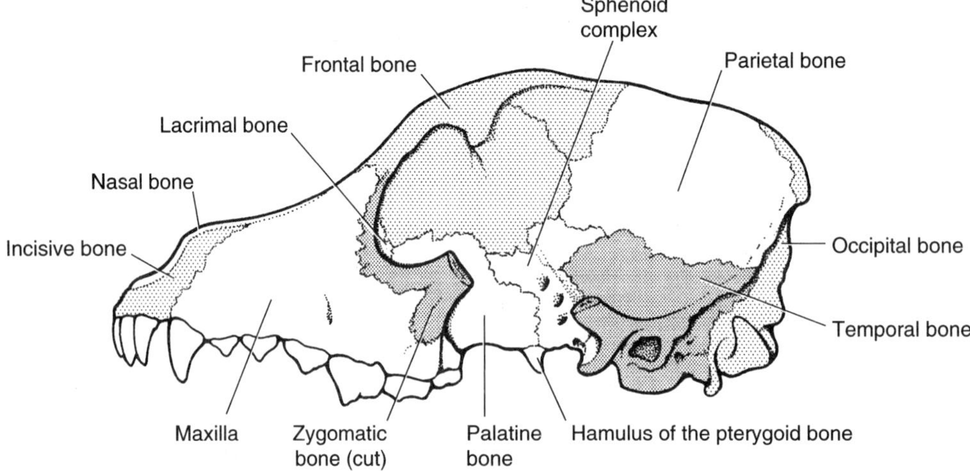

Figure 8–2. The bones of the skull, lateral view. The mandible and zygomatic arch have been removed.

(1) The **ventral orbital crest** is a roughly horizontal line demarcating the junction of the orbit with the pterygopalatine fossa. This variably prominent line is located approximately halfway down the medial wall of the combined orbital and pterygopalatine regions.

(2) The **hamulus of the pterygoid bone,** a small but striking, caudally directed, hook-like projection from the caudal region of the pterygoid bone, is a prominent feature of the caudal region of the medial wall of the pterygopalatine fossa. In the intact state, the tendon of a pharyngeal muscle passes over the hamulus, using a part of the hooked region to adjust its course.

(3) Foramina

(a) Rostral region

(i) The pterygopalatine fossa narrows in its rostral extremity to terminate at the **maxillary foramen.** The maxillary foramen is the entrance into the rostrally directed **infraorbital canal,** which houses the maxillary nerve and artery as they course rostrally before becoming the infraorbital nerve and artery.

(ii) The **sphenopalatine** and **caudal palatine foramina** are also located in the rostral part of the pterygopalatine fossa, somewhat ventral to the maxillary foramen.

(b) Caudoventral region. In the caudoventral region, the medial wall of the pterygopalatine fossa presents several major foramina. From rostral to caudal these are the:

(i) Optic canal, which transmits the optic nerve (cranial nerve II)

(ii) Orbital fissure, which transmits the oculomotor nerve (cranial nerve III), the trochlear nerve (cranial nerve IV), the ophthalmic component of the trigeminal nerve (cranial nerve V_1), and the abducent nerve (cranial nerve VI), as well as the external ophthalmic vein

(iii) Rostral alar foramen, which transmits the maxillary artery, a tributary of the maxillary vein, and the maxillary component of the trigeminal nerve (cranial nerve V_2).

(iv) Caudal alar foramen, which transmits the maxillary artery and a tributary of the maxillary vein

(4) The **alar canal** is a bony canal extending from the caudal alar foramen to the rostral alar foramen.

(a) The **maxillary artery** enters the caudal alar foramen, traverses the entire length of the alar canal, and exits via the rostral alar foramen.

(b) The **round foramen** opens into the alar canal from the interior of the cranial cavity. The relation of the round foramen and the alar canal can be likened to an inverted and slightly skewed capital "T."

(i) The **maxillary component of the trigeminal nerve (cranial nerve V_2)** enters the alar canal via the round foramen, turns cranially, and then exits the canal via the rostral alar foramen. Thus, the alar canal transmits the maxillary artery through its full length, and the maxillary nerve through only part of its length.

(ii) The round foramen also conducts a **vein from the cavernous sinus** into the alar canal.

3. **Caudal to the orbital region (neurocranium).** The **parietal** and **temporal bones** as well as **part of the frontal bones and sphenoid complex** form most of this skull region. To a minor degree, **part of the occipital bone** contributes to the caudal lateral aspect of the skull. Most of the lateral neurocranium is convex in outline; in spite of this fact, the region is referred to as the **temporal fossa.** The lateral and ventrolateral walls of much of the cranial cavity are slightly roughened for attachment of the temporal muscle. The ventrolateral part of the neurocranium is complex, being uneven in form, and having several prominent projections.

   a. The **temporal bone** has three portions.

   (1) The **squamous part of the temporal bone** in this region is modified into the **zygomatic process of the temporal bone.** The **retroarticular process** is an extension from the zygomatic process of the temporal bone that effectively deepens the mandibular fossa for articulation of the mandible.

   (2) The **tympanic part of the temporal bone** is also located in the ventrolateral part of the neurocranium. Portions of its external surface are modified into the **tympanic bulla,** an easily recognizable, bubble-shaped elaboration. The **external acoustic meatus** is the opening into the tympanic bulla. In the intact state, the meatus is closed by the tympanic membrane (eardrum), and its borders provide the attachment site for the cartilage of the ear canal.

   (3) The **petrous part of the temporal bone** is just deep to the tympanic bulla. However, this portion of the temporal bone is not visible on the external surface of the skull.

   b. The **mastoid process** is a small and indistinct elevation of bone situated just rostral to the tympanic bulla. Despite the tiny size and inconspicuous appearance of this structure, it is significant in that this region is the site of origin or insertion for several muscles of the head and neck.

   c. The **paracondylar process** is an elongate projection of bone extending ventrally from the skull caudal to the tympanic bulla and lateral to the occipital condyle.

   d. **Foramina.** Two foramina are present in this region of the skull.

   (1) The **stylomastoid foramen** provides passageway for the facial nerve (cranial nerve VII).

   (2) The **retroarticular foramen** transmits the large temporomandibular vein that drains the cranial cavity.

B. Dorsal surface of the skull (excluding the mandible). Again, the orbits provide a prominent demarcation between the rostral (viscerocranium) and caudal (neurocranium) regions of the skull.

1. **Rostral to, and including, the orbital region (the viscerocranium).** The dorsal surface of the facial region is formed from portions of the **incisive, maxillary, nasal,** and **temporal bones** (Figure 8–3).
2. **Caudal to the orbital region (the neurocranium).** The braincase is ovoid in a rostral—caudal direction when viewed dorsally, and is convex over most of its surface.

   a. The **external occipital protuberance** is a median, triangular projection that marks the most dorsocaudal extent of the skull (see Figure 8–3).

   b. The **sagittal crest** is a midline, rostrally directed ridge of bone continuing rostrally from the external occipital protuberance. Development of the crest varies consider-

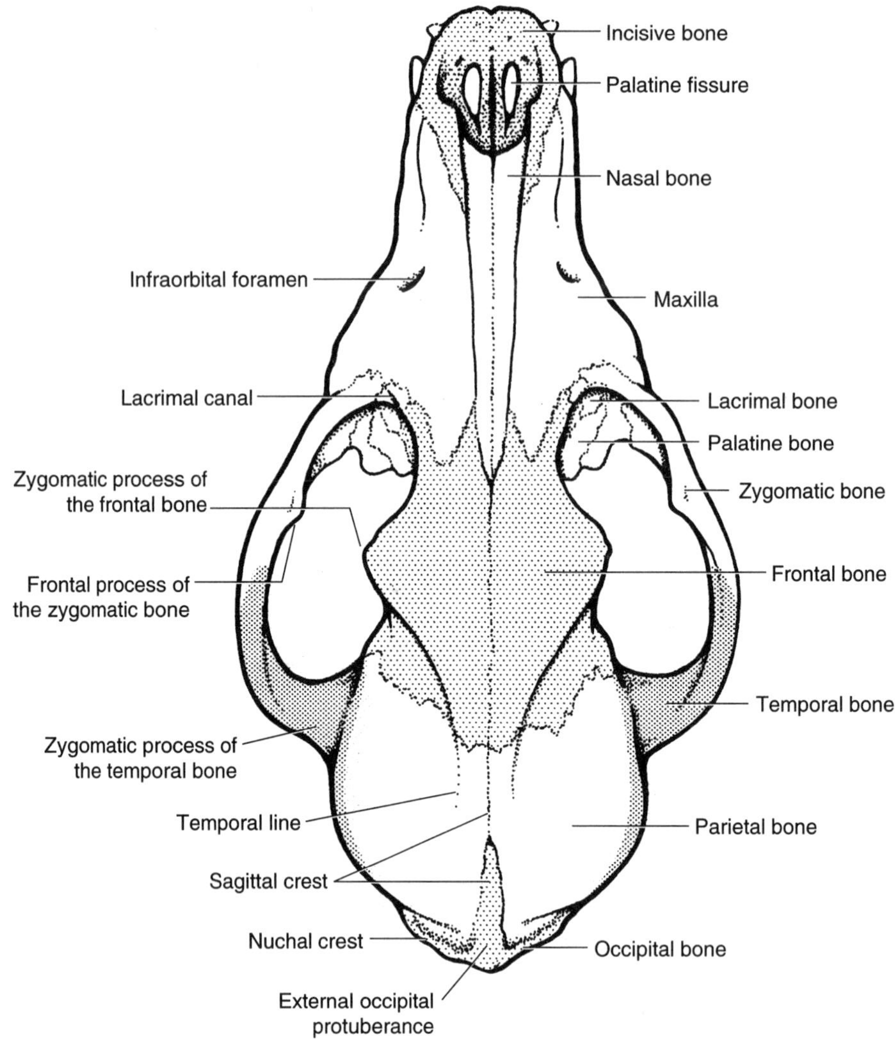

Figure 8–3. The bones of the skull, dorsal view. In the dorsal view, the facial region is widest where the zygomatic processes of the temporal bone extend laterally; from this point, the skull narrows rostrally to its most narrow dimension at the rostral end of the nasal region. The nasal aperture, rimmed by the incisive and nasal bones, and the orbit are prominent from the dorsal view.

ably with age, breed, and sex, being most prominent in adult male dogs of breeds with heavy head musculature.

c. The **nuchal crest** is a variably developed ridge of bone that extends laterally from each side of the external occipital protuberance. This ridge (or the general region when the ridge is poorly developed) demarcates the junction of the dorsal and caudal regions of the skull.

C. **Ventral surface of the skull (excluding the mandible).** Again, the orbits provide a prominent demarcation between the viscerocranium and neurocranium.

1. **Rostral to, and including, the orbital region (the viscerocranium).** The horizontal parts of the **nasal, palatine,** and **maxillary bones** largely form the ventral surface of the facial region.

a. Hard (bony) palate. The nasal, palatine, and maxillary bones contribute to the formation of the hard palate. The hard palate bears several openings (Figure 8–4). Each of these is paired.

(1) The **palatine fissure** is a relatively large, elongate oval opening lying between the canine teeth. Anastomoses between the palatine and the infraorbital and nasal vessels pass through this opening.

(2) The **major palatine foramen** lies medial to the carnassial teeth (see IV A 3). Branches of the major palatine vessels and nerve pass through this foramen.

(3) The **minor palatine foramen** lies just caudal to the major palatine foramen. As with the major palatine foramen, branches of the major palatine vessels and nerve pass through the minor palatine foramen.

b. Choanal region. The choanal region extends from the caudal end of the hard palate (the **choanal border**) to the junction with the neurocranium.

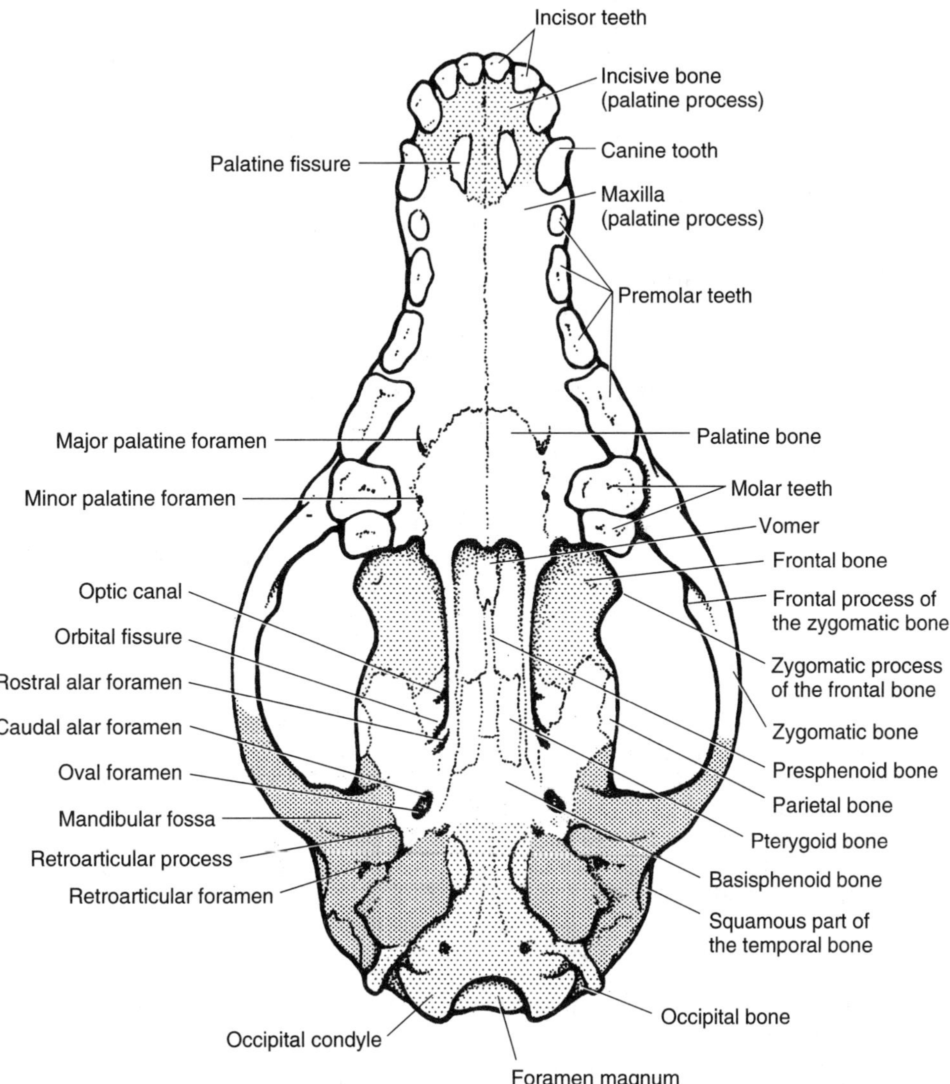

Figure 8–4. Ventral surface of the skull.

(1) The **choanal region** is bounded dorsally by the floor of the cranial cavity, and laterally by the palatine and pterygoid bones. In the prepared skull, the choanal region is open ventrally, but in the intact state the ventral wall is formed by the soft palate.

(2) The **choanal border** is formed by bone, while the **choanae** themselves are the spaces bordered by the bone. In the intact state, the choanae lead from the nasal cavity into the nasopharynx.

c. **Maxillary and incisive bones.** The full dorsal arcade of **teeth** is visible on the ventral view of the skull. The incisive bone carries the incisors, while the maxilla carries the canine, premolar, and molar teeth.

d. **Zygomatic arches.** As in all other views, the zygomatic arches are prominent on the ventral view of the skull.

2. **Caudal to the orbital region (the neurocranium).** Aside from a triangular, relatively smooth zone forming its central area, the ventral neurocranial region is complex in that it bears numerous foramina and elevations or depressions for muscle attachment. Each structure described here, except the foramen magnum, is paired.

a. **Mandibular fossa.** Where the squamous part of the temporal bone projects from the skull, its form is modified to produce the transversely elongate mandibular fossa, which articulates with the mandible. This fossa is deepened by the **retroarticular process,** which extends ventrally and cranially from the fossa.

(1) The **oval foramen** lies just caudal to the opening of the caudal alar foramen and medial to the mandibular fossa (see Figure 8–4). It transmits the mandibular branch of the trigeminal nerve (cranial nerve V_3) and an emissary vein from the cranial cavity.

(2) The **retroarticular foramen** lies, as the name suggests, just caudal to the retroarticular process. It transmits the large temporomandibular articular vein that drains the cranial cavity.

b. **Tympanic bulla.** The tympanic bulla is a "bubble" of bone that projects ventrally from the skull and houses the middle ear.

(1) The **musculotubal canal** is a tiny opening at the rostromedial edge of the tympanic bulla that is shielded ventrally by a tiny shelf of bone (the muscular process). The auditory tube passes through this canal.

(2) The **foramen lacerum,** another tiny opening, lies just medial to the musculotubal canal. A loop of the internal carotid artery passes through this foramen.

(3) The **tympanooccipital fissure** is an elongate oval opening at the caudomedial edge of the tympanic bulla. It transmits the glossopharyngeal nerve (cranial nerve IX), the vagus nerve (cranial nerve X), and the spinal accessory nerve (cranial nerve XI).

(4) The **external acoustic meatus** lies on the lateral edge of the tympanic bulla. In the intact state, this opening is closed by the tympanic membrane, which conducts sound to the middle ear.

(5) The **stylomastoid foramen** lies on the lateral edge of the tympanic bulla, just caudal to the external acoustic meatus. This foramen transmits the facial nerve (cranial nerve VII).

(6) The **hypoglossal canal** is a round foramen that lies just caudal to the tympanooccipital fissure. The hypoglossal nerve (cranial nerve XII) exits the skull through this foramen.

c. **Occipital condyle.** The occipital condyle is a rounded, elongate structure oriented obliquely from a caudomedial to a craniolateral direction (see Figure 8–4). The two occipital condyles provide sites for articulation of the skull with the atlas.

d. **Paracondylar process.** The paracondylar process is an elongate projection of bone that extends ventrally from the skull caudal to the tympanic bulla and lateral to the occipital condyle.

e. **Foramen magnum.** The foramen magnum is the **opening through which the spinal cord passes.**

D. **Caudal surface of the skull (excluding the mandible).** The caudal surface of the skull is also referred to as the **nuchal surface.** Most of the nuchal surface of the skull (excluding the mandible) is roughened for attachment of the dorsal neck musculature.

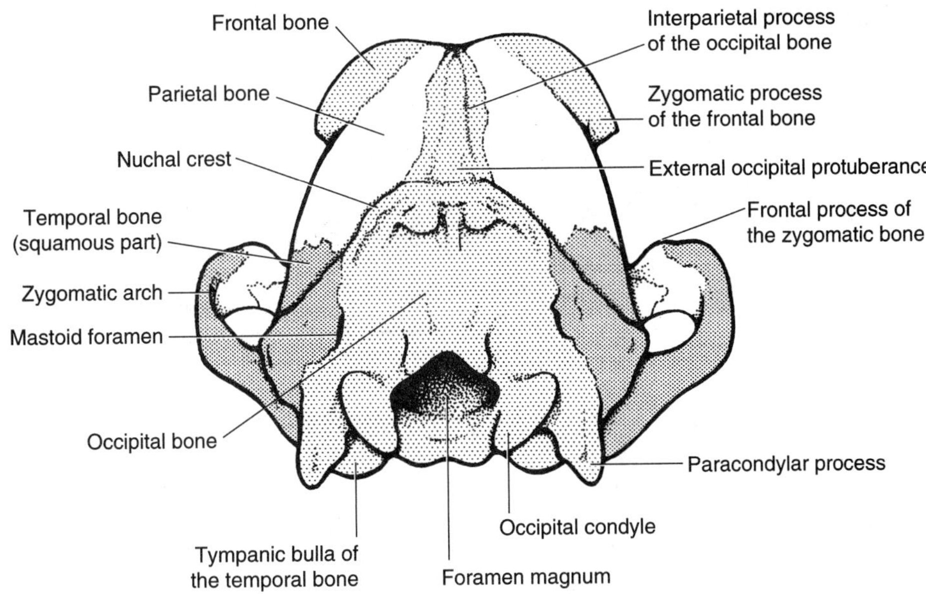

Figure 8–5. Caudal view of the skull. Note the foramen magnum, the large midline opening situated between the occipital condyles through which the spinal cord passes.

1. The form of the nuchal surface is roughly **triangular,** with the apex formed by the dorsally positioned **external occipital protuberance,** and the base of the triangle oriented ventrally (Figure 8–5). The lateral borders of the triangular area are formed by the **nuchal crests.**
2. The **occipital condyles** are rounded, elongate structures oriented obliquely from a caudomedial to a craniolateral direction.
3. The **paracondylar processes** are elongated projections of bone that extend ventrally from the skull caudal to the tympanic bullae and lateral to the occipital condyles.

E. **Rostral surface of the skull (excluding the mandible).** Due to its shape, the skull does not actually have a rostral surface. Its appearance from the rostral aspect is marked mainly by the prominent nasal aperture, incisor and canine teeth, orbits, frontal region, and zygomatic arches.

F. **Mandible** (Figure 8–6). The mandible is composed of two essentially identical halves, joined rostrally on the midline at the **mandibular symphysis,** which, in dogs, is fibrous. Caudal to the mandibular symphysis, the two halves of the mandible are separated by the **intermandibular space.** This space is more narrow rostrally than caudally, so that together the halves of the mandible describe a "V" shape.

1. The **body** of the mandible, the elongate horizontal portion, bears the entire inferior arcade of teeth, including the incisor, canine, premolar, and molar teeth.
   a. The **lateral mandibular surface** is smooth and presents multiple **mental foramina** at its rostral end, near the premolars and canine teeth. These foramina transmit the mental branches of the inferior alveolar vessels and nerves. Typically, one mental foramen is considerably larger than the others.
   b. The **medial mandibular surface** is also largely smooth, except at its most rostral end near the canine and incisor teeth, where it is roughened for articulation with its fellow. The large **mandibular foramen,** which transmits the inferior alveolar vessels and nerve, is located at the caudal end of the medial mandibular surface.

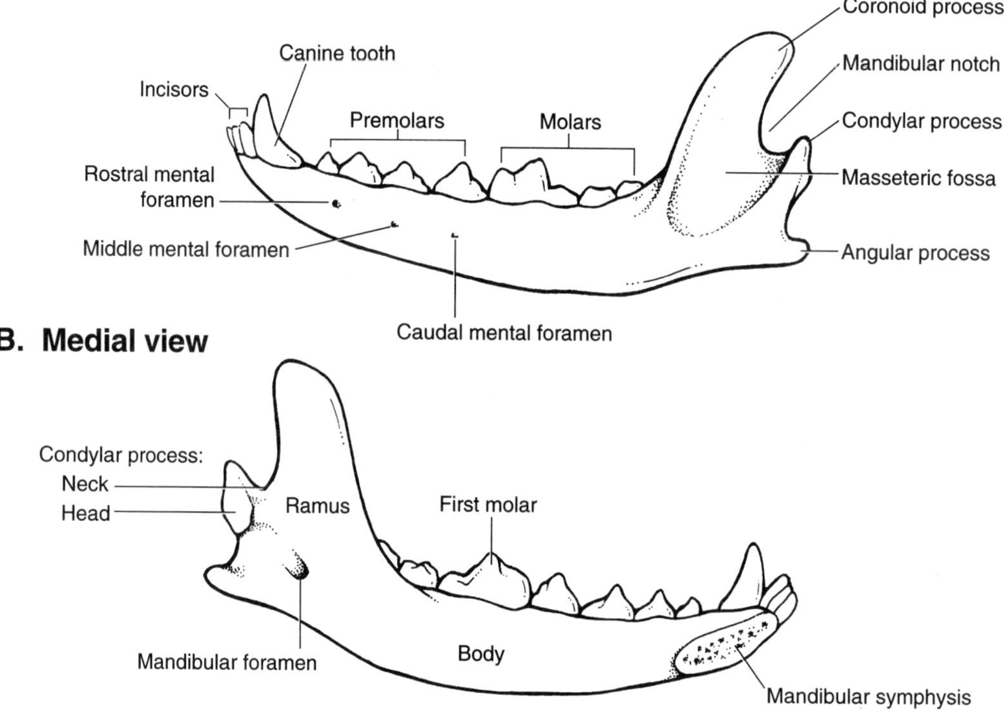

Figure 8–6. The mandible, lateral and medial views.

2. The **ramus** is the vertical extension of the caudal region of the mandible.
   a. The dorsal extremity of the ramus ends in the rounded **coronoid process.**
      (1) The deep **masseteric fossa,** which provides access to the masseter muscle, is located on the lateral surface of the coronoid process. A shallower, unnamed depression is located on its medial surface and provides access for the temporal and pterygoid muscles.
      (2) In the intact state, the coronoid process projects into the **temporal fossa,** dividing the fossa into a lateral and medial area.
   b. The **condylar process** projects caudally from the mandibular ramus. The condylar process is the structure by which the mandible articulates with the remainder of the skull at the mandibular fossa.
   c. The **angular process,** a small, often hook-shaped projection from the caudoventral extremity of the mandible, provides attachment for the digastricus muscle.

G. Cavities of the skull

1. **Nasal cavity.** The nasal cavity, contained within the rostral portion of the facial bones, is considered part of the respiratory tract.
   a. The **nasal septum** is a vertical plate, cartilaginous in the rostral region and bony in the caudal region.
      (1) The nasal septum separates the nasal cavity into the right and left **nasal fossae** (i.e., symmetrical halves of the cavity). The nasal fossae extend from the opening of the nasal aperture to the choanae (Figure 8–7A).
      (2) The **vomeronasal organ,** a paired structure lying in the rostroventral portion of the nasal septum, functions in both kin recognition and sexual behavior by its reception of pheromones.

(a) Each vomeronasal organ opens into the **incisive duct,** which connects the oral and nasal cavities. The **Flehman response** refers to the behavior of dogs (and other animals) in which the upper lip is curled to facilitate access to the incisive duct and delivery of air (containing pheromones) to the vomeronasal organ.

(b) The paired incisive ducts open on each side of the incisive papillae, a small median elevation just caudal to the incisor teeth located in the oral cavity.

b. Conchae. The nasal fossa is largely filled by conchae ("shells"), which are delicate, paper-thin scrolls of bone covered (in the intact state) with a richly vascular mucous membrane. In life, passage of inspired air over these membranes serves to warm and moisten the incoming air. The conchae are named according to their point of attachment to the wall of the nasal cavity (Figure 8–7B).

(1) The **dorsal nasal concha** attaches dorsally along the lateral wall of the nasal cavity.

(2) The **ventral nasal concha** attaches relatively ventrally along the lateral nasal cavity wall. This is the largest and most intricate of the conchae.

(3) The **ethmoidal nasal conchae (ethmoidal labyrinth)** of the dog nearly fill the caudal half of the nasal cavity. These conchae develop as a rostral outgrowth of the ethmoid bone and are covered by mucosa containing sensory endings of the olfactory nerve. The size of these chonchae in the dog attest to the importance of the sense of smell in this species.

c. Meati. The presence of the chonchae in the nasal cavity divides the cavity into recognizable spaces (see Figure 8–7A).

(1) The **dorsal nasal meatus** lies between the nasal bone and the dorsal concha.

(2) The **middle nasal meatus** lies between the dorsal and ventral chonchae.

(3) The **ventral nasal meatus** lies between the ventral concha and the floor of the nasal cavity (i.e., the hard palate).

(4) The **common nasal meatus** is best appreciated from a transverse section (see Figure 8–7B), where it is readily recognizable as a median longitudinal space along the nasal septum that communicates with the other three meati.

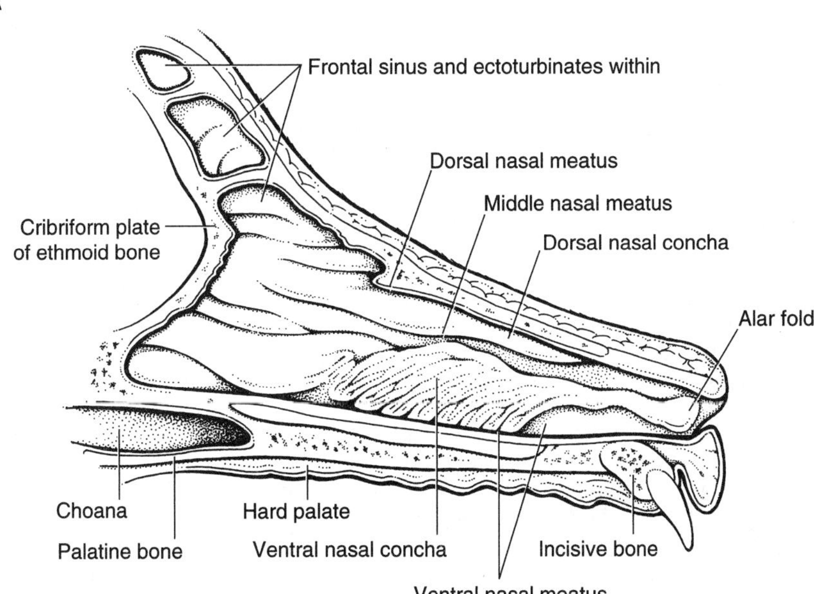

Figure 8–7. Nasal cavity, conchae, and meati. (*A*) Lateral view. (Modified with permission from Anderson WD: *Atlas of Canine Anatomy*. Baltimore, Williams & Wilkins, 1994, p 223.) (*continued*)

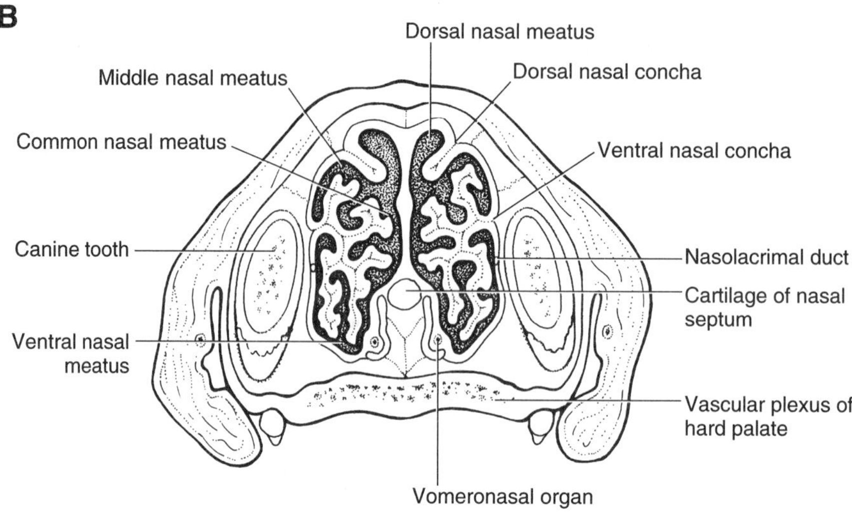

Figure 8–7—*continued* (*B*) Transverse section. (Modified with permission from Evans HE, deLahunta A: *Miller's Guide to the Dissection of the Dog,* 4th ed. Philadelphia, WB Saunders, 1996, p 266.)

Canine Clinical Correlation

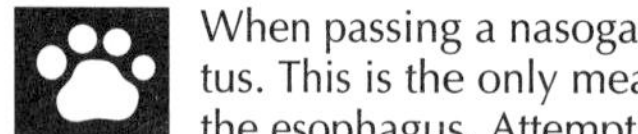

When passing a nasogastric tube, the nasal cavity is accessed through the ventral nasal meatus. This is the only meatus that communicates caudally with the nasopharynx and thence to the esophagus. Attempts to pass the tube through the middle or dorsal meati would only result in damage to the delicate chonchae and their very vascular membrane, causing significant damage to the air passageway and marked epistaxis (nosebleed).

2. **Paranasal sinuses.** The paranasal sinuses are air-filled spaces in the skull that lie between the external and internal layers (diploë) of the skull's facial bones. The paranasal sinuses communicate with the space of the nasal cavity (though that communication may take place through a rather small opening). The reason for the development of the paranasal sinuses has been debated for many years without complete resolution; however, the prevailing opinion is that sinuses serve to lighten the weight of the skull. Lending plausibility to this theory is the fact that the paranasal sinuses in dogs are much less well-developed than the paranasal sinuses in larger, heavier-headed animals such as domestic herbivores. The size and extent of the paranasal sinuses is notably affected by the shape of the skull.
   a. **Maxillary recess.** The maxillary recess is a lateral diverticulum of the nasal cavity that is situated rostral to the orbit, caudal to the infraorbital foramen.
      (1) This space must technically be termed a recess rather than a proper sinus in the dog because it lies between two bones, rather than between the layers of a single bone. The maxillary recess of the dog occupies a similar position to the true maxillary sinus of other species.
      (2) The infraorbital canal, along with its vessels and nerves, passes over the lateral surface of the region of the maxillary recess. The recess extends over the roots of the last upper premolar and the molars.
   b. **Frontal sinus.** The frontal sinus lies between the two layers of the frontal bone. This sinus is relatively variable in size, even among individuals of the same breed. The si-

Canine Clinical Correlation

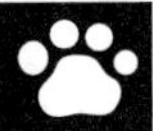

The roots of the upper cheek teeth lie in close proximity to the maxillary recess, and the bone separating the teeth from the sinus is relatively thin. Thus, tooth root abscesses may erode the bony partition and establish a purulent sinusitis within the maxillary recess. In such cases, drainage is difficult to safely establish through a lateral approach to the recess, due to the course of the infraorbital canal in the region of the maxillary recess. Thus, drainage is best approached by removal of the carnassial tooth, which allows drainage into the mouth.

nus is divisible into lateral and medial parts. Interestingly, a portion of the frontal sinus extends into the zygomatic arch.

c. **Sphenoid sinus.** The sphenoid sinus lies within the presphenoid bone and has little clinical significance.

3. **Cranial cavity**
   a. **Walls.** The walls of the cranial cavity are contributed to by several bones:
      (1) **Dorsal wall.** The "roof" of the skull is termed the **calvaria,** and is formed mainly by the **frontal** and **parietal bones.**
      (2) **Lateral wall.** The lateral wall is formed mainly from the **temporal, parietal,** and **frontal bones,** and to a lesser degree, from the **sphenoid** and **occipital bones.**
      (3) **Ventral wall.** The "base" of the skull is formed from the **sphenoid** and **basioccipital bones.**
      (4) **Rostral wall.** The rostral wall is formed from the **cribriform plate of the ethmoid bone.**
      (5) **Caudal wall.** The caudal wall is formed from the **occipital bones.**
   b. **Contours.** The dorsal, lateral, cranial, and caudal internal walls of the cranial cavity are, for the most part, smooth. The interior **ventral wall** of the cranial cavity is sculpted into complex regions referred to as the **cranial fossae**.
      (1) The **rostral cranial fossa** is relatively narrow and dorsal, and lies rostral to the optic canals. This region houses the olfactory tracts, olfactory bulbs, and frontal lobes of the brain (i.e., the rostral part of the cerebrum).
         (a) Its cranial border is marked by the **cribriform plate,** a sieve-like area of bone perforated by a myriad of tiny holes providing passage for the olfactory nerves and blood vessels.
         (b) The **optic canals** lead rostrally from the floor of the rostral cranial fossa outward to the pterygopalatine fossa.
      (2) The **middle cranial fossa** is situated more ventrally in the skull than the rostral fossa, and houses much of the cerebrum. The middle cranial fossa extends from the optic canals to the **hypophyseal region.**
         (a) The **hypophyseal fossa** and the **sella turcica,** located in the hypophyseal region, are bony structures supporting the hypophysis cerebri (pituitary gland).
         (b) Features of note within the middle cranial fossa include the **orbital fissures** and the **round** and **oval foramina.**
      (3) The **caudal cranial fossa** houses the cerebellum, the pons, and the medulla oblongata, and extends from the hypophyseal region to the foramen magnum. The floor of the caudal cranial fossa presents numerous structures, the most significant being the:
         (a) **Canal for the trigeminal nerve**
         (b) **Internal acoustic meatus**
         (c) **Cerebellar fossa**
         (d) **Petrous part of the temporal bone**
         (e) **Jugular foramen,** which transmits cranial nerves IX, X, and XI and the sigmoid venous sinus to the externally located tympanooccipital fissure
         (f) **Hypoglossal canal,** which transmits cranial nerve XII

III. HYOID APPARATUS. The hyoid apparatus, the bony support of the tongue, is discussed in Chapter 12 V.

IV. TEETH

A. Types

1. **Incisors** are small teeth adapted to cutting. In the upper arcade, these teeth are seated in the incisive bone, and in the lower arcade, they are seated in the mandible.
2. **Canines** are robust, long, pointed, and slightly curved teeth that are adapted to piercing and grasping prey or food. The upper canine teeth are seated in the maxilla and the lower ones are seated in the mandible.
3. **Premolars and molars.** The term **"cheek teeth"** is used to refer to premolars and molars as a group.
   a. **Premolars** are relatively small, and are adapted to assist the canine teeth with grasping.
      (1) In the upper arcade, these teeth are seated in the maxilla, and in the lower arcade, they are seated in the mandible.
      (2) The **upper fourth premolars** are the largest teeth of the upper arcade. They mesh with the corresponding teeth of the lower arcade in such a way as to make them particularly effective in shearing. These teeth are referred to as **carnassial** or **sectorial teeth of the upper jaw.**
   b. **Molars** are quite variable in size and form. The molars are adapted to chewing or shearing.
      (1) The upper molars are seated in the maxilla, and the lower ones are seated in the mandible.
      (2) The **first lower molar teeth** are particularly large, and mesh with the upper fourth premolars in such a way as to make them particularly effective in shearing. These teeth are referred to as the **carnassial** or **sectorial teeth of the lower jaw.**

B. The dental formula

1. **Naming convention.** The dental formula is written in an abbreviated form.
   a. The **number of teeth** on **one side** of the upper and lower arcade is indicated. Thus, the number of teeth in each group must be doubled to arrive at the correct number for that arcade.
   b. The **names of the teeth** are abbreviated using the first letter of the type of tooth. Thus, I = incisor, C = canine, P = premolar, and M = molar.
2. **Deciduous formula.** There are no deciduous molars. The deciduous formula is as follows:
   a. **Upper arcade:** I-3, C-1, P-3
   b. **Lower arcade:** I-3, C-1, P-3
   c. **Total:** 2 (I 3/3, C 1/1, P 3/3), for a total of **28 deciduous teeth**
3. **Permanent formula**
   a. **Upper arcade:** I-3, C-1, P-4, M-2
   b. **Lower arcade:** I-3, C-1, P-4, M-3
   c. **Total:** 2 (I 3/3, C 1/1, P 4/4, M 2/3), for a total of **42 permanent teeth**

C. Structure.

The teeth of the dog are **brachyodont** in nature, in that the portion projecting above the gumline is relatively short (as compared with the teeth of some herbivores). All teeth of the dog grow only until they are fully erupted, in contrast to the continually erupting teeth of herbivores.

1. The **root** is the portion of the tooth embedded in the alveolus (socket). Ready knowledge of the numbers of roots of each tooth is important during dental extractions. The number of roots varies according to the type and position of the tooth:
   a. **Incisors** and **canine teeth.** All incisors and canine teeth have **one** root.
   b. **Upper arcade of cheek teeth**

(1) The first tooth has one root.
(2) The next two teeth have two roots each.
(3) The next three teeth have three roots each.

c. Lower arcade of cheek teeth
(1) The first tooth and the last tooth have one root.
(2) All the remaining teeth have two roots.

2. The **neck** is a mildly constricted region of the tooth at the juncture of the embedded root and the free portion projecting above the gum. The prominence of the neck varies considerably among the types of teeth.
3. The **crown** is that part of the tooth that projects freely above the gum line into the mouth.

D. Composition

1. **Substances.** Mammalian teeth are comprised of three substances:
   a. **Enamel,** the hardest substance in the body, covers the entire surface of the portion of the tooth that projects into the mouth (i.e., the crown). Enamel is white.

Canine Clinical Correlation

Enamel, an acellular substance, is unable to repair itself following fracture.

   b. **Dentine** is a hard, yellowish-white osseous substance that lies entirely deep to the enamel and forms the body of the tooth.
   c. **Cement,** which is similar to bone, anchors the tooth within its alveolus in the skull. The neck and root of the tooth are covered by cement.
2. **Dental pulp** fills the **dental cavity,** which extends into each major elevation of the crown, as well as into each root. The dental cavity opens at an **apical foramen** at the base of each root. The pulp is composed of marginated odontoblasts and a delicate connective tissue containing rich vascular, lymphatic, and nervous plexuses.

Canine Clinical Correlation

Estimating age in dogs. Examining the teeth for eruption and wear can be used to estimate a dog's age.

- **Young dogs.** Up to the age of 6–7 months, the age of a dog can be estimated quite reliably by noting the eruption of the teeth (Table 8–2).

TABLE 8–2. Approximate Eruption Times for Deciduous and Permanent Teeth

Deciduous Teeth	*Time of Eruption*	*Permanent Teeth*	*Time of Eruption*
I1	4 weeks	I1	3 months
I2	5 weeks	I1	4 months
I3	6 weeks	I3	5 months
C1	3–5 weeks	C1	6 months
P1	. . .	P1	4–5 months
P2	5–6 weeks	P2	5–6 months
P3	5–6 weeks	P3	5–6 months
P4	5–6 weeks	P4	5–6 months
		M1	4–5 months
		M2	6–7 months
		M3	6–7 months

C = canine; I = incisor; M = molar; P = premolar.

- **Older dogs.** The age of older dogs may be roughly estimated by examining the teeth for wear. However, this method is much less accurate than aging by tooth eruption, because of the tremendous variability in rate and pattern of wear once the teeth have erupted. Differences in diet, environment, and behavior affect the wear of the teeth, and render exact aging of adult dogs an art at best. However, some broad generalizations regarding the status of the teeth at various ages can be made (Table 8–3).

TABLE 8–3. Aging Dogs by Tooth Wear

Age	*Status of Teeth*
6–7 months	Permanent dentition in
1.5 years	Cusps worn off lower I1
2.5 years	Cusps worn off lower I2
3.5 years	Cusps worn off upper I1
4.5 years	Cusps worn off upper I2
6 years	Cusps worn off upper and lower I3
7 years	Occlusal surface of lower I1 elliptical and worn
8 years	Occlusal surface of lower I1 inclined forward
9–10 years	Occlusal surface of lower I2 and upper I3 elliptical
12 years	I1 begin to fall out
16 years	Incisors lost
20 years	Canines lost

I = incisor.

Chapter 9

Vasculature of the Head

I. ARTERIES OF THE HEAD

A. Overview

1. Two arteries are mainly responsible for delivering arterial blood to the head and associated structures, including the brain.
   a. The **common carotid artery** delivers most of the arterial blood to the head. It, or its branches, form the primary route for delivery of blood to the **external structures** of the head, as well as supplying a considerable amount of blood to the **interior of the cranial cavity** and associated structures.
   b. The **basilar artery** is the main vessel supplying blood to the brain (see Chapter 13 VI A 1 a).
2. **Flow of arterial blood to the head** (Figure 9–1)
   a. The **central channel** of arterial blood flow to the head is:
      (1) Common carotid artery
      (2) External carotid artery
      (3) Maxillary artery
      (4) Infraorbital artery
   b. Numerous **branches** arise from each of these arteries to supply successive regions of the head. From caudal to cranial, these are:
      (1) The **common carotid artery** branches into the cranial thyroid artery, internal carotid artery, and external carotid artery.
      (2) The **external carotid artery** branches into the:
         (a) **Occipital artery**
         (b) **Cranial laryngeal artery**
         (c) **Lingual artery**
         (d) **Facial artery**
         (e) **Caudal auricular artery**
         (f) **Superficial temporal artery**
         (g) **Maxillary artery**
      (3) The **maxillary artery** terminates by branching into the **infraorbital artery** and the common trunk of the **sphenopalatine** and **caudal palatine arteries.**
3. The origins and the areas supplied by the major arteries of the head are summarized in Table 9–1.

B. Common carotid artery.

Common carotid artery. The common carotid artery is paired, with the pair of arteries arising from the brachiocephalic trunk within the thoracic cavity. The arteries ascend through the neck to reach the head. The branching pattern of each is similar; therefore, the branching is described in the singular form throughout this section.

1. The **cranial thyroid artery** actually arises within the cranial region of the neck, but is mentioned here for the sake of completeness. The cranial thyroid artery leaves the common carotid artery at about the level of the larynx, and supplies:
   a. The thyroid and parathyroid glands
   b. The pharyngeal muscles
   c. The larynx
   d. Parts of the trachea and esophagus
   e. Parts of the ventral neck musculature
2. Slightly caudal to the base of the ear, the **common carotid artery terminates** by dividing into the **internal carotid artery** and the **external carotid artery.**

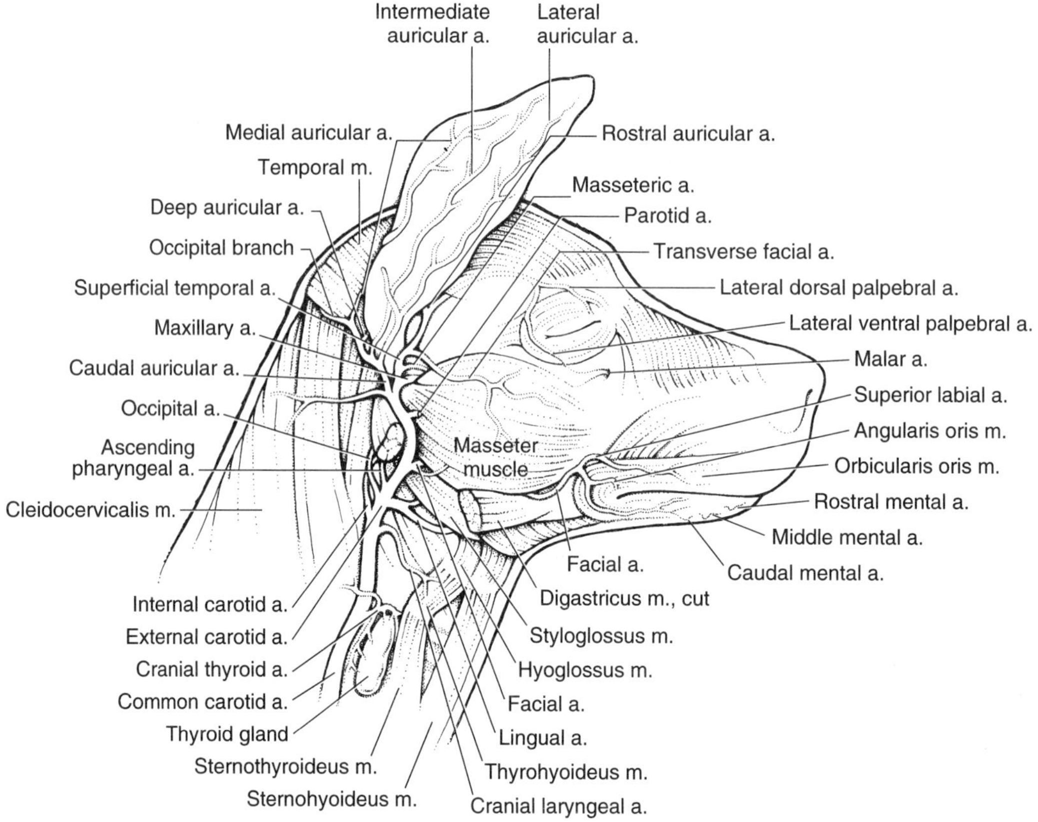

Figure 9–1. Branches of the common and external carotid arteries, and related structures.

a. The **internal carotid artery** ascends obliquely from the common carotid and is directed medially as it passes across the pharyngeal region *en route* to the cranial cavity. It gives no branches prior to its entrance to the skull through the small petroccipital fissure. Just prior to entering the fissure, the artery passes over the surface of the cranial cervical ganglion. After passing through the petroccipital fissure, the internal carotid artery enters the carotid canal, which lies deep in the tympanooccipital fissure, and passes rostrally. A curious feature of the course of the internal carotid artery is its exit from the carotid canal via the foramen lacerum, at which point it makes a 180-degree turn, loops back on itself, and reenters the carotid canal. Upon reentering the carotid canal, the internal carotid artery passes rostrally along the floor of the cranial cavity, through the cavernous sinus, and dorsally out of the sinus to enter the cerebral arterial circle supplying the **brain** (see Chapter 13 VI A 1 b). The **carotid sinus,** a baroreceptor (i.e., a structure sensitive to changes in blood pressure), is a bulbous enlargement of varying prominence at the origin of the internal carotid artery. This structure is sometimes large and conspicuous, and at other times may be unnoticeable.

b. The **external carotid artery** continues obliquely cranially in the same straight course that the common carotid artery took leading into it, continuing the main channel of arterial flow to the head (see Figure 9–1).

C. External carotid artery. The external carotid artery has several branches (see Figure 9–1).

1. The **occipital artery** branches dorsally from the external carotid near the origin of the internal carotid, passing lateral to the internal carotid. It passes craniodorsally into the occipital region of the head and supplies the **caudal skull musculature** and some portions of the **meninges.**

2. The **cranial laryngeal artery** is a small branch leaving the ventral surface of the external carotid, also close to the origin of the internal carotid artery. It supplies an adjacent ventral neck muscle (the **sternomastoideus**), the **pharyngeal muscles,** and the **larynx.**
3. The **lingual artery** is usually the largest branch of the external carotid. It branches ventrally from the parent artery and passes ventrocranially, medial to the digastricus.

TABLE 9–1. Summary of the Major Arteries of the Head

Artery	Origin	Structures Supplied
Internal carotid artery	Termination of common carotid	Brain
External carotid artery	Termination of common carotid	
Occipital artery	Branch of external carotid	Caudal skull muscles, meninges
Cranial laryngeal artery	Branch of external carotid	Neck muscles, pharyngeal muscles, larynx
Lingual artery	Branch of external carotid	Tongue, hyoid, tonsil, pharynx
Facial artery	Branch of external carotid	Sublingual muscles; skin, subcutis, and muscles of the face
Caudal auricular artery	Branch of external carotid	Parotid and mandibular salivary glands; regional skin, subcutis, and muscle, ear cartilage
Superficial temporal artery	Termination of external carotid	Masseter and temporal muscles, parotid salivary glands, eyelids, regional skin and subcutis
Maxillary artery	Termination of external carotid	
Mandibular region		Temporomandibular joint, meninges, temporal and masseter muscles, lower arcade of teeth, regional skin and subcutis
Pterygoid region		None
Pterygopalatine region		Pterygoid and temporal muscles, lacrimal gland, cheek, hard and soft palates, eye
Inferior alveolar artery	Mandibular region of maxillary artery	Lower arcade of teeth; skin and subcutis of the chin (mental) region
External opthalmic artery	Pterygopalatine region of maxillary artery	Eye
Infraorbital artery	Termination of maxillary artery	Upper lip; regional muscles, skin and subcutis, vibrissae, teeth of the upper arcade
Sphenopalatine artery	Termination of maxillary artery	Palate and structures of the nasal cavity
Major palatine artery	Termination of maxillary artery	Bony and soft tissues of hard palate

a. The lingual artery is closely paralleled by the hypoglossal nerve through much of its course.
b. In addition to supplying the **tongue,** the lingual artery also sends branches that supply the **hyoid, palatine tonsil,** and **pharyngeal muscles.**

4. The **facial artery** typically arises near the mandibular angle, and passes medial to the digastricus. It courses rostrally along the side of the face medial to the masseter muscle, and gives rise to several large branches (as well as to some smaller branches that are not discussed here) *en route* to its termination.
   a. The **sublingual artery** typically arises from the facial artery medial to the ventral mandibular body, and then runs rostrally parallel to the bone. It supplies the muscles ventral to the tongue (i.e., the **mylohyoideus, digastricus, genioglossus,** and **geniohyoideus**), and is accompanied by a satellite vein and the mylohyoid nerve.
   b. The **inferior labial artery** typically arises from the facial artery near the commissure of the lips and courses rostrally along the ventral border of the lower lip. It terminates as the **superior labial artery,** which runs rostrally along the dorsal border of the upper lip and ramifies over the cheek and nose. The superior labial artery supplies mainly the **orbicularis oris** and the **levator nasolabialis.**

5. The **caudal auricular artery** typically arises in almost a directly dorsal direction from the external carotid at the base of the ear and courses caudally around the ear. It may be covered by the parotid salivary gland in the early part of its course, and then by the caudal auricular musculature in the latter part of its course. The caudal auricular artery has several named branches (which will not be detailed here) that supply the **skin, subcutis,** and **various muscles** of the region, as well as the **parotid** and **mandibular salivary glands** and the **ear cartilage.**
6. The **termination of the external carotid artery** is marked by its uneven division into the smaller **superficial temporal artery** and the much larger **maxillary artery** (see I D). The superficial temporal artery typically arises just rostral to the base of the auricular cartilage and courses almost directly dorsally into the temporal region. It has several named branches (which will not be detailed here) that supply the **masseter** and **temporal muscles, parotid salivary gland, eyelids,** and the **skin** and **subcutis** of the region.

D. Maxillary artery. The maxillary artery forms the main continuation of flow from the external carotid artery (Figure 9–2). It continues rostrally ventral to the retroarticular process and then turns directly dorsally for a short distance, before turning rostrally again to pass through the alar canal.

1. **Regions.** A regional approach simplifies consideration of the many branches of the large maxillary artery.
   a. The **mandibular portion of the maxillary artery** extends from the continuation of the maxillary from the external carotid to the entrance of the maxillary into the alar canal via the caudal alar foramen.
      (1) This segment of the maxillary artery closely follows the contour of the retroarticular process and gives rise to several named branches that supply the **temporomandibular joint capsule,** the **temporal** and **masseter muscles,** and the **meninges.**
      (2) The **inferior alveolar artery** is one named branch of the mandibular portion of the maxillary artery that is commonly encountered in dissections and clinically, and will therefore be described in some detail here.
         (a) This artery enters the mandibular foramen on the medial side of the mandible and courses rostrally in the mandibular canal. It sends twigs to the **apical foramina of the roots of the lower arcade of teeth,** as well as to the **mandible** itself.
         (b) Typically, three branches are given from the inferior alveolar artery. Each one exits one of the mental foramina on the rostral lateral mandibular surface (see Figure 9–1).
   b. The **pterygoid portion of the maxillary artery** enters the caudal alar foramen, passes through the alar canal, and exits the canal rostrally at the rostral alar foramen (see Figure 9–2). This region gives off no branches.

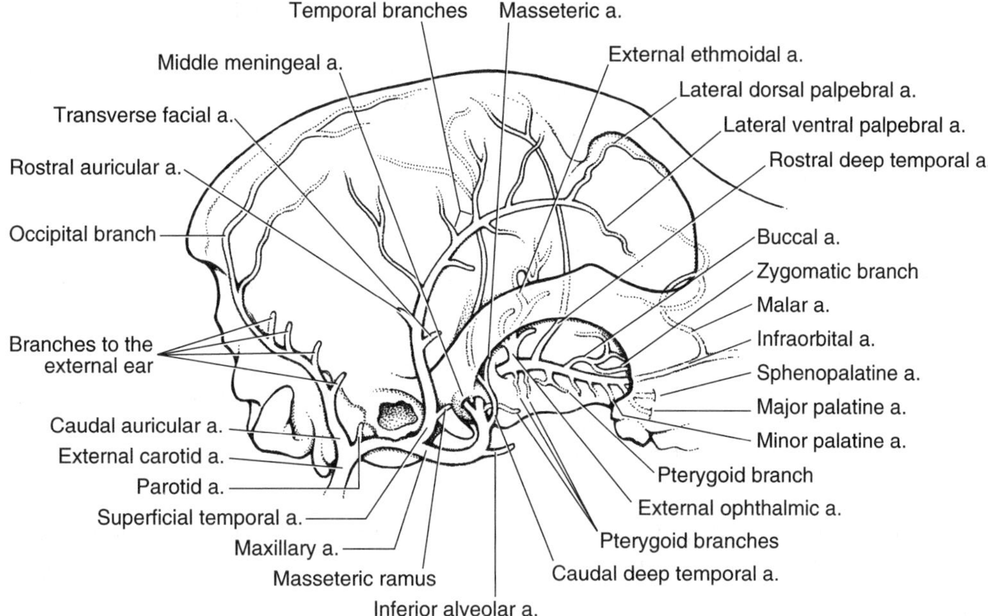

Figure 9–2. Termination of the external carotid artery and the course and branches of its terminal vessels, the superficial temporal artery and the maxillary artery.

c. The **pterygopalatine portion of the maxillary artery** lies on the lateral surface of the pterygoid muscles within the pterygopalatine fossa, as the name suggests (see Figure 9–2).

(1) The pterygopalatine portion of the maxillary artery gives off several named branches, some of which are not commonly observed or encountered clinically, that supply the **pterygoid** and **temporal muscles,** the **lacrimal gland,** the **cheek** and the **hard** and **soft palates.**

(2) The **external ophthalmic artery** typically arises from the pterygopalatine portion of the maxillary artery immediately after exiting the alar canal. The external ophthalmic artery supplies structures of the **orbit** as well as certain internal and external structures of the **eye** (see Chapter 15 VII A 2 a).

2. The **termination of the maxillary artery** is marked by its fairly even division into the infraorbital artery and the common trunk of the sphenopalatine and palatine arteries (see Figure 9–2).

a. The **infraorbital artery** forms the main continuation of the maxillary artery into the rostral regions of the head. The infraorbital artery continues directly rostrally from the maxillary artery and enters the maxillary foramen, along with the maxillary nerve. It passes rostrally through the infraorbital canal together with the maxillary nerve (which becomes the infraorbital nerve).

(1) While in the canal, the infraorbital artery provides branches to the **roots of the upper arcade of teeth.**

(2) After exiting the infraorbital foramen, the infraorbital artery terminates by dividing into the **dorsal** and **lateral nasal arteries,** which supply the **regional skin, subcutis,** and **muscles,** as well as the **vibrissae.**

b. The **common trunk of the sphenopalatine and major palatine arteries** arises as the second part of the termination of the maxillary artery just rostral to the maxillary foramen.

(1) The **sphenopalatine artery,** a large artery, passes into the sphenopalatine foramen (just dorsal to the caudal palatine foramen) and then passes rostrally, supplying

part of the **palate** as well as structures within the **nasal cavity,** including the nasal septum and conchae.

(2) The **major palatine artery** passes through the caudal palatine foramen and supplies the **soft** and **bony tissues** of the **hard palate.**

II. VEINS OF THE HEAD

A. Overview

1. **Pattern.** Most of the deeper named arteries of the head are accompanied by satellite veins of the same name that follow a similar course (Figure 9–3). However, significant variations from this general pattern exist in the more superficial veins as the veins become larger and merge to form the largest tributaries of the external jugular vein.
2. **Flow of venous blood from the head.** The **external jugular vein,** the final common pathway for venous return from the head (exclusive of much of the cranial cavity) forms from the confluence of the **linguofacial** and **maxillary veins.** (The venous drainage of the cranial cavity is discussed in Chapter 13 VI B).

B. Linguofacial vein.

The **lingual vein** becomes confluent with the **facial vein** to form the **linguofacial trunk,** which then forms the external jugular vein by becoming confluent with the maxillary vein.

1. **Lingual vein.** The lingual vein is largely similar in course to the artery of the same name, except at its termination, where it joins the facial vein. The **hyoid venous arch** is an unpaired vein that has no companion artery. This vein lies superficial to the basihyoid

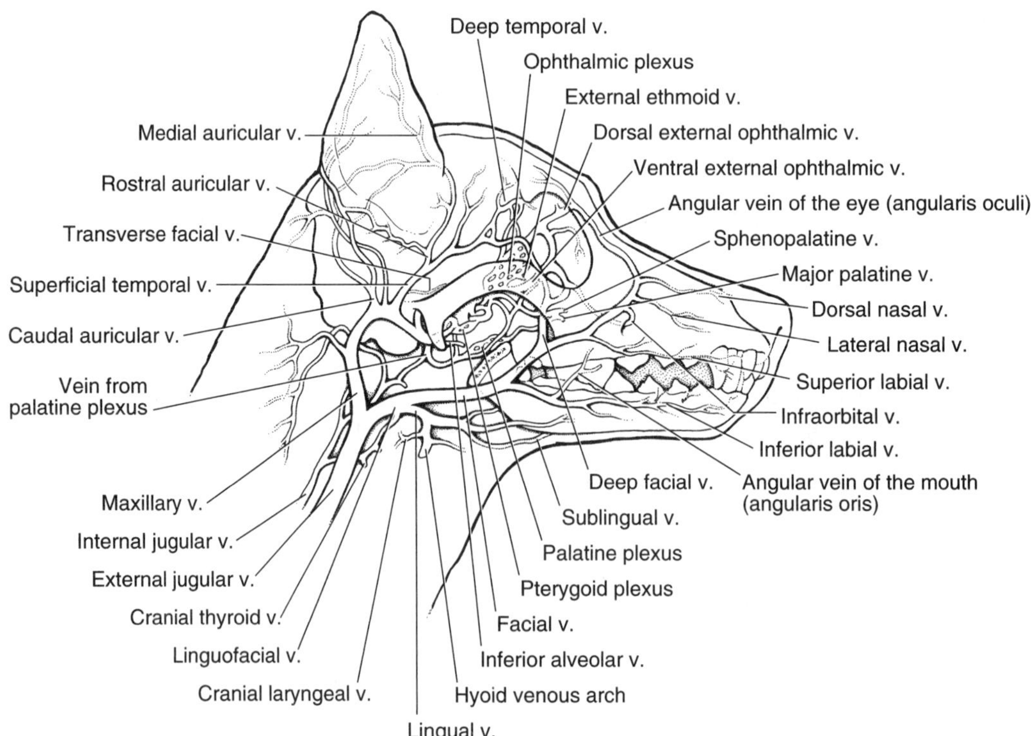

Figure 9–3. Major superficial veins of the head.

bone just deep to the skin, and usually links the two lingual veins. In addition, the hyoid venous arch typically receives other tiny tributaries from surrounding structures.

2. **Facial vein**
   a. **Course.** The facial vein differs from the course of the artery of the same name in two major respects:
      (1) While the termination of the facial artery lies at the superior labial artery, the facial vein forms more dorsally on the face where the dorsal nasal vein joins the angular vein of the eye (angularis oculi).
      (2) The facial artery is a direct branch from the major artery of the neck (i.e., the external carotid artery), but the facial vein does not directly join the major neck vein (i.e., the external jugular vein). Rather, it becomes confluent with the lingual vein.
   b. Tributaries of the facial vein include the following.
      (1) The **angular vein of the eye (angularis oculi)** is a large vein lacking valves that lies along the rostral edge of the orbit. It passes rostrally to approximately midway between the rostral edge of the orbit and the nose, where it receives the dorsal and lateral nasal veins before turning caudoventrally and becoming the facial vein. [Caudally, it becomes the dorsal ophthalmic vein; see II C 7 b (1)].
      (2) The **infraorbital vein** traverses the infraorbital canal along with the infraorbital artery and nerve. Rostrally, the infraorbital vein enters the facial vein, while caudally it is continuous with veins within the orbital region.
      (3) The **angular vein of the mouth (angularis oris)** is a short, small vein that forms in the region of the commissure of the lips and enters the facial vein.
      (4) The **deep facial vein,** which has no companion artery, forms in the rostroventral region of the orbit, and courses ventrally, roughly through the rostral end of the pterygopalatine fossa. It terminates in the facial vein at the ventral edge of the attachment of the zygomatic arch with the skull. The deep facial vein receives as tributaries the sphenopalatine, infraorbital, and (inconstantly) the major palatine arteries.

C. Maxillary vein. In its course, the maxillary vein differs considerably from the artery of the same name. It forms from the merger of veins of the pterygopalatine plexus and the small vein within the alar canal, and receives several small tributaries in the region of the pterygopalatine fossa (e.g., from the cavernous sinus, other cranial cavity sinuses, and meninges). Other larger tributaries received by the maxillary vein include the following.

1. The **vein from the palatine plexus** connects the palatine plexus with the maxillary vein. The **palatine plexus** (see Figure 9–3) is a loosely organized meshwork of tiny veins within the substance of the soft palate.
   a. The **hard palate** drains into another, poorly defined plexus that then drains into the palatine plexus.
   b. The **soft palate** drains directly into the venous palatine plexus.
2. The **temporomandibular articular vein** is a large vein that more than doubles the size of the maxillary vein. The temporomandibular articular vein drains a significant amount of blood from the interior of the cranial cavity.
3. The **inferior alveolar vein** emerges from the mandibular foramen on the medial surface of the mandible and drains into the maxillary vein.
4. The **deep temporal** and **masseteric veins** drain the musculature medial to the mandible.
5. The **superficial temporal vein** is a satellite of the artery of the same name.
6. The **caudal auricular vein** is a satellite of the artery of the same name.
7. The **pterygoid plexus** (see Figure 9–3) lies on the medial wall of the pterygopalatine fossa near the alar canal.
   a. This plexus is considered to be the **origin of the maxillary vein.** A small vein departs from the pterygoid plexus, enters the rostral alar foramen, and traverses the foramen adjacent to the maxillary artery and nerve. This vein then exits the caudal alar foramen to rejoin the maxillary vein caudal to the alar canal.
   b. The pterygoid plexus communicates with the **ophthalmic plexus** (see Figure 9–3). The ophthalmic venous plexus lies within the periorbita and is formed by the breaking up

of the **dorsal external ophthalmic vein** as it passes medial to the level of the zygomatic arch. In its course caudally, the plexus coalesces back into a single vein just rostral to the orbital fissure. This vein enters the orbital fissure, passes through it, and then enters the cavernous sinus.

(1) The **angular vein of the eye (angularis oculi)** passes caudally to the dorsomedial edge of the orbit, where it disappears from view as it **becomes the dorsal external ophthalmic vein.** (Rostrally, it becomes the facial vein.)

(2) The **ventral external ophthalmic vein** arches ventrally from the dorsal external ophthalmic vein to pass more ventrally along the caudal orbital region. This vein terminates by joining the ophthalmic venous plexus.

III. LYMPHATIC VESSELS OF THE HEAD (Figure 9–4)

A. **Afferent lymphatic vessels** drain essentially three generalized areas of the head and face. A **lymphocenter** consists of one or several lymph nodes that consistently occur in and receive lymphatic drainage from a characteristic area.

1. The **parotid lymphocenter** receives lymphatic vessels arising in the:
   - **a.** Skin of the lateral cranial region and the caudal half of the dorsal area of the muzzle
   - **b.** Temporal, masseter, and zygomatic muscles as well as the muscles of the ear
   - **c.** The mandible and the nasal, frontal, parietal, zygomatic, and temporal bones
2. The **mandibular lymphocenter** receives lymphatic vessels arising in essentially all regions of the head not drained by the parotid lymphocenter. Considerable overlap is present between these two areas of drainage. Drainage to the mandibular lymphocenter arrives from the palate, tongue, oral floor, and pharynx.
3. The **retropharyngeal lymphocenter** receives lymphatic vessels arising in the deep structures of the head. Importantly, the retropharyngeal lymphocenter also receives the efferent lymphatics of the parotid and mandibular lymphocenters. Regions and structures drained by the retropharyngeal lymphocenter include the:

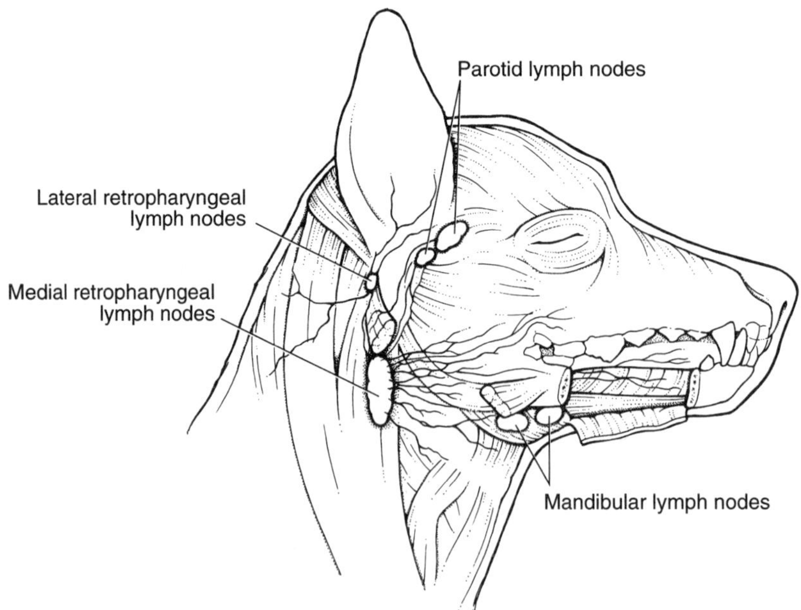

Figure 9–4. Lymph nodes of the head.

a. Tongue and the walls of the oral, nasal, and pharyngeal regions
b. Salivary glands
c. Deep parts of the external ear
d. Larynx
e. Esophagus
f. Parotid and mandibular lymphocenters

B. Efferent lymphatic vessels

1. The **parotid lymphocenter** sends its efferent vessels to the retropharyngeal lymphocenter.
2. The **mandibular lymphocenter** also sends its efferent vessels to the retropharyngeal lymphocenter.
3. Efferents of the **retropharyngeal lymphocenter** are large vessels leaving the caudal pole of the medial retropharyngeal lymph nodes as the **right** and **left tracheal ducts.**

Chapter 10

Innervation of the Head

I. INTRODUCTION

A. Cranial nerves provide both motor and sensory innervation to most head structures.

1. **Characteristics**
   a. The cranial nerves are set apart from the spinal nerves in that they are **adjoined to the brain** (either by entering it or exiting from it) rather than the spinal cord, and they **enter or leave the brain or brain stem through foramina of the skull.**
   b. All of the cranial nerves are **paired.**
   c. The cranial nerves may be **sensory, motor,** or **sensorimotor.**
   d. In many cases, the cranial nerves **carry autonomic nerve fibers** with them. Both sympathetic and parasympathetic fibers accompany certain cranial nerves.
      (1) **Parasympathetic fibers** are associated with the following cranial nerves:
         (a) Oculomotor nerve (cranial nerve III), to the head
         (b) Facial nerve (cranial nerve VII), to the head
         (c) Glossopharyngeal nerve (cranial nerve IX), to the head
         (d) Vagus nerve (cranial nerve X), to the cervical, thoracic, and abdominal viscera
      (2) **Sympathetic fibers** are variably associated with the following cranial nerves:
         (a) Glossopharyngeal nerve (cranial nerve IX)
         (b) Vagus nerve (cranial nerve X)
         (c) Accessory nerve (cranial nerve XI)
         (d) Hypoglossal nerve (cranial nerve XII)
2. **Naming convention.** All of the cranial nerves are named as well as numbered.
   a. Most cranial nerves bear names descriptive of their function or descriptive of some other feature of the nerve.
   b. The numbers assigned to the cranial nerves indicate their location (rostral to caudal) on the brain (see Chapter 13, Figure 13–2). By convention, Roman numerals rather than Arabic ones are used to designate the cranial nerves.

Canine Clinical Correlation

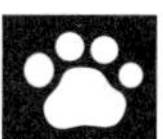

The cranial nerve examination is an integral part of a complete neurologic examination. Because the position of each cranial nerve on the brain stem is known, functional deficits can provide clues regarding the affected part of the brain. Identification of a functional deficit is relatively straightforward, because each cranial nerve is associated with a specific function, and all can be fairly easily and directly tested.

B. Spinal nerves. Despite the overwhelming contribution made by the cranial nerves to innervation of the head, the more caudal regions of the head as well as much of the ear also receive sensory innervation via branches of the **second cervical nerve,** a spinal nerve.

II. CRANIAL NERVES

A. Olfactory nerve (cranial nerve I)

1. **Function.** The olfactory nerve provides the sense of **smell** (i.e., it is a special visceral afferent nerve). It is wholly **sensory** in nature.

2. **Course.** What is commonly referred to as "the" olfactory nerve is actually the conceptual, functional, and anatomic grouping of many individual olfactory nerves.
   a. Receptors of the olfactory nerve are distributed thickly over the surface of the mucosa that covers the ethmoidal labyrinth (ethmoid concha) and dorsal part of the nasal septum. Fibers from these olfactory cells form small bundles that separately pierce the ethmoid bone via the cribriform plate to **enter** the rostral extremity of the cranial cavity.
   b. After passing through the cribriform plate, these fibers collect together to form the **olfactory bulb** (see Chapter 13, Figure 13–2), which in turn continues caudally into the brain.

B. Optic nerve (cranial nerve II)

1. **Function.** The optic nerve provides the sense of **sight** and is wholly **sensory.**
2. **Course**
   a. The optic nerve's fibers originate as a collection of axons exiting the retina at the optic disk.
   b. The optic nerve **enters** the skull at the optic canal.
   c. At the **optic chiasm,** the two optic nerves meet and approximately 75% of the fibers of each optic nerve cross to the other side. The optic nerves then continue as the **optic tracts,** ascending the lateral surface of the diencephalon to terminate at the lateral geniculate body.

C. Oculomotor nerve (cranial nerve III)

1. **Function.** The oculomotor nerve is **motor** only.
   a. **Movement of the eyeball.** The oculomotor nerve carries **general somatic efferent fibers** that are motor to several extraocular muscles (see Chapter 15 VI C 1).
   b. **Constriction of the pupil.** The oculomotor nerve also carries **general visceral efferent (parasympathetic) fibers** that contribute to the innervation of the **ciliary muscles** (which control the thickness of the lens) and the **pupillary sphincter.**

2. **Course.** The somatic and parasympathetic fibers **leave** the brain stem close together, course rostrally (still close together), and exit the brain stem at the **orbital fissure** (along with the trochlear, ophthalmic, and abducent nerves). The oculomotor nerve appears on the ventral brain stem approximately halfway along the length of the piriform lobe, and close to the midline.
   a. The **somatic fibers** divide into two nerves on entering the orbit, the **dorsal** and **ventral branch** (see Chapter 15 VI C 1).
   b. The **parasympathetic fibers** continue slightly rostrally and terminate at the **ciliary ganglion.** The **short ciliary nerves** arise from the ciliary ganglion and supply the pupillary sphincter and the ciliary muscle.

D. Trochlear nerve (cranial nerve IV)

1. **Function.** The trochlear nerve, which is **motor** only, carries **general somatic efferent fibers** to the **dorsal oblique muscle** (one of the extraocular muscles); therefore; it is also concerned with **movement of the eyeball.**
2. **Course.** The trochlear nerve **exits** the cranial cavity at the **orbital fissure** (along with the oculomotor, ophthalmic, and abducent nerves). The trochlear nerve is unique among the cranial nerves in three respects:
   a. It is the only cranial nerve to exit the dorsal brain stem surface, becoming visible on the ventral surface of the brain stem just at the caudal brim of the piriform lobe. (Its dorsal origins are hidden in the intact brain, even from a dorsal view.)
   b. It is the only cranial nerve to cross the brain entirely to innervate the contralateral side.
   c. It is the smallest cranial nerve and only innervates one structure.

E. Trigeminal nerve (cranial nerve V).
As the name suggests, the trigeminal nerve has three major divisions, each of which is named and itself subdivides into named branches (Figure 10–1).

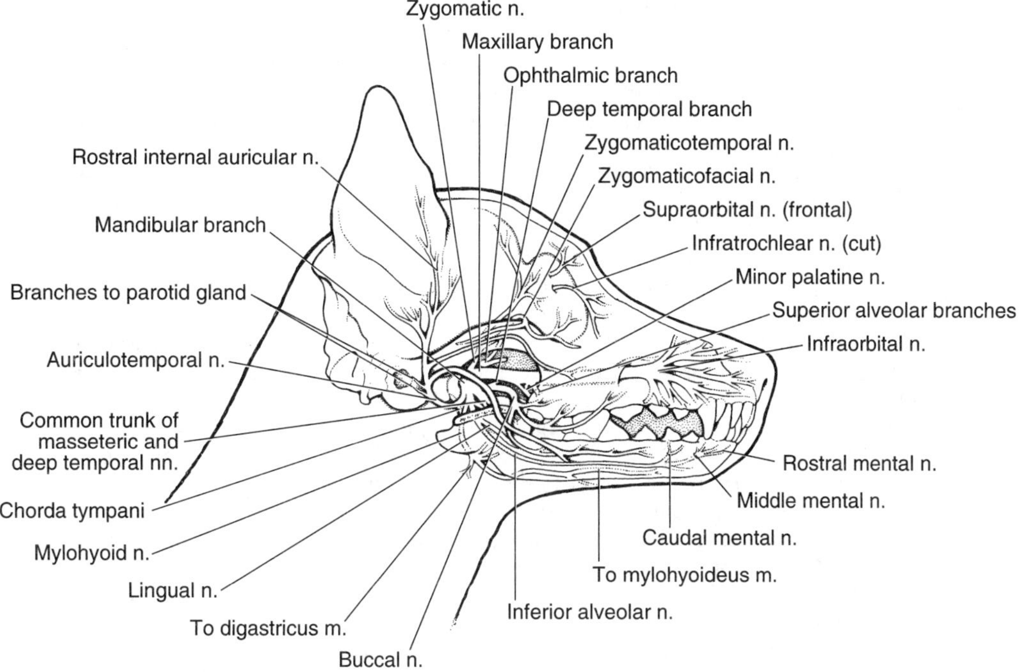

Figure 10–1. The trigeminal nerve (cranial nerve V) has three branches: the ophthalmic division (cranial nerve V_1), the maxillary division (cranial nerve V_2), and the mandibular division (cranial nerve V_3). The subnumbering corresponds to the position of the innervated area on the head, from dorsal to ventral.

1. **Function.** The trigeminal nerve is **motor to the muscles of mastication** and **sensory to the skin and deeper face.** It supplies a vast amount of the head's innervation entirely on its own.
2. **Divisions**
   a. The **ophthalmic division of the trigeminal nerve (cranial nerve V_1)** distributes to the **eye** and **adnexa.** It is **sensory** only, and divides into three named branches:
      (1) The **frontal nerve,** sensory to the supraorbital and supratrochlear regions
      (2) The **lacrimal nerve,** sensory to the lacrimal gland, deeper structures of the eye, and a region of skin adjacent to the lateral angle of the eye
      (3) The **nasociliary nerve,** which branches into the:
         (a) **Infratrochlear nerve,** sensory to the structures and face near the medial angle of the eye
         (b) **Long ciliary nerve,** sensory to the sensitive tissues of the globe, including the cornea
         (c) **Ethmoidal nerve,** sensory to the nasal mucosa
   b. The **maxillary division of the trigeminal nerve (cranial nerve V_2)** is distributed to the **maxillary region** of the face. It is **sensory** only.
      (1) **Branches** of the maxillary division of the trigeminal nerve include the:
         (a) **Zygomatic nerve,** which divides into the:
            (i) **Zygomaticotemporal nerve,** sensory to an area over much of the temporal muscle (dorsal to the zygomatic arch and rostral to the external ear)
            (ii) **Zygomaticofacial nerve,** sensory to an area of skin over much of the zygomatic arch and the lower eyelid
         (b) **Pterygopalatine nerve,** which divides into the:
            (i) **Lesser palatine nerve,** sensory to the soft palate
            (ii) **Greater palatine nerve,** sensory to the hard palate

(iii) **Caudal nasal nerve,** sensory to the ventral nasal cavity, the maxillary sinus, and the palate

(2) The **infraorbital nerve** is the continuation of the maxillary nerve within the infraorbital canal (see Figure 10–1). The infraorbital nerve innervates the upper arcade of teeth (while in the canal) and the rostral muzzle and nose (after exiting the canal at the infraorbital foramen).

(a) The upper dental arcade is supplied by the **caudal, middle,** and **rostral superior alveolar branches,** which are given off while the nerve is inside the infraorbital canal.

(b) On exiting the infraorbital foramen, the infraorbital nerve divides into three general bundles of nerves that supply the areas suggested by their names: the **external** and **internal nasal,** and **superior labial branches.**

c. The **mandibular division of the trigeminal nerve (cranial nerve V_3)** is distributed to the region surrounding the **mandible.** It is both **motor** and **sensory,** and itself detaches many named branches.

(1) **Motor branches** of the mandibular nerve include the:

(a) **Masticator nerve,** motor to the rostral belly of the digastricus muscle

(b) **Masseteric nerve,** motor to the masseter muscle

(c) **Deep temporal nerves,** motor to the temporalis muscle

(d) **Deep pterygoid nerves,** motor to the medial and lateral pterygoid muscles

(e) **Tensor tympani nerve,** motor to the muscle of the same name

(f) **Tensor veli palatini nerve,** also motor to the muscle of the same name:

(2) **Sensory branches** of the mandibular nerve include the following:

(a) The **buccal nerve** is sensory to the mucosa of the cheek. [Do not confuse the buccal nerve, a sensory branch of the mandibular nerve, with the dorsal and ventral buccal branches of the facial nerve (cranial nerve VII), which are motor].

(b) The **auriculotemporal nerve** is sensory to the skin over much of the external ear and external ear canal, as well as the temporal region, and gives off many branches.

(i) The **transverse facial nerve** supplies a narrow strip of skin extending to the angle of the mouth.

(ii) The **nerve of the external acoustic meatus** is a sensory branch.

(iii) The **ramus to the tympanic membrane** is also a sensory branch.

(iv) Several **parotid branches** carry postganglionic parasympathetic fibers to the parotid salivary gland.

(v) The **rostral auricular nerves** are sensory to a small region immediately at the base of the ear, as well as to a large part of the ventral aspect of the temporalis muscle and the zygomatic arch.

(vi) The **communicating branches to the facial nerve (cranial nerve VII)** join the dorsal buccal branch of the facial nerve to provide skin sensation over approximately the same field for which the dorsal buccal branch of the facial nerve provides motor innervation.

(c) The **lingual nerve** is general sensory to the oropharyngeal mucosa and rostral two thirds of the tongue, as well as special sensory (i.e., supplying taste) to the rostral two thirds of the tongue.

(i) The **sublingual nerve** carries sensory fibers from the mucosa of the oral floor and also participates in delivering postganglionic parasympathetic fibers to the sublingual salivary glands.

(ii) The lingual nerve **communicates with the hypoglossal nerve (cranial nerve XII)** before dividing into its terminal branches within the substance of the tongue.

(d) The **inferior alveolar nerve** enters the mandibular foramen and is distributed to the lower arcade of teeth. The **mental nerves** are the termination of the inferior alveolar nerve as it exits the mental foramina.

(3) **Motor and sensory branches.** The **mylohyoid nerve,** which is usually a branch of the inferior alveolar nerve (but may arise from the mandibular nerve itself) has both motor and sensory components, being motor to the mylohyoideus muscle

and the rostral belly of the digastricus muscle, and sensory to the skin of the lower lip and cheek and an area of the intermandibular region.

3. **Course.** The trigeminal nerve is visible on the ventral surface of the brain stem, just at the junction of the pons and the trapezoid body. The trigeminal nerve leaves the brain stem and enters the trigeminal canal within the cranial cavity. Within the trigeminal canal lies the large trigeminal ganglion. Immediately distal to the trigeminal ganglion, the nerve exits the canal and divides into its three named branches.
   a. The **ophthalmic nerve (cranial nerve V_1)** is composed of sensory fibers from the eyelids and globe, the nasal mucosa, and the skin of the nose. It enters the cranial cavity via the orbital fissure (in company with the oculomotor, trochlear, and abducent nerves) and has three named branches within the periorbita. For ease of discussion, the course of these branches will be described from the orbital fissure outward (superficially), but it must be kept in mind that the fibers (being sensory) are actually traveling in the opposite direction.
      (1) The **frontal nerve** passes rostrally within the lateral surface of the periorbita, becomes subcutaneous near the orbital ligament, and terminates as the supraorbital and supratrochlear nerves.
      (2) The **lacrimal nerve** passes rostrally along the lateral rectus muscle to supply the lacrimal gland. It carries (postganglionic) parasympathetic fibers from the pterygopalatine ganglion.
      (3) The **nasociliary nerve** passes rostrally along the medial surface of the retractor bulbi, one of the extraocular muscles.
         (a) On the way to the pupillary dilators and other smooth muscles of the orbit, the nasociliary nerve dispatches a communicating branch (postganglionic sympathetic fibers) to the ciliary ganglion. It also dispatches several long ciliary nerves, which are general sensory to the globe.
         (b) The nasociliary nerve terminates by dividing into the **infratrochlear nerve** and **ethmoidal nerve.** The latter exits the orbit and reenters the cranial cavity via the rostral ethmoidal foramen, passes rostrally through the cribriform plate, and then divides again into medial and lateral branches. The medial and lateral branches of the ethmoidal nerve are sensory to parts of the nasal cavity. The medial branch terminates as the cutaneous external nasal branches, innervating the skin of the nasal vestibule.
   b. The **maxillary nerve (cranial nerve V_2)** is composed of sensory fibers from the lower eyelid, nasal mucosa, upper arcade of teeth, upper lip, and nose, as well as postganglionic parasympathetic axons to the lacrimal, nasal, and palatine glands.
      (1) The maxillary nerve exits the cranial cavity by first passing through the round foramen and into the alar canal. It turns sharply rostrally within the canal, traverses its section of the alar canal in a rostral direction, and exits the canal via the rostral alar foramen.
      (2) It then courses rostrally along the surface of the medial pterygoid muscle and gives rise to three branches within the pterygopalatine fossa.
         (a) The **zygomatic nerve** divides into the zygomaticotemporal and zygomaticofacial nerves [see 2 b (1)(a)].
         (b) The **pterygopalatine nerve** receives fibers from the pterygopalatine ganglion, and then gives off its own branches (the major and minor palatine nerves and the caudal nasal nerve). The caudal nasal nerve, actually the continuation of the pterygopalatine nerve, turns and enters the nasal cavity by way of the sphenopalatine foramen to supply sensation to part of the nasal cavity and postganglionic parasympathetic fibers to the nasal glands.
      (3) The **infraorbital nerve** is the continuation of the maxillary nerve after the caudal nasal nerve departs the parent trunk. The infraorbital nerve enters the maxillary foramen, passes through the infraorbital canal, and then exits the canal via the infraorbital foramen.
   c. The **mandibular nerve (cranial nerve V_3)** is composed of sensory fibers from the buccal cavity, tongue, lower arcade of teeth, lower lip, much of the skin of the head, and

the mucosa of part of the external ear canal, as well as motor fibers to the muscles of mastication and some related muscles. The mandibular nerve exits the cranial cavity via the oval foramen, giving rise to its several major branches (see II E 2 c).

F. Abducent nerve (cranial nerve VI)

1. **Function.** The abducent nerve is composed mainly of **motor** (general somatic efferent) fibers to the lateral rectus and retractor bulbi muscles of the eye.
2. **Course.** The abducent nerve is visible on the ventral surface of the brain stem just caudal to the medial edge of the trigeminal nerve, at the rostral edge of the trapezoid body. It exits the cranial cavity at the orbital fissure (along with the oculomotor, trochlear, and ophthalmic nerves).

G. Facial nerve (cranial nerve VII)

1. **Function.** The facial nerve is **sensory** to the rostral two thirds of the **tongue** and **motor** to all of the muscles of **facial expression**.
   a. The **sensory component** of the facial nerve is involved with both general sensation and the special sense of taste (special visceral afferent).
      (1) The **general sensory component** includes the **lateral internal auricular nerve,** sensory to the nonosseous part of the external ear canal, the **middle internal auricular nerve,** sensory to the skin on the rostral concave region of the pinna, and the **caudal internal auricular nerve,** sensory to the caudal convex region of the pinna.
      (2) The **special sensory component** is relatively small, but nonetheless quite important in that it is the **chorda tympani,** the nerve carrying **taste sensation** to the rostral two thirds of the tongue. The chorda tympani joins the lingual nerve in the deep facial region.
   b. The **motor component** sends many branches:
      (1) The **stapedius nerve,** motor to the muscle of the same name
      (2) The **caudal auricular nerve,** motor to the platysma muscle on the dorsum of the neck
      (3) The **digastric branch,** motor to the caudal belly of the digastricus muscle
      (4) The **cervical branch,** motor to the parotidoauricularis and sphincter colli
      (5) The **dorsal** and **ventral buccal branches,** motor to the muscles of the cheek, lips, and lateral nose
      (6) The **auriculopalpebral nerve,** motor to the rostral ear muscles and several superficial facial muscles in the ocular region
         (a) The **auricular branch** supplies muscles at the rostral ear base.
         (b) The **palpebral branch** forms a plexus between the ear and the eye and innervates several regional facial muscles.
   c. **Portions.** The facial nerve is actually composed of a facial component and an intermediate component. Immediately on exiting the brain stem at the lateral extremity of the trapezoid body, the two components come together. From this point onward, the nerve so formed is referred to in this discussion (and in most texts), as simply the "facial nerve."
      (1) The **facial component** is the portion **motor** to the muscles of facial expression.
      (2) The **intermediate nerve** is a visceral nerve having **sensory** and **parasympathetic motor functions.** The parasympathetic motor fibers innervate the lacrimal gland, mandibular salivary gland, sublingual salivary gland, and the glands of the lingual, buccal, and nasal mucosae.

2. **Course**
   a. The facial nerve exits the cranial cavity by way of the **internal acoustic meatus** of the petrous temporal bone. As it passes toward this meatus, the facial nerve accompanies the vestibulocochlear nerve (cranial nerve VIII); the two nerves are invested in a common dural sheath.
   b. The facial nerve then parts company with the vestibulocochlear nerve, and enters the **facial canal** of the petrous temporal bone.

(1) The facial canal makes a sharp turn toward the stylomastoid foramen. Within the facial canal, the corresponding bend in the facial nerve is referred to as the **genu** (*genu-*, "knee") of the facial nerve. An indistinct swelling of the nerve, the **geniculate ganglion,** is located at the genu of the facial nerve.

(a) The **major petrosal nerve,** which carries the **parasympathetic component of the facial nerve,** leaves the facial nerve at the geniculate ganglion, runs in the tiny petrosal canal of the petrous temporal bone, and is shortly joined by the deep petrosal nerve.

(b) The **deep petrosal nerve** arrives from the cranial cervical ganglion (and thus carries sympathetic fibers), joining the major petrosal nerve to form the **nerve of the pterygoid canal.** The nerve of the pterygoid canal carries both sympathetic and parasympathetic nerves to the lacrimal and nasal mucosal glands.

(2) The facial nerve continues in the facial canal after giving off the major petrosal nerve. In the midst of its course, the facial canal has an opening into the cavity of the middle ear. (The facial canal then continues onward past this opening.)

(a) The stapedial nerve arises from the facial nerve in this region.

(b) The chorda tympani also departs from the facial nerve in this general area. The chorda tympani crosses the tympanic cavity and emerges at the petrotympanic fissure. Upon exiting the skull, the chorda tympani joins company with the lingual nerve.

(3) Within the facial canal, the facial nerve continues onward toward the stylomastoid foramen, through which it exits the skull. From this point on, this portion of the facial nerve is often referred to as the "free" part of the facial nerve. Shortly after emerging from the stylomastoid foramen, the free part of the facial nerve is joined by the auricular branch of the vagus nerve (cranial nerve X), and is likely distributed to the external ear canal along with the vagus nerve.

(a) **Initial branches.** Most of the initial branches from the free part of the facial nerve are smaller and relatively deeply situated. These branches include the:

(i) Unnamed **motor branches to the caudal auricular muscles**

(ii) **Caudal auricular nerve** supplying the platysma muscle on the dorsum of the neck (this branch is not deep)

(iii) **Digastric branch** supplying both the caudal belly of the digastricus muscle and the stylohyoid muscle

(iv) **Caudal, middle,** and **lateral internal auricular nerves,** sensory to the skin of the various regions of the ear

(b) **Superficial branches** (Figure 10–2). From this portion onward, the facial nerve is more superficial. Three major branches are present in this superficial region.

(i) The **cervical branch** is the smallest of these three, and passes superficial to the mandibular salivary gland. It ends by joining a ventral branch of the second cervical nerve.

(ii) The **dorsal** and **ventral buccal branches** of the facial nerve pass rostrally over the superficial surface of the masseter muscle. The dorsal buccal branch often is less collected than the ventral, commonly being observed as a network of fibers rather than a single prominent channel. In such cases, the parotid duct, which passes between the two branches, may be mistaken for the dorsal buccal branch.

(iii) The **auriculopalpebral nerve** climbs steeply up the lateral side of the face just rostral to the base of the ear, and shortly thereafter divides into the palpebral branch and the auricular branch.

H. Vestibulocochlear nerve (cranial nerve VIII)

1. **Function.** The vestibulocochlear nerve is **sensory** only. In keeping with the nerve's dual function, it has a dual composition.

   a. The **vestibular nerve** provides **positional information** to the brain regarding the position of the head relative to the pull of gravity, and **motion sense** (as related to linear and angular acceleration).

   b. The **cochlear nerve** is involved with **hearing.**

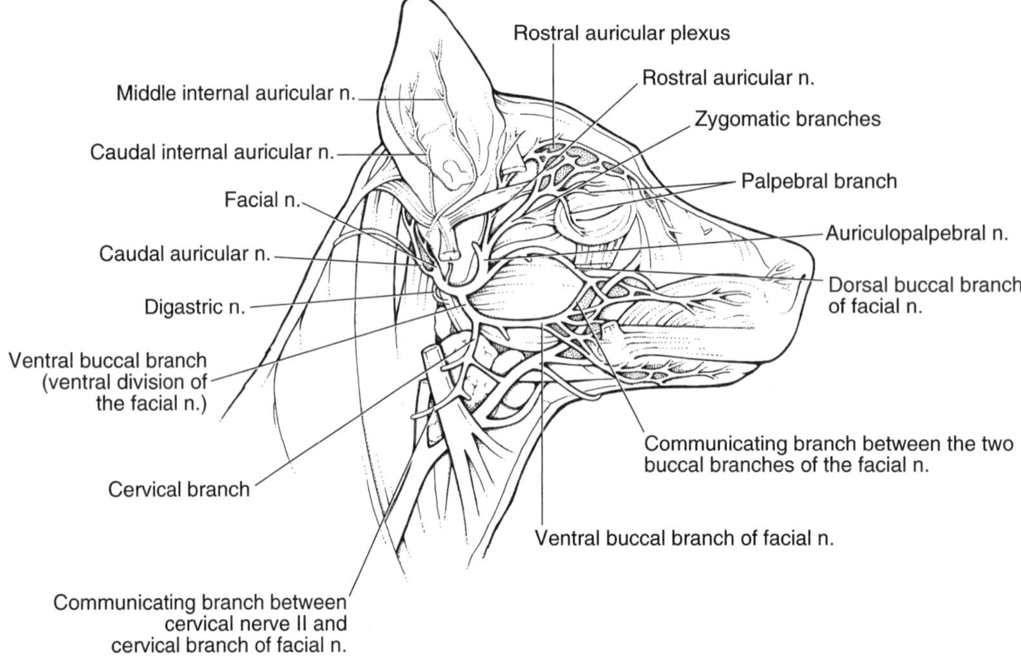

Figure 10–2. The superficial branches of the facial nerve.

2. **Course.** The vestibulocochlear nerve never leaves the skull, because it originates within the inner ear, which is housed in the petrous portion of the temporal bone within the cranial cavity, and passes directly into the medulla oblongata. The vestibulocochlear nerve is located near the craniolateral edge of the trapezoid body, just caudal to the trigeminal nerve (cranial nerve V) and lateral to the facial nerve (cranial nerve VII).

I. Glossopharyngeal nerve (cranial nerve IX)

1. **Function.** The glossopharyngeal nerve is **motor** and **sensory.**
   a. **Motor components**
      (1) The glossopharyngeal nerve carries **visceral motor** (i.e., **parasympathetic**) **fibers** to the **parotid** and **zygomatic salivary glands** and the **glands** and **vasculature of the tongue.**
      (2) The glossopharyngeal nerve provides **motor innervation** to the **stylopharyngeus muscle** (by itself) and **other pharyngeal musculature** (together with branches from the vagus nerve).
   b. **Sensory components** of the glossopharyngeal nerve include:
      (1) **General sensory** output from the caudal third of the **tongue** and the **pharyngeal mucosa**
      (2) **Special sensory** output from the caudal third of the tongue (taste)
      (3) **Baroreceptors** in the carotid bulb and **chemoreceptors** in the carotid body
2. **Course**
   a. The glossopharyngeal nerve surfaces on the medulla in a nearly direct rostrocaudal line with the origins of cranial nerves X and XI, and passes in close company with them to the jugular foramen (the intracranial side of the passage that opens externally at the tympanooccipital fissure).
   b. At approximately the level of the tympanooccipital fissure, the **tympanic nerve** leaves the glossopharyngeal nerve.

(1) The tympanic nerve enters the tympanic (middle ear) cavity and carries parasympathetic (i.e., visceral motor) fibers to the tympanic plexus.

(2) The minor petrosal nerve leaves the plexus, and travels to the otic ganglion, where its fibers synapse. Postganglionic parasympathetic fibers leave the otic ganglion to travel with the auriculotemporal nerve to the parotid and zygomatic salivary glands.

c. The glossopharyngeal nerve exits the skull via the tympanooccipital fissure (together with cranial nerves X and XI) and gives of the following branches:

(1) The **branch to the carotid sinus,** which carries chemoreceptors to the carotid body and baroreceptors to the carotid sinus

(2) A motor **branch to the stylopharyngeus muscle**

d. The glossopharyngeal nerve terminates by dividing into the lingual and pharyngeal branches.

(1) The **lingual branch** (not to be confused with the lingual nerve, a sensory branch of the mandibular nerve) enters the tongue near and on a similar course with the lingual artery and hypoglossal nerve.

(a) The lingual branch is sensory to the caudal third of the tongue and the palatine tonsil.

(b) It is motor (via parasympathetic nerves) to the vasculature and glands within the tongue and the glands of the soft palate. It is also motor to the levator veli palatini muscle.

(2) The **pharyngeal branch** joins the vagus nerve in providing parasympathetic fibers to the **pharyngeal plexus.**

(a) The sympathetic component of the pharyngeal plexus arrives from the cranial cervical ganglion.

(b) Autonomic fibers leave the pharyngeal plexus to innervate the caudal pharyngeal muscles and pharyngeal mucosa.

J. Vagus nerve (cranial nerve X)

1. Function. The vagus nerve is **motor** and **sensory,** carrying parasympathetic (i.e., visceral efferent) innervation to the palate, pharynx, larynx, trachea, esophagus, thoracic viscera, and abdominal viscera. Most of the vagus nerve (approximately 80%) is composed of **general visceral sensory fibers:** very few nociceptive fibers are present because the main manner in which pain can be registered from the viscera is by the perception of stretch.

a. Motor components of the vagus nerve include:

(1) The **pharyngeal ramus,** which leaves the vagus and participates with the glossopharyngeal nerve in the formation of the **pharyngeal plexus,** which then disperses motor fibers to the caudal pharyngeal muscles and cranial esophagus

(2) a **portion of the cranial laryngeal nerve,** which in addition to its sensory function is also motor to the cricothyroideus muscle

(3) The **caudal laryngeal nerve** (i.e., the continuation of the recurrent laryngeal nerve), which is motor to all laryngeal muscles except the cricothyroideus (which is innervated by the cranial laryngeal nerve)

(4) The portions of the **cardiac nerves** carrying preganglionic parasympathetic axons

(5) Motor nerves to the **bronchial smooth musculature**

(6) Motor nerves to the **wall of the gastrointestinal tract**

b. Sensory components of the vagus nerve include:

(1) The **auricular branch,** which joins the facial nerve and supplies sensory innervation to the nonosseous portion of the external ear canal

(2) The **proximal** and **distal vagal ganglia,** associated with sensory cells of the visceral organs

(3) A **portion of the cranial laryngeal nerve,** which in addition to its motor function is also sensory to the laryngeal mucosa and taste buds of the epiglottis

(4) The **pararecurrent laryngeal nerves,** which are branches of the recurrent laryngeal nerves supplying sensory innervation to the trachea and esophagus

(5) **Visceral efferent fibers** from the **visceral organs**

2. **Course.** The field of distribution of the vagus nerve is the widest of all cranial nerves, extending from the head through the neck and thorax, and into the abdomen as far caudally as the left colic flexure.
   a. The vagus nerve leaves the medulla and passes through the **jugular foramen** in company with the glossopharyngeal nerve (cranial nerve IX) and the accessory nerve (cranial nerve XI). The jugular foramen is simply a foramen on the interior of the cranial cavity that leads to a short channel within the skull. The channel exits the skull by means of the tympanooccipital fissure. Two features of importance related to the vagus nerve are present at the level of the jugular foramen:
      (1) The **auricular branch** of the vagus nerve leaves its parent nerve near the entrance of the vagus into the jugular foramen and courses laterally with the facial nerve through the facial canal in the petrous temporal bone to be distributed as **general sensory** to the skin of the **external ear canal.**
      (2) The **proximal vagal ganglion** lies within the jugular foramen. This ganglion is the first of two **sensory** ganglia of the vagus nerve, functioning in general sensory **input from the viscera of the body cavities.**
   b. The vagus nerve then exits the skull from its proximal ganglion via the **tympanooccipital fissure,** still in company with cranial nerves IX and XI. As with the jugular foramen, several important features concerning the vagus nerve are associated with the tympanooccipital fissure.
      (1) The **pharyngeal branch** leaves the vagus nerve just as the vagus exits the skull. The pharyngeal branch is joined by the communicating branch from the glossopharyngeal nerve (cranial nerve IX) to form the **pharyngeal plexus,** which innervates the caudal pharyngeal muscles and esophagus. The pharyngeal branch then continues into the pharynx, to innervate the **cricopharyngeus muscle** and **part of the cervical esophagus.**
      (2) The **distal vagal ganglion,** which is the second of the two visceral **sensory** ganglia of the vagus nerve, lies on the vagus nerve just as it leaves the tympanooccipital fissure. The **cranial laryngeal nerve** detaches from the vagus at the level of the distal vagal ganglion, and shortly divides into internal and external branches.
         (a) The **internal branch** is sensory only, and provides the **internal laryngeal mucosa** with general sensation and the **taste buds of the epiglottis** with special sense. These taste buds are important in the reflex closure of the glottis when the epiglottis is stimulated by water or other fluids.
         (b) The **external branch** is sensory and motor, providing motor innervation to the **cricothyroideus muscle** and sensory innervation to the **pharyngeal mucosa.**
   c. The vagus nerve parts company with cranial nerves IX and XI shortly after leaving the tympanooccipital fissure and lies very close to the **cranial cervical ganglion,** part of the sympathetic nervous system. Distal to this **sympathetic** ganglion, the vagus nerve and sympathetic trunk become closely associated and pass through the neck invested in a common epineurium as the **vagosympathetic trunk.** The vagosympathetic trunk courses through the neck as one of the components of the carotid sheath.
      (1) The vagus nerve is mainly carrying parasympathetic fibers caudally along the neck, *en route* to the thorax and abdomen.
      (2) The sympathetic trunk is mainly carrying sympathetic fibers cranially along the neck, *en route* to the head and neck.
   d. The vagus nerve and the sympathetic trunk separate near the thoracic inlet, where the vagus separates from the vagosympathetic trunk just cranial to the middle cervical ganglion. The vagus then passes ventral to the subclavian artery (very close to the ansa subclavia) and on caudally through the thorax related to the trachea and esophagus.
      (1) The **cardiac branches** of the vagus nerve arise directly from the parent nerve in this general area, and course directly to the heart.
      (2) The **recurrent laryngeal nerves,** right and left, also detach from the vagus nerve in this area. Each recurrent laryngeal nerve:
         (a) Departs from the vagus near the heart and arches around one of the great arteries of the heart

(i) The left recurrent laryngeal nerve arches around the aorta.

(ii) The right recurrent laryngeal nerve arches around the right subclavian artery.

(b) Reascends the neck along the trachea to attain the level of the larynx, where each terminates as the appropriate caudal laryngeal nerve

(i) Each caudal laryngeal nerve innervates all of the **muscles** on its respective side **of the larynx,** except the cricothyroideus (which is supplied by the cranial laryngeal nerve).

(ii) This seemingly unnecessary course from the brain to the internal thorax and back again to the larynx is explained by the fact that the heart initially develops in the ventral neck. During that time, the caudal laryngeal nerves take a direct lateral course into the larynx, growing in a straight path through the developing aortic arches to the larynx. However, as the heart "descends" into the thoracic cavity later in development, the caudal laryngeal nerves are trapped by the arteries, and are pulled caudally with them to become the recurrent laryngeal nerves.

e. At the **pulmonary hilus,** the vagus nerve provides **branches to the bronchi.**

f. The vagus nerves pass on to the lateral surface of the esophagus, where each vagus nerve divides into a **dorsal** and a **ventral vagal branch.** Thus, there is a total of four vagal branches, one dorsal and one ventral from the left vagus nerve, and one dorsal and one ventral from the right vagus nerve.

(1) These vagal branches course caudally along the lateral surface of the esophagus to approximately the level of the diaphragm. Each vagal branch then passes slightly medially and unites with its fellow of the same name, to form a similarly named vagal trunk, which occupies the appropriate surface of the esophagus (i.e., the right and left dorsal vagal branches unite to form the dorsal vagal trunk, which runs on the dorsal surface of the esophagus, and the right and left ventral vagal branches unite to form the ventral vagal trunk, which runs on the ventral surface of the esophagus).

(2) The vagal trunks pass the diaphragm through the esophageal hiatus in contact with the esophagus. After passing into the abdomen, the **ventral vagal trunk** is distributed to the **stomach** and **liver.** After passing the diaphragm, the **dorsal vagal trunk** passes through (but does not synapse in) the celiac plexus, and has its fibers distributed to the various **abdominal viscera.** By means of distribution along with the abdominal arteries, the fibers of the vagus nerve are distributed to essentially all of the abdominal viscera as far caudally as the left colic flexure.

K. Accessory nerve (cranial nerve XI)

1. **Function.** The accessory nerve is the only cranial nerve that **does not take part in innervation of head structures.** Rather, it supplies **motor** innervation to several **ventral neck muscles** (i.e., parts of the **sternocephalicus muscle,** the **cleidomastoideus muscle,** and the **cleidocervicalis muscle)** and the **trapezius muscle** on the back.

2. **Course**

a. The accessory nerve has a dual origin, from the brain stem and from the cervical spinal cord.

(1) The **cranial (brain stem) roots** emerge directly from their brain stem nuclei.

(2) The **caudal (spinal) root.** The rootlets from the first seven or eight spinal cord segments emerge from the lateral surface of the cord, pass cranially, and coalesce to form this named root, which in turn passes cranially through the foramen magnum to join the root from the brain stem.

b. The cranial and caudal roots progress together for a very limited time, entering the jugular foramen and passing through the stylomastoid foramen along with cranial nerves IX and X.

(1) During the course related to these two foramina, the cranial root departs from the accessory nerve and joins the vagus nerve (as the internal branch of the accessory nerve).

(2) The spinal root then continues as the "accessory nerve" described in gross

anatomy. This portion is sometimes referred to as the "external branch of the accessory nerve."

c. On exiting the skull, the accessory nerve divides into dorsal and ventral branches.
   (1) The dorsal branch innervates the cleidomastoideus, cleidocephalicus, omotransversarius, and the trapezius.
   (2) The ventral branch innervates the sternocephalicus.

L. Hypoglossal nerve (cranial nerve XII)

1. **Function.** The hypoglossal nerve is **motor** only, to the **intrinsic muscle of the tongue,** the **extrinsic muscles of the tongue** (i.e., the **hyoglossus, styloglossus,** and **genioglossus**), and the **geniohyoideus.**
2. **Structure.** The hypoglossal nerve exits fairly directly from the cranial cavity via the hypoglossal canal. It courses rostroventrally (lateral to the external carotid artery and medial to the mandibular salivary gland) and comes into close contact with the lingual artery as it enters the tongue. Within the tongue, it forms the cervical loop where it communicates with the ventral branch of the first cervical nerve. (Variations in the detail of this structure commonly occur.)

III. SPINAL NERVES.

Although the cranial nerves provide most of the sensory innervation for the head, a large portion of the pinna as well as the caudal-most region of the head receive sensory innervation from **named branches of the second cervical nerve, a spinal nerve.**

A. Greater occipital nerve.

The greater occipital nerve arises from the dorsal branch of the second cervical nerve and is:

1. **Motor** to several muscles of the caudal region of the head
2. **Sensory** to most of the skin covering the dorsal region of the temporal muscle and most of the convex (dorsal) surface of the pinna

B. Transverse cervical nerve.

The transverse cervical nerve arises from the ventral branch of the second cervical nerve. It is **sensory** to the skin over the caudal mandibular border and laryngeal region.

C. Great auricular nerve.

The great auricular nerve arises from the ventral branch of the second cervical nerve and is **sensory** to the skin over most of the convex (dorsal) surface of the pinna (overlapping considerably with the area innervated by the greater occipital nerve) and much of the concave (ventral) surface of the pinna (overlapping considerably with the area innervated by the facial nerve).

Chapter 11

The Face

I. SUPERFICIAL FACE.

I. SUPERFICIAL FACE. The superficial face is the region of the face on a level superficial to the zygomatic arch.

A. Surface features

1. **Skin of the face.** The skin of the face is haired over essentially its entire surface, except for the very edges of the lips and eyelids, the bare skin of the nose, and much of the internal surface of the pinna.
   a. **Facial hair.** The character of facial hair varies widely among breeds, being relatively fine and short in many breeds, but also wiry in some and long enough to obscure the eyes in others. The hair on the external ear may be approximately the same in length, shorter than, or longer than the hair that covers the rest of the face and body.
   b. **Tactile hairs (vibrissae;** see Chapter 2 I C 3) protrude well beyond the margins of the face.
      (1) Vibrissae are anchored deep in the subcutis. The base of each tactile hair is surrounded by a venous sinus. Motion of the blood within the sinus amplifies the movement of the basal hair shaft, greatly increasing the sensitivity of the hair.
      (2) Vibrissae are associated mainly with the eyes and the rostral-most area of the mouth.
         (a) The greatest number of tactile hairs are located on the **upper lip,** where they are arranged roughly in four rows. These are the longest of the tactile hairs.
         (b) An additional set of relatively long tactile hairs (one pair on each side) is usually located on the **cheek near the angle of the mouth.**
         (c) A small number of relatively long vibrissae are located **dorsal to the eye.**
         (d) Typically, a small number of shorter tactile hairs are found on the **lower lip** and **chin.**
2. **External nose (nasal plane).** The nasal plane forms the most rostral end of the muzzle. It is the region of thickened, hairless skin that surrounds and extends beyond the borders of the **nostrils.** The **philtrum** is a prominent vertical groove on the rostral-most surface of the nasal plane that bisects the space between the nostrils and extends onto the most rostral portion of the upper lip.
   a. **Skin.** A roughened, polygonal pattern characterizes the skin of the nasal plane. The unique nature of the nasal plane's patterning from one dog to the next allows identification of dogs using a "noseprint," much the way fingerprints are used to identify humans.
   b. **Cartilage** supports the external nose. The presence of the cartilages and associated muscles imparts a considerable degree of mobility to the nasal plane.
      (1) The unpaired **septal cartilage** is vertical and median in position, and separates the large, single cavity of the **nasal fossa** into the paired right and left **nasal cavities.**
      (2) The paired **dorsolateral nasal cartilages** are large and support most of the dorsal and lateral regions of the nose. These cartilages follow the curved (scrolled) lateral edge of the nostrils' walls.
      (3) The paired **ventrolateral nasal cartilages** support the ventral nasal wall and part of the ventrolateral nasal wall, but contribute little to the immediately recognizable external form of the nose.
      (4) The paired **accessory cartilages** are small cartilages that lie under the skin of the ventrolateral region of the nose, adjacent to the philtrum.
   c. **Ligaments.** The paired **lateral nasal ligaments** attach the dorsolateral nasal cartilage to the rostral edge of the nasal bones.
   d. **Nasal vestibule.** The nasal vestibule, formed by portions of the cartilage and skin of

the nasal plane, extends from the nostrils caudally to the entrance of the bony nasal cavity. The nasal vestibule receives the openings of various ducts and glands. The serous secretions of these glands moisten the nasal plate, which itself is devoid of glands, and are responsible for the proverbial "cold, wet nose of a healthy dog."

(1) The **nasolacrimal duct** conveys the secretions of the lacrimal gland and opens into the nasal vestibule near the rostral end of the alar fold.

(2) The **lateral nasal gland** opens by a duct on the dorsolateral nasal wall. (The gland itself also lies within the lateral wall of the nose.) The secretions of the lateral nasal gland apparently have a role in social behavior, leading to the common practice of nose-to-nose sniffing when dogs meet.

(3) **Minor nasal glands** are scattered throughout the vestibule and open directly onto the skin of the nasal vestibule.

3. Mouth

a. Oral fissure. The oral fissure is the space between the lips.

b. Angle of the mouth. The junction between the upper and lower lips, also referred to as the **commissure of the lips,** is positioned relatively far caudally (in relation to the orbit) along the side of the muzzle. Because of the highly mobile nature of the upper and lower lips, the dog can draw the angle of the mouth even further caudally than in the resting position, until essentially all of the teeth are exposed. Alternatively, the angle of the mouth can be drawn as far rostrally as the incisors (e.g., when howling).

4. Eyes. The **palpebral fissures** are the spaces between the eyelids.

5. External ear. The pinna (auricle) and the ear canal form the external ear.

a. The **pinna (auricle)** is the portion of the ear that is visible externally. The **auricular cartilage** is elastic in nature, and supports most of the pinna.

(1) Form. The rostral surface of the auricular cartilage is concave and its caudal contour is convex, thus forming a natural "scoop" for sound waves. The size and shape of the auricular cartilage determine the form of the ear. Marked breed variation is present, from the small, erect ears of dogs such as huskies, to the partially erect ears of breeds such as collies, to the fully dependent ears of breeds such as basset hounds.

Canine Clinical Correlation

Over the years, humans have sought to alter the appearance of the ears in some breeds for cosmetic or other reasons. The erect ears of some breeds (e.g., Doberman pinschers, Great Danes, boxers, schnauzers) are cosmetic mutilations of naturally dependent ears. Although some contend that ear cropping promotes healthy ears by increasing air flow (and thus decreasing the frequency of otitis externa), breeds with partially erect ears that do not undergo ear cropping display no significant increase in the incidence of otitis externa. Furthermore, it is not common practice to crop the ears of breeds such as cocker spaniels, which are prone to such infections.

(2) Regions. The pinna has two main regions, the **concha** and the **scapha,** which share a peripheral border (i.e., the medial and lateral borders of the **helix,** the free margin of the pinna). The **anthelix,** a prominent, transverse ridge of tissue lying in the proximal portion of the conchal cavity, separates the concha and the scapha (Figure 11–1).

(a) The **concha** is the most proximal, strongly curved portion of the pinna (i.e., the portion closest to the head). The **conchal cavity** is rostrally directed and concave and is most defined in breeds with erect or semi-erect ears. It is relatively sparsely haired, and has several elevations of cartilage defined within it (see Figure 11–1):

(i) The **tragus** is a thickened plate of auricular cartilage positioned almost at the midpoint of the ventral border of the external ear.

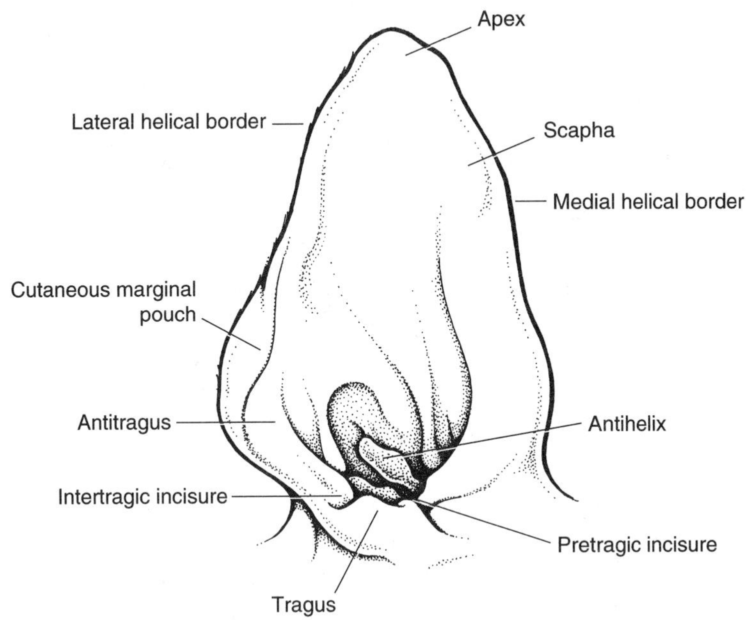

FIGURE 11–1. External ear, lateral view. Because the auricular cartilage may be wholly, partly, or not at all erect, appreciation of the named regions of the auricular cartilage is best achieved if any dependent portion of the pinna is laid out into what would be an erect position before attempting to identify the structures of the pinna.

- **(ii)** The **pretragic incisure** is a groove that separates the tragus (laterally) from the beginning of the medial helical border (medially).
- **(iii)** The **antitragus** is an elongate elevation of auricular cartilage that extends laterally from the tragus and marks the beginning of the lateral helical border.
- **(iv)** The **intertragic incisure** separates the antitragus (laterally) from the tragus (medially).

(b) The **scapha** is the more distal, flattened portion of the pinna.

(3) The **cutaneous marginal pouch** is a small pocket of integument, located on the lateral helical border at approximately the junction of the conchal and scaphal regions. No function has been ascribed to the cutaneous marginal pouch.

(4) The **apex** is the free distal edge of the pinna, where the medial and lateral borders of the helix meet.

b. The **ear canal** is mainly cartilaginous, but also has a bony portion.

(1) The **cartilaginous portion of the ear canal** represents the tubular, lateral portion of the auricular cartilage. The **annular cartilage,** a small, tubular piece of cartilage that is interposed between the medial edge of the auricular cartilage and the skull, increases the mobility of the external ear by joining the external ear's main portion with its deepest portion. The course of the external ear canal is roughly "L"-shaped. From the pinna, the cartilaginous portion of the ear canal heads ventromedially, making an almost 90-degree turn at the level of the external acoustic meatus to head directly medially toward the skull.

(2) The **bony portion of the external ear canal** is short, and essentially represents an extension of bone from the external acoustic meatus of the skull on the lateral aspect of the tympanic bulla. This portion of the ear canal meets with the annular cartilage to complete the channel from the pinna to the middle ear.

Canine Clinical Correlation

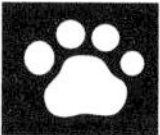

The "L"-shaped course of the external ear canal has advantages and disadvantages.

- On the positive side, the sharp turn of the canal at its ventral-most limit minimizes the risk of tympanic membrane rupture as a result of gentle probing. Conscientious clients can often be taught to clean the dog's external ear canal, and they may even be entrusted to administer medications relatively deep in the ear canal.
- On the negative side, the abrupt angle of the external ear canal makes drainage of material from the ear as well as circulation of air through the canal somewhat problematic. In breeds with dependent ear forms (and especially in those with dependent ear forms and relatively large amounts of hair in the external ear canal), the stage is set for the development of **chronic otitis externa.** This condition can be extremely painful to the dog as well as dangerous to its general health. Treatment for chronic otitis externa involves surgical removal of the lateral wall of the vertical portion of the ear canal (ear canal ablation), which effectively opens the horizontal portion directly to the exterior, thereby facilitating natural aeration and drainage of the ear canal.

B. Superficial structures just deep to the skin

1. **Superficial salivary glands.** Two of the four salivary glands are superficial. (The remaining two—the sublingual salivary gland and the zygomatic salivary gland—are structures of the deep face and are discussed in II B 2.)

   a. The **parotid salivary gland** surrounds the base of the external ear, hence its name ("para-otid," condensed to "parotid").

      (1) **Appearance.** The parotid salivary gland resembles the letter "V" (Figure 11–2) and is thickest at the apex of the "V," with the two arms becoming progressively thinner as they move away from the base. The gland is dark in color and is marked by coarse lobations that are visible through the capsule.

      (2) **Parotid duct.** The duct of the parotid salivary gland leaves the ventral region of the gland and runs rostrally, parallel and closely applied to the fibers of the masseter muscle (see Figure 11–2). The parotid duct opens on a papilla situated at the caudal margin of the upper fourth premolar tooth. **Accessory parotid salivary glands** are sometimes present along the parotid duct. These may vary in size from quite small to up to 1 centimeter long. Their ducts open into the parotid ducts.

Canine Clinical Correlation

The opening of the parotid duct opposite the upper carnassial tooth on each side results in the introduction of copious amounts of saliva into the mouth at this point. Food particles tend to accumulate relatively early in this region, resulting in tartar buildup. For the health of the teeth and gingiva, as well as of the dog itself, regular removal of this buildup by brushing the teeth of the dog by the client or by periodic veterinary dental cleaning is strongly advised.

   b. The **mandibular salivary gland** is a large oval salivary gland situated between the linguofacial and maxillary veins, just caudal to the mandibular angle (see Figure 11–2).

      (1) **Appearance.** The mandibular salivary gland is pale in color and more compact than the parotid salivary gland, with its lobules not as prominently separated. The particularly stout capsule of the gland renders the lobules even less visible on superficial dissection.

      (2) **Mandibular duct.** The duct of the mandibular salivary gland leaves the rostromedial surface of the gland and courses rostrally under the oral mucosa.

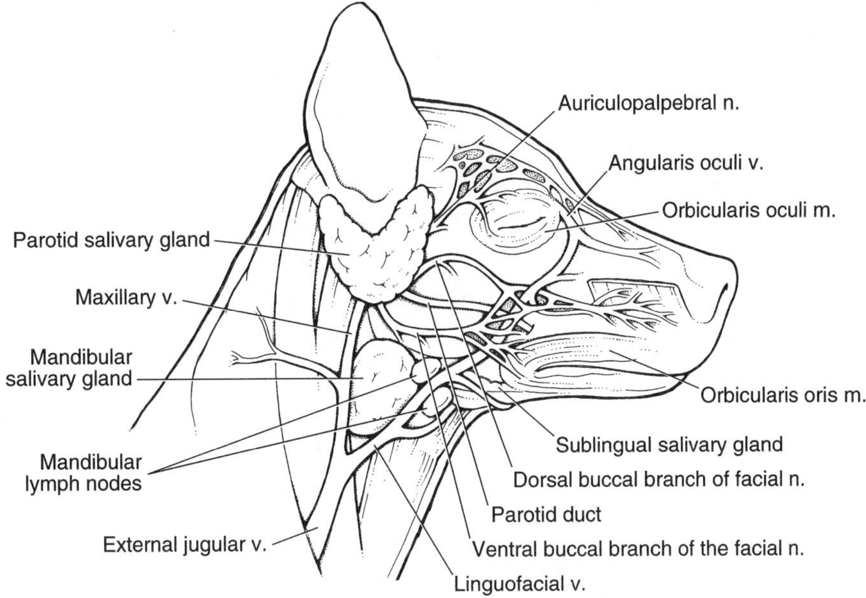

FIGURE 11–2. Superficial structures of the head. During dissection, the parotid duct can be mistaken for the dorsal buccal branch of the facial nerve.

Canine Clinical Correlation

Knowledge of the location of the salivary glands and their ducts becomes important in the surgical treatment of **sialocele,** a condition in which a discontinuity in a major salivary duct occurs, resulting in cyst-like accumulations of saliva in the adjacent tissues. Treatment of these lesions involves removal of the glands and their ducts. The anatomic relations of the numerous structures in the superficial face are complex, and surgical texts often recommend review of the anatomy before surgery is performed.

2. **Superficial lymph nodes**
   a. The **mandibular lymph nodes** form the consistent part of the **mandibular lymphocenter.** (The deeper buccal lymph nodes comprise the other portion of this lymphocenter; however, the buccal lymph nodes are inconstant, and are, in fact, rather rare.)
      (1) The mandibular lymph nodes typically number two, but some individuals have as many as five.
      (2) The mandibular lymph nodes are uneven in size and positioned ventral to the mandibular angle, associated with the linguofacial vein (see Figure 11–2). Most typically, a smaller node lies dorsal to the vein and a larger one lies ventral to it.
   b. The **parotid lymph nodes** compose the **parotid lymphocenter.**
      (1) The parotid lymph nodes typically number from one to three.
      (2) The parotid lymph nodes are uneven in size and positioned rostral to the rostral edge of the parotid salivary gland, in the region of the base of the ear.
3. **Superficial musculature** (Figure 11–3). The muscles of the face move the skin, lips, cheeks, eyelids, nose, and ear (Table 11–1). Most of these movements are associated with eating, drinking, or intra- and interspecific communication. The muscles of facial expression are extremely thin and delicate; frequently, they are removed with the skin during dissection. The slight substance of these muscles belies the degree of mobility they provide to facial structures!

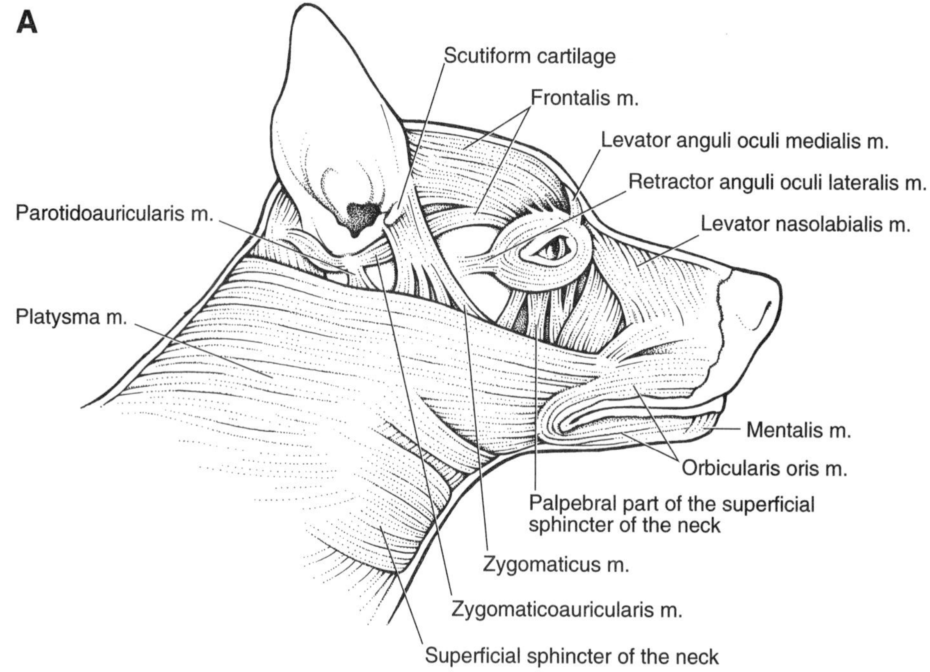

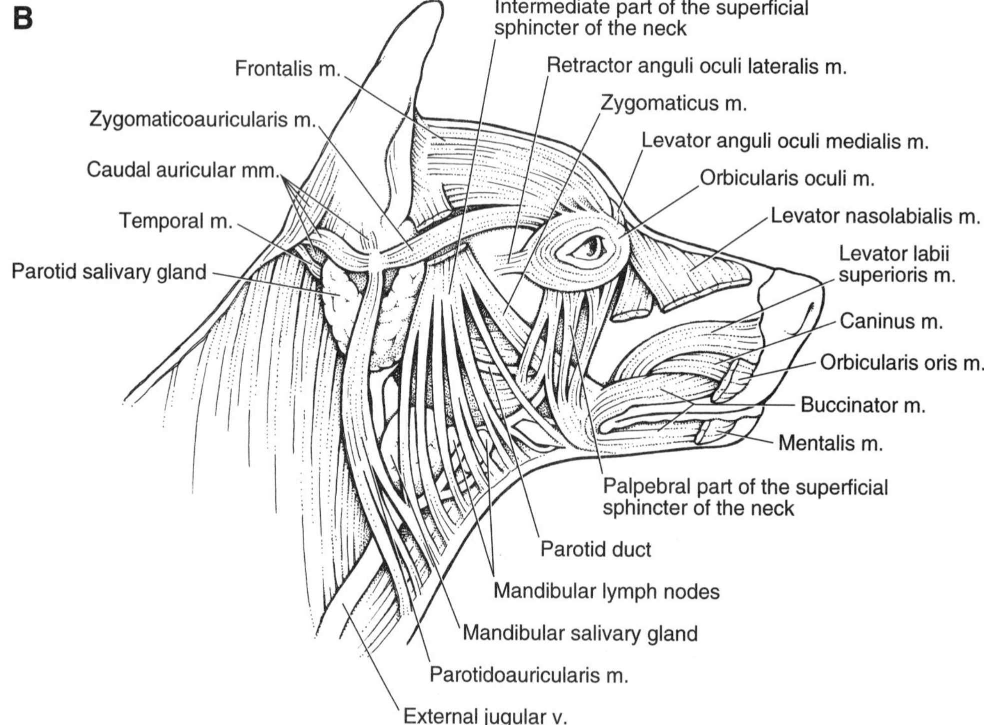

FIGURE 11–3. (*A*) Superficial layer of the superficial head muscles, lateral view. (*B*) Deeper layer of the superficial head muscles, lateral view. (*continued*)

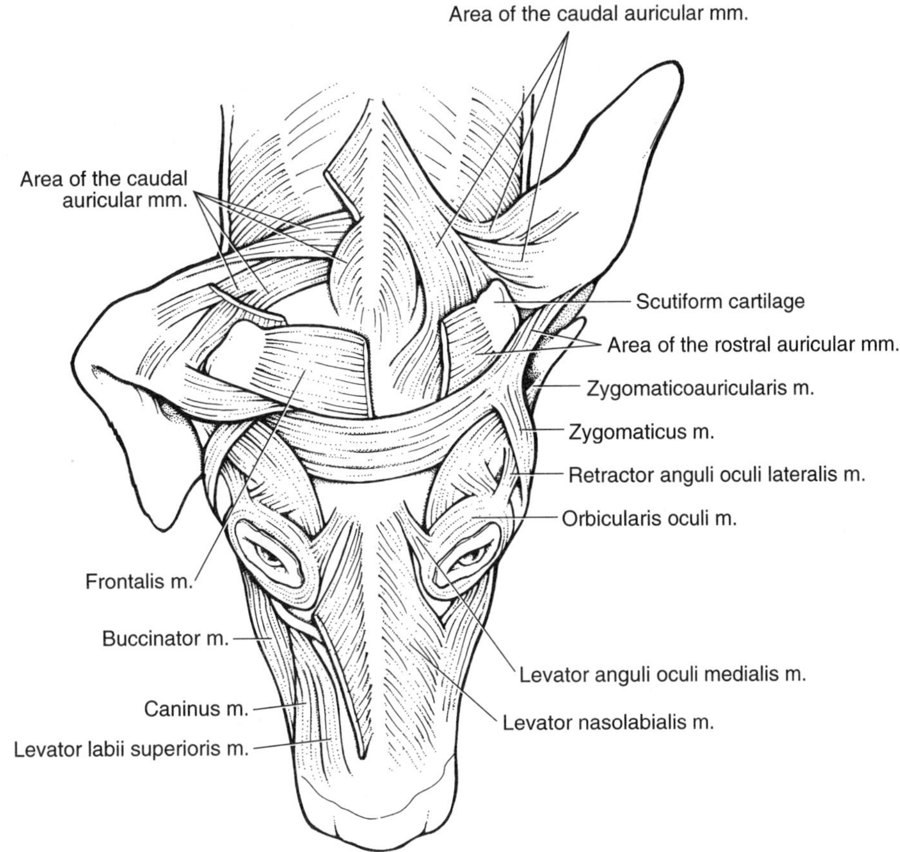

FIGURE 11–3.—*continued* (*C*) Superficial muscles of the head, dorsal view. (*C* modified with permission from Evans HE, 1993, *Miller's Anatomy of the Dog,* 3e. Philadelphia, WB Saunders, p 1045.)

a. Muscles of the neck

(1) The **superficial sphincter of the neck** is a delicate muscle best developed in the laryngeal region (see Figure 11–3A). It is the most superficial of the muscles on the face and neck.

(2) The **deep sphincter of the neck** is divided into several parts, including the muscles of the cheek, lips, and external ear (see I B 3 b–c and f).

(a) The **intermediate part of the deep sphincter of the neck** (see Figure 11–3B) is usually considered separately from its other portions. The intermediate part of the deep sphincter of the neck consists of fine strands sweeping from the ventral midline up toward the base of the ear, where they end on the **scutiform cartilage,** a small, boot-shaped piece of cartilage that is associated with the rostral auricular muscles. Contraction of the deep sphincter of the neck draws the external ear ventrally and somewhat cranially.

(b) The **palpebral part of the deep sphincter of the neck** (see Figure 11–3A&B) consists of several delicate strands that extend from the ventral midline to the lower eyelid. Contraction of the palpebral part of the deep sphincter of the neck depresses the lower eyelid.

b. Muscles of the cheek

(1) The **platysma** is a relatively well-developed sheet of muscle that originates from the dorsal raphe of the neck (see Figure 11–3A). The platysma sweeps cranially

TABLE 11–1. Muscles of the Superficial Face

Muscle	Action	Innervation*
Platysma	Draws the angle of the mouth caudally	Dorsal and ventral buccal branches and the caudal auricular branches of the facial nerve
Levator nasolabialis	Dilates nostrils, raises upper lip	Auriculopalpebral branch of the facial nerve
Orbicularis oris	Closes lips by drawing them together in an "O" shape	Dorsal and ventral buccal branches of the facial nerve
Maxillonasolabialis		
Levator labii superioris	Raises upper lip, dilates nostrils	Dorsal buccal branch of the facial nerve
Caninus	Raises upper lip	Dorsal buccal branch of the facial nerve
Buccinator	Draws the cheek inward against the teeth	Dorsal and ventral buccal branches of the facial nerve
Zygomaticus	Draws the angle of the mouth caudally, draws the external ear cranially and ventrally	Auriculopalpebral branch of the facial nerve
Mentalis	Stiffens the apical regions of the lower lip	Ventral buccal branch of the facial nerve
Orbicularis oculi	Closes the palpebral fissure	Auriculopalpebral branch of the facial nerve
Retractor anguli oculi lateralis	Draws the lateral palpebral angle caudally	Auriculopalpebral branch of the facial nerve
Levator anguli oculi medialis	Raises the upper lid and erects hairs of the eyebrow	Auriculopalpebral branch of the facial nerve
Levator palpebrae superioris	Raises the eyelid	Oculomotor nerve (cranial nerve III)
Frontalis	Draws the scutular cartilage forward, raises eyebrows	Auriculopalpebral and temporal branches of the facial nerve
Rostral auricular muscles	Turn the conchal fissure rostrally, stabilize the pinna and make the ear rigid, stabilize the scutular cartilage	Temporal branch of the facial nerve
Caudal auricular muscles	Pull the scutular cartilage ventrically, tense the nasal and frontal fascia, turn the conchal fissure rostrally, turn the conchal fissure laterally or caudally, stabilize the scutular cartilage, erect the concha	Caudal auricular branches of the facial nerve

continued

TABLE 11–1. Muscles of the Superficial Face

Muscle	Action	Innervation*
Ventral auricular muscle (parotidoauricularis)	Draws the external ear caudally and ventrally	Cervical branch of the facial nerve

*With a single exception (the levator palpebrae superioris), the muscles of facial expression are innervated by named branches of the facial nerve (cranial nerve VII).

from the region of the base of the ear to the ventral midline, and rostrally as far as the lips. The action of the platysma is to draw the angle of the mouth caudally.

(2) The **buccinator** (see Figure 11–3B) is a thin, wide sheet of muscle that forms the noncutaneous substance of the cheek. The buccinator attaches to the mandible and maxilla in the region of the alveolar margins of the teeth, and then fills the substance of the cheek itself between the outer skin and the inner oral mucosa. Contraction of the buccinator draws the cheek inward against the teeth.

c. **Muscles of the lips**

(1) The **platysma** is the most superficial muscle of the face. The relation of the platysma to the lips is discussed in I B 3 b (1).

(2) The **levator nasolabialis,** also in the most superficial facial muscle layer (see Figure 11–3A–C), covers the lateral surface of the nasal bone and maxilla, just deep to the skin. Contraction of the nasolabialis causes dilatation of the nostrils and raises the upper lip.

(3) The **orbicularis oris** lies deep to the platysma and levator nasolabialis (see Figure 11–3A–C). It lies with its fibers running longitudinally around the opening of the mouth; contraction of this muscle closes the lips by drawing them together into the shape of an "O."

(4) The **maxillonasolabialis** is a specialization of the dorsal part of the orbicularis oris. It is divided into two portions, both of which lie deep to the levator nasolabialis.

(a) The **levator labii superioris** (see Figure 11–3B) is the more dorsal portion. This muscle lies over the maxilla, originating near the infraorbital foramen and inserting into the upper lip and lateral edge of the nose. It raises the upper lip and dilates the nostrils.

(b) The **caninus** (see Figure 11–3B) is the more ventral portion of the maxillonasolabialis (i.e., of the upper portion of the orbicularis oris). The origin of the caninus is similar to that of the levator labii superioris, but the caninus inserts only into the upper lip. Contraction of the caninus raises the upper lip.

(5) The **zygomaticus** (see Figure 11–3A&B) is a rostral portion of the deep sphincter of the neck. This muscle crosses the zygomatic arch as it sweeps from the rostral edge of the scutiform cartilage, passes deep to the palpebral part of the deep sphincter of the neck, and terminates by intermingling with the fibers of the orbicularis oris. The zygomaticus draws the angle of the mouth caudally and the external ear cranially and ventrally.

(6) The **mentalis** (see Figure 11–3A&B) is essentially a subdivision of the ventral part of the buccinator. The mentalis arises at the alveolar border of the canine teeth and passes ventrally toward the midline, meeting and fusing with its fellow from the opposite side. Contraction of the mentalis stiffens the apical region of the lower lip.

c. **Muscles of the nose.** The widening of the nostrils during sniffing or scenting is achieved largely by the action of the intrinsic muscles of the nose on the lateral edges of the dorsolateral and accessory cartilages. The **levator nasolabialis** and the **levator labii superioris** are described in and I B 3 c (2) and I B 3 c (4) (a), respectively.

d. **Muscles of the eyelids**
   (1) The **orbicularis oculi** (see Figure 11–3A–C) surrounds the palpebral fissure, much as the orbicularis oris surrounds the lips. Contraction of the orbicularis oculi closes the palpebral fissure.
   (2) The **retractor anguli oculi lateralis** (see Figure 11–3A–C) passes directly caudally from the lateral palpebral angle to blend with the temporal fascia. The action of the lateral retractor is to draw the lateral palpebral angle caudally, thereby assisting in closing the eye.
   (3) The **levator anguli oculi medialis** (see Figure 11–3A–C) passes directly from the medial palpebral angle to attach to the frontal bone. The action medial retractor raises the upper lid and erects the hairs of the eyebrow.
   (4) The **levator palpebrae superioris** arises deep within the orbit and inserts into the upper eyelid. Contraction of the levator of the upper lid raises the eyelid.
   (5) The **palpebral part of the deep sphincter of the neck** is deep to the platysma. This muscle depresses the lower eyelid.

e. **Muscles of the forehead.** The **frontalis** (see Figure 11–3A–C) is a thin sheet of muscle overlying the temporal bone. A portion of the rostral region of this muscle attaches to the orbital ligament. Contraction of the frontalis draws the scutular cartilage forward and raises the eyebrows.

f. **Muscles of the external ear.** The pinnae can be moved in many directions, to become erect, face forward, face caudally, or to flatten against the head. Each pinna can be moved independently of the other, even so that one ear is facing rostrally and the other is facing caudally! The muscles of the ear can be grouped into one of three major groups, the rostral, caudal, and ventral auricular muscles.
   (1) The **rostral auricular muscles** (see Figure 11–3C) form a group of seven muscles that lie on the forehead caudal to the orbit; these muscles converge toward the auricular cartilage. The names, which need not be listed here, are descriptive of the muscles' attachments. These seven muscles act to:
      (a) Turn the conchal fissure rostrally
      (b) Stabilize the pinna and make the ear rigid
      (c) Stabilize the scutular cartilage
   (2) The **caudal auricular muscles** (see Figure 11–3C) are the largest group of external ear muscles, most of which arise on the dorsal median raphe of the head. Again, the names will not be detailed here, but they are descriptive of the muscles' attachments. This group consists of twelve muscles, which group into sets that act to:
      (a) Support the scutular cartilage
      (b) Turn the conchal fissure in several directions
      (c) Erect the concha
   (3) The **ventral auricular muscle** is the **parotidoauricularis** (see Figure 11–3A&B), the caudal-most portion of the deep sphincter of the neck. The parotidoauricularis covers the parotid gland as it sweeps from its ventral midline origin to the base of the ear. Contraction of the parotidoauricularis draws the external ear caudally and ventrally.

4. **Vasculature.** The major arteries and veins of the superficial face are merely listed here for the sake of completeness; more detail is provided in Chapter 9.
   a. **Arteries.** Major arteries of the superficial face include the:
      (1) **Facial artery** (a branch of the external carotid artery)
      (2) **Caudal auricular artery** (a branch of the external carotid artery)
      (3) **Superficial temporal artery** (a termination of the external carotid artery)
      (4) **Infraorbital artery** (the continuation of the maxillary artery)
      (5) **Mental artery** (the continuation of the inferior alveolar artery)
   b. **Veins.** Major veins of the superficial face include the:
      (1) **Maxillary vein**
      (2) **Caudal auricular vein**
      (3) **Rostral auricular vein**

(4) **Angular vein of the eye (angularis oculi)**
(5) **Dorsal nasal vein**
(6) **Facial vein**
(7) **Inferior labial vein**
(8) **Lingual vein**

5. **Innervation.** The nerves innervating the superficial facial region are merely mentioned here; more detail is provided in Chapter 11. Major nerves of the superficial face include the following.
   a. **Facial nerve (cranial nerve VII).** In the superficial face, nearly all of the branches of the facial nerve are **motor.** (A single branch is sensory to the skin of much of the pinna.) The motor branches include the:
      (1) **Dorsal** and **ventral buccal branches** (not to be confused with the buccal nerve)
      (2) **Auriculopalpebral nerve** [not to be confused with the auriculotemporal nerve, a sensory branch of the mandibular division of the trigeminal nerve (cranial nerve V_3)]
      (3) **Rostral auricular nerve**
      (4) **Palpebral branches**
   b. **Mandibular division of the trigeminal nerve (cranial nerve V_3).** The superficial branch of the mandibular division of the trigeminal nerve in the superficial facial region, the **auriculotemporal nerve,** is **sensory.**
   c. **Maxillary division of the trigeminal nerve (cranial nerve V_2).** The superficial branch in this region, the **infraorbital nerve,** is **sensory.**

II. DEEP FACE.

The deep face is the region of the face on a level deep to the zygomatic arch.

A. Regions of the deep face

1. The **temporal fossa** is the region along the lateral and ventrolateral walls of much of the cranial cavity where the bones are roughened for muscular attachment, and the space immediately adjacent to it. The term "fossa" is not descriptive, because the region is actually convex.
2. The **pterygopalatine fossa** lies ventral to the orbit.

B. Related structures.

Most of the structures in the following discussion are discussed in more detail in other chapters. They are merely summarized here for the sake of completeness.

1. **Temporomandibular joint.** The **temporomandibular joint** is formed at the juncture of the mandibular fossa of the temporal bone and the condylar process of the mandible. The joint is synovial, and an **articular disc,** essentially a meniscus, is present between the two bones.
2. **Salivary glands**
   a. The **sublingual salivary gland** has two regions.
      (1) **Monostomatic portion.** The caudal portion of the sublingual salivary gland is referred to as the monostomatic portion, because a single duct (the **major sublingual duct**) leads from it to the sublingual papilla.
         (a) The monostomatic portion of the sublingual salivary gland is closely associated at its caudal extremity with the mandibular salivary gland. The same capsule invests both glands, and the contour of each gland fits the other. Thus, distinguishing between the two glands may be difficult, but generally the monostomatic portion of the sublingual gland is slightly darker in color than the mandibular salivary gland. Furthermore, the monostomatic portion of the sublingual gland is roughly triangular in shape, whereas the mandibular salivary gland is ovoid.
         (b) The major sublingual duct leaves the rostromedial surface of the monostomatic portion of the sublingual salivary gland and courses adjacent to the

mandibular duct of the mandibular salivary gland. Despite the close association between the monostomatic portion of the sublingual gland and the mandibular salivary gland, their ducts are separate throughout their length.

(2) The **polystomatic portion** of the sublingual salivary gland is present as a group of glands of varying size and prominence.

(a) These glands are positioned rostral to the monostomatic part of the gland, alongside the body of the tongue. The glands that compose the polystomatic portion of the sublingual salivary gland can be quite large, and may extend rostrally almost to the angle of the mouth.

(b) The polystomatic portion of the gland is so named because each small gland opens directly onto the floor of the mouth, rather than into a common duct or the sublingual duct.

b. The **zygomatic salivary gland,** sometimes referred to as the **orbital salivary gland,** lies deep to the zygomatic arch, in the ventral region of the orbit against the periorbita. It actually forms part of the orbital floor.

(1) **Appearance.** The capsule is poorly developed and the lobules are quite distinct.

(2) **Ducts.** The zygomatic salivary gland has multiple ducts:

(a) A **major duct** that opens caudal to the parotid duct

(b) Two to four **minor ducts** that open caudal to the major duct

3. **Lymph nodes.** The **retropharyngeal lymph nodes** are sometimes considered structures of the deep face, although they actually lie in the cranial region of the neck.

a. The **medial retropharyngeal lymph node** is constant in its occurrence, and is the largest lymph node of the head and cervical region. (In a 40-pound dog, the node would be approximately 50 mm long and 20 mm wide!)

(1) This elongate lymph node lies deep to the wing of the atlas.

(2) The medial retropharyngeal lymph node receives lymphatic drainage from:

(a) All deep head structures having lymphatics (e.g., the tongue, salivary glands, deeper parts of the external ear, and walls of the oral, nasal, and pharyngeal regions)

(b) Other deep structures of the neck (e.g., the esophagus and larynx)

(c) The parotid and mandibular lymph nodes

b. The **lateral retropharyngeal lymph nodes** are inconstant, being found in approximately 33% of dogs. When present, the lateral retropharyngeal lymph nodes are less than one fifth the size of the medial retropharyngeal lymph node. They lie at approximately the level of the external acoustic meatus and receive lymphatics from immediately neighboring structures.

4. **Musculature** (Table 11–2)

a. **Muscles of mastication.** The temporal fossa contains the muscles of mastication, entirely or in part. The muscles of mastication are those associated with **closing the jaw** (i.e., **raising the mandible).** Two of these muscles, the temporal and the masseter, have superficial as well as deep portions.

(1) The **masseter muscle** forms most of the mass of the lateral facial region caudal to the angle of the mouth, and is thus palpable subcutaneously. It is covered by a stout fascial layer that is so thick, it appears white in the fresh state.

(a) **Position.** The masseter muscle lies lateral to the mandibular ramus in the space ventral to the zygomatic arch. In general, it may be regarded as **passing from the zygomatic arch to the lateral side of the coronoid process and ventral border of the mandible.**

(b) **Regions.** The masseter is divisible into three regions, based on fiber direction.

(i) The **superficial portion** forms the largest part of the muscle. It originates from the ventral border of the rostral half of the zygomatic arch, courses caudoventrally, and inserts mainly on the ventrolateral surface of the mandible. Some fibers continue around the ventral and lateral mandibular border to insert on the ventromedial mandibular surface and the tendinous raphe that separates the masseter and medial pterygoid muscles.

(ii) The **middle portion** is the weakest part, although it is still a muscle of

TABLE 11–2. Summary of Attachments, Actions, and Innervation of the Muscles of Mastication and the Digastricus Muscle

Muscle	Origin	Insertion	Action	Innervation
Temporal	Parietal bone; also frontal and occipital bones	Coronoid process	Raises the mandible	Temporal nerve (branch of CN V_3)
Masseter				
Superficial part	Zygomatic arch	Ventrolateral mandible	Raises the mandible	Masseteric nerve (branch of CN V_3)
Middle part	Zygomatic arch	Masseteric fossa	Raises the mandible	Masseteric nerve
Deep part	Zygomatic arch and shared origin with temporal muscle	Masseteric fossa	Raises the mandible	Masseteric nerve
Medial pterygoid	Pterygopalatine fossa	Angular process of mandible	Raises the mandible	Pterygoid nerve (branch of CNV_3)
Lateral pterygoid	Pterygopalatine fossa	Mandibular condyle	Raises the mandible	Pterygoid nerve
Digastricus				
Caudal belly	Paracondylar process	Tendinous intersection	Opens the mouth	Mandibular nerve (branch of CN V_3)
Rostral belly	Tendinous intersection	Ventral mandibular border	Opens mouth	Facial nerve (CN VII)

CN V_3 = mandibular division of the trigeminal nerve (cranial nerve V), CN VII = facial nerve.

considerable strength. It originates medial to the superficial part of the masseter on the zygomatic arch, courses ventrally, and inserts on the ventral margin of the masseteric fossa.

(iii) The **deep portion,** another relatively small but powerful part, originates from the maxillary skull region and the medial zygomatic arch, courses caudoventrally, and inserts on the caudal part of the masseteric fossa.

(c) Innervation. The masseter muscle is innervated by the **masseteric branch of the mandibular nerve.**

(d) Vascularization. The masseter receives blood from the **masseteric branch of the maxillary artery.**

(2) The **temporal muscle,** the largest and strongest muscle of the head, covers much of the dorsal and lateral surfaces of the skull, and thus is palpable subcutaneously. It is also covered by a thick, white fascial layer. It extends from the bony wall of the temporal fossa to the coronoid process of the mandible.

(a) Course. The temporal muscle originates along a broad surface of the lateral skull, covering most of the surface of the parietal bones and also attaching to parts of the temporal, frontal, and occipital bones. It courses rostroventrally within the temporal fossa, dorsal and medial to the zygomatic arch, and inserts on the coronoid process of the mandible, along its dorsal border and the greatest part of its medial surface.

(b) Innervation. The temporal muscle is innervated by the **deep temporal nerves** of the mandibular nerve.

(c) Vascularization. The temporal muscle receives arterial blood from the **rostral** and **caudal deep temporal arteries,** which are **branches of the maxillary artery.**

(3) The **medial pterygoid muscle** is very deeply situated and extends from the ventral part of the pterygoid and palatine bones to the angular process of the mandible.
   (a) **Course.** The medial pterygoid muscle originates on the wall of the pterygopalatine fossa, from the lateral surfaces of the pterygoid, palatine, and sphenoid bones. It courses caudolaterally and inserts on the angular process of the mandible, as well as on the tendinous raphe separating the medial pterygoid from the superficial part of the masseter.
   (b) **Innervation.** The medial pterygoid muscle is innervated by the **pterygoid nerves of the mandibular nerve.**
   (c) **Vascularization.** The medial pterygoid muscle receives its blood supply from **small branches of neighboring arteries.**

(4) The **lateral pterygoid muscle** is also deeply situated but markedly smaller than the medial pterygoid muscle. It extends from a small part of the sphenoid bone (just dorsal to the medial pterygoid muscle) to the medial surface of the mandibular condyle.
   (a) **Course.** The lateral pterygoid muscle originates from a small fossa on the sphenoid bone just ventral to the ventral group of foramina in the pterygopalatine fossa (i.e., the optic canal, orbital fissure, and alar canal). It courses ventrolaterally and caudally to insert medially on the mandibular condyle, just ventral to its articular surface.
   (b) **Innervation.** The lateral pterygoid muscle is innervated by the **pterygoid nerves of the mandibular nerve.**
   (c) **Vascularization.** The lateral pterygoid muscle is supplied by **small branches of neighboring arteries.**

b. **Digastricus muscle.** The digastricus **opens the mouth.** It is partially positioned medial to the parotid and mandibular salivary glands.
   (1) **Bipartite muscle.** A faint tendinous intersection located at approximately the middle part of the muscle distinguishes the rostral belly from the caudal belly. In other species, including humans, the "two-bellied" classification is more applicable in that the dividing region is quite narrow and distinctly formed like a tendon, clearly dividing the muscle into two bellies. Although not immediately visible as a bipartite muscle in the dog, the dual innervation of the digastricus muscle attests to its bipartite nature.
      (a) The **rostral belly** develops from the same region as the muscles of mastication (i.e., the first branchial arch); therefore, it is **innervated by the mandibular nerve.**
      (b) The **caudal belly** develops from the same region as the muscles of facial expression (i.e., the second branchial arch); therefore, it is **innervated by the facial nerve.**
   (2) **Course.** The caudal belly of the digastricus muscle originates from the paracondylar process and courses rostrally to insert on the caudal part of the ventral border of the mandible.
   (3) **Vascularization.** Arterial blood arrives from **adjacent arteries.**

5. **Vasculature.** The major arteries and veins of the deep face are listed here for the sake of completeness; more detail is provided in Chapter 9.
   a. **Arteries.** The **maxillary artery** carries most of the blood through and to the deep face. Its branches in this region are the:
      (1) **Inferior alveolar artery,** which supplies the lower arcade of teeth
      (2) **Caudal deep temporal artery,** which supplies the temporal muscle
      (3) **Middle meningeal artery,** which supplies the interior of the cranial cavity
      (4) **External ophthalmic artery,** which supplies the structures of the periorbita, with smaller branches to the interior of the cranial cavity and the ethmoidal labyrinth
      (5) **Descending palatine artery,** with its branches, the:
         (a) **Minor palatine artery**
         (b) **Major palatine artery**
         (c) **Sphenopalatine artery**

b. Veins. Major veins of the deep face include the:

(1) **Dorsal** and **ventral external ophthalmic veins,** draining the orbital region

(2) **Deep facial vein,** forming mainly from the continuation of the ventral external opthalmic vein

(3) **Pterygoid venous plexus,** lying just ventral to the alar canal and closely associated with the second part of the maxillary artery

(4) The **palatine venous plexus,** lying within the substance of the soft palate

6. Innervation. The nerves innervating the deep face are merely mentioned here; more detail is provided in Chapter 10. Major nerves of the deep face include the following:

a. The **maxillary division of the trigeminal nerve (cranial nerve V_2)** has the following major branches in the deep face:

(1) The **zygomatic nerve,** to the lacrimal gland and eyelids

(2) The **pterygopalatine ganglion,** which contains cell bodies of the postganglionic parasympathetic neurons supplying the lacrimal, nasal, and palatine glands

(3) The **pterygopalatine nerve,** which has three branches of its own, the:

(a) **Major palatine nerve**

(b) **Minor palatine nerve**

(c) **Caudal nasal nerve**

(4) The **infraorbital nerve,** which is the continuation of the maxillary division of the trigeminal nerve through the pterygopalatine fossa

b. The **mandibular division of the trigeminal nerve (cranial nerve V_3)** has the following major branches in the deep face:

(1) The **masseteric nerve,** motor to the masseter muscle

(2) The **deep temporal nerves,** motor to the temporal muscle

(3) The **medial** and **lateral pterygoid nerves,** motor to those muscles

(4) The **buccal nerve,** sensory to the mucosa and skin of the cheek

(5) The **lingual nerve,** sensory to the rostral two thirds of the tongue

(6) The **inferior alveolar nerve,** sensory to the lower arcade of teeth

(7) The **mylohyoid nerve,** mainly motor (to the mylohyoideus and digastricus muscles)

(8) The **auriculotemporal nerve,** sensory to the skin at the base of the ear and temporal region

Chapter 12

The Oral Cavity, Pharynx, Larynx, and Associated Structures

I. ORAL CAVITY

A. General considerations

1. **Functions.** Although the functions of the mouth intuitively include **prehension** and **mastication** of food, oral structures also play a role in other important activities, such as **providing an alternate** or **supplemental airway, facilitating intra-** and **interspecific communication** (by facial posturing), **defense,** and **vocalization.**
2. **Form**
   a. The **wide gape** of the mouth in the dog is related to its role as a predator—the ability to open the mouth wide permits the use of the teeth in **securing prey.** The wide gape also permits **rapid consumption of large pieces of food** without extensive mastication, as wild canids commonly do when feeding at carcasses.

Canine Clinical Correlation

Oral inspection and surgery, as well as procedures such as prophylactic dental cleaning, are greatly facilitated by the ready access to even the remote recesses of the mouth afforded by the wide gape in the dog. Other animals, such as horses, are only able to open their mouths to a small degree.

   b. The oral cavity is **elongate** in all but brachycephalic breeds.

B. Oral vestibule.

Oral vestibule. The oral vestibule (Figure 12–1) is the space bounded laterally by the cheeks and lips and medially by the teeth and gums that contains the openings of certain salivary glands.

1. **Cheeks and lips.** The conformation of the cheeks and lips varies considerably with breed, being relatively close and tight in some breeds (e.g., German shepherds), moderately loose in others (e.g., Cocker spaniels), and frankly redundant and pendulous, with the commissure of the lips hanging well below the ventral border of the mandible, in others (e.g., Saint Bernards, bassett hounds).

Canine Clinical Correlation

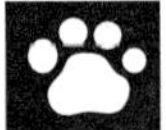

The generous amount of space in the oral vestibule (even in dogs with relatively "close" cheeks) allows for the convenient oral administration of small to moderate amounts of liquids. Tipping the dog's head upward while holding the mouth gently closed and placing the liquid in the caudal region of the vestibule results in a funneling effect as the liquid flows through the interdental spaces and into the oral cavity at a rate convenient for the dog to swallow.

   a. The **cheeks** are quite mobile. The dog can draw them as far rostrally as the level of the canine teeth and as far caudally as the level of the carnassial teeth.
   b. The **lips** are long, and the angle of the mouth (commissure of the lips) is placed relatively far caudally.

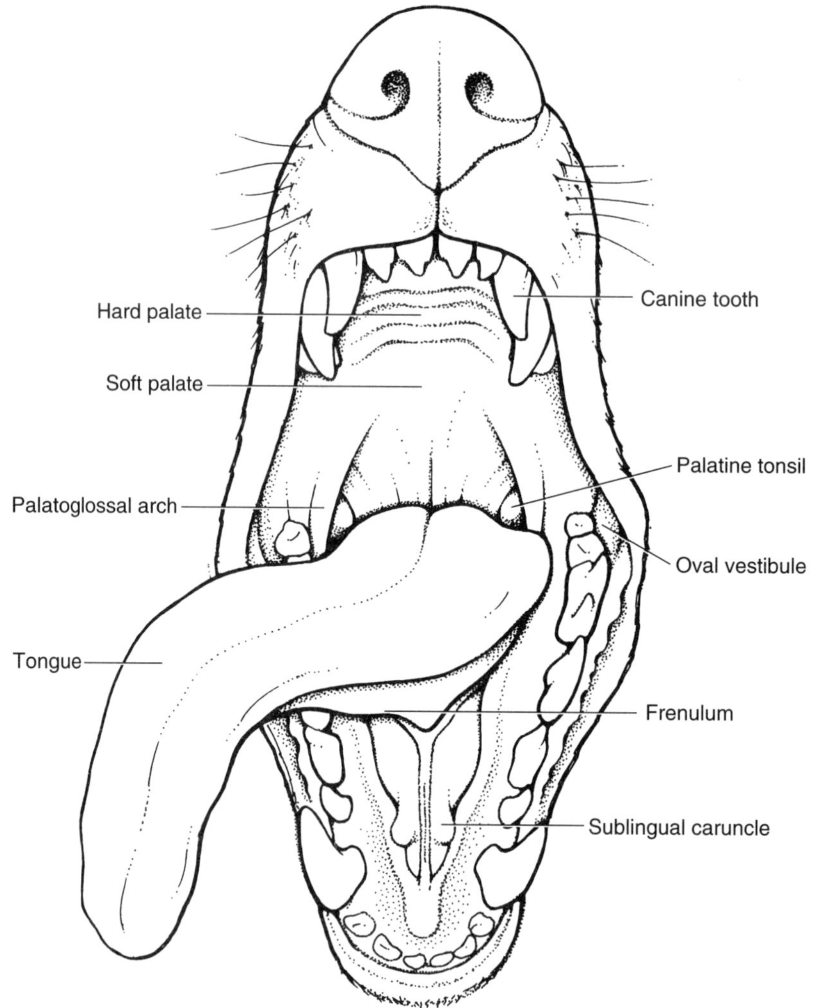

FIGURE 12–1. Rostral view of the oral vestibule and oral cavity proper.

(1) The lips are smooth and hairless along their free margins (i.e., nearest the mouth). This hairless border is generally most pronounced on the lower lip. On both the upper and lower lip, the border is relatively narrow through most of the length of each lip, but widens into a broad area near the angle of the mouth.

(2) The lower lip possesses blunted papillae on its free (upper) edge nearest the angle of the mouth.

2. Salivary gland openings

a. The **parotid duct** (from the parotid salivary gland) opens into the oral vestibule on the **parotid papilla,** a small elevation of tissue lateral to the last upper premolar (carnassial tooth).

b. The **main duct of the zygomatic salivary gland** opens into the oral vestibule on a small papillary mucosal elevation a short distance caudal to the parotid papilla. A low ridge of mucosa extends between the openings of the parotid and main zygomatic salivary gland ducts.

c. The **accessory ducts of the zygomatic salivary gland** are usually seen as one to four small openings on the oral mucosa of the vestibule, directly caudal to the main duct.

C. **Oral cavity proper.** The oral cavity proper is the region containing the teeth, tongue, and openings of certain salivary glands. It is bounded dorsally by the hard palate, ventrally by the mucosa reflected from the tongue covering the mylohyoideus muscle as it forms a sling for the tongue, laterally and rostrally by the teeth and gums, and caudally by the palatoglossal arches (see Figure 12–1).

1. The **roof of the oral cavity** is formed by the **hard palate,** which divides the oral cavity ventrally from the nasal cavity dorsally.
   a. **Structure**
      (1) The hard palate consists of a **bony shelf** (formed by contributions from the maxillary, palatine, and incisive bones) a relatively thick and tough **mucosal covering,** and a layer of heavy **connective tissue** between the bone and the oral surface of the mucosa.
      (2) The oral surface of the hard palate's mucosa is marked by several (six to ten) transverse ridges **(rugae).** The rugae are generally arched as they pass from one side of the palate to the other, with the concave side of the arch facing caudally. Rugae presumably assist in retaining food within the mouth prior to swallowing.
   b. **Vasculature**
      (1) **Arterial supply.** The main arterial supply arrives through the **major palatine artery** (a terminal branch of the maxillary artery). The **minor palatine artery** (a late branch of the maxillary artery) supplies a much smaller part of the hard palate, and a portion of the adjacent soft palate as well.
      (2) **Venous drainage** departs through the **palatine plexus,** which drains through the vein of the palatine plexus to the maxillary vein.
   c. **Innervation** is provided by terminal branches of the maxillary nerve, as follows:
      (1) The **major palatine nerve,** which follows the course of the same-named artery
      (2) The **minor palatine nerve,** which also follows the course of the same-named artery
      (3) The **accessory palatine nerve,** a small branch of the major palatine nerve that supplies the caudal part of the hard palate

2. The **floor of the oral cavity** is covered by loose mucosa continuous with that on the ventral surface of the tongue, and is marked mainly by two structures.
   a. The **sublingual fold** is a slightly raised longitudinal elevation in the mucosa along the sides of the tongue. This fold, which is much more prominent in living animals than in embalmed specimens, is produced by the underlying, rostrally directed course of the **mandibular** and **major sublingual ducts,** which lead from the mandibular and monostomatic portions of the sublingual salivary glands, respectively.
   b. The **sublingual caruncle** (see Figure 12–1) is a paired elevation positioned on each side of the frenulum (the rostral fold of mucosa attaching the tongue to the floor of the mouth). The sublingual caruncle is typically laterally compressed and may appear to be more of a fold than a papilla. The mandibular and major sublingual ducts open into the oral cavity at the sublingual caruncle.

II. TONGUE.

The tongue largely fills the oral cavity, and extends caudally beyond the oral cavity into the oropharynx.

A. Overview

1. **Regions** (Figure 12–2)
   a. The **root** of the tongue is its widest, most caudal portion, where it is attached by its extrinsic muscles to the basihyoid bone. This region of the tongue lies within the oropharynx.
   b. The **body** of the tongue extends rostrally from the root and is attached to the floor of the oral cavity. It is thick and triangular in cross-section.
      (1) The **frenulum** (see Figure 12–1) is the free edge of the oral mucosal fold extending from the floor of the oral cavity to the ventral midline of the body of the tongue.

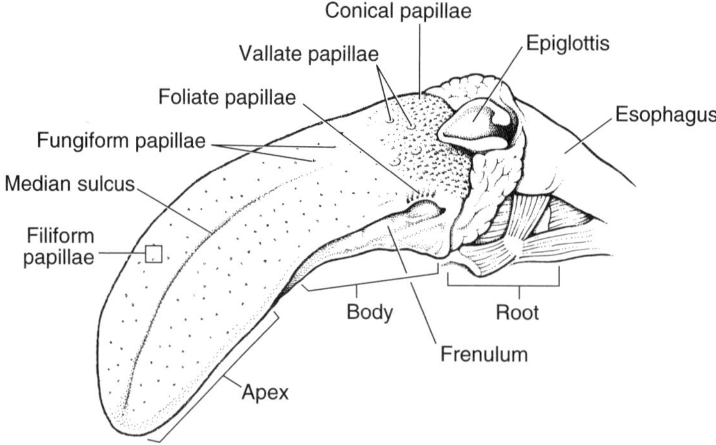

FIGURE 12–2. Dorsolateral view of the tongue, showing the regions of the tongue and the distribution of the lingual papillae.

(2) The **palatoglossal arches (folds)** are paired elevations of mucosa that extend from the caudal region of the body of the tongue caudodorsally to the cranial region of the soft palate. These arches are most prominent when the tongue is protruded some distance from the mouth (see Figure 12–1).

c. The **apex** of the tongue is the free, rostral-most portion of the tongue not attached by the frenulum. It is relatively thin and flattened and is the most dextrous portion of the tongue. The **lyssa,** an unpaired, tapered, rod-shaped structure composed of skeletal muscle and fat and encapsulated by a thick connective tissue capsule, is situated on the median plane in the rostral part of the tongue's apex. It extends from near the free apical edge of the tongue caudally to approximately the rostral edge of the genioglossus muscle and is thought to act as a stretch receptor for the tongue. The lyssa receives its own blood supply and innervation.

2. **External appearance.** In dogs, the tongue is markedly elongate.

a. **Dorsal surface**

(1) The mucosa that covers the dorsal surface of the tongue is greatly roughened by **papillae,** which project upward from the surface. The stratified squamous epithelium covering the papillae is markedly thickened and cornified, providing protection from the constant abrasive action of foodstuffs passing through the mouth.

(2) A **median sulcus** extends longitudinally along the rostral midline of the tongue from its tip to nearly its base, dividing it into symmetric right and left halves (see Figure 12–2).

b. **Lateral** and **ventral surfaces.** In stark contrast to the mucosa of the dorsal surface, the mucosa of the lateral and ventral surfaces is smooth to the point of being slick in the live animal.

3. **Embryologic development.** A brief review of the embryologic origins of the tongue facilitates understanding of certain aspects of the structure and innervation of this organ (Table 12–1).

B. **Lingual papillae** entirely cover the dorsal surface of the tongue.

1. **General considerations**

a. **Structure.** Lingual papillae consist of a **dermal core** covered by **stratified squamous cornified epithelium.**

b. **Types.** Several forms of papillae exist, each with a characteristic field of distribution over the dorsal lingual surface. Papillae that possess taste buds are generally fewer in number than those with a strictly mechanical function.

TABLE 12–1. Embryologic Development and Innervation of the Tongue

	Branchial Arch Derivation	**Mucous Membrane Derivation**	**General Sensory Innervation**	**Taste Innervation**
Rostral two thirds	First and second	Oral ectoderm of stomodeum	Lingual nerve	Facial nerve via chorda tympani
Caudal third	Third	Oral endoderm of foregut	Glossopharyngeal nerve	Glossopharyngeal nerve

2. **Papillae without taste buds**
   a. **Filiform papillae** function in **protection of the tongue, retention of food or water on the tongue,** and in **grooming.**
      (1) **Appearance.** Grossly, filiform papillae appear **small** and **conical,** although subgrossly they possess a central conical core accompanied by secondary and tertiary serrations. They are exceptionally heavily cornified.
      (2) **Distribution.** They are the **smallest,** but also the **most numerous** and **widespread,** of the lingual papillae. They are distributed evenly over the **rostral two thirds of the tongue's dorsum,** in a manner so that the tips of the cones point caudally (see Figure 12–2).
      (3) **Innervation.** The dermal cores of the filiform papillae receive branches of the **lingual nerve** (a branch of the mandibular nerve, cranial nerve V_3). They function in general sensory perception but not in taste.
   b. **Conical papillae** function in **protection of the tongue** and **retention of food or water on the tongue.**
      (1) **Appearance.** Conical papillae are relatively large; their conical form is plain to the naked eye. These papillae are well-cornified.
      (2) **Distribution.** The conical papillae are distributed over the **caudal third** of the tongue's dorsum, in a manner so that the tips of the cones point caudally.
         (a) A range of overlap with the filiform papillae is present.
         (b) The conical papillae are more numerous, denser, and relatively smaller in the rostral regions of their field, and fewer, larger, and more sparse caudally.
      (3) **Innervation.** The dermal core of the conical papillae receives branches of the **glossopharyngeal nerve** (cranial nerve IX). These papillae also function in general sensory perception but not taste.
   c. **Marginal papillae** are present in **suckling puppies** and function to improve the seal of the tongue around the nipple when nursing. These papillae, which are located along the lateral margins of the apex and body of the tongue, are lost when the puppy changes from a liquid to a solid diet.

3. **Papillae with taste buds**
   a. **Fungiform papillae** are **protective** and **gustatory** in function.
      (1) **Appearance.** Fungiform papillae look, as the name suggests, like tiny mushrooms. They are shorter and broader than the filiform papillae, and are much less heavily cornified. The markedly thinner layer of cornified epithelium of the fungiform papillae allows the red color of the underlying vasculature to show through, giving the fungiform papillae a darker appearance than the filiform papillae in the living dog.
      (2) **Distribution.** The fungiform papillae are **relatively small,** and are the **second most numerous** of the lingual papillae. They are scattered over the **rostral two thirds** of the tongue's dorsum (see Figure 12–2).
         (a) Fungiform papillae are most numerous at the tip and along the lateral surfaces of the tongue, where they are smaller than in other locations. Rarely, a few may be located caudal to the vallate papillae.
         (b) Each fungiform papilla is generally closely surrounded by several, taller fili-

form papillae (see Figure 12–2). This arrangement promotes the retention of a small pool of saliva around each fungiform papilla, which facilitates the taste function of the fungiform papilla by keeping dissolved substances in immediate proximity to the fungiform papilla's taste buds.

(3) **Innervation.** The dermal cores of the filiform papillae receive branches of the **lingual nerve** (a branch of the mandibular nerve, cranial nerve V_3), as well as branches of the **chorda tympani** (a branch of the facial nerve, cranial nerve VII).

(a) The **lingual branches** provide general sensation.

(b) The **chorda tympani** provides special sensory innervation (taste) to those fungiform papillae that possess taste buds. (Not all of the fungiform papillae are provided with taste buds). The chorda tympani also provides some mechanoreceptors and temperature receptors.

b. **Vallate (circumvallate) papillae** are **gustatory** in function.

(1) **Appearance.** Individual vallate papillae average 1.5–2.5 mm in diameter, making them the largest of the lingual papillae. These papillae are lightly cornified.

(a) **Simple vallate papillae** consist of an outer rim of tightly packed, modified (larger and broader) conical papillae surrounding a round elevated internal (primary) papilla. The rim of conical papillae effectively produces a gutter (moat) around the central papilla. The dorsal surface of the central papilla also possesses a central depression with a secondary papilla projecting upward through it; thus, the simple vallate papillae possess two moats.

(b) **Complex vallate papillae** possess two to four individual simple vallate papillae inside the moat formed by the rim of modified conical papillae.

(2) **Distribution.** The vallate papillae are the sparsest of the lingual papillae; typically four are present, although the number may range from three to six. They are located where the **rostral two thirds of the tongue meets the caudal third** (i.e., at the junction of the ectodermal and endodermal derivatives, respectively).

(a) When an even number of vallate papillae is present, the papillae are symmetrically arranged in a "V" shape on each side of the median sulcus, with the point of the "V" projecting caudally.

(b) When there is an odd number, the arrangement is asymmetrical.

(3) **Innervation.** The dermal core of the vallate papilla receives branches of the **glossopharyngeal nerve.** These branches provide both general sensation as well as special sense (taste). Taste buds are positioned on the surface of the primary papilla, and sometimes on the walls of the moat as well.

c. **Foliate papillae** are **gustatory** in function.

(1) **Appearance.** Foliate papillae are not as well developed in dogs as in some other species. They appear as **a group of roughly rectangular folds separated from each other by deep crypts.** The folds are positioned with their long axes roughly perpendicular to the mandible.

(a) The papillae follow each other sequentially like the leaves of a book, hence their name. Papillae in the central region of the group are best developed and their associated crypts are the deepest, while the papillae at the rostral and caudal end of each series are smaller and more poorly defined.

(b) Foliate papillae are relatively lightly cornified.

(2) **Distribution.** The foliate papillae are present only on a small area on the lateral surface of the tongue immediately rostral to the palatoglossal fold (see Figure 12–2).

(3) **Innervation.** The dermal core of the foliate papilla receives branches of the **glossopharyngeal nerve.** These branches provide both general sensation as well as special sense (taste). The taste buds of the foliate papillae are positioned on the surface of the folds within the walls of the crypts.

C. Glands

1. **Gustatory glands** are serous salivary glands associated with the bases of the crypts between the foliate papillae.
2. **Serous salivary glands** are intermingled with the bundles of the intrinsic lingual muscles.

3. **Mucoserous salivary glands** are plentiful in the submucosa over the caudal third of the tongue, and also in the lateral lingual margins.

D. **Musculature** (Table 12–2). The musculature of the tongue consists of a myriad of intrinsic muscles with the substance of the tongue itself, as well as various extrinsic muscles attaching the tongue to surrounding structures. These muscles combine to impart a remarkable degree of mobility to the tongue; the tongue is capable of movements of both considerable strength as well as agility, as required by its numerous and varied roles (e.g., prehension, manipulation of food within the mouth, swallowing, lapping, grooming, positioning during panting to facilitate heat loss, and vocalization).

1. **Intrinsic muscles.** The intrinsic lingual muscles act to stiffen the substance of the tongue, as well as to shape it into the variety of forms necessary for prehension, mastication, bolus formation, swallowing, grooming, vocalization, and panting.
   a. **Four major groups.** The intrinsic muscles of the tongue are numerous and run in many directions within the substance of the tongue. On careful examination, four major groups of muscles can be demonstrated. Each of these four groups is bilateral in distribution.
      (1) The **superficial longitudinal fibers** lie immediately deep to the mucosa on the dorsum of the tongue, and occupy approximately the dorsal half of the depth of the tongue (Figure 12–3).
         (a) Rostrally, these fibers are grouped in widely spaced bundles, which are thickest near the midline and thinnest at the lateral margins of the tongue.
         (b) Caudally, the superficial longitudinal fibers are more robust and closely packed, forming two symmetrical, dense masses on each side of the **lingual septum,** a longitudinal fibrous structure that extends the greatest part of the length of the tongue and provides an attachment site for many of the intrinsic tongue muscles.
      (2) The **deep longitudinal fibers** occupy the ventral half of the lingual substance (see Figure 12–3). These fibers are fewer and more poorly organized than their superficial counterparts. They are best organized in the apical region of the tongue, where they form a compact mass surrounding the lyssa.
      (3) The **transverse fibers,** as their name suggests, are oriented mainly transversely to the long axis of the tongue.
         (a) These fibers attach to the lingual septum within the central region of the

TABLE 12–2. Summary of Attachments, Actions, and Innervation of the Lingual Muscles

Muscle	Origin	Insertion	Action	Innervation
Intrinsic muscles	Lingual substance	Lingual substance	Manifold shape changes	Hypoglossal nerve
Extrinsic muscles				
Genioglossus (3 bundles)	Medial mandible near mandibular symphysis	Dorsal lingual substance from lyssa caudally	Depress and protrude the tongue	Hypoglossal nerve
Styloglossus (3 heads)	Stylohyoid bone	Mid-lingual substance from lyssa caudally	Depress and retract the tongue	Hypoglossal nerve
Hyoglossus	Basihyoid bone (mainly)	Root and caudal third of the tongue	Depress and retract tongue	Hypoglossal nerve

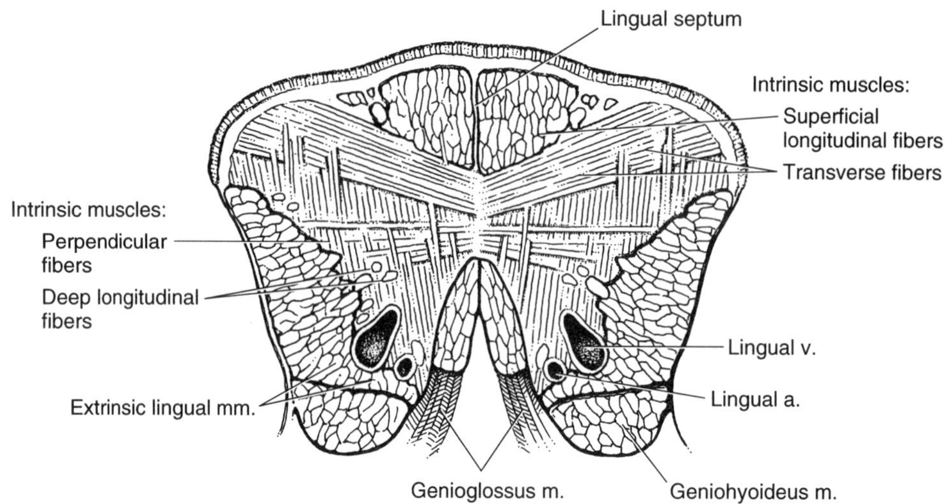

FIGURE 12–3. Transverse section of the tongue demonstrating the intrinsic musculature.

tongue, and pass laterally in a fan-shaped arrangement to the lateral and some dorsal surfaces of the tongue.

(b) The transverse fibers are intricately interwoven with the perpendicular lingual fibers throughout most of the central lingual region. This network is located between the superficial and deep longitudinal fibers (see Figure 12–3).

(4) The **perpendicular fibers** are oriented with their long axes perpendicular to the long axis of the tongue (see Figure 12–3). These fibers are most dense in the ventral half of the tongue, but do extend into the more dorsal half, where they intermingle with the transverse lingual fibers.

b. Innervation. The intrinsic muscles of the tongue are all **innervated** by the **hypoglossal nerve.**

2. Extrinsic muscles. Like the intrinsic lingual muscles, are all paired.

a. Genioglossus (*genio,* "chin;" *-glossus,* "tongue"). The apex of the genioglossus, a triangular muscle (Figure 12–4), is attached to the medial mandibular surface just caudal to the mandibular symphysis. From this origin, the genioglossus fans dorsocaudally.

(1) Regions. Three distinct regions are visible in the genioglossus as it fans upward.

(a) The **vertical bundle** is a broad band of fibers that inserts into the rostral portion of the ventral tongue from the caudal edge of the lyssa to approximately halfway down the length of the tongue. In the resting position, its fibers are indeed essentially vertical. The role of the vertical bundle of the genioglossus is to **depress the rostral half of the tongue** caudal to the lyssa.

(b) The **oblique bundle** is narrower than the vertical bundle, and is positioned with its relatively long fibers passing obliquely dorsocaudally to attach to the ventral surface of the caudal region of the tongue. The role of the oblique bundle of the genioglossus is to **protrude the tongue.**

(c) The **straight bundle** lies lateral to the other two bundles, with its fibers essentially parallel to the mandibular body. The straight bundle inserts into the caudal third of the tongue, the basihyoid bone, and the ceratohyoid bone. The straight bundle of the genioglossus **depresses and protrudes the tongue.**

(2) Innervation. The **hypoglossal nerve** innervates all parts of the genioglossus.

b. Styloglossus. The styloglossus, the most laterally positioned of the extrinsic muscles of the tongue, is flat and strap-shaped. It is narrow at its origin from the skull, but then it widens and thins as it approaches and inserts into the tongue (see Figure 12–4).

(1) **Regions.** The styloglossus has three subdivisions. All arise from specific regions of the stylohyoid bone, and insert into particular areas of the tongue.

(2) **Action.** The action of the styloglossus muscle varies according to whether the bundles contract individually or in concert.

(a) Individually, the bundles depress the region of the tongue into which they insert.

(b) In concert, the bundles of the styloglossus draw the tongue caudally.

(3) **Innervation.** The **hypoglossal nerve** innervates the styloglossus. The portion of the styloglossus that is visible behind the angle of the mandible closely parallels the course of the hypoglossal nerve in this area, with the nerve running just ventral to the muscle.

c. **Hyoglossus.** The hyoglossus, a wide, flat, and relatively short muscle, originates mainly on the ventrolateral surface of the basihyoid bone and inserts in the root and caudal two thirds of the tongue (see Figure 12–4).

(1) **Action.** The hyoglossus **retracts** and **depresses the tongue.**

(2) **Innervation** of the styloglossus arrives through the **hypoglossal nerve.**

E. Vasculature

1. Arterial supply

a. The **lingual artery,** an early branch of the external carotid artery, is the principal source of blood to the tongue. The right and left lingual arteries anastomose freely in the substance of the tongue, and the branches of the lingual artery form capillary retes among the lingual muscle fibers.

(1) **Course.** The lingual artery leaves the external carotid artery shortly after the external carotid artery gives rise to the occipital artery, and passes rostrally, medial to the hyoglossus muscle and lateral to the genioglossus muscle. After passing rostral to the hyoglossus muscle, the lingual artery is joined by the hypoglossal nerve, which accompanies the artery to the tip of the tongue.

(2) **Structures supplied.** During its rostral course to the apex of the tongue, the lingual artery gives off branches to both the **extrinsic** and **intrinsic tongue musculature.** It also supplies branches to the **hyoid** and **pharyngeal muscles,** as well as to the **palatine tonsil.**

b. The **sublingual artery,** a branch of the facial artery, is not a major arterial supply for the tongue.

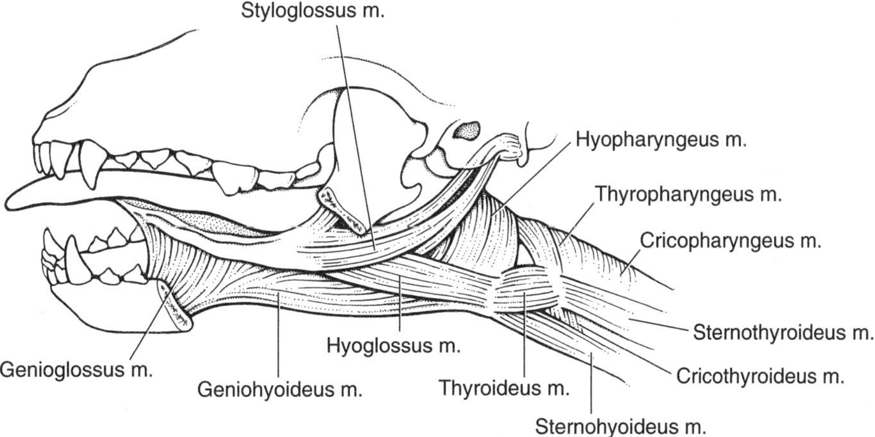

FIGURE 12–4. Extrinsic tongue musculature. (Modified with permission from Evans HE, 1993, *Miller's Anatomy of the Dog,* 3e. Philadelphia, WB Saunders, p 285.)

(1) **Course.** The sublingual artery arises from the facial artery and passes rostrally along the medial and ventral border of the mandible.

(2) **Structures supplied.** The sublingual artery mainly supplies the **mylohyoid** and **digastricus muscles.** Small branches of the sublingual artery may supply the **genioglossus** and **geniohyoideus muscles.** In addition, the sublingual artery anastomoses with the lingual artery, and thus potentially supplies a small amount of blood to the **lingual substance.**

2. **Venous drainage.** The **lingual vein** originates in the tip of the tongue and courses caudally in close association with the lingual artery and hypoglossal nerve. It becomes superficial just caudal to the caudal edge of the mylohyoideus muscle, where it receives the sublingual vein. The lingual vein then becomes confluent with the facial vein, forming the linguofacial vein, which joins the maxillary vein in the rostral part of the neck to form the external jugular vein.

Canine Clinical Correlation

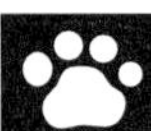

The lingual vein lies directly under the thin substance of the mucosa on the ventral lingual surface. If absolutely necessary during anesthesia, this vein can be used as a site for venipuncture. However, the loose connective tissue surrounding the vein promotes formation of large hematomas should technique not be perfect, so routine use of the vessel for this purpose is not advisable.

3. **Arteriovenous anastomoses.** Numerous arteriovenous anastomoses are present in the dog's tongue, positioned superficially along the lingual dorsum. They are particularly prominent in the apical region, still numerous in the body, and least numerous in the root of the tongue. The superficial position of the arteriovenous anastomoses, as well as their abundance in the rostral lingual regions, facilitates heat dissipation during panting.

F. **Innervation.** Nerves supplying the tongue are **all cranial nerves:** the **lingual nerve** (a branch of the mandibular division of the trigeminal nerve), the **chorda tympani** (a branch of the facial nerve), the **glossopharyngeal nerve,** and the **hypoglossal nerve.**

1. **General sensory innervation** (touch, pain, temperature)
   a. The **lingual nerve** supplies general somatic afferent innervation to the rostral two thirds of the lingual mucosa.
   b. The **glossopharyngeal nerve** supplies general somatic afferent innervation (as well as taste) to the caudal third of the lingual mucosa.
2. **Special sensory innervation** (taste)
   a. The **chorda tympani** supplies taste innervation (as well as touch and temperature innervation) to the rostral two thirds of the tongue.
   b. The **glossopharyngeal nerve** supplies taste innervation (as well as general sensation) to the caudal third of the lingual mucosa.
3. **Motor innervation**
   a. The **hypoglossal nerve** innervates all of the muscles of the tongue.
   b. The **glossopharyngeal nerve** carries secretory and vasodilator (general visceral efferent) fibers to the lingual glands in the caudal lingual region.

III. PHARYNX.

PHARYNX. The pharynx is a soft-walled chamber situated caudal to the bone-bordered nasal and oral cavities, and rostral to the entrance to the esophagus and trachea. Air and food or water pass caudally through the pharynx to either the trachea or esophagus, respectively.

Canine Clinical Correlation

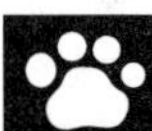

In brachycephalic breeds, the soft palate extends sufficiently far caudally to protrude into the airway and interfere with breathing. Resection of a portion of the soft palate is often performed in such instances; however, the amount resected must be carefully judged, because a soft palate of insufficient length can cause difficulties with swallowing as well as nasal breathing.

A. Structure

1. **Walls.** The walls of the pharynx are largely composed of a thin mucosal layer supported by an underlying musculofascial layer.
2. **Muscles.** Deep to the pharyngeal mucosa, skeletal muscle covers the greatest part of the lateral and dorsal walls of the pharynx (Table 12–3). Most of these muscles meet on the dorsal midline of the pharynx at a prominent **mid-dorsal fibrous raphe.** Each of these muscles is paired.
   a. **Shorteners and constrictors.** Together, the pterygopharyngeus and the palatopharyngeus serve to **shorten and constrict the rostral part** of the pharynx.
      (1) The **pterygopharyngeus,** the more dorsal of these muscles, arises on the pterygoid bone and passes caudodorsally to insert on the mid-dorsal raphe.
      (2) The **palatopharyngeus,** the more ventral of these two muscles, is more poorly developed. This muscle passes from the soft palate caudodorsally to insert on the mid-dorsal raphe.
   b. **Constrictors.** The constrictors attach at some fixed point on the lateral pharyngeal wall or adjacent structure, and their fibers pass dorsally and then medially to arch over the dorsal surface of the pharynx to meet the fibers of the fellow muscle on the other side.
      (1) The **hyopharyngeus** (the **middle pharyngeal constrictor)** arises from the hyoid apparatus and passes along the lateral wall and roof of the pharynx at a level roughly even with the basihyoid bone. The hyopharyngeus **constricts** the **midportion** of the pharynx.

TABLE 12–3. Summary of Attachments, Actions, and Innervation of the Pharyngeal Muscles

Muscle	Origin	Insertion	Action	Innervation
Pterygopharyngeus	Hamulus of pterygoid bone	Mid-dorsal raphe	Constricts and shortens rostral pharynx	Glossopharyngeal nerve, vagus nerve
Palatopharyngeus	Soft palate	Mid-dorsal raphe	Constricts and shortens rostral pharynx	Glossopharyngeal nerve, vagus nerve
Hyopharyngeus	Thyro- and ceratohyoid bones	Mid-dorsal raphe	Constricts the midportion of the pharynx	Glossopharyngeal nerve, vagus nerve
Thyropharyngeus	Thyroid cartilage	Mid-dorsal raphe	Constricts the caudal portion of the pharynx	Glossopharyngeal nerve, vagus nerve
Cricopharyngeus	Cricoid cartilage	Mid-dorsal raphe	Constricts the caudal portion of the pharynx	Glossopharyngeal nerve, vagus nerve
Stylopharyngeus	Stylohyoid bone	Dorsolateral pharyngeal wall	Dilates, elevates, and protracts the pharynx	Glossopharyngeal nerve, vagus nerve

(2) The **thyropharyngeus** and the **cricopharyngeus** (the **caudal pharyngeal constrictors)** arise from the thyroid laryngeal cartilage and cricoid laryngeal cartilage, respectively. These muscles pass along the lateral wall and roof of the pharynx over the larynx and serve to **constrict** the **caudal regions** of the pharynx.

c. **Dilator.** The **stylopharyngeus,** a relatively weak muscle arising from the stylohyoid bone, passes rostrally and fans out to insert into the lateral pharyngeal wall.

3. **Soft palate.** The soft palate, which continues caudally from the caudal end of the hard palate, divides the respiratory portion of the pharynx dorsally from the digestive portion of the pharynx ventrally.

a. **Composition of the soft palate**

(1) **Epithelial covering.** The soft palate is covered with stratified squamous epithelium on its ventral surface, where it is continuous with the epithelium of the hard palate, and respiratory epithelium on its dorsal surface, where it is continuous with the nasal cavity.

(2) **Palatine glands,** seromucous glands that open directly onto the surface of the soft palate, form the main bulk of the substance of the soft palate. The number of palatine glands varies; they are most numerous in the rostral regions of the soft palate, where the number of openings per square centimeter may be as high as 200!

(3) A robust **tendinous aponeurosis** lies beneath the dorsal mucosa, giving strength to the general structure of the palate.

b. **Musculature of the soft palate**

(1) The **palatinus** lies dorsal to the layer of palatine glands. Each member of the pair lies adjacent to its mate on each side of the median plane.

(a) **Action.** The palatinus shortens the soft palate.

(b) **Innervation.** The **glossopharyngeal nerve** and **vagus nerve** innervate the palatinus.

(2) The **tensor veli palatini** is a very small muscle that arises near the indistinct mastoid process of the skull (rostral to the tympanic bulla), extends cranioventrally over the wall of the pharynx (past the hamulus of the pterygoid bone), and inserts by radiating rostrally into the cranial region of the palate.

(a) **Action.** The tensor veli palatini laterally stretches the palate between the pterygoid bones.

(b) **Innervation.** The **mandibular division of the trigeminal nerve (cranial nerve V_3)** innervates the tensor veli palatini.

(3) The **levator veli palatini,** another very small muscle, also arises from the indistinct mastoid process of the skull. This muscle extends caudoventrally and passes between the pterygopharyngeus and the palatopharyngeus muscles to insert by radiating widely into the substance of the caudal parts of the soft palate.

(a) **Action.** The levator veli palatini elevates the caudal regions of the soft palate.

(b) **Innervation.** The **glossopharyngeal** and **vagus nerves** innervate the levator veli palatini.

c. **Vasculature of the soft palate**

(1) **Arterial supply**

(a) The **minor palatine artery,** a branch of the maxillary artery, is the main arterial supply to the soft palate.

(b) The **ascending pharyngeal** and **major palatine arteries** contribute a small amount of blood to the soft palate.

(2) **Venous drainage** of the soft palate is through the extensive **palatine plexus,** which is the caudal continuation of the much smaller venous plexus of the hard palate.

(3) **Lymphatic drainage** from the soft palate passes to the medial retropharyngeal lymph node.

d. **Innervation of the soft palate**

(1) **Sensory innervation** is provided mainly by the **minor palatine branch of the maxillary nerve (cranial nerve V_2).** The **glossopharyngeal nerve (cranial nerve IX)** is sensory to a small portion of the caudal soft palate.

(2) **Motor innervation** to the muscles of the soft palate arrives through the **mandibular division of the trigeminal nerve (cranial nerve V_3),** the **glossopharyngeal nerve (cranial nerve IX),** and the **vagus nerve (cranial nerve X).**

B. **Regions.** The pharynx is divided into three portions.

1. **Nasopharynx.** The nasopharynx conducts air from the nasal cavity to the laryngopharynx.
   a. **Position.** The nasopharynx may be thought of as the **space dorsal to the soft palate.**
      (1) The **nasal choanae** form the cranial border.
      (2) The **palatopharyngeal arches,** paired elevations of mucosa produced by the underlying palatopharyngeus muscle, form the caudal border. Because the elevation of the arch is formed by the muscle beneath it, this structure can be difficult to appreciate in the embalmed dog.
      (3) The **base of the skull** forms the dorsal boundary.
      (4) The **soft palate** forms the ventral boundary.
   b. **Associated structures**
      (1) The **intrapharyngeal ostium** is an open space, marked by the continuation of the nasopharynx past the caudal edge of the soft palate, where it enters into a common area with the oro- and laryngopharynges.
      (2) The **pharyngeal opening of the auditory tube** is positioned far dorsally in the lateral wall of the nasopharynx. The opening, a narrow slit, lies approximately at the level of the mid-rostral to caudal extent of the soft palate. The auditory tube extends from the nasopharynx to the middle ear and provides a means of pressure equalization—the pharyngeal opening is surrounded by muscle bundles that permit dilatation or closure of the orifice, thus permitting air to enter or leave the tube and equalizing pressure on each side of the tympanic membrane.
      (3) The **pharyngeal tonsil** is a grossly visible collection of aggregated lymphoid tissue in the mucosal layer of the pharynx. The mucosal layer of the nasopharynx is provided with a **typical respiratory epithelium,** complete with abundant mucous glands and lymphoid tissue. The lymphoid tissue of the mucosal layer is varied in form, being scattered in some areas and organized into masses in others.
         (a) The pharyngeal tonsil contributes to the ring of lymphoid tissue surrounding the entrance to the deeper parts of the respiratory and digestive systems. This collection of lymphoid tissue is strategically placed to encounter the antigenic load arriving to the respiratory and gastrointestinal tracts (in the form of nonsterile inspired air and nonsterile ingesta).
         (b) Because of its location (i.e., at the entrance to the nasopharynx), the pharyngeal tonsil can obstruct normal air flow if it becomes excessively enlarged.

2. **Oropharynx.** The oropharynx conducts ingested materials from the oral cavity to the esophageal opening.
   a. **Position.** The oropharynx may be thought of as the **space ventral to the soft palate.**
      (1) The **palatoglossal folds** form the cranial border.
      (2) The **caudal border of the soft palate** and the **base of the epiglottis** form the caudal boundary.
      (3) The **soft palate** forms the dorsal border.
      (4) The **root of the tongue** forms the ventral border.
      (5) The **tonsillar fossa** of the palatine tonsil forms the lateral border.
   b. **Associated structures**
      (1) The **palatine tonsil,** a prominent feature of the lateral oropharyngeal wall, contributes to the ring of lymphoid tissue surrounding the entrance into the deeper parts of the respiratory and digestive systems.
         (a) **Structure**
            (i) A fusiform **superficial** portion that protrudes from the lateral oropharyngeal wall comprises the vast bulk of the tonsil. The superficial part of the palatine tonsil lies in a depression known as the **tonsillar fossa.** A fold of mucosa termed the **semilunar (tonsillar) fold** covers the medial surface of the palatine tonsil.

Canine Clinical Correlation

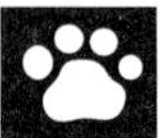

In healthy adult dogs, the palatine tonsil is effectively hidden from view during oral examination. In young dogs, as well as in adult dogs suffering from tonsillitis, the palatine tonsil commonly protrudes from the tonsillar fossa into the oropharyngeal region.

(ii) A smaller **deep** portion is recessed into the submucosa. This region is typically absent in young dogs.

Canine Clinical Correlation

When performing a palatine tonsillectomy, both the superficial and deep portions must be completely removed to effect a successful surgery. The position of the lingual nerve and the mandibular and major sublingual ducts just lateral to the palatine tonsil must be considered to avoid inadvertent damage to these important structures during the surgery.

(b) **Vasculature**
   (i) The **arterial supply** to the palatine tonsil arrives mainly through the **tonsillar artery,** a branch of the facial artery.
   (ii) The **venous drainage** from the palatine tonsil flows into the **palatine venous plexus.**
   (iii) **Lymphatic drainage.** The **medial retropharyngeal lymph node** receives the efferent lymphatics from the palatine tonsil.

(2) The **lingual tonsil** is composed of lymphoid tissue so diffuse that it cannot be appreciated by the unaided eye. The lingual tonsil also contributes to the ring of lymphoid tissue guarding the deeper regions of the respiratory and digestive tracts.

(3) The **isthmus of the fauces** is **the short region adjoining the oral cavity with the oropharynx.** The term "fauces" refers to the lateral oropharyngeal wall. Boundaries of the isthmus of the fauces are the soft palate dorsally, the palatoglossal arches laterally, and the tongue ventrally.

3. **Laryngopharynx.** The laryngopharynx conducts inspired air from the nasopharynx to the laryngeal opening and ingested material from the oropharynx to the esophagus.
   a. **Position.** The laryngopharynx may be thought of as the **space dorsal to the larynx.**
      (1) The **intrapharyngeal ostium** forms the rostral border.
      (2) The **pharyngoesophageal limen,** a prominent annular ridge of mucosa surrounding the pharynx at the junction of the laryngopharynx with the esophagus, forms the caudal border.
   b. **Associated structures.** The **cranial portions of the larynx** occupy the greatest part of the floor of the laryngopharynx.

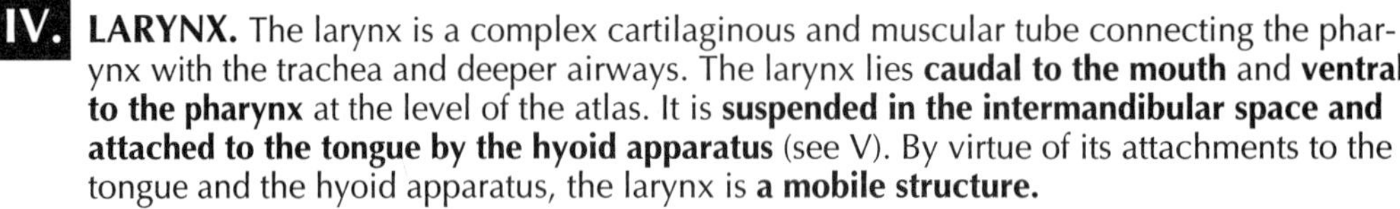

IV. LARYNX.

LARYNX. The larynx is a complex cartilaginous and muscular tube connecting the pharynx with the trachea and deeper airways. The larynx lies **caudal to the mouth** and **ventral to the pharynx** at the level of the atlas. It is **suspended in the intermandibular space and attached to the tongue by the hyoid apparatus** (see V). By virtue of its attachments to the tongue and the hyoid apparatus, the larynx is **a mobile structure.**

A. Laryngeal cartilages

1. **Overview.** The cartilaginous skeleton of the canine larynx consists of six cartilages.
   a. **Major laryngeal cartilages.** Four of the six cartilages are large and form the vast majority of the laryngeal skeleton.

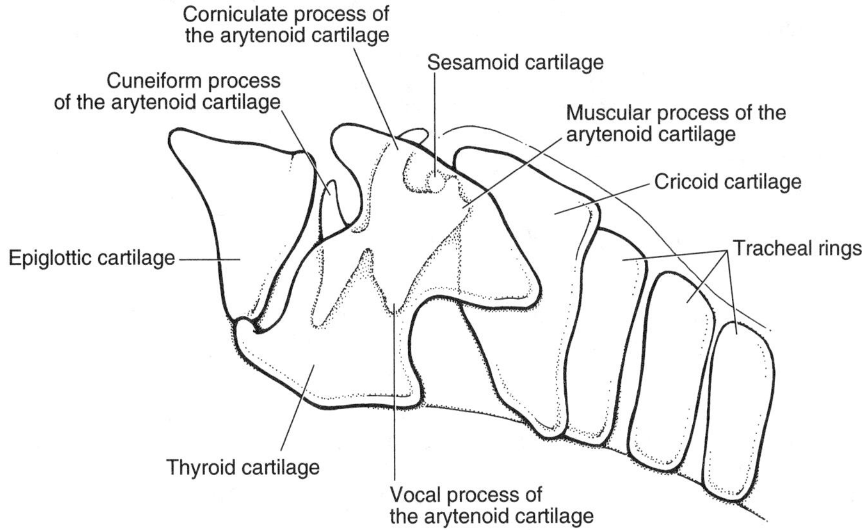

FIGURE 12–5. The laryngeal cartilages, articulated.

(1) Three of these cartilages form a fairly continuous passage from rostral to caudal. In that order, these are the **epiglottic, thyroid,** and **cricoid cartilages** (Figure 12–5).

(2) The fourth of the large cartilages, the **arytenoid cartilage,** is located relatively dorsally, overlapping a large portion of the thyroid cartilage and articulating at a small point with the cricoid cartilage. **The arytenoid cartilage is the only paired cartilage of the canine larynx.**

b. Minor laryngeal cartilages. Two of the six cartilages are small, and have little practical significance. These are the **interarytenoid** and **sesamoid cartilages.**

2. **Epiglottic cartilage.** The epiglottic cartilage forms the core of the **epiglottis,** which is the epiglottic cartilage together with its native mucosal covering.
   a. The epiglottic cartilage is the sole laryngeal cartilage formed of **elastic cartilage.**
   b. It consists of a small **stalk** and a large, roughly spoon-shaped **blade.**
      (1) The **stalk** is anchored between the basihyoid bone/lingual root and the thyroid cartilage, and is attached to each of these structures.
      (2) The **blade** is pointed at its rostral (apical) end, convex on its rostral (oral) surface (i.e., the surface that faces the oral cavity), and concave on its dorsocaudal (aboral) surface (i.e., the surface that faces the trachea).

3. **Thyroid cartilage.** The thyroid cartilage is the largest of the laryngeal cartilages.
   a. The thyroid cartilage is formed of **hyaline cartilage.** It may become calcified with advancing age, or even ossified in spots in particularly old dogs, a fact that must be kept in mind when viewing radiographs of older dogs.
   b. The thyroid cartilage consists of **right** and **left laminae** that are continuous ventrally but open dorsally, so that in cross-section, the thyroid cartilage is roughly "U"-shaped. Each lamina possesses a **rostral** and **caudal cornu (horn)** at its rostral and caudal extremities. The **rostral** and **caudal thyroid notches** separate the cornu from the body of the lamina.
      (1) The **oblique line,** a poorly defined edge oriented obliquely along the laminae, demarcates the attachment of the **sternothyroid muscle.**
      (2) The **cricothyroid ligament** spans the caudal thyroid notch and connects the thyroid cartilage to the cricoid cartilage. The **cranial laryngeal nerve** and the **cranial laryngeal artery** pass through the rostral thyroid notch.

Canine Clinical Correlation

The internal cavity of the larynx can be conveniently accessed without damaging the cartilage (e.g., to obtain a transtracheal wash) by passing through the cricothyroid ligament.

(3) The **laryngeal prominence** is a slight elevation on the ventral midline of the thyroid cartilage. Although not visible externally (as it is in humans as the "Adam's apple"), it is palpable.
(4) The rostral border of the thyroid cartilage is smooth and slightly convex. The **thyrohyoid membrane** joins the rostral border of the thyroid cartilage to the basihyoid bone.

4. **Cricoid cartilage.** The cricoid cartilage is the only laryngeal cartilage that forms a complete ring. Thus, when the larynx is viewed dorsally, the wall of the closed dorsal surface is formed by the cricoid cartilage.
   a. The cricoid cartilage is also formed of **hyaline cartilage,** and like the thyroid cartilage, is subject to calcification with age.
   b. The cricoid cartilage consists of the **dorsal lamina,** a broad region several times wider than its most ventral region, and the **arch,** which passes ventrally from the lamina to meet its fellow from the other side. In its ventral course, the arch progressively and markedly narrows, so that on the ventral-most surface it is but a fraction of the width of the lamina.
      (1) Two pairs of **articular facets** are present on the cricoid cartilage, generally in the region of the rostral cornu of the thyroid cartilage.
         (a) The more rostral of these is for the arytenoid cartilages.
         (b) The more caudal set is for the caudal cornu of the thyroid cartilage.
      (2) Both sets of articular sites form true **synovial joints** between the respective cartilages.

5. **Arytenoid cartilage.** The arytenoid cartilage, a paired structure, is the most irregular of the laryngeal cartilages, possessing numerous named projections. The arytenoid cartilages are **positioned largely medial to the thyroid lamina,** so that approximately half of the cartilage is hidden when viewed from the lateral surface.
   a. The arytenoid cartilage is also formed of **hyaline cartilage.**
   b. Prominent features of the arytenoid cartilage include the following.
      (1) The **cuneiform process,** the most rostral part of the arytenoid cartilage, is roughly triangular and is connected to the caudal regions of the arytenoid cartilage by a narrow stalk.
         (a) The ventral portion of the cuneiform process is enclosed within the **aryepiglottic fold.**
         (b) The **ventricular ligament** and **ventricularis muscle** attach to the cuneiform process.
      (2) The **corniculate process** is narrow and somewhat pointed, and curved gently caudally.
      (3) The **muscular process** is a thick, rounded process on the caudal border of the arytenoid cartilage. The **cricoarytenoideus dorsalis muscle** attaches here.
      (4) Paired **articular facets** on the caudodorsal extremity of the arytenoid cartilage are the site of articulation with the cricoid cartilage.
      (5) The **vocal process** is a stout ventral projection from the main portion of the arytenoid cartilage. The **vocal ligament ("vocal cord")** and **vocalis muscles** attach here.

6. **Sesamoid cartilage.** The sesamoid cartilage is a small, ovoid nugget of cartilage positioned between the arytenoid cartilages just cranial to the cricoid lamina. It is interposed in the midregion of the transverse arytenoid muscle.

7. **Interarytenoid cartilage.** The interarytenoid cartilage is small and disk-shaped. It lies in

the same general location as the sesamoid cartilage, but in a more superficial position (caudodorsal to the transverse arytenoid muscle rather than within it).

B. Interior of the larynx

1. **Laryngeal mucosa.** The laryngeal mucosa is well-provided with **mucous glands** as well as **lymphoid aggregations.** The epithelium of the laryngeal mucosa varies with the region of the larynx.
   a. **Stratified squamous epithelium** is positioned near the entrance to the larynx (where some risk of abrasion from swallowed foodstuff exists) and along the edges of the various mucosal folds that move against each other as they are approximated during normal laryngeal movements.
   b. **Pseudostratified ciliated** (i.e., **respiratory**) **epithelium** is located throughout the remainder of the larynx, in keeping with its respiratory function. Interestingly, the respiratory epithelium near the vocal folds may undergo squamous metaplasia associated with chronic coughing, clearly an adaptive response.
2. **Laryngeal cavity.** The laryngeal cavity may be considered to be composed of three successive regions, described relative to the vocal folds. From rostral to caudal, these are the laryngeal vestibule, the glottis, and the infraglottic cavity.
   a. The **laryngeal vestibule** (not to be confused with the laryngeal ventricle) is the antechamber of the larynx, extending from the laryngeal entrance to the vocal folds.
      (1) The **laryngeal entrance (aditus laryngis)** is marked by several structures protruding to some degree through the laryngeal mucosa. The laryngeal entrance is bordered **rostrally** by the **epiglottis, caudally** by the **corniculate processes of the arytenoid cartilage,** and **laterally** by the **aryepiglottic folds** (Figure 12–6).
         (a) The **aryepiglottic folds** are extensions of mucosa that begin at the corniculate process of the arytenoid cartilage (most caudal), extend rostrally over the cuneiform process, and progress rostrally to the epiglottis. The projection of the tips of the corniculate and cuneiform processes dorsally under the mucosa produces small, focal elevations in the mucosa referred to as the **corniculate** and **cuneiform tubercles,** respectively. A deep, smooth notch separates the two.
         (b) The **piriform recesses** are shallow troughs located lateral to each aryepiglottic fold. Fluids *en route* to the esophagus bypass the larynx by funneling through these channels.

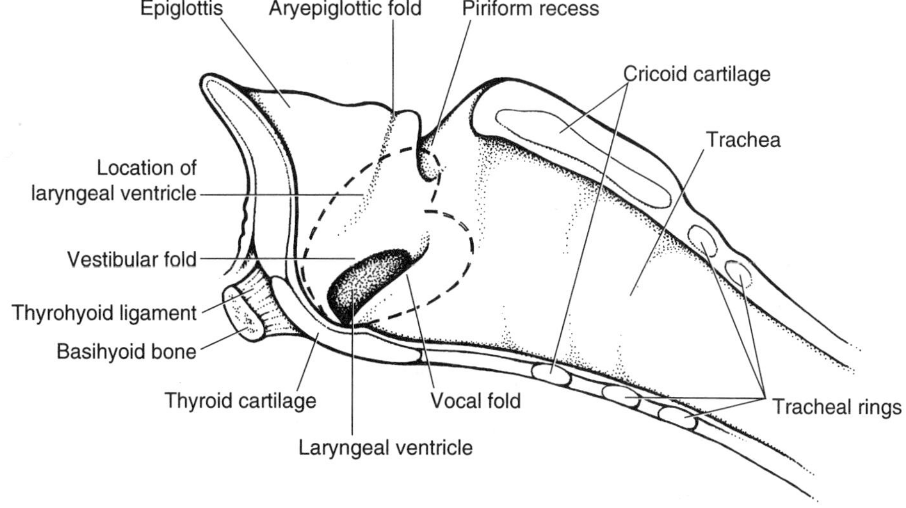

FIGURE 12–6. Lumen of the larynx.

(2) The **vestibular fold** is a fold of mucosa that extends from the ventral margin of the cuneiform process of the arytenoid cartilage to the thyroid cartilage.

(3) The **laryngeal ventricle** is a small, blind sac formed by an outpocketing of the laryngeal mucosa.

(a) The entrance to the laryngeal ventricle is provided by a rectangular opening bordered by the vestibular fold cranially and the vocal ford caudally. Under normal circumstances, the entrance to the laryngeal ventricle is always open.

(b) The saccule of the ventricle is positioned between the thyroid cartilage and the vocal and vestibular folds.

Canine Clinical Correlation

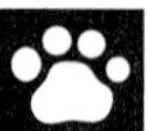

In brachycephalic dogs with elongation of the soft palate and associated breathing difficulties, the negative pressure created by the effort to move air through the obstructed airway may lead to eversion of the saccules of the laryngeal ventricles into the laryngeal vestibule. The saccules then swell, exacerbating the respiratory difficulty. In such instances, surgical intervention involves removal of the saccules of the laryngeal ventricle as well as soft palate resection.

b. The **glottis,** the narrowest portion of the laryngeal cavity, consists of the paired arytenoid cartilages dorsally and the paired vocal folds laterally and ventrally. The **rima glottidis** is the actual space between the two sides of the glottis (*rima,* "cleft"). The **vocal folds** are formed by mucosa covering the vocalis muscle and the vocal ligament as they extend from the vocal process of the arytenoid cartilage to the thyroid cartilage. The vocal fold may be distinguished from the vestibular fold by its more caudal level, more medial positioning, and longer length.

Canine Clinical Correlation

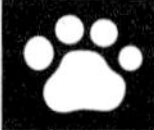

Distinction between the vocal and vestibular folds is important when performing debarking surgery, in which the vocal folds are severed. When correctly performed, this procedure results in marked diminution (though not obliteration) of the dog's ability to vocalize. However, should the vestibular folds be transected in error, the dog's voice is not affected.

c. The **infraglottic cavity** extends caudally from the glottis to the cranial edge of the trachea. It essentially assumes the form of the surrounding cricoid cartilage.

C. Musculature. Both **extrinsic** and **intrinsic muscles** are related to the larynx. The extrinsic muscles (with the exception of the sternothyroideus) use the larynx as a base from which to exert influence on other structures, rather than effecting change on the larynx itself. The intrinsic muscles, which both arise from and insert on the larynx, affect only the larynx itself.

1. Extrinsic muscles attach to the sternum, pharynx, and hyoid apparatus.

a. Laryngeal muscles attaching to the sternum. The **sternothyroideus** is a thin, strap-like muscle that arises from the sternal manubrium and passes cranially deep to the sternohyoideus muscle to insert on the lateral thyroid lamina.

(1) **Action.** The sternothyroideus draws the larynx, hyoid apparatus, and tongue caudally.

(2) **Innervation.** The sternothyroideus is innervated by ventral branches of the **cervical nerves.**

b. Laryngeal muscles attaching to the pharynx include the **thyropharyngeus** and **cricopharyngeus** (see III A 2 b (2); Table 12–3). These muscles constrict the caudal portion of the pharynx.

c. **Laryngeal muscles attaching to the hyoid apparatus.** The **thyrohyoideus** connects the lamina of the thyroid cartilage to the thyrohyoid bone of the hyoid apparatus.
   (1) **Action.** The thyrohyoideus retracts the hyoid apparatus.
   (2) **Innervation** is via the hypoglossal nerve.

2. **Intrinsic muscles** (Table 12–4)
   a. **Superficial laryngeal muscles.** The **cricothyroideus** is the only member of this group. The cricothyroideus extends between the arch of the cricoid cartilage and the lateral thyroid lamina.
      (1) **Action.** The cricothyroideus draws the cricoid and arytenoid cartilages caudally, thereby tensing the vocal folds.
      (2) **Innervation.** The cricothyroideus is innervated by the **cranial laryngeal nerve.**
   b. **Deep laryngeal muscles** include the **cricoarytenoideus dorsalis,** the **cricoarytenoideus lateralis,** the **thyroarytenoideus,** the **arytenoideus transversus,** and the **hyoepiglotticus.** These muscles are situated more deeply among the laryngeal cartilages, with much of the substance of many of them lying deep to the thyroid lamina. They all **attach to the arytenoid cartilage** and as a group are **innervated** by the **caudal laryngeal nerve.**

TABLE 12–4. Summary of Attachments, Actions, and Innervation of the Intrinsic Laryngeal Muscles

Muscle	Origin	Insertion	Action	Innervation
Cricothyroideus	Lateral cricoid cartilage	Caudal–medial thyroid cartilage	Tenses vocal cords	Caudal laryngeal nerve (branch of vagus nerve)
Cricoarytenoideus dorsalis	Cricoid lamina	Muscular process of the arytenoid cartilage	Opens the glottis	Cranial laryngeal nerve (branch of vagus nerve)
Cricoarytenoideus lateralis	Craniolateral cricoid cartilage	Muscular process of the arytenoid cartilage	Closes the glottis	Cranial laryngeal nerve
Thyroarytenoideus				
Main mass	Internal midline of the thyroid cartilage	Arytenoid cartilage	Constricts the glottis to relax vocal cord	Cranial laryngeal nerve
Vocalis	Internal midline of the thyroid cartilage	Vocal process of the arytenoid cartilage	Relaxes vocal cord	Cranial laryngeal nerve
Ventricularis	Cuneiform process of the arytenoid cartilage	Interarytenoid cartilage	Constricts the glottis to dilate laryngeal ventricle	Cranial laryngeal nerve
Arytenoideus transversus	Muscular process of the arytenoid cartilage	Interarytenoid cartilage	Constricts the glottis to adduct vocal folds	Cranial laryngeal nerve
Hyoepiglotticus	Ceratohyoid bone	Midline of the epiglottis	Depresses epiglottis	Cranial laryngeal nerve

(1) The **cricoarytenoideus dorsalis** arises along the full length of the cricoid lamina (i.e., its dorsal surface), passes cranioventrally as the fibers converge, and inserts on the muscular process of the arytenoid cartilage. The dorsal cricoarytenoid muscle **dilates the glottis.**

(2) The **cricoarytenoideus lateralis** arises along the lateral and cranial surface of the cricoid cartilage, passes craniodorsally, and inserts on the muscular process of the arytenoid cartilage. The lateral cricoarytenoid muscle **closes the glottis.** (It is interesting to note that this strong adductor of the glottis is innervated by the same nerve that innervates the cricoarytenoideus dorsalis, the strong abductor of the glottis!)

Canine Clinical Correlation

Forced closure of the glottis against expired air leads to adduction of the vocal folds and results in increased intrathoracic (and thereby intraabdominal) pressure, which assists functions such as coughing, defecation, micturition, and parturition. The increased intrathoracic pressure produced by closure of the glottis also stabilizes the entire thoracic cage by forcing its walls outward, effecting more efficient and powerful action of the muscles attaching to the ribs.

(3) The **thyroarytenoideus** has a **main mass,** as well as two additional portions, the **vocalis** and **ventricularis muscles.**

(a) The **main mass** of the thyroarytenoideus arises along the internal ventral midline of the thyroid cartilage, passes caudodorsally, and inserts on the muscular process of the arytenoid cartilage.

(b) The **vocalis,** the medial division of the thyroarytenoideus, lies beneath the vocal fold. It arises on the internal ventral midline of the thyroid cartilage medial to its parent muscle mass, dorsally and slightly caudally, and inserts on the vocal process of the arytenoid cartilage. The **vocal ligament ("vocal cord")** is attached to the cranial border of the vocalis muscle and can be distinguished from the muscle by its lighter color. The vocalis **relaxes the vocal cord by drawing the arytenoid cartilage ventrally.**

(c) The **ventricularis,** the cranial division of the thyrohyoideus, lies beneath the vestibular fold. In the dog, it arises from the cuneiform (rather than the thyroid) cartilage, passes dorsally, and inserts on the interarytenoid cartilage. The ventricularis **constricts the glottis** and, by virtue of its positioning medial to the laryngeal ventricle, likely assists in dilating this structure.

(4) The **arytenoideus transversus** arises on the muscular process of the arytenoid cartilage, passes toward the median plane, and inserts on the interarytenoid cartilage. This muscle **constricts the glottis** and **abducts the vocal folds.**

(5) The **hyoepiglotticus** is a small muscle bundle that arises from the ceratohyoid bone, passes medially, turns dorsally on reaching the midline, and passes further dorsally to insert on the ventral midline of the epiglottis. The hyoepiglotticus **depresses the epiglottis.**

D. Vasculature

1. **Arterial supply.** The **cranial laryngeal artery,** a branch of the external carotid artery, passes through the rostral thyroid notch and is the main source of blood to the larynx.
2. **Venous drainage** of the larynx is provided by the **cranial laryngeal vein,** the companion to the same-named artery, and the **unpaired laryngeal vein,** a tiny vein that drains into the cranial laryngeal vein.

E. Innervation.

The larynx is **entirely supplied by the vagus nerve,** by means of two named branches.

1. The **cranial laryngeal nerve** departs directly from the vagus nerve and divides into an **in-**

ternal branch (sensory from the internal mucosa cranial to the vocal folds) and an **external branch** (motor to the cricothyroideus muscle).

2. The **caudal laryngeal nerve** is the **terminal segment** of the **recurrent laryngeal nerve.** This nerve is motor to all of the intrinsic laryngeal muscles except the cricothyroideus.

V. HYOID APPARATUS.

The hyoid apparatus suspends the tongue and larynx from the skull in the intermandibular space. Skeletal attachments of the hyoid apparatus are to the mastoid region of the skull proximally and to the thyroid cartilage distally.

A. Cartilage and bones.

The hyoid apparatus is composed of a set of diminutive (yet strong) bones assembled by synchondroses (see Chapter 8, Figure 8–1). The cartilage and all of the bones of the hyoid apparatus (except the basihyoid bone) are paired.

1. The **tympanohyoid cartilage,** a small bit of cartilage at the proximal-most part of the hyoid apparatus, attaches the apparatus to the indistinct mastoid process of the skull. Its name is derived from its proximity to the tympanic bulla.
2. The **stylohyoid bone,** one of the longer bones of the hyoid apparatus, extends from the tympanohyoid cartilage proximally to the epihyoid cartilage distally, inclining cranioventrally. It is rod-shaped (*stylo,* "pole") and distinctly bowed toward the midline.
3. The **epihyoid bone,** also a relatively long bone in the hyoid apparatus, extends from the stylohyoid cartilage proximally to the ceratohyoid cartilage distally. It is slightly more ventrally inclined than the stylohyoid bone and can be thought of as sitting "upon" the central region of the hyoid apparatus, hence its name (*epi-,* "upon").
4. The **ceratohyoid bone,** the shortest of the hyoid bones, extends from the epihyoid cartilage proximally to the basihyoid cartilage distally, turning sharply caudally from the epihyoid bone and articulating with it at nearly a right angle. The ceratohyoid bone is noticeably tapered from its proximal to distal end, somewhat resembling a horn (*cerato,* "horn").
5. The **basihyoid bone** is rather stout compared with the remaining hyoid bones, and is noticeably bowed ventrally. It is situated transversely across the midline, within the substance of the base of the tongue, and articulates with the thyrohyoid and ceratohyoid bones of both sides. It is named for its position within the base of the tongue.
6. The **thyrohyoid bone,** another long bone of the hyoid apparatus, extends caudodorsally from the basihyoid bone at an angle approximately parallel to the epihyoid bone, and attaches to the cranial cornu of the thyroid cartilage of the larynx. It is named for its attachment to the thyroid cartilage.

B. Musculature

Musculature (Table 12–5). The hyoid apparatus is provided with several small muscles that attach at sites on or near the hyoid apparatus itself. In addition, it has some muscles with attachments to sites relatively distant on the body, such as the sternum.

1. **Short muscles**
   a. The **thyrohyoideus** originates on the thyroid cartilage, and sends its fibers obliquely cranioventrally to the thyrohyoid bone.
   b. The **ceratohyoideus** is a small, flat triangular muscle interposed between the ceratohyoid and thyrohyoid bones. This muscle has little clinical significance.
   c. The **jugulohyoideus** is a very short band of muscle that extends between the paracondylar process (formerly known as the "jugular process") to the tympanohyoid cartilage. Again, this muscle is seldom encountered clinically.
   d. The **stylohyoideus** is a thin, elongate muscle that extends between the proximal stylohyoid bone and the lateral edge of the basihyoid bone.
2. **Long muscles**
   a. The **mylohyoideus** is a flat sheet of muscle that bridges the intermandibular space. With its fellow from the opposite side of the body, the mylohyoideus forms a sling to support the tongue. Although most of the muscle inserts on a fibrous median raphe, the most caudal fibers attach to the basihyoid bone, and the muscle is thus considered together with the other hyoid muscles.

b. The **geniohyoideus** is a robust, elongate muscle extending from the rostroventral extremity of the mandible (*genio,* "chin") directly caudally to the basihyoid bone.

c. The **sternohyoideus,** the longest of the hyoid muscles, originates on the manubrium of the sternum. The muscle is flat and strap-like, and attaches rostrally to the basihyoid bone.

TABLE 12–5. Summary of Attachments, Actions, and Innervations of the Hyoid Muscles

Muscle	Origin	Insertion	Action	Innervation
Thyrohyoideus	Lamina of thyroid cartilage	Thyrohyoid bone	Retracts hyoid apparatus (and tongue)	Hypoglossal nerve
Ceratohyoideus	Thyrohyoid bone	Ceratohyoid bone	Draws the two bones closer	Glossopharyngeal nerve
Jugulohyoideus	Paracondylar process	Tympanohyoid cartilage and stylohyoid bone	Draws the stylohoid bone caudally	Facial nerve
Stylohyoideus	Tympanohyoid cartilage and stylohyoid bone	Lateral edge of the basihyoid bone	Raises the stylohyoid bone	Facial nerve
Mylohyoideus	Medial mandibular border	Median raphe and basihyoid bone	Raises the oral floor; draws the hyoid apparatus and tongue caudally	Hypoglossal nerve
Geniohyoideus	Rostral–ventral mandible	Basihyoid bone	Draws the hyoid apparatus and tongue rostrally	Hypoglossal nerve
Sternohyoideus	Sternal manubrium	Basihyoid bone	Draws the basihyoid bone and tongue caudally	Cervical spinal nerves, sometimes the hypoglossal nerve

C. **Vasculature. Arterial supply** to the structures of the hyoid apparatus arrives mainly through the **hyoid branches of the lingual artery.**

VI. MECHANISM OF NASAL BREATHING, DEGLUTITION, AND VOCALIZING

A. **Nasal breathing** and **deglutition (swallowing).** The configuration of the airway and digestive pathway within the pharynx is curious, in that the two pathways completely cross each other. In other words, the airway begins relatively dorsally in the nasal cavity, but must pass ventrally to attain the trachea, and the digestive pathway begins ventrally in the oral cavity, but must pass dorsally to attain the esophagus.

1. **Nasal breathing.** In the normal resting position, the caudal edge of the soft palate lies ventral to the epiglottis. This positioning closes the airway dorsal to the soft palate off from the oropharynx below, and provides a pathway for air to flow uninterrupted from the nasal cavity through the nasopharynx to the laryngeal opening.
2. **Deglutition.** The following events do not necessarily occur in a stepwise fashion.

- **a.** The tongue forms a bolus of ingesta, and the piston motion of the root of the tongue pushes the bolus caudally out of the oral cavity and into the oropharynx. The soft palate is elevated dorsally to occlude the passage into the choanae.
- **b.** The pharyngeal dilator (stylopharyngeus muscle) widens the rostral part of the pharynx to receive the bolus of food.
- **c.** The pharyngeal shorteners/constrictors (the palatopharyngeus and pterygopharyngeus muscles) draw the pharynx onto and over the bolus.
  - **(1)** The larynx is drawn cranially and the epiglottis partially closes over the laryngeal opening, protecting the deeper airway from entrance of ingesta.
  - **(2)** The vocal folds are adducted, further protecting the tracheal entrance.
- **d.** The middle and caudal pharyngeal constrictors (i.e., the hyopharyngeus, thyropharyngeus, and cricopharyngeus muscles) contract in a rostrocaudal direction.
  - **(1)** **Solids** are carried directly over (dorsal to) the laryngeal entrance and into the esophagus.
  - **(2)** **Fluids** are deflected laterally by the epiglottis, and are diverted into the piriform recesses. From the piriform recesses, they flow laterally around the larynx into the esophagus.
- **e.** The pharyngeal constrictors, shorteners, and dilator relax, and the soft palate and epiglottis return to their normal positions (i.e., those associated with nasal breathing).

B. **Vocalization.** Although the larynx produces the basic sounds of vocalization, other structures of the throat and mouth modify the sounds into their final form.

1. Passage of air over the vocal folds causes the folds to passively vibrate, producing sound.
2. The character of the sound is partly affected by the degree of tension on (and thus the thickness and length of) the vocal fold. Therefore, the action of the various laryngeal muscles affects the sound. Studies have suggested that coarse adjustments to vocalizations are made by the action of the cricothyroideus muscle, and fine adjustments are made by the action of the vocalis muscle.

Chapter 13

The Brain and Associated Structures

I. INTRODUCTION.

INTRODUCTION. This discussion presents an overall review of the most salient features grossly visible from the surface of the entire brain and of the brain stem with the cerebral hemispheres removed, as well as the vasculature of these structures. No attempt is made to follow nerve tracts within the brain in detail, or to provide a detailed discussion of structures visible on cut section of the brain.

A. Embryologic development of the brain.

Embryologic development of the brain. Brief review of the ontogenic progression of brain development provides insight into why certain regions of the brain are often considered together, when grossly they appear so disparate.

1. The brain originates as a series of **three fluid-filled enlargements (brain vesicles)** at the cranial end of the neural tube. From rostral to caudal these are the:
   - a. **Prosencephalon (forebrain)**
   - b. **Mesencephalon (midbrain)**
   - c. **Rhombencephalon (hindbrain)**
2. The prosencephalon and metencephalon each divide into two regions that remain recognizable into the definitive form. Only the mesencephalon remains undivided. Thus, from rostral to caudal, **five regions** are recognized:
   - a. **Telencephalon,** which in its definitive form, forms the **cerebral hemispheres**
   - b. **Diencephalon,** which in its definitive form is the **"interbrain"** (i.e., the **epithalamus, thalamus,** and **hypothalamus)**
   - c. **Mesencephalon,** which remains undivided and undergoes very little change
   - d. **Metencephalon,** which in its definitive form, is the **pons** and **cerebellum**
   - e. **Myelencephalon,** which in its definitive form, is the **medulla oblongata**

B. Brain tissue.

Brain tissue. The tissue of the brain is roughly divided into regions of **cell bodies** and regions of **cell processes.**

1. **Cell bodies**
   - a. **Grey matter** is tissue that contains mainly cell bodies of neurons, where those cell bodies are fairly diffusely spread. The **cortex** is the grey matter covering the surface of the cerebrum and cerebellum.
   - b. A **nucleus** is a localized, dense collection of neuronal cell bodies deeper within the substance of the brain.
2. **Cell processes** form **white matter** (i.e., tissue containing mainly the axonal cell processes of neurons). White matter is often collected into prominent groups or paths of axons (often referred to as **"tracts").**

C. Surface organization of the brain.

Surface organization of the brain. Grossly, the brain has three recognizable portions: a centrally positioned **brain stem,** which developmentally is partially overgrown dorsally by two expanded portions, the **cerebrum** rostrally, and the **cerebellum** caudally (Figure 13–1).

1. **Cerebrum.** The cerebrum is the largest portion of the brain, and is derived embryologically from the **telencephalon** (i.e., the rostral derivative of the prosencephalon).
   - a. **Location.** The cerebrum fills the majority of the rostral and middle cranial fossae. The **frontal, temporal, parietal,** and **occipital lobes** may be loosely described as the general regions of the brain lying deep to the bones of the same name. However, this approach is of limited practical use, because in domestic mammals, these divisions are somewhat arbitrarily defined and do not have a functional significance as strong as that in humans.

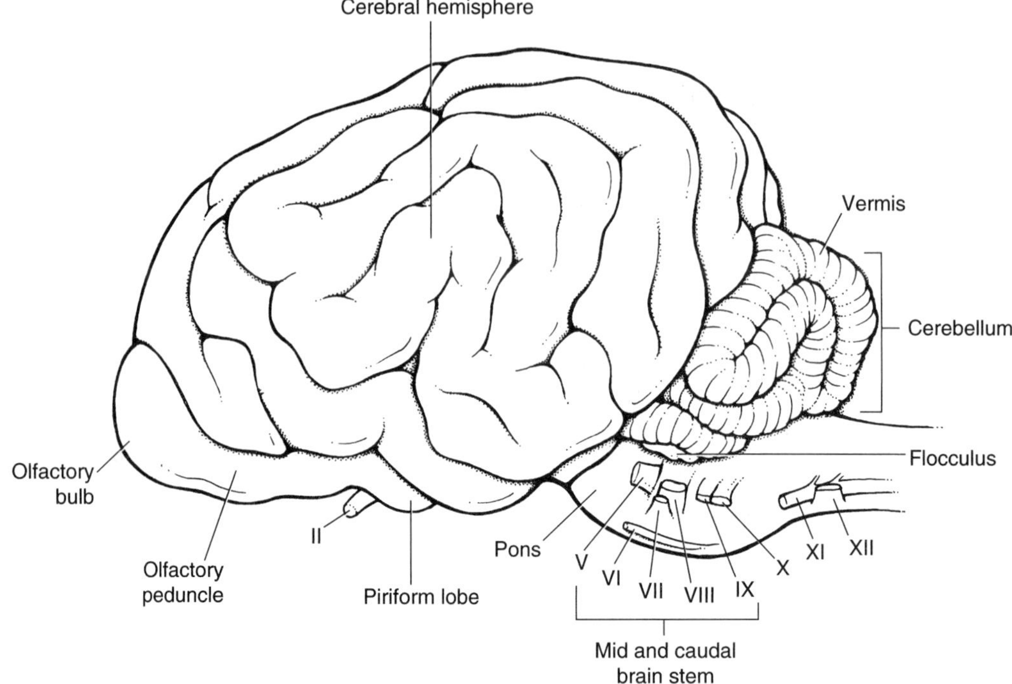

FIGURE 13–1. Gross appearance of the brain, lateral view. *Roman numerals* correspond with the cranial nerves that are visible on this view: *II* = optic nerve, *V* = trigeminal nerve, *VI* = abducent nerve, *VII* = facial nerve, *VIII* = vestibulocochlear nerve, *IX* = glossopharyngeal nerve, *X* = vagus nerve, *XI* = accessory nerve, *XII* = hypoglossal nerve.

b. **Function.** Phylogenetically the most recently developed portion of the brain, the cerebrum is concerned with higher functions (i.e., it is not necessary to the maintenance of vegetative life).

2. **Cerebellum.** The cerebellum is much smaller than the cerebrum, and is derived embryologically from the **metencephalon** (i.e., the cranial derivative of the rhombencephalon).
   a. **Location.** The cerebellum is nestled at the caudal part of the cerebrum. It fills the majority of the caudal cranial fossa.
   b. **Function.** The cerebellum is concerned with **coordination of movement.** Like the cerebrum, it is not necessary to the maintenance of vegetative life.

3. **Brain stem.** The brain stem is a segmented portion of the brain. From rostral to caudal, the segmented portions of the brain stem are the:
   a. **Diencephalon ("interbrain"),** composed of the **epithalamus, thalamus,** and **hypothalamus** (Inclusion of the diencephalon here is morphologic only.)
   b. **Mesencephalon**
   c. **Pons** (i.e., the ventral portion of the metencephalon)
   d. **Myelencephalon (medulla oblongata)**

II. FOREBRAIN.

The embryologic forebrain develops into the **cerebrum,** which therefore includes the forebrain's derivatives, the telencephalon and the diencephalon. The **telencephalon** is represented in the definitive form by the **cerebral hemispheres,** and the **diencephalon** is represented in the definitive form by the **thalamic structures** (i.e., the thalamus, metathalamus, subthalamus, epithalamus, and hypothalamus).

A. Telencephalon (cerebral hemispheres)

1. **Surface organization.** The cerebral hemispheres are paired, symmetrical, ovoid structures that cover most of the dorsal and lateral surfaces of the brain stem. They comprise the largest part of the brain that is visible externally.
   a. The **longitudinal cerebral fissure** is a deep cleft that separates the right and left cerebral hemispheres. In the intact state, the **falx cerebri,** an elongated fold of the dura mater, extends into the longitudinal cerebral fissure and separates the two hemispheres.
   b. The **transverse fissure** is a deep cleft that separates both cerebral hemispheres from the cerebellum.
   c. The **gyri** and **sulci** are all named, but individual names will not be given in this text.
      (1) **Gyri** (singular, gyrus) are convoluted elevations on the surface of the hemispheres that serve to increase surface area and thus increase the number of neurons that may reside in the brain.
      (2) **Sulci** (singular, sulcus) are grooves that exactingly follow the curves of the gyri, separating the gyri from one another.

2. **Phylogenetic regions.** The cerebral hemispheres may be divided into three regions, based on phylogenetic age and function.
   a. The **paleopallium** is of truly ancient phylogenetic origin.
      (1) The paleopallium retains its ancestral function mainly with regard to olfaction. Portions of the paleopallium visible from the intact surface include the olfactory bulb, olfactory peduncle, medial olfactory tract, and the piriform lobe.
      (2) During development, the paleopallium is largely overgrown by the dorsal and caudal expansion of the higher telencephalon; therefore, it occupies a relatively ventral position in its final form. The paleopallium is separated from the remainder of the cerebral hemispheres by the rhinal sulcus.
   b. The **archipallium** is of intermediate phylogenetic age.
      (1) This region of the cerebrum originally dealt with the correlation of olfactory perception with other types of sensory perception. However, in modern mammals, the archipallium has acquired other functions, such as the coordination of emotional and behavioral responses to various forms of stimuli.
      (2) No part of the archipallium is visible from the external surface.
   c. The **neopallium** is, phylogenetically speaking, the newest part of the brain. The neopallium is the portion of the telencephalon that, during development, undergoes the dramatic growth and dorsocaudal expansion over the underlying brain stem. All of the portions of the brain visible in a dorsal view, as well as the majority of what is visible laterally, compose the neopallium.

3. **Composition**
   a. The **cerebral cortex** is the **superficial grey matter** of the cerebral hemispheres. In the cerebral cortex, the neuronal cell bodies are relatively diffusely placed.
      (1) This layer is composed of six recognizable cellular layers.
      (2) Although the term "cerebral cortex" technically refers only to the grey matter of the cerebrum, the term is often used to refer to the cerebrum as a whole, grey and white matter together.
   b. The **associated white matter** is deep to the cortex.
      (1) Three **general types of white matter** tracts are recognized:
         (a) **Association fibers** pass between cortical regions within the same hemisphere.
         (b) **Commissural fibers** connect corresponding regions in the two hemispheres.
         (c) **Projection fibers** either pass into or out of the hemisphere from sites near or distant.
      (2) **Specific named regions** of white matter exist.
         (a) The **corona radiata** is the collection of white matter tracts radiating among and interconnecting the various areas of cortical grey matter. On the cut surface, stained or unstained, the corona radiata is visible as the white matter areas within the core of, and just deep to, the various gyri over the dorsal and lateral surface of the hemispheres.

(b) The **corpus callosum** is the largest commissure in the brain. It links the left and right hemispheres into a single functioning unit.

(c) The **internal capsule** is composed of projection fibers passing from the hemisphere to the brain stem, as well as fibers passing to the basal nuclei. A very wide band of white matter, the internal capsule is plainly visible on a stained or unstained cut section as it passes ventromedially between the caudate nucleus medially and the claustrum, putamen, and pallidum laterally.

c. Basal ganglia (deep grey matter) are specific nuclei positioned deeply in the base of the cerebral hemispheres. In the basal ganglia, the neuronal cell bodies are collected into more focal, often grossly visible collections.

4. Anatomic areas

a. Olfactory region (rhinencephalon). The olfactory region of the brain is the oldest phylogenetic region of the cerebrum (i.e., the paleopallium).

(1) The **olfactory bulb,** nestled against the cribriform plate, is the most rostral part of the olfactory region (see Figure 13–1, Figure 13–2). The multitudinous axons of the **olfactory nerve (cranial nerve I),** as well as fibers from the vomeronasal organ, pass through the plate and then aggregate to form the olfactory bulb.

(2) The **olfactory peduncle** continues caudally from the olfactory bulb (see Figure 13–2), and ends at a structure of variable prominence termed the **olfactory tubercle.** The olfactory bulb and peduncle are both hollow, containing the fluid-filled **olfactory ventricle,** which in some individuals may retain a patent connection to the remainder of the ventricular system (see V A 1).

(3) The **medial olfactory tract,** not visible on a surface view, travels deeply from the olfactory peduncle to the septal nuclei.

(4) The **lateral olfactory tract** passes from the olfactory lobe to the piriform lobe (see Figure 13–2), as well as to other nuclei and ganglia.

(5) The **piriform lobe** (see Figure 13–1, 13–2) is a large, pear-shaped (hence its name), and plainly visible lobe on the ventral surface of the brain. It is involved in many functions related to olfaction.

(6) The **rostral commissure** is a white matter tract connecting the right and left sides of the rhinencephalon.

b. Corpus striatum. The corpus striatum is a region of the ventrolateral wall of the cerebral hemisphere that becomes greatly thickened as a result of the development of several large nuclei within it.

(1) Most of the **basal nuclei** are located in the corpus striatum. Nuclei in this region are related to **vision** as well as **execution of voluntary movement** and include the:

(a) Caudate nucleus

(b) Lentiform nucleus (composed of the **putamen** and **pallidum)**

(c) Claustrum

(2) The name of this area is derived from its striated (striped) appearance on cut section. The striped appearance is imparted by the alteration of its several grey matter bodies with their associated white matter tracts.

c. Amygdala (amygdaloid body). The amygdala is a collection of six major nuclei, the names of which need not be enumerated here, positioned deeply and fairly centrally in the hemispheres, dorsal to the paleopallium. These nuclei receive input from the rhinencephalon, hippocampus, and hypothalamus, and they send output to those regions, as well as to other regions of the brain.

d. Septum. The septum, a roughly midline region in the rostral part of the brain (in the general area of the rostral extent of the corpus callosum), lies ventral to the corpus callosum and houses the septal nuclei. The **septal nuclei** receive input from the medial olfactory tract and also connect with the hypothalamus and hippocampus.

e. Hippocampal formation. The hippocampal formation is essentially the archipallium.

(1) The hippocampal formation consists of **two gyri** (the cingulate and supracallosal gyri), the **hippocampus proper,** and the **fornix.** These components actually become folded inward by the expanding cerebral hemispheres and come to lie en-

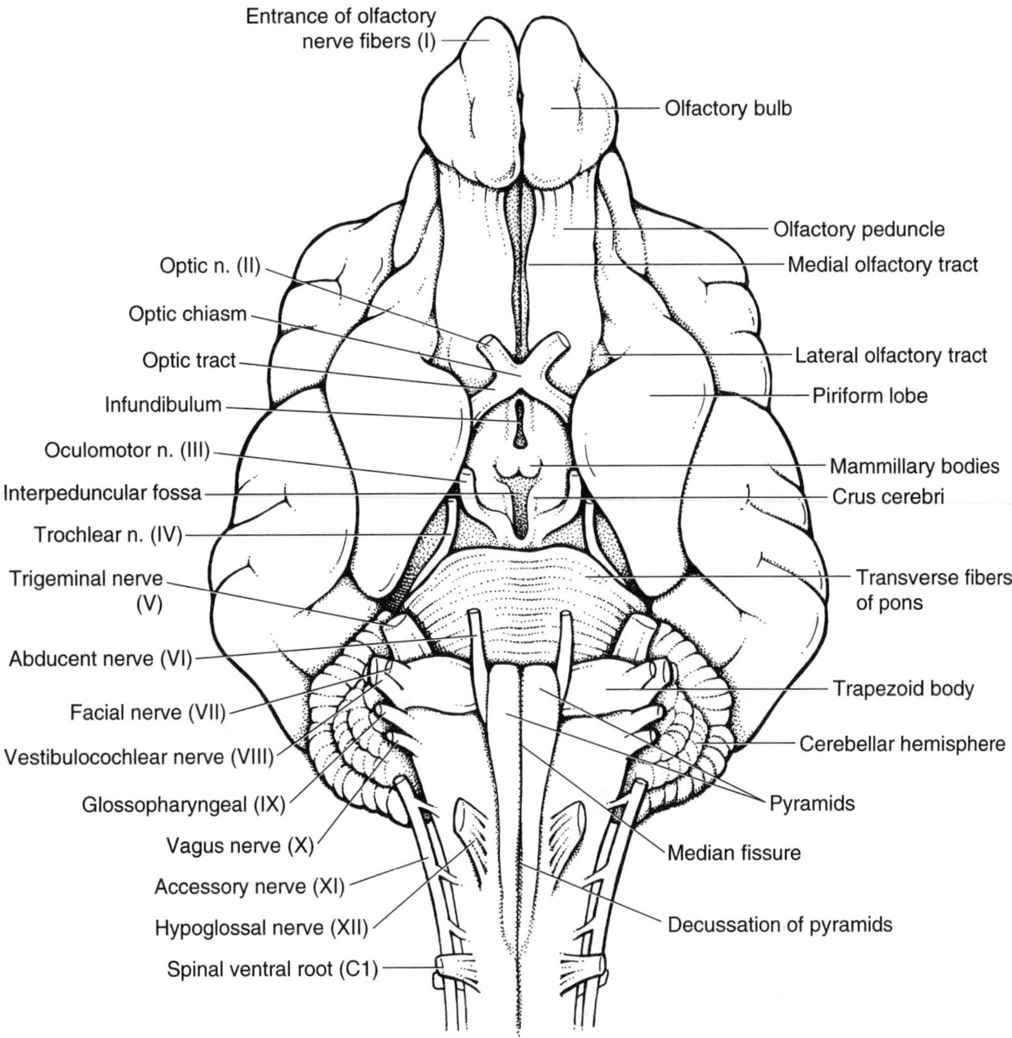

FIGURE 13–2. Ventral view of the brain. *CN* = cranial nerve.

tirely deep to the surface of the brain. The folding, together with the expansion of the hemispheres, causes all parts of the formation to assume a semicircular form that essentially surrounds most of the thalamus, with the caudal ends of the semicircle more widely spaced than the rostral ends (Figure 13–3).

(2) Consideration of the path of information through the formation assists in conceptualization of the positioning of its parts.
   - **(a)** Input enters the rostral part of the **gyri** and passes through them to the ventral and caudal regions of the hippocampus.
   - **(b)** Information passes through the grey matter substance of the **hippocampus proper** in a ventral to dorsal direction.
   - **(c)** Outflow from the hippocampus proper enters its white matter tract, the **fornix.**
   - **(d)** Impulses pass through the fornix to enter the **hypothalamus,** terminating on the **mammillary body.**

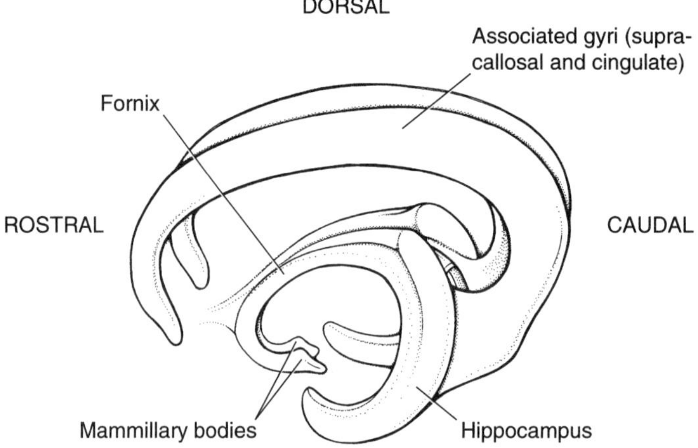

FIGURE 13–3. The hippocampal formation, lateral view.

f. "Limbic system". The "limbic system" is a rather nebulous region of the brain, more of a functional unit than an anatomic unit.

(1) The limbic system includes numerous, diverse structural contributions from the rhinencephalon, other regions of the cerebral hemispheres, and the brain stem. The name, "limbic system," is derived from the shape of its components, which form a curved border around the diencephalon (*limbus* = border), having been displaced there by the massive expansion of the developing cerebral hemispheres.

(2) The limbic system functions in coordinating emotional and behavioral responses to numerous forms of physical and psychic stimuli. It further plays a role in appetite, thirst, libido, anger, fear, and instinctive behavior.

5. Functional areas within the cerebral cortex can be broadly classified into two groups.

a. According to connections

(1) Cortical areas **communicating with the brain stem or spinal cord** are active in relatively low-level information processing, having to do largely with **vegetative functions.**

(2) Cortical areas **communicating only with other cortical regions** form the **association cortex** and function in higher information processing. These areas are associated with **intelligence.** Approximately 20% of the neopallium of the dog is composed of association fibers.

b. According to function. Cortical areas may also be classified based on the actual function they perform. In domestic animals, these functional regions are not as clearly associated with grossly visible lobes of the brain as they are in humans.

(1) The **olfactory area** lies in the piriform lobe of the rhinencephalon, on the ventral surface of the brain.

(2) The **motor area** occupies a region on the craniodorsal and craniolateral surface of the hemisphere (i.e., surrounding the cruciate sulcus), and functions in execution of voluntary movement and posture.

(3) The **premotor area** lies just rostral to the motor area, and programs patterns of movement, sending this information to the motor area.

(4) The **supplementary motor area** also lies close to the motor area (rostral to the cruciate sulcus) and functions in planning more extensive series of movements.

(5) The main **somesthetic area** is positioned on the craniolateral surface of the hemisphere just caudal to the motor area (along the coronal and ansate gyri). This area functions in perception of tactile and kinesthetic information as well as some nociperception (pain perception).

(6) The **gustatory area (taste)** is positioned adjacent to the somesthetic area.

(7) The main **auditory area** is positioned dorsolaterally on the caudal half of the hemisphere.
(8) The **vestibular area** lies adjacent to the auditory area, a logical location given the close association of these two functions in the inner ear.
(9) The main **visual area** lies dorsomedially along the caudal half of the brain (along the caudal half of the marginal gyrus).

B. Diencephalon. The diencephalon forms the most rostral limit of the brain stem, and is composed of the large thalamus, the metathalamus, and the much smaller hypothalamus, epithalamus, and subthalamus. Among these five parts, only the hypothalamus is visible externally.

1. **Thalamus**
   a. **Location.** The thalamus is by far the largest part of the diencephalon. In the definitive form, it comprises a large central mass of tissue connected across the midline and extending to a moderate degree on either side.
   b. **Function.** The thalamus is composed of almost three dozen nuclei, and serves mainly as a **major relay center.** Input of almost any kind to the cerebral cortex first passes through the thalamus. The thalamus receives and/or processes the following types of information:
      (1) All sensory input, except for olfactory input
      (2) Output from the basal nuclei that is then relayed to the motor cortex
      (3) Feedback from motor pathway control systems
      (4) Information from cerebellar regulation pathways
      (5) Information from the reticular activating system (which functions in the maintenance of wakefulness)

2. **Metathalamus.** The metathalamus is composed of the lateral and medial geniculate bodies.
   a. The **lateral geniculate body** (Figure 13–4) projects laterally from the caudodorsal surface of the thalamus. The lateral geniculate body contains the **lateral geniculate nucleus** and is involved with **vision.**
      (1) The lateral geniculate body receives input from the **optic tract** and sends output through the **optic radiations** to the visual cortex.
      (2) The lateral geniculate body has connections with the **rostral colliculus** of the midbrain, which is involved in reflexive movements of the eye.
   b. The **medial geniculate body** (see Figure 13–4) is situated caudoventral to the lateral geniculate body, and it forms the caudal limit of the diencephalon. The medial geniculate body contains the **medial geniculate nucleus** and is involved with **auditory function.** The medial geniculate body receives input from the **caudal colliculus** and also sends output to the **caudal colliculus** of the midbrain and the **cerebral cortical auditory areas.**

3. **Subthalamus.** The subthalamus contains the **subthalamic nuclei** and some other small structures, which are sometimes included among the basal nuclei.

4. The **epithalamus** is a very small structure located on the dorsal midline of the thalamus, consisting of the pineal gland and the habenula.
   a. The **pineal gland** is a tiny endocrine gland that produces melatonin as well as secretions affecting sexual activity.
   b. The **habenula** contains the nuclei and has a tract associated with it. The habenula appears to function in producing visceral responses, particularly in association with smell.

5. **Hypothalamus.** The hypothalamus is situated on the ventral surface of the thalamus.
   a. **Surface structures.** The hypothalamus presents several surface structures of note.
      (1) The **optic nerve** passes into the brain at the rostral end of the hypothalamus, and the **optic chiasm** crosses the ventral surface of the hypothalamus at its rostral extent (see Figure 13–2, 13–4).

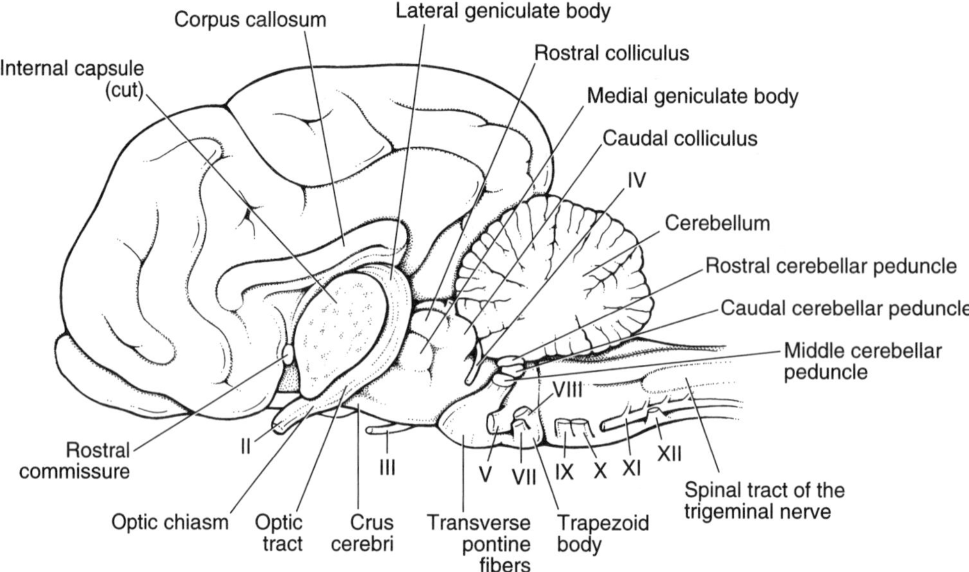

FIGURE 13–4. Lateral view of the brain with the left cerebral hemisphere and the left half of the cerebellum removed. *Roman numerals* indicate cranial nerves: *II* = optic nerve, *III* = oculomotor nerve, *IV* = trochlear nerve, *V* = trigeminal nerve, *VII* = facial nerve, *VIII* = vestibulocochlear nerve, *IX* = glossopharyngeal nerve, *X* = vagus nerve, *XI* = accessory nerve, *XII* = hypoglossal nerve.

(2) The **tuber cinereum** is located between the optic chiasm rostrally and the mammillary bodies caudally.

(3) The **hypophysis** is comprised of the **neurohypophysis** and the **adenohypophysis.**

- **(a)** The **neurohypophysis,** the neural portion of the hypophysis (pituitary gland), arises from the tuber cinereum.
  - **(i)** The neurohypophysis is composed of the **infundibulum,** a stalk-like extension of the hypothalamus, and the **neural lobe,** its main portion.
  - **(ii)** The neurohypophysis secretes oxytocin and antidiuretic hormone.
- **(b)** The **adenohypophysis,** a glandular structure, forms from an evagination from the pharynx. The adenohypophysis secretes several trophic hormones that control the major endocrine axes.

(4) The **mammillary bodies** are small, paired, round elevations at the caudal end of the hypothalamus, just rostral to the infundibulum (see Figure 13–2).

- **(a)** Each mammillary body, despite its small size, contains at least three nuclei.
- **(b)** The mammillary bodies function in affective (emotional) behavior.

b. Functions. The hypothalamus has **numerous diverse functions,** that can be divided into two major groups:

(1) Regulation of the endocrine system, via the hypophysis

(2) Regulation of many visceral and behavioral functions, such as:

- **(a)** Thermoregulation, appetite, the sleep—wake cycle
- **(b)** Major affective behaviors, such as pleasure, rage, escape
- **(c)** Control of the autonomic nervous system (ANS) as related to gastrointestinal, respiratory, cardiovascular, and urinary function

III. MIDBRAIN.

The **ventral surface** of the midbrain, or mesencephalon, is **visible externally** in the intact brain, where its **crura cerebri** are plain (see Figure 13–2). The **dorsal surface** is entirely hidden in the intact state by the cerebral hemispheres (see Figure 13–4).

The midbrain is organized into two layers, the dorsally positioned tectum, and the ventrally positioned cerebral peduncles.

A. **Tectum.** Two pairs of rounded eminences, the rostral and caudal colliculi, are visible on the dorsal surface of the tectum. The term **"corpora quadrigemina"** is sometimes used to refer to all four of the colliculi together.

1. The **rostral colliculi** (singular, colliculus) are adjacent to each other on each side of the midline (Figure 13–5).
   a. The rostral colliculi are **relay posts in the visual pathway.** In addition, they play a role in **visual reflexes** [e.g., the palpebral response (blinking), pupillary adjustment, orientation of the eyes and head toward an abrupt visual stimulus].
   b. The rostral colliculi are linked to the lateral geniculate bodies (which also have a role in visual function) by a not-prominent tract of fibers, the **brachium of the rostral colliculus.**
2. The **caudal colliculi** lie just caudal to the rostral colliculi, but are more lateral and thus more widely spaced across the midline (see Figure 13–5). The caudal colliculi are joined to each other by a stout commissure.
   a. The caudal colliculi integrate the **auditory pathways.** In addition, they play a role in the **auditory reflexes** (e.g., orientation of the ears and head toward an abrupt auditory stimulus).
   b. A prominent **brachium of the caudal colliculus** joins each caudal colliculus to the ipsilateral medial geniculate bodies (which, not unexpectedly, also have a role in auditory function).
   c. The **trochlear nerve (cranial nerve IV)** is unique among the cranial nerves in that it is the only cranial nerve to leave the brain by its dorsal surface, adjacent to the caudal colliculus (see Figures 13–4, 13–5). The nerve then courses laterally and ventrally to reach the ventral surface of the brain stem before making its way to the orbital fissure.

B. **Cerebral peduncles** (paired right and left) form the ventral part of the mesencephalon (see Figure 13–5). Each cerebral peduncle is itself composed of, from dorsal to ventral, the tegmentum, the substantia nigra, and the crus cerebri.

1. The **tegmentum** forms the main substance of the mesencephalon.
   a. A considerable portion of the **reticular formation** is located in the tegmentum.
   b. The **nuclei of several cranial nerves** are positioned in the tegmentum, including the:
      (1) Motor nucleus of the oculomotor nerve (cranial nerve III)
      (2) Parasympathetic nucleus of the oculomotor nerve (cranial nerve III)
      (3) Motor nucleus of the trochlear nerve (cranial nerve IV)
   c. The **red nucleus,** which functions in motor activity, is also located in the tegmentum.
2. The **substantia nigra** is a dark lamina associated with control of voluntary movement.
3. The **crura cerebri** (see Figures 13–2, 13–4) are formed of fibers traveling from the cerebral cortex to the spinal cord. These fibers are continuations of fibers in the internal capsule (see Figure 13–4).
   a. The **interpeduncular fossa** (see Figure 13–2) is the small triangular space between the two crura cerebri. The derivation of the name, "interpeduncular fossa," becomes plain when one considers that the crura cerebri are part of the cerebral peduncle.
   b. The **oculomotor nerve (cranial nerve III)** exits the brain at the medial edge of the crus cerebri (see Figure 13–4).

IV. HINDBRAIN.

The hindbrain consists of two regions, the more rostral metencephalon (i.e., the pons and cerebellum), and the more caudal myelencephalon (i.e., the medulla oblongata).

A. **Metencephalon.** The metencephalon is sharply divided into dorsal and ventral parts, these being the cerebellum and the pons, respectively (see Figure 13–1).

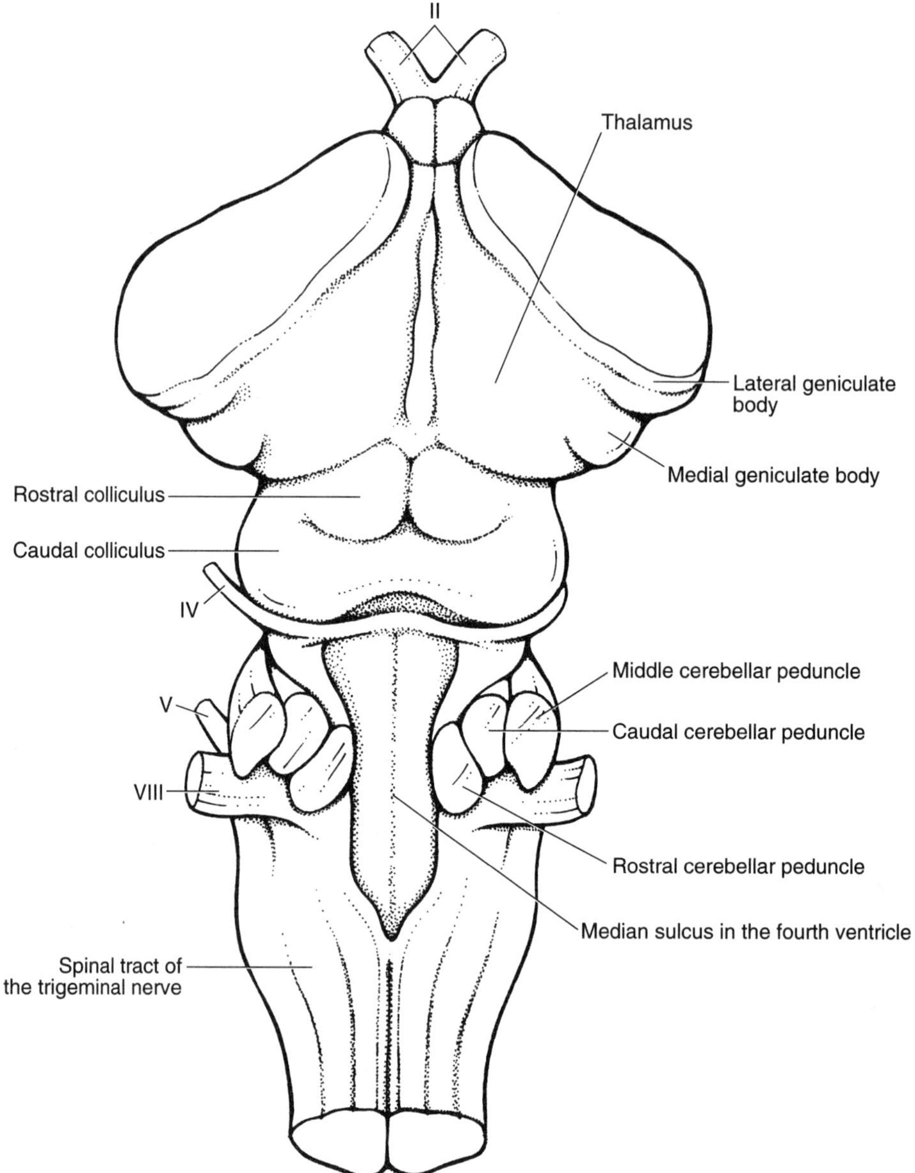

FIGURE 13–5. Isolated brain stem, dorsal view. Several structures of the midbrain are clearly visible, including the caudal and rostral colliculi and the cerebellar peduncles. The peduncles are positioned roughly in a linear arrangement from lateral to medial. *Roman numerals* indicate cranial nerves: *II* = optic nerve, *IV* = trochlear nerve, *V* = trigeminal nerve, *VIII* = vestibulocochlear nerve.

1. Cerebellum

a. Functions

(1) Coordination of posture and movement is the primary function of the cerebellum. In order to promote smooth and effective movement, the cerebellum continually compares motor command input with ongoing proprioceptive and tactile input to permit instantaneous adjustments of speed and direction.

(2) Regulation of muscle tone is also a role played by the cerebellum.

(3) **Maintenance of equilibrium.** The cerebellum is essential to equilibrium maintenance.

b. **Surface organization.** The cerebellum is a hemispherical mass of tissue perched atop the brain stem just caudal to the cerebrum. It is separated from the cerebrum by the **transverse cerebral fissure,** into which projects the **tentorium cerebelli,** a fold of dura mater. The surface of the cerebellum is roughened by a multitude of folds.

(1) **Regions.** The cerebellum presents three regions which, though immediately recognizable grossly, have little to do with functional relations. These regions are the:

(a) **Vermis,** the relatively narrow median ridge

(b) **Two cerebellar hemispheres,** which are larger and paired

(2) **Lobes.** The lobation pattern is more representative of functional regions of the cerebellum. A series of transverse ridges divides the cerebellum into **lobes, lobules,** and then **folia.** These divisions are named down to and including each individual lobule, but only the names of the larger lobes are of interest here.

(a) The **flocculonodular lobe** is the smallest, caudally placed lobe. This region is the most phylogenetically ancient portion of the cerebellum, and hence can be referred to as the **paleocerebellum.**

(b) The **rostral lobe** is still very old, but not as ancient as the flocculonodular lobe. It is referred to as the **archicerebellum.**

(c) The **caudal lobe** is, phylogenetically, the most recent lobe and can be termed the **neocerebellum.**

c. **Composition.** The overall arrangement of the grey and white matter of the cerebellum is essentially similar to that of the remainder of the brain.

(1) The bulk of the **grey matter** is positioned **superficially,** although the superficial layer is thinner than in the cerebrum.

(2) The **white matter** is positioned **deeply.** This region of white matter is referred to as the **medulla of the cerebellum.**

(3) Additional grey matter collections, the **cerebellar nuclei,** are individually named, but that detail will not be presented here.

d. **Cerebellar peduncles.** The cerebellar peduncles attach the cerebellum to the brain stem (see Figures 13–4, 13–5). Three pairs of peduncles are present, the rostral, middle, and caudal. Confusion can quickly develop if an attempt is made to relate the names of the peduncles to their position on the brain stem: **the cerebellar peduncles are named for the position of origin of the tracts contained within them, rather than according to their surface placement.**

(1) The **rostral cerebellar peduncle** arises in the **midbrain.** This peduncle conveys largely (though not exclusively) efferent fibers, from the cerebellum to the brain stem.

(2) The **middle cerebellar peduncle** arises in the **pontine nuclei** on the contralateral side of the brain stem. The fibers leave their home side, pass ventrally under the brain stem as the **transverse fibers of the pons,** and then enter the cerebellar hemisphere on the contralateral side as the middle cerebellar peduncle. This peduncle conveys exclusively afferent fibers.

(3) The **caudal cerebellar peduncle** communicates with the medulla and conveys largely afferent fibers.

2. **Pons.** The pons is divided into two regions, the dorsal tegmentum of the pons, and the ventral transverse fibers of the pons.

a. The **tegmentum of the pons** (not to be confused with the tegmentum of the mesencephalon!) contains numerous structures, many of which will not be detailed here. Prominent features of the pontine tegmentum include the:

(1) **Pontine reticular nuclei**

(2) **Nuclei and tracts associated with the trigeminal nerve (cranial nerve V).** The trigeminal nerve exits the brain stem at the caudolateral aspect of the transverse pontine fibers (see Figure 13–2). The following nuclei and tracts are associated with the trigeminal nerve and located in the pontine tegmentum:

(a) The nuclei of the spinal tract of the trigeminal nerve
(b) The pontine sensory nuclei of the trigeminal nerve
(c) The motor nuclei of the trigeminal nerve

b. The **transverse fibers of the pons** are ventrally situated, and demarcated clearly at the superficial level from the remainder of the brain stem (see Figure 13–2). Although the superficial distinction between the transverse pontine fibers and the medulla oblongata is plain, more deeply, the communications between the pons and the medulla oblongata are very extensive, blurring the distinction considerably. The transverse pontine fibers originate in the pontine nuclei of one cerebellar hemisphere and cross to the contralateral side to enter the cerebellum as the middle cerebellar peduncle.

c. The **longitudinal fibers of the pons** are the continuation of the fibers from each crus cerebri (which in turn originated in the corona radiata of the cerebral hemispheres). Some longitudinal fibers synapse on the pontine nuclei, while others pass directly through to the pyramids.

B. **Myelencephalon (medulla oblongata).** The medulla extends from the transverse pontine fibers to the site of origin of the first cervical spinal nerve, at which point the medulla continues as the spinal cord. A large number of tracts, general nuclei, and cranial nerve nuclei are located within the medulla.

1. **Surface organization**
   a. **Trapezoid body** (see Figures 13–2, 13–4). The trapezoid body is a transverse band of fibers at the caudal edge of the transverse pontine fibers. These fibers are **continuous with the vestibulocochlear nerve (cranial nerve VIII)** and **the cochlear nuclei.** Thus, the trapezoid body has auditory function.
   b. **Pyramids** (see Figure 13–2). The pyramids are paired sets of longitudinal fibers on the ventral surface of the myelencephalon, just caudal to the pons and superficial to the trapezoid body. The fibers of the pyramids are the continuation of the longitudinal fibers of the pons, which become superficial again caudal to the transverse pontine fibers.
   c. **Decussation of the pyramids.** This is the region where the pyramids eventually disappear from view (see Figure 13–2). Here, the fibers disperse into the substance of the spinal cord, where they continue as various corticospinal tracts. Most of the fibers **cross the midline** (i.e., they **decussate) to continue on the opposite side of the body from their point of origin,** which explains why the left side of the brain controls the right side of the body, and vice versa.
2. **Composition.** The medulla contains:
   a. **Gray matter nuclei** (relay, cranial nerve, reticular formation, and cerebellar projection nuclei, among others)
   b. **White matter tracts,** including cranial nerve fibers, connections with the cerebellum, and fibers traversing and terminating in the medulla
   c. The **reticular formation,** intermixed grey and white matter
3. **Internal features.** Prominent internal features include, but are not limited to, the following structures.
   a. **Rostral region**
      (1) Dorsal and ventral trapezoid nuclei
      (2) Motor nuclei of the abducent nerve (cranial nerve VI)
      (3) Dorsal and ventral cochlear nuclei [associated with the vestibulocochlear nerve (cranial nerve VIII)]
   b. **Midregion**
      (1) Motor nucleus of the facial nerve (cranial nerve VII)
      (2) Parasympathetic nucleus of the facial nerve (cranial nerve VII)
      (3) Four vestibular nuclei
   c. **Caudal region**
      (1) Reticular formation
      (2) Olivary nucleus, associated with posture

(3) Parasympathetic nucleus of the vagus nerve (cranial nerve X)
(4) Motor nucleus of the hypoglossal nerve (cranial nerve XII)
(5) Nucleus ambiguus
(6) Solitary tract, containing visceral afferent axons

d. At the junction with the spinal cord

(1) Fasciculus cuneatus and medial cuneate nucleus, which function in discriminatory touch and kinesthesia from the thoracic limb and neck
(2) Fasciculus gracilis and nucleus gracilis, which function in discriminatory touch and kinesthesia from the caudal half of the body
(3) Spinal tract of the trigeminal nerve (cranial nerve V), which conveys input regarding nociception, temperature, and crude touch from the face, nasal cavity, oral cavity, and teeth

V. VENTRICULAR SYSTEM

V. VENTRICULAR SYSTEM (Figure 13–6). The central regions of the brain possess a system of fluid-filled cavities derived from the central canal of the primitive neural tube. This ventricular system contains the cerebrospinal fluid essential to the health of the central nervous system (CNS; see Chapter 4 II A 3).

A. Lateral ventricles

1. The lateral ventricles are curved in the form of a half circle within the substance of the cerebral hemispheres (see Figure 13–6). A rostral and a caudal extension are present, with the rostral extension possibly joining the fluid space within the olfactory bulb peduncle (i.e., the olfactory bulb cavity).
2. Each hemisphere contains one lateral ventricle, and the two lateral ventricles communicate with the third ventricle by way of the **interventricular foramen.**

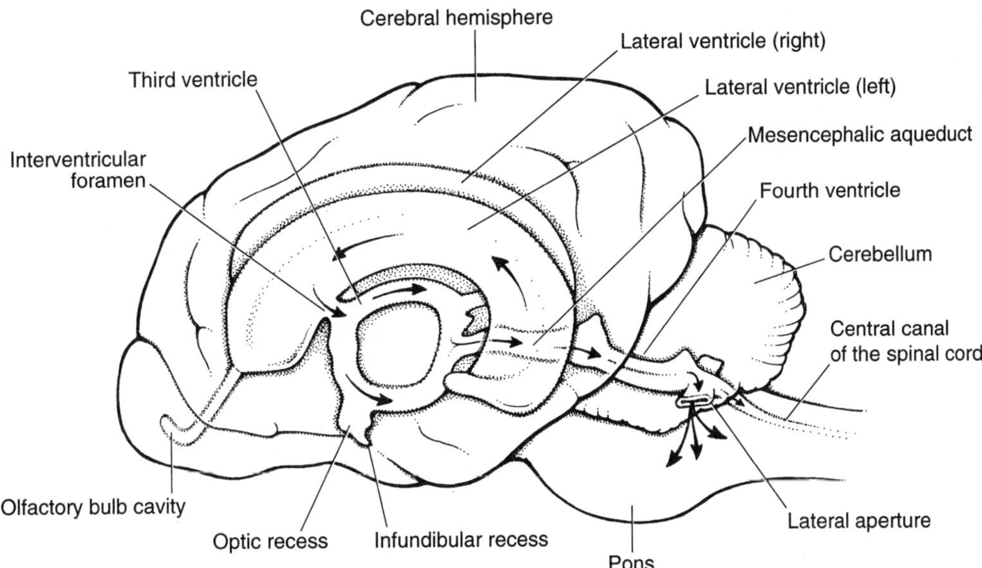

FIGURE 13–6. The ventricular system. *Arrows* indicate the flow of cerebrospinal fluid. Cerebrospinal fluid is produced by the choroid plexuses, capillary tufts that extend through the roofs and sides of the ventricles in several places, including the floor of the lateral ventricles and the roof of the third and fourth ventricles. The cerebrospinal fluid flows through the ventricles and directly into the central canal of the spinal cord or through the lateral apertures into the subarachnoid space. (Modified with permission from Evans HE, 1993, *Miller's Anatomy of the Dog,* 3e. Philadelphia, WB Saunders, p 825.)

B. Third ventricle. The third ventricle lies within the diencephalon. It is ring-shaped, with the interthalamic adhesion occupying the central space of the ring (see Figure 13–6). The third ventricle communicates caudally with the mesencephalic aqueduct.

C. Mesencephalic aqueduct. The mesencephalic aqueduct is the equivalent of a "ventricle" of the mesencephalon. Because the mesencephalon does not change drastically during development from its original tubular form, the mesencephalic aqueduct is a simple tube that connects the third ventricle rostrally with the fourth ventricle caudally (see Figure 13–6).

D. Fourth ventricle. The fourth ventricle lies within the pons (ventral to the cerebellum), and extends into the medulla oblongata. The fourth ventricle is incompletely closed dorsally, where it is roofed by the caudal medullary velum.

1. From the medulla oblongata, the fourth ventricle becomes continuous with the **central canal of the spinal cord** at the level of the foramen magnum, allowing cerebrospinal fluid to flow caudally into the central canal of the spinal cord.
2. The fourth ventricle also communicates with the subarachnoid space at the paired **lateral apertures.** Cerebrospinal fluid flows into the subarachnoid space through these apertures.

Canine Clinical Correlation

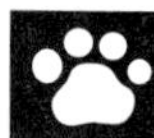

When production of cerebrospinal fluid exceeds resorption, the pressure in the ventricles of the brain can increase to the extent that the expanding ventricular spaces compress the overlying brain parenchyma, causing cell loss, which can lead to clinical signs. This condition is known as **hydrocephalus.** When caused by mechanical obstruction of flow, the site most usually obstructed is the mesencephalic aqueduct, due to its narrow tubular nature.

VI. VASCULATURE OF THE BRAIN

A. Arterial supply. The arterial supply to the brain is delivered mainly through two arterial structures, the **arterial circle of the brain,** which supplies all of the cerebrum and the rostral cerebellum, and the **basilar artery,** which provides major amounts of blood directly to the arterial circle of the brain, as well as supplying the major artery to the caudal cerebellar regions (Figure 13–7).

1. **Arterial circle of the brain.** The arterial circle of the brain is located on the ventral surface of the hypothalamus. **Sources of arterial blood to the circle** include the **basilar artery** and the **internal carotid arteries.**
   a. **Basilar artery.** The basilar artery forms as the cranial continuation of the ventral spinal artery (coursing along the ventral midline of the spinal cord) after the right and left vertebral arteries join the flow. The basilar artery courses along the ventral midline of the brain stem from the region of the decussation of the pyramids to the rostral edge of the transverse pontine fibers.
      (1) **Sources.** The basilar artery is supplied by the:
         (a) Small, unpaired **ventral spinal artery**
         (b) Large, paired **vertebral arteries,** which bring the bulk of the blood to the basilar artery
      (2) **Branches.** The basilar artery divides into the paired **caudal communicating arteries** just at the rostral edge of the transverse pontine fibers. The right and left caudal communicating arteries travel rostrally to anastomose with the other vessels of the circle.
   b. **Internal carotid arteries.** The right and left internal carotid arteries also supply blood to the arterial circle of the brain. The internal carotid arteries are one of the terminal branches of the external carotid artery.

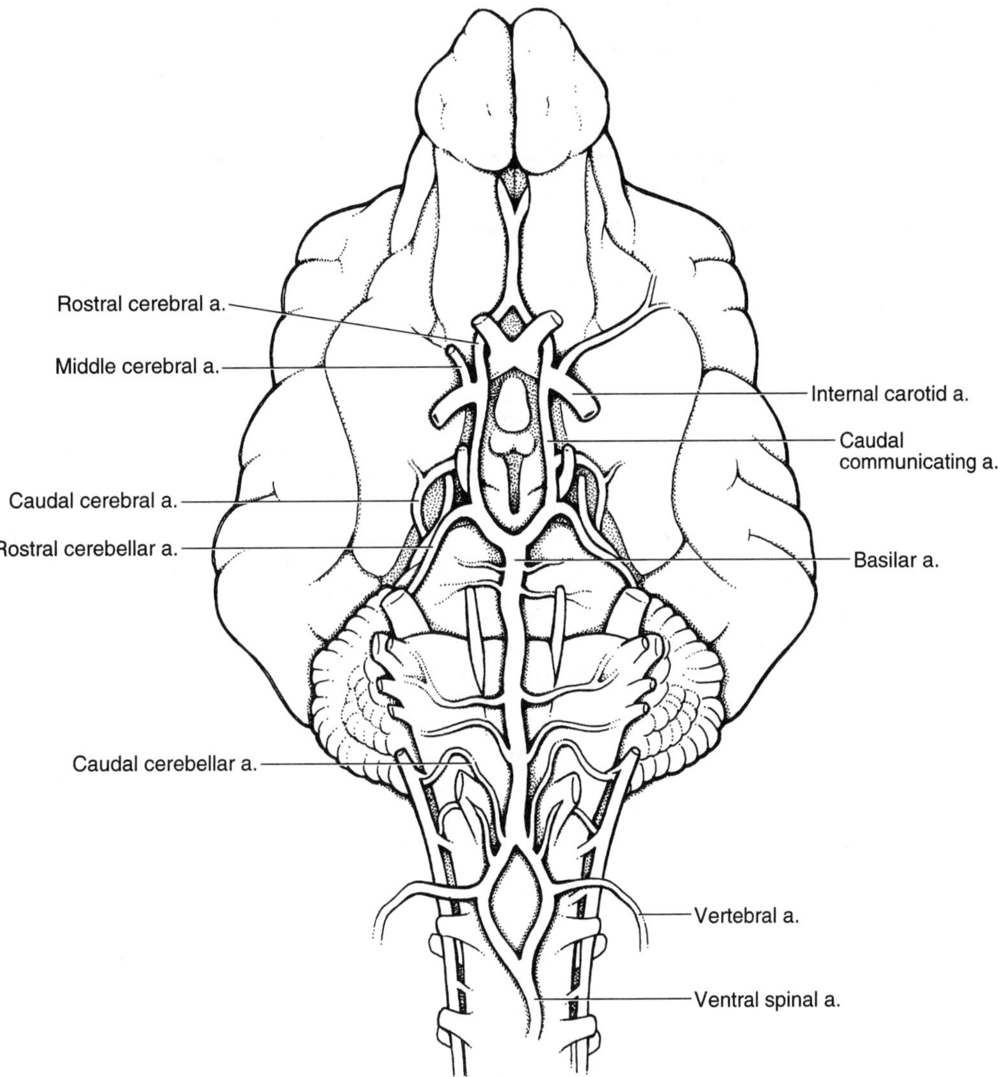

FIGURE 13–7. Arterial supply of the brain.

(1) Course. The internal carotid arteries approach the skull by a convoluted course, involving (in part):

   (a) Entrance to the skull via the caudal carotid foramen

   (b) Momentary exit from the skull through the foramen lacerum, followed by immediate return to the skull by the same foramen

   (c) Perforation of the external dural layer and passage through the cavernous sinus

   (d) Perforation of the internal dural layer and entrance to the subarachnoid space

(2) Branches. On penetrating the arachnoid membrane, the internal carotid divides into two branches, one passing rostrally and one caudally. (Note that the internal carotid is sometimes described as trifurcating; however, one of those "branches" is more conveniently thought of as arising from the arterial circle.)

   (a) The **rostral cerebral artery** passes forward and anastomoses with its fellow from the other side.

(b) The **caudal communicating artery** is the name given to the caudally directed branch of the internal carotid artery, as well as to the branches of the basilar artery. This point of possible confusion can be allayed by noting that the two vessels eventually become continuous. The caudal communicating artery anastomoses with the rostrally directed branch of the basilar artery and provides numerous small, direct **rostral hypophyseal arteries** on its course past the hypophysis.

2. **Arterial supply to the cerebrum** is supplied by three of the four paired branches of the arterial circle.
   a. **Rostral cerebral artery.** The rostral cerebral artery can be considered a continuation of the same-named artery from the internal carotid, as well as a branch of the arterial circle.
      (1) **Areas supplied.** The rostral cerebral artery supplies both the **cortex and medulla of the region of the frontal lobes.**
      (2) **Course.** The rostral cerebral artery leaves the arterial circle at its rostral end (rostral to the optic chiasm) and passes toward the longitudinal fissure. In the region of the optic nerve, it joins its fellow from the opposite side to form a single vessel that courses rostrally for some distance. Eventually, it separates and passes dorsally (as two separate rostral cerebral arteries, one on each side) into the longitudinal fissure between the two frontal lobes. From the longitudinal fissure, it turns caudally and passes along the dorsal surface of the corpus callosum, giving off numerous substantial branches in its path.
      (3) **Branches.** Notable branches of the rostral cerebral artery include the:
         (a) **Internal ophthalmic artery,** a small artery that passes rostrally along the optic nerve to anastomose with the external ophthalmic artery to supply the globe of the eye
         (b) **Internal ethmoid artery,** which anastomoses with the external ethmoid artery, and passes rostrally through the cribriform plate to supply the ethmoturbinates and part of the nasal septum
   b. **Middle cerebral artery.** The middle cerebral artery is the **largest vessel supplying the brain.**
      (1) **Areas supplied.** The middle cerebral artery supplies the **entire lateral surface of the brain.**
      (2) **Course.** The middle cerebral artery arises from the arterial circle of the brain at the level of the hypothalamus and courses laterally over the ventral surface of the olfactory peduncle, just rostral to the piriform lobe.
      (3) **Branches.** The middle cerebral artery provides the **choroid artery** to the choroid plexus of the lateral ventricle.
   c. **Caudal cerebral artery.** The caudal cerebral artery is easily distinguished from the neighboring rostral cerebellar artery because the oculomotor nerve (cranial nerve VIII) crosses the ventral surface of the caudal cerebral artery.
      (1) **Areas supplied.** The caudal cerebral artery supplies the:
         (a) **Medial surface of the caudal cerebral hemisphere**
         (b) **Diencephalon**
         (c) **Rostral parts of the mesencephalon**
      (2) **Course.** The caudal cerebral artery arises from the basilar artery's portion of the caudal communicating branch at the caudal edge of the hypophysis, just rostral to the oculomotor nerve (cranial nerve VIII). It then courses caudodorsally, following the optic tract, to approach the longitudinal fissure from the caudal direction. It enters the longitudinal fissure and passes cranially on the dorsal surface of the corpus callosum, as a sort of a mirror image of the rostral cerebral artery.

3. **Arterial supply to the cerebellum**
   a. **Rostral cerebellar artery.** The rostral cerebellar artery is the fourth (and last) large branch of the arterial circle of the brain.
      (1) **Areas supplied.** The rostral cerebellar artery supplies the **caudal half of the mesencephalon** and the **rostral cerebellar regions.**

(2) **Course.** The rostral cerebellar artery departs from the caudal third of the arterial circle and passes dorsally and caudally along the ventral surface of the mesencephalon to disappear from view in the angle formed by the caudal edge of the piriform lobe and the transverse pontine fibers.

b. **Caudal cerebellar artery.** The caudal cerebellar artery is the only major artery to the brain that arises directly from the basilar artery.

(1) **Areas supplied.** The caudal cerebellar artery courses dorsally to supply the **caudal cerebellar regions.**

(2) **Course.** The caudal cerebellar artery leaves the basilar artery caudal to the trapezoid body and halfway caudally along the pyramids. It passes directly laterally, disappearing after it passes caudally to the root of the vagus nerve (cranial nerve X).

B. Venous drainage

1. **Venous sinuses** are specialized structures that provide the major route of venous drainage for many cranial structures. They receive the venous drainage from the **brain** and **skull** and deliver this blood to the **maxillary vein, internal jugular vein, vertebral veins,** and **vertebral venous plexuses.**

a. **Structure.** The venous sinuses have **neither muscle in their walls, nor valves.**

b. **Location.** The venous sinuses are located between the external and internal layers of particular areas of the dura mater and within certain bony canals of the skull.

c. **Arrangement.** The venous sinuses are organized into a dorsal grouping and a ventral grouping (Figure 13–8). All of the sinuses freely communicate with each other (because they have no valves).

(1) **Dorsal venous sinuses**

(a) The **dorsal sagittal sinus** forms at the confluence of the right and left rhinal veins. It is located just ventral to the sagittal suture of the skull, and extends from the margin of the cribriform plate over the dorsal surface of the brain along and within the attached side of the falx cerebri. It terminates by passing through a foramen in the occipital bone (i.e., the foramen impar), where it joins the right and left transverse sinuses in a region called the **confluence of the sinuses.**

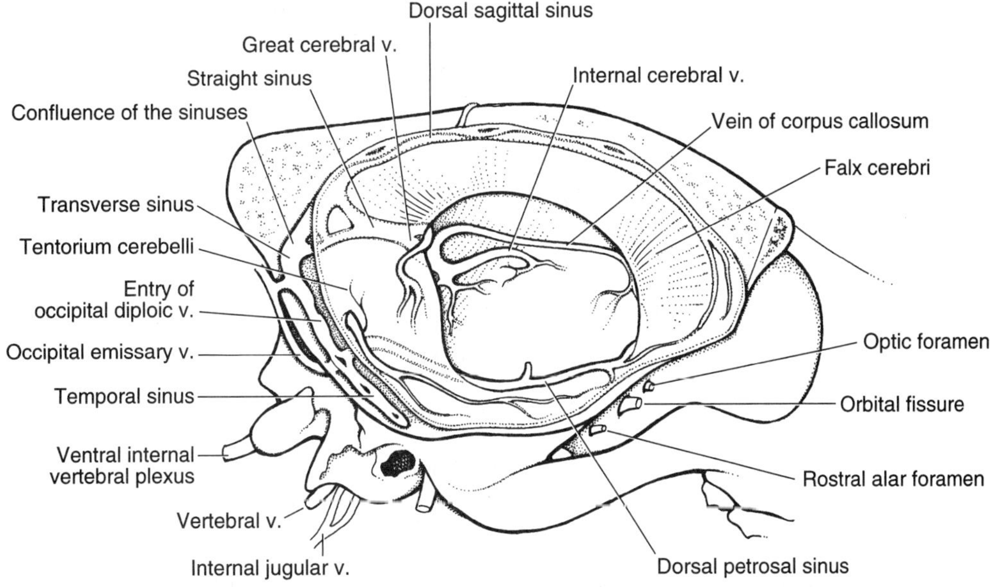

FIGURE 13–8. Dural venous sinuses and veins of the brain. (Modified with permission from Evans HE, 1993, *Miller's Anatomy of the Dog,* 3e. Philadelphia, WB Saunders, p 709.)

(b) The **straight sinus** lies along the caudal border of the falx cerebri, near the tentorium cerebelli. It is formed by the confluence of the great cerebral vein and the vein of the corpus callosum, and usually terminates by entering the dorsal sagittal sinus near its termination. Alternatively, it can follow an independent course to the confluence of the sinuses.

(c) The **transverse sinuses** form caudodorsally, at the most caudal extent of the cranial region, in the region of the confluence of the sinuses. They pass laterally in the transverse canal of the skull, and then leave the canal to continue in the transverse groove. They terminate at the end of the transverse groove by dividing into the temporal and sigmoid sinuses.

(2) **Ventral venous sinuses**

(a) The **temporal sinuses** form as a continuation of the transverse sinuses, essentially continuing in the same general path as the transverse sinuses and then turning ventrally. They pass between the petrous and squamous parts of the temporal bone and terminate after passing through the retroarticular foramen as the **retroarticular vein,** which in turn enters the **maxillary vein.**

(b) The **sigmoid sinuses** form as the caudoventral continuation of the transverse sinuses. They extend in a sigmoid course along the base of the cranial cavity in the region of the petrous temporal bone. After passing through the tympanooccipital fissure, the sigmoid sinuses divide and continue as the **internal jugular vein** and the **vertebral vein.**

(c) The **basilar sinus** forms as the continuation of the **condyloid vein** as that vein leaves the sigmoid sinus through the condyloid canal. The basilar sinus continues caudally from the condyloid canal on the ventral surface of the brain stem until it becomes the **vertebral venous plexus** on the ventral surface of the spinal cord.

(d) The **dorsal petrosal sinuses** are the **caudal extensions of the basal vein of the cerebrum.** They course along the lateral surface of the pyramids and terminate by entering the **temporal sinus.**

(e) The **ventral petrosal sinuses** form at the caudal end of the cavernous sinus and extend to the ventral end of the sigmoid sinus. They lie in the petroccipital canal, thus essentially representing a continuation of the cavernous sinus.

(f) The **cavernous sinuses** form at the **orbital fissure** by confluence of the ophthalmic plexus and extend along the floor of the cranial cavity to the petroccipital fissure. They terminate by passing into the petroccipital fissure, where they are continued as the **ventral petrosal sinuses.**

(i) The cavernous sinuses **communicate freely with each other** by means of the rostral and caudal **intercavernous sinuses.**

(ii) The lumen of the cavernous sinuses houses the **middle meningeal artery,** the **anastomotic branch of the external ophthalmic artery,** and part of the **internal carotid artery.**

2. **Veins**

a. **General considerations**

(1) Some arteries of the brain have satellite veins sharing their names, but an additional set of veins is present that has no arterial parallel.

(2) Like the venous sinuses, the veins of the brain have neither valves nor muscle in their walls.

(3) The veins of the brain empty into the dural venous sinuses.

b. **Veins of the cerebrum**

(1) The **dorsal cerebral veins** are **paired,** but not always symmetrical, and may be variable in number (from one to four). They drain nearly the entire cortex of the cerebrum, and terminate in the **dorsal sagittal sinus.**

(2) The **ventral cerebral vein** is unpaired and drains most of the cortex of the temporal lobe. The ventral cerebral vein terminates in the **dorsal petrosal sinus.**

(3) The **great cerebral vein** is unpaired and provides the **sole drainage route for the deep veins of the cerebrum.** It terminates in the **straight sinus.**

(a) The great cerebral vein occupies the triangular space between the vermis and the two cerebral hemispheres.

(b) It receives the:

(i) **Vein of the corpus callosum** (from the dorsal surface of the corpus callosum)

(ii) **Internal cerebral veins** (a cluster of veins from the dorsal regions of the mesencephalon)

c. **Veins of the cerebellum**

(1) The **dorsal cerebellar veins,** which are **paired,** are positioned in the fissures between the vermis and the cerebellar hemispheres. They terminate in the **transverse sinus.**

(2) The **ventral cerebellar veins** are **paired,** minute veins positioned between the cerebellar hemispheres and the medulla. They terminate variably among individuals, either into the **sigmoid** or the **basilar sinus.**

d. **Veins of the pons.** The **pontine veins** are **paired.** They are positioned transversely on the ventrolateral surface of the pons, and they terminate in the **sigmoid sinus.**

e. **Veins of the medulla.** The **medullary veins** are **paired** and positioned longitudinally on the ventrolateral surface of the medulla, lateral to the pyramids. They terminate in the **basilar sinuses.**

f. **Veins of the diploë.** The **diploic veins** drain the cancellous bone—filled space between the internal and external tables of the skull (in areas where this space, the diploë, is developed).

(1) The **frontal diploic vein,** which may be double, drains rostrally into the **angular vein of the eye** and caudally into the **sagittal sinus** or a **dorsal cerebral vein.**

(2) The **parietal diploic vein,** which may also be double, drains into the **sagittal sinus.**

(3) The **occipital diploic vein,** which may be double or even triple, drains into the **transverse sinus.**

Chapter 14

The Ear

I. INTRODUCTION

A. Structure of the ear. The ear is composed of three parts. From superficial to deep, as well as from most evolutionarily advanced to primitive, these are the external, middle, and inner ear.

1. The **external ear** consists of the portion of the ear that is visible from the surface (the pinna) and the ear canal, which leads from the surface to the tympanic membrane (eardrum).
2. The **middle ear** consists of the small cavity within the petrous part of the temporal bone medial to the tympanic membrane, together with the structures contained within the cavity.
3. The **inner ear** consists of a delicate, tiny, and intricate system of closed membranous ducts and cavities housed within the petrous part of the temporal bone.

B. Functions of the ear. Although the sense of hearing is of course correctly associated with the ear, this organ also plays a critical role in maintaining balance.

1. **Hearing.** The ear transduces mechanical energy (in the form of sound waves) into electrical energy (in the form of nerve impulses), and transmits that information to the brain. The external, middle, and inner ear play a role in hearing.
2. **Balance.** The ear delivers information to the brain on the position and movement of the head as related to gravitational pull, thus giving the animal positional information about its head and body. Only the inner ear is involved with balance.

II. EXTERNAL EAR. The external ear is discussed in detail in Chapter 11 I A 5.

A. Pinna. The pinna is the portion of the ear that is visible externally. The pinna is supported by the auricular cartilage, and provided with three groups of muscles, the **rostral, caudal,** and **ventral auricular muscles.** These muscles are capable of directing the pinnae independently of each other in multiple directions to facilitate sound capture.

B. Ear canal. For most of its length, the ear canal is cartilaginous, but the most proximal part, immediately adjacent to the skull, includes a few millimeters of bony ring.

III. MIDDLE EAR (Figure 14–1)

A. The **tympanic membrane** is a thin, semi-transparent membrane situated at the lumen of the external acoustic meatus, separating the external ear from the middle ear. The tympanic membrane is attached around its circumference to the temporal bone by the tympanic ring.

1. The tympanic membrane is positioned at an angle to the ear canal, so that its dorsal margin is more lateral than its ventral one.
2. The tympanic membrane is drawn into a somewhat concave profile along its external surface by the attachment of the malleus to the central region of the membrane. The **umbo** is the point on the eardrum most indented by this attachment.

B. The **tympanic cavity** can be divided into three portions.

1. The **epitympanic recess** is the smallest and the most dorsal of the three chambers.

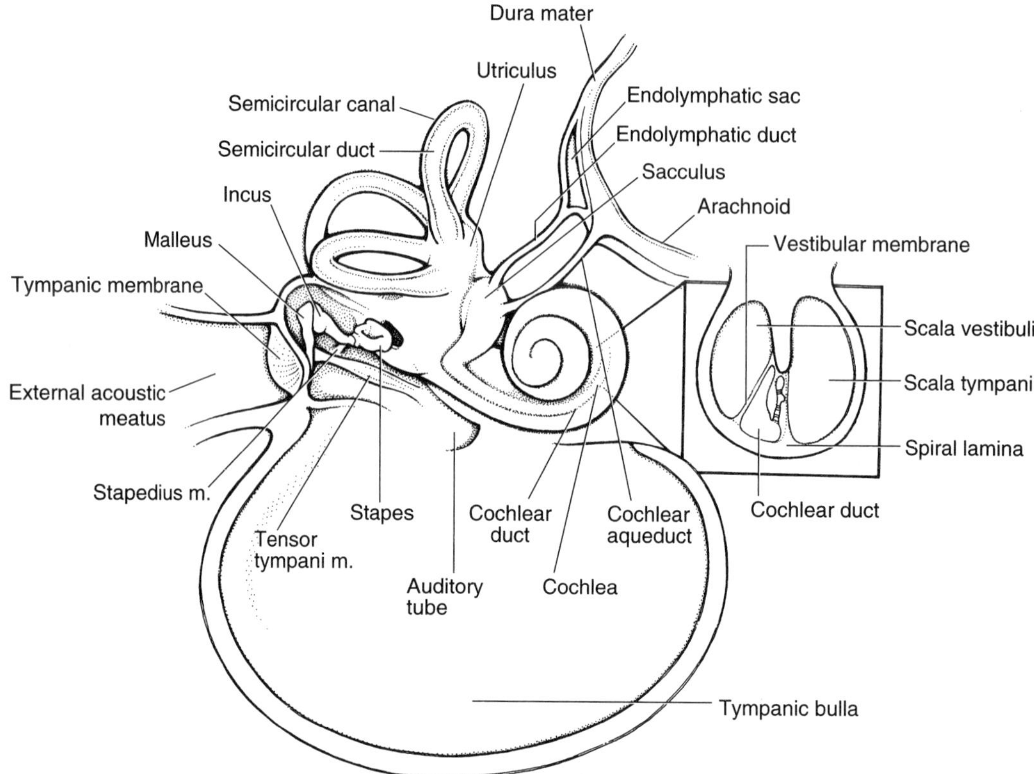

FIGURE 14–1. Schematized drawing of the middle and inner ear. *Inset.* The relation of the bony and membranous labyrinths of the cochlear region results in essentially three chambers within the cochlea, two bony and one membranous. The cochlear duct (which is membranous) is entirely enclosed within the spiral or cochlear canal (which is bony). The bony spiral lamina together with the cochlear duct divide the internal chamber of the cochlea. Thus, a cross-section through a turn of the cochlea reveals a bony-walled chamber ventrally (the scala tympani), which contains perilymph, a membrane-bound chamber centrally (the cochlear duct), which contains endolymph, and a bony-walled chamber dorsally (the scala vestibuli), which contains perilymph. Therefore, both membranes of the cochlear duct are contacted on essentially all sides by fluid (endolymph internally and perilymph externally), a critical factor in the functioning of the inner ear. (Modified with permission from Dellmann H-D, Carithers JR: *NVMS Cytology and Microscopic Anatomy.* Baltimore, Williams & Wilkins, 1996, p 359.)

It contains the **auditory ossicles (bones of the middle ear)** and their **associated muscles.**

a. The **auditory ossicles** are the **malleus,** the **incus,** and the **stapes.** These three tiny bones form a short chain passing along the dorsally positioned epitympanic recess, and function to physically connect the tympanic membrane with the inner ear (see Figure 14–1). A set of ligaments attaches the auditory ossicles to each other and to surrounding structures. These ligaments are descriptively named for these attachments (e.g., "lateral ligament of the malleus"), but the names will not be given here.

(1) The **malleus,** named for its supposed resemblance to a hammer, is the most lateral of the three bones and the one that is adjacent to the tympanic membrane. The largest of the auditory ossicles, the malleus has several identifiable parts and regions, not all of which require mention here.

(a) The **manubrium** (or handle) is the elongated part that is embedded in the fibrous layer of the eardrum, as are certain other bony processes.

Canine Clinical Correlation

A pale streak (the **stria mallearis)** passing dorsocaudally from the umbo is visible during otoscopic examination; this is representative of the area of attachment of the manubrium to the eardrum.

(b) A **tiny hook** on the muscular process of the malleus provides the insertion point for the tensor tympani muscle.

(c) The **head** of the malleus articulates with the next bone in the chain, the incus.

(2) The **incus** is considerably smaller than the malleus. The incus, originally named for its supposed resemblance to an anvil, consists of a body with two tapering, diverging crura extending away from it. The body of the incus articulates with the head of the malleus, while the long crus of the incus articulates with the next bone in the chain, the stapes.

(3) The **stapes** ("stirrup") is the smallest bone in the entire body. The head of the stapes articulates with the long crus of the incus, and its base (or footplate) closes the vestibular window. A minute muscular process, which provides an attachment site for the stapedius muscle, is present on the caudal crus of the stapes.

b. The **muscles** of the middle ear are two in number, and are minute in size. These muscles tense or firm the tympanic membrane and bony chain, reducing their movement as a protective measure against excessive vibration caused by either low-range frequencies or the sudden onset of a loud sound.

(1) The **tensor tympani** attaches to the malleus, at the hook on the muscular process. This muscle is innervated by the mandibular division of the trigeminal nerve (cranial nerve V_3). Although it may seem odd that a muscle of the middle ear is innervated by the nerve responsible for innervating the muscles of mastication, when one understands that the malleus is derived from the mandible in lower vertebrates, the logic becomes plain: when the muscle associated with that bone migrated to its new destination along with the bone, the muscle retained its original innervation.

(2) The **stapedius** attaches to the stapes, at the muscular process. This muscle is innervated by the facial nerve (cranial nerve VII).

2. The **midportion** of the tympanic cavity (the **"tympanic cavity proper")** is the region adjoining the tympanic membrane. In fact, the tympanic membrane forms a large portion of the cavity's lateral wall. The midportion of the tympanic cavity receives the **opening of the auditory tube** (from the nasopharynx) in its rostral portion and communicates with the inner ear by way of the **vestibular (oval)** and **cochlear (round) windows.**

Canine Clinical Correlation

Pressure equalization on both sides of the tympanic membrane, a protective function, is afforded by the connection between the auditory tube and the nasopharynx. Momentary opening of the tube, such as occurs when swallowing or yawning, allows this equalization of pressure.

a. The **promontory** is an elevation in the medial wall of the tympanic cavity, opposite the tympanic membrane, that houses the cochlea of the inner ear.

b. The **tympanic plexus,** formed mainly from the glossopharyngeal nerve (cranial nerve IX), lies on the promontory and innervates the tympanic membrane.

c. The **chorda tympani (tympanic nerve)** crosses the tympanic cavity proper *en route* to joining the lingual nerve. The chorda tympani carries taste fibers from the facial nerve to the rostral tongue; therefore, this nerve really has nothing to do with the function of the ear.

d. The **tensor tympani** and the **tensor veli palatini** have attachments in the tympanic cavity proper.

3. The **ventral portion** of the tympanic cavity is the **tympanic bulla,** the ventrally expanded "bubble" of bone visible from the external surface of the skull. The function of the tympanic bulla is unclear, but it has been theorized that the tympanic bulla aids in perception of sounds at both the very high and the very low ranges of the scale.

IV. INNER EAR.

Although balance and hearing are very different functions, the inner ear's role in both activities involves the movement of fluid within a set of minuscule ducts.

A. Terminology. The inner ear is essentially composed of two parts, a membranous labyrinth and a bony labyrinth; the two parts are similar in overall form, because the membranous labyrinth actually resides within the bony labyrinth. Confusion can arise as a result of the similarity of names among many of the structures involved. However, a general rule of thumb is that the term **"ducts"** refers to parts of the **membranous labyrinth,** and the term **"canals"** refers to parts of the **bony labyrinth.** The term **"aqueduct"** is also used to describe **bony structures.** (The similarity between "aqueduct" referring to bone and "duct" referring to membranous structures is admittedly unfortunate, but not insurmountable.)

B. Membranous labyrinth. The membranous labyrinth is a set of intricately structured, interconnecting, membrane-bound sacs and channels.

1. **Overview**

a. **Regions.** There are two general regions of the membranous labyrinth, which correspond with the two functions of the inner ear. The two general labyrinthine regions are necessarily interconnected because, although they serve different functions, the mechanism behind the initial step in each of their functions is the same: both are connected to the vestibular window, which is the site where mechanical stimuli are introduced into both parts of the membranous labyrinth. These general labyrinthine regions are each composed of a dilated saccular region and at least one duct (see Figure 14–1).

(1) The **utriculus** and **semicircular ducts** are associated with **balance.**

(2) The **sacculus** and **cochlear duct** are associated with **hearing.**

(3) The **ductus reuniens** is a small channel that extends between the sacculus and the utriculus.

b. **Endolymph,** a clear dialysate of blood formed from vessels in specialized regions of the membranous labyrinth, fills all parts of the membranous labyrinth.

(1) Endolymph mediates the function of the membranous labyrinth, in that mechanical impulses initiated by waves in the fluid stimulate various types of receptors within the two general regions of the membranous labyrinth. Waves in the fluid can be induced by movement of the head (as is the case with movements affecting balance) or they can result from the transmission of sound waves (as is the case with hearing).

(2) The **endolymphatic duct,** a blind-ended channel that extends from the sacculus into the epidural space and terminates at the expanded endolymphatic sac, is believed to play a role in resorption of endolymph.

2. **Balance.** The **utriculus** and **semicircular ducts** are involved with balance.

a. The **utriculus** is an expanded region of the membranous canal situated at the base of the semicircular ducts, forming a common area to which they all connect.

(1) The **macule** ("spot") is a sensory region in the wall of the utriculus that generates information related to the **position of the head relative to gravity** and transmits this information to the brain via the vestibulocochlear nerve (cranial nerve VIII). The macula is covered with a gelatinous layer containing **statoconia** (calcium

carbonate crystals). Deformation of sensory hairs on specialized cells is brought about by positional changes in the statoconia.

(2) The surface of the gelatinous layer is bathed by the endolymph within the utriculus.

b. The **semicircular ducts** are three horseshoe-shaped ducts that extend outward from the utriculus. The ducts are oriented at roughly right angles to each other, with one designated **anterior,** one designated **posterior,** and one designated **lateral.** (This is one of the few places where the terms "anterior" and "posterior" are used in veterinary anatomy.)

(1) The **ampullae** are dilations present at one end of each semicircular duct.

(2) The **crista** is a sensory structure contained within each ampulla (for a total of three, one in each ampulla). Sensory "hairs" present on the surface of the crista are deflected by motions in the endolymph caused by motions of the head (i.e., by rotational inertia of the fluid). These impulses are conveyed to the brain by the vestibular part of the vestibulocochlear nerve (cranial nerve VIII), where they are interpreted as information related to movement of the head.

3. **Hearing.** The **sacculus** and **cochlear duct** are related to hearing.

a. The **sacculus** is an expanded region situated at the base of the cochlear duct. A sensory **macule,** similar to the one in the wall of the utriculus, is present within the wall of the sacculus and functions in balance.

b. The **cochlear duct** arises from the sacculus and passes outward from it in an extended spiral (see Figure 14–1).

(1) The cochlear duct is essentially a membranous tube with a roof and a floor.

(a) The **floor (base)** of the tube is formed by the **basilar membrane.** The basilar membrane separates the cavity of the cochlear duct from the corresponding cavity of the cochlea itself (i.e., the scala tympani).

(b) The **roof** of the tube is formed by the **vestibular membrane,** which separates the cavity of the cochlear duct from the corresponding cavity of the cochlea itself (i.e., the scala vestibuli).

(2) The **spiral organ (organ of Corti)** is the extremely specialized region within the cochlear duct that transduces mechanical energy (i.e., fluid waves) into electrical energy (i.e., nervous impulses) for transmission to the brain.

(a) As with the crista ampullaris, the mechanism involves deflection of sensory hair cells. These nerve impulses are transmitted to the brain via the cochlear portion of the vestibulocochlear nerve (cranial nerve VIII).

(b) The **tectorial membrane,** an awning-like membrane extending over the surface of the hair cells, responds to fluid waves in the endolymph, contacting the hair cells and causing them to "fire."

C. **Bony labyrinth.** The bony labyrinth is a closed bony chamber that entirely encloses and protects the delicate membranous labyrinth (see Figure 14–1). The bony labyrinth is only slightly larger than the membranous labyrinth, and thus closely follows the contour of its membranous counterpart.

1. **Overview**

a. **Regions.** Just as the membranous labyrinth is composed of regions related to balance and to hearing, so is the bony labyrinth. These regions are the **semicircular canals** and the **cochlea,** respectively. In addition, a third region, the **vestibule,** encloses both the utriculus and the sacculus of the membranous labyrinth.

b. **Perilymph** fills the small amount of space between the external surface of the membranous labyrinth and the internal surface of the bony labyrinth. Perilymph is believed to be elaborated by fine blood vessels in the periosteum of the bony labyrinth.

2. **Vestibule.** The vestibule is the central portion that encloses both the utriculus and the sacculus of the membranous labyrinth (see Figure 14–1). Two openings are present in its lateral walls, and two small bony channels lead toward its medial walls.

a. **Openings**

(1) The **vestibular window** receives the stapes (in the intact state).

(2) The **cochlear window** is covered by a membrane (sometimes called the **sec-**

ondary tympanic membrane) that functions to dissipate fluid waves. The cochlear window opens at the base of the cochlea into the air-filled middle ear cavity.

b. Channels (see Figure 14–1)

(1) The **vestibular aqueduct,** which houses the endolymphatic duct, extends from the vestibule to the caudal surface of the petrous temporal bone.

(2) The **cochlear aqueduct** leads from the cochlea to the space adjacent to the dura mater; it drains perilymph into the epidural space.

3. Semicircular canals. The semicircular canals house the semicircular ducts, and follow the contour of the ducts so closely that each semicircular canal also has an ampulla corresponding to that of the enclosed membranous structure. The semicircular canals are designated anterior, posterior, and lateral to match the ducts within them.

4. Cochlea. The cochlea encloses the cochlear duct, and from the external surface very strongly **resembles a snail shell.** The cochlea projects ventrorostrally, with its base positioned dorsally and its apex pointed ventrally (see Figure 14–1).

a. The **modiolus** is a central hollow core of bone around which the "snail shell" turns. The **spiral ganglion,** a collection of ganglion cells housed within the modiolus, receives input from the sensory cells in the cochlear duct. Nerve fibers from the cells of the spiral ganglion wind around the modiolus and collect at the base of the cochlea to form the **cochlear nerve.** The modiolus is perforated by many small holes, which transmit branches to the cochlear nerve.

b. The **spiral canal** is the actual lumen of the cochlea. The spiral canal spirals around the modiolus.

c. The **spiral lamina** is a shelf of bone that extends outward from the modiolus, following the turns of the spiral canal like the threads of a corkscrew. The spiral lamina extends outward about half the distance across the open space of the cochlea and follows the spiral canal from "top to bottom," thereby partially bisecting the canal into two portions, one more dorsal and one more ventral (see Figure 14–1). This subdivision of the space inside the spiral turns of the cochlea is completed by the basilar and vestibular membranes of the cochlear duct.

(1) The **scala vestibuli** is the space within the bony cochlea that lies **dorsal to the bony spiral lamina.** The scala vestibuli is bounded ventrally by the bone of the cochlea and dorsally by the combined length of the bony spiral lamina and the vestibular membrane portion of the cochlear duct.

(a) The scala vestibuli begins at the base of the cochlea near the **vestibular window,** hence the "vestibuli" portion of its name.

(b) The scala vestibuli becomes continuous with the upward turns of the cochlea at the **helicotrema,** a small opening at the apex of the cochlea.

(2) The **scala tympani** is the space within the bony cochlea that lies **ventral to the bony spiral lamina.** The scala tympani is bounded ventrally by the combined length of the bony spiral lamina and the membranous basilar membrane of the cochlear duct, and dorsally by the bone of the cochlea.

(a) The scala tympani begins at the apex of the cochlea at the communication with the scala vestibuli, and spirals upward to the base of the "snail shell."

(b) It terminates at the **cochlear window,** which is covered in the intact state by the **secondary tympanic membrane** (hence the "tympani" in the name of the scala tympani).

D. Vascularization

1. **Arterial supply** to the labyrinth is provided almost exclusively by the tiny **labyrinthine artery,** which arrives through the internal acoustic meatus.
2. **Venous drainage** is by two channels, one each draining along the vestibular and cochlear aqueducts.

E. Innervation is via the vestibulocochlear nerve (cranial nerve VIII).

1. **Balance.** The **vestibular nerve** passes from the semicircular ducts.
2. **Hearing.** The **cochlear nerve** passes from the cochlea.

V. MECHANISM OF HEARING

A. External ear. The pinna collects sound and funnels it through the external ear canal to the middle ear.

B. Middle ear. The tympanic membrane vibrates in response to the sound waves carried on the air. This vibration is transmitted to the chain of auditory ossicles, where it is amplified by a factor of approximately 20 by the time it reaches the end of the chain. The stapes, the last bone in the chain of auditory ossicles, moves against the membrane covering the vestibular window, which transfers the energy (still mechanical in form) to the inner ear.

C. Inner ear. The inner ear is the site where the mechanical impulses produced by the sound waves (received by the tympanic membrane and transmitted to the vestibular window) are transformed into electrical, nervous impulses that can be interpreted by the brain.

1. The mechanical energy from the movement of the stapes against the vestibular window is transferred to the perilymph filling the vestibule. Because fluids are incompressible, the sound wave is transferred through the fluid in wave form. The waves are propagated through the perilymph, and enter the scala vestibuli of the cochlea.
2. As the waves move downward through the perilymph in the scala vestibuli, the movement of the fluid is transferred to the vestibular membrane.
   a. As the vestibular membrane vibrates, it moves against the endolymph within the cochlear duct.
   b. The waves pass through the endolymph, and impinge on the tectorial membrane of the cochlear duct. Deflection of the tectorial membrane by these waves causes the tectorial membrane to contact the hair cells, which vibrate. **This is the point at which the actual transduction of mechanical energy to electrical (nervous) energy actually takes place.**
   c. The cells of the spiral organ then transmit the nervous impulse to the brain via the cochlear nerve.
3. The fluid waves continue along the length of the scala vestibuli to the apex of the cochlea. They then pass from the scala vestibuli to the scala tympani (via the helicotrema).
   a. Transference of the sound waves across the basilar membrane (which forms one boundary of the scala tympani) into the endolymph of the cochlear duct and through the endolymph to the tectorial membrane stimulates the hair cells of the spiral organ again, resulting in a multifaceted stimulation of the spiral organ. This multifaced stimulation of the spiral organ contributes to the richness of the impulses directed to the brain.
   b. The fluid waves pass along the full length of the scala tympani until they reach the termination of this bony channel at the cochlear window, which is closed by the secondary tympanic membrane. The secondary tympanic membrane vibrates in accordance with those waves, allowing the energy to pass through the membrane and to be dissipated in the air space of the middle ear cavity.

Chapter 15

The Eye

I. INTRODUCTION.

INTRODUCTION. The term "eye" is often taken to mean simply the eyeball, but most correctly refers to much more than that single structure. In terms of a whole organ, the eye includes the globe, the adnexa, and the orbit.

A. The **globe (eyeball, bulbus oculi)** includes only the structures contained within the sclera.

B. The **adnexa (associated structures)** include the:

1. **Lacrimal apparatus,** which provides the tear film that provides nutrients to and protects the cornea
2. **Extraocular muscles,** which provide motion to the globe
3. **Eyelids (palpebrae),** which protect the eye both physically and by moving the nutritive tear film over the cornea
4. **Nictitating membrane (third eyelid)**
5. **Vessels and nerves within the orbit**

C. The **orbit** protects and supports the globe and its associated structures. The orbit is provided with two sets of fascia that support and protect the eye and adnexa.

II. GLOBE

A. Topography of the globe. Several descriptive terms are used to indicate particular sites on the globe. These descriptors are useful for describing adnexal structures in relation to the eyeball, as well as for describing the locations of lesions. The terms are illustrated and defined in Figure 15–1.

B. Tunics. The globe is composed of three concentric sheaths of tissue: the fibrous, vascular, and nervous tunics.

1. **Fibrous tunic.** The fibrous tunic is composed of very dense collagenous and elastic tissue, and the fibrocytes that produce those fibers.
   - **a. Functions.** The fibrous tunic:
     - **(1)** Gives the eye its shape and stiffness by resisting the pressure of the internal fluid media
     - **(2)** Protects the internal vascular and light-sensitive portions of the eye from the environment
     - **(3)** Refracts light and conducts light rays to the retina
     - **(4)** Provides a site for attachment of the extraocular muscles
   - **b. Regions.** The fibrous tunic has two portions, the more posterior **sclera** and the more anterior **cornea** (Figure 15–2). The **limbus** is the border where the sclera and cornea meet.
     - **(1)** The **sclera** is the white portion of the eye, covering approximately 75% of the globe's surface. The sclera is largely smooth over most of its external surface.
       - **(a)** The **area cribrosa** is a focal region just ventral to the posterior pole where the fibers are less densely packed, allowing the many fascicles of retinal nerves to exit the globe to coalesce and form the optic nerve (see Figure 15–2).
         - **(i)** Foramina, through which the short posterior ciliary vessels (which supply the ciliary body and iris) enter the globe, are present along the periphery of the area cribrosa.

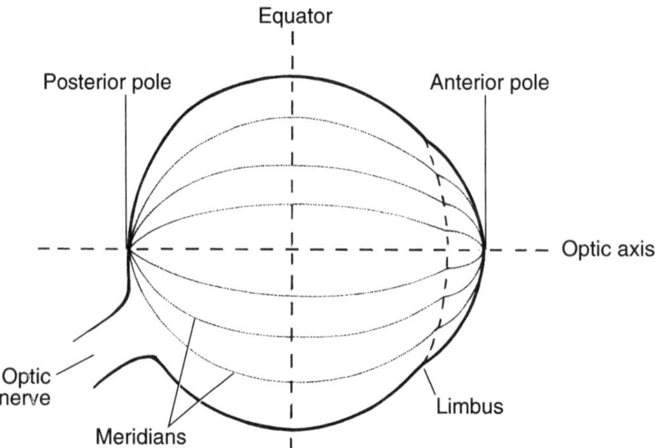

FIGURE 15–1. Topography of the globe. The *anterior pole* is the highest point on the cornea. The *posterior pole* is the point on the posterior scleral surface directly opposite the anterior pole. Note that this is a positional reference point only, and does not correspond to the exit point of the optic nerve. The *optic axis* is a straight line that passes through both poles (i.e., through the center of the globe rather than over its external surface). The *equator* is an imaginary line around the globe that is equidistant from the poles. A *meridian* is any line passing from pole to pole over the surface of the globe (rather than through its interior) that intersects the equator at right angles.

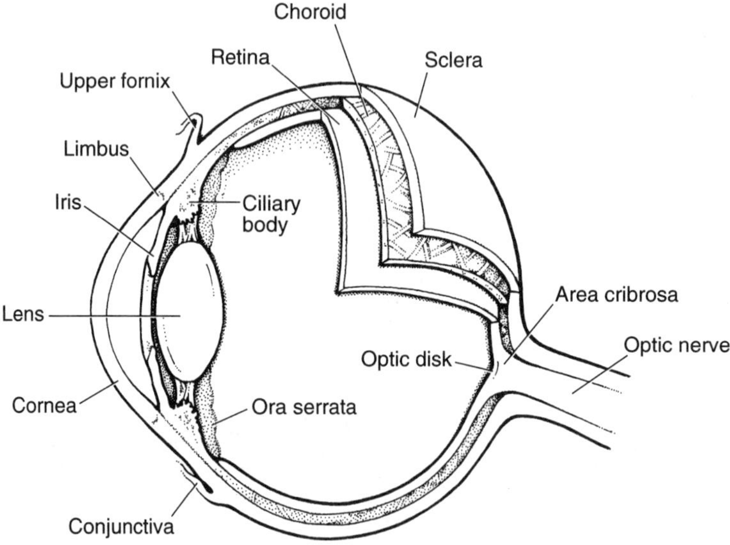

FIGURE 15–2. Schematic drawing of a midsagittal section through the globe. Note the three tunics, the sclera, choroid, and retina, and the three chambers (the anterior chamber, posterior chamber, and vitreous chamber). The anterior chamber extends from the cornea to the anterior surface of the iris. The posterior chamber extends from the posterior iridial surface to the lens, and is the smallest of the three ocular chambers. The vitreous chamber extends from the zonule and posterior lens capsule to the retina in all directions and is the largest of the three chambers. (Modified with permission from Dellmann H-D: *Textbook of Veterinary Histology,* 4th ed. Baltimore, Williams & Wilkins, 1993, p 314.)

(ii) The dura mater of the optic nerve becomes continuous with the outer scleral layers in the region of the area cribrosa.

(b) The sclera gives attachment to the extraocular muscles in the region anterior to the equator.

(2) The **cornea** (see Figure 15–2), the clear portion of the eye, forms approximately 25% of the anterior segment of the fibrous tunic. The curvature of the cornea is more acute than that of the sclera; therefore, the cornea projects anteriorly from the sclera.

(a) **Histologic layers.** The cornea is classically described as having five histologic layers. Four of these layers are present in the dog. The central of these is the **substantia propria,** which is composed of collagenous fibers and is continuous with the substance of the sclera.

(b) **Transparency of the cornea,** necessary for vision, is achieved both by:

(i) **Structural features,** including the particular lamellar structure of the fibers within the substantia propria, as well as the absence of vessels, pigment, or large myelinated nerve fibers

(ii) The **active pumping of fluid** out of the substantia propria by the layers on each side of the propria

(c) **Vascularization.** The cornea is normally **avascular** (although it may acquire vascularization in some disease states). Nutritive substances arrive through capillary loops at the limbus, via the tear film provided by the lacrimal apparatus, and via the aqueous humor.

(d) **Innervation** of the cornea is essential to its normal function; denervation produces degenerative changes. The **long ciliary nerves** (see VI E 1 c) enter the cornea at the limbus and lose their myelin sheaths before progressing into the cornea. Free nerve endings are present in the cornea, which make it exquisitely sensitive.

Canine Clinical Correlation

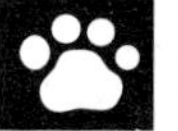

The **corneal reflex** (i.e., closure of the eye when the cornea is touched) is used to estimate the plane of anesthesia. In moderate planes of anesthesia, the palpebral reflex (closure of the eye when the eyelids are touched) is lost, but the corneal reflex remains. Loss of the corneal reflex is indicative of a very deep and potentially dangerous plane of anesthesia.

2. **Vascular tunic.** The vascular tunic lies just internal to the fibrous tunic. The term "uvea" (Latin, *grape*) is sometimes used in reference to the vascular tunic; indeed, the round form and dark color of the vascular tunic are somewhat reminiscent of a grape. The vascular tunic is composed of three continuous regions. From posterior to anterior (and also from simpler to more complex in structure), these are the choroid, ciliary body, and iris (see Figure 15–2). All three regions are extremely vascular and heavily pigmented.

a. The **choroid,** which consists of a dense meshwork of blood vessels (i.e., the **choriocapillaris)** embedded in heavily pigmented connective tissue, covers the posterior hemisphere of the globe, except over the area cribrosa. The choroid:

(1) **Provides nutrients and oxygen** to the avascular retina

(2) **Limits light scatter.** The pigment in the choroid absorbs light scatter inside the eye under conditions of bright lighting.

(3) **Improves vision in low-light situations.** The **tapetum lucidum** is a structure of the choroid that is adapted to increasing light intensity under low-lighting situations. An **avascular** region of the otherwise thickly vascularized choroid, the tapetum lucidum is positioned in the dorsal region of the fundus (i.e., those regions of the eye visible on ophthalmic examination). In dogs, the tapetum lucidum contains rod-shaped crystals that refract incoming light. When a light is shined into the eye

of a dog at night, the resulting greenish "eye shine" results from the light refracting off the tapetum.

b. The **ciliary body** is the portion of the vascular tunic rostral to the termination of the choroid and caudal to the iris; it forms from a thickening of the choroid that is raised inward into the posterior chamber of the eye. The ciliary body both suspends the lens within the eye, and acts to change the thickness of the lens (accommodation).

(1) The **ciliary processes** extend from the base of the ciliary body inward toward the lens. When viewed from the caudal surface, this series of folds forms a ring around the anterior region of the eye, reminiscent of the gills of a mushroom. The ciliary folds tend to alternate tall and short. The taller folds are **major processes** and the shorter folds are **minor processes.**

(2) The **zonule** is a meshwork consisting of fibers that originate at the bases (not the tips) of the ciliary processes, extend outward alongside and covering the processes, and extend beyond their tips to attach around the equator of the lens.

(a) The **anterior zonular fibers** are best developed. These originate from the ciliary part of the retina (see II B 3 c), just anterior to the ora serrata, and are directed anteriorly. In their course, the anterior zonular fibers cover the surface of the major ciliary processes, which offer them support. The anterior zonular fibers insert on the anterior lens capsule.

(b) The **posterior zonular fibers** originate on the tips of the minor ciliary processes as well as in the "valleys" between the ciliary processes. These fibers are directed posteriorly, and insert on the posterior lens capsule. The grid formed by the anterior and posterior fibers adds strength to the lens' supportive function.

(3) Ciliary muscles are smooth muscle bundles that originate on the sclera and attach to the base of the ciliary body.

c. The **iris** is the most anterior and also the smallest segment of the vascular tunic. It is a thin, flat circular structure projecting axially from its attachment to the ciliary body (see Figure 15–2). The periphery of the iris is continuous with the ciliary body.

(1) Melanin granules within the iris are responsible for **eye coloration.** Melanin is the only pigment present in the iris.

(a) Dark eyes possess densely packed melanin granules in both the stroma and posterior layers of the iris.

(b) Light brown or **yellowish eyes** possess melanin granules also, but fewer of them, and less densely packed.

(c) Blue eyes result when pigment is present only in the posterior layer. Differences in the absorption and reflection of light by the iridial tissues and by the pigmented layer of the iris cause the blue color to develop. In other words, blue eyes are not caused by an absence of pigment (in which case the eye would be reddish-pink, as in albinos), but by a relative scarcity and particular distribution of the pigment.

(2) The **pupil** is a central opening in the iris of variable size. In dogs, the pupils are round. A reciprocal set of smooth muscles allow the pupil to adjust the amount of light that reaches the interior of the eye. Both sets of muscles receive both parasympathetic and sympathetic innervation (Table 15–1).

(a) The **pupillary dilator** is arranged radially within the iris, so that contraction draws the pupil open and admits more light to the eye. Sympathetic tone contracts the muscle, while parasympathetic tone inhibits its contraction.

(b) The **pupillary constrictor (sphincter)** is arranged circumferentially around the pupil, so that contraction draws the pupil closed. Parasympathetic tone contracts the muscle, while sympathetic tone inhibits its contraction.

3. Nervous tunic. The **retina** is the innermost layer of the globe. The retina originates from an outgrowth of the diencephalon and retains that connection in the definitive form by means of the optic nerve. The retina extends from the optic disk to the pupil, and is described as having three parts and a divisionary zone.

a. The **optical part of the retina (pars optica retinae)** is the largest part. The optical part

TABLE 15–1. Innervation of the Pupillary Musculature

Pupillary muscle	Nature	Origin of Fibers	Location of Ganglion or Plexus	Nerve Delivering Fibers
Dilator	Sympathetic	Cavernous plexus	Cavernous sinus	Long ciliary nerves
Sphincter	Parasympathetic	Ciliary ganglion	Medial orbital wall	Short ciliary nerves

covers the internal surface of the eye over approximately two thirds of the posterior globe's inner surface, which is the area where light can reach. This region of the retina is relatively thick; it is composed of ten layers of cells.

(1) Pigment. Except for the area of the retina overlying the tapetum lucidum, the optical part of the retina is deeply pigmented, which, together with the pigment within the choroid, renders the interior of the eye very dark and gives the pupil its black color.

(2) Light-sensitive cells. The optical part of the retina achieves the wondrous event of changing light energy into chemical energy and then into electrical energy in the form of nerve impulses to the brain. Curiously, the light-sensitive cells are layer nine out of ten (counting from the vitreous body toward the sclera) so that the light must penetrate eight layers of cells before reaching the light-sensitive one. The nervous impulses are then carried on axons back through those eight cellular layers before collecting into the nerve fascicles that leave the globe.

Canine Clinical Correlation

Rods (specialized for black and white vision) comprise approximately 95% of the photoreceptors in the dog's retina. Thus, for many years, dogs were thought to have black and white vision. However, recent studies have shown that two types of cells are present in the retina, and that dogs in fact possess dichromat color vision. In dichromat color vision, stimuli can be distinguished on the basis of wavelength (blues from greens, yellows, and reds) and on the basis of spectral energy (blues, yellows, and browns from grays or whites).

(3) Optic disk. The optic disk is the area where the many nerve fibers from the retina collect, become myelinated, and leave the globe to continue as the optic nerve.

- **(a)** The optic disk, a prominent feature during fundoscopic examination, appears white because of the myelin sheaths of the nerve fibers.
- **(b)** No photoreceptors are present in the disk, which represents the **"blind spot"** of the eye.

(4) Central area (area centralis). The central area is the region dorsal and slightly lateral to the optic disk where the receptor cells are thickest. Thus, this is an area of particularly acute vision.

b. The **ora serrata** marks the boundary between the visual (optical) part and nonvisual (ciliary and iridial) parts of the retina. The optic part of the retina is about four times the thickness of the "blind" part (pars ceca retinae); thus, the abrupt change in thickness produces the recognizable ridge that is the ora serrata.

c. The **ciliary part of the retina (pars ciliaris retinae)** begins where the optical part of the retina abruptly thins to a **bilayered epithelium that covers the ciliary body.** This portion of the retina **produces the aqueous humor** via active secretion.

d. The **iridial part of the retina (pars iridica retinae)** is a bilayered epithelial layer covering the posterior surface of the iris. The outer layer of the iridial part of the retina gives origin to the iridial musculature.

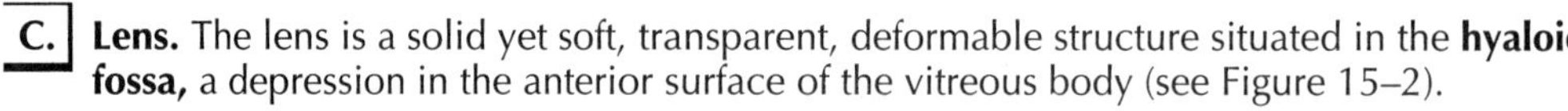

C. Lens. The lens is a solid yet soft, transparent, deformable structure situated in the **hyaloid fossa,** a depression in the anterior surface of the vitreous body (see Figure 15–2).

1. **Landmark points** on the lens are described, similar to the globe as a whole, as the anterior pole, posterior pole, and equator.
2. **Structure**
   - a. The lens is composed of elongate **epithelial cells (lens fibers)** that are oriented regularly into concentric sheets. The epithelial cells continue to proliferate throughout life. Older cells are compressed toward the center of the lens and are then covered superficially by the younger lenticular cells that displaced them. Thus, the lens is composed of many superimposed layers (i.e., it is **lamellar).**

Canine Clinical Correlation

The lens fibers toward the center of the lens undergo progressive condensation and dehydration with advancing age. This tends to give the eyes of older dogs a hazy, bluish color. Care must be taken to distinguish this **lenticular sclerosis,** which is a normal feature of aging, from **cataracts,** which always indicate a pathologic process.

   - b. An **elastic capsule** envelops the lens. The lens is **avascular** in adult dogs. Nutrients diffuse across the lens capsule from the aqueous and vitreous bodies; wastes diffuse across in the opposite direction.
3. **Function.** The lens **brings images into focus on the retina.** The ciliary processes, zonules, and ciliary muscles alter the shape of the lens to change the distance at which objects are focused; this process is called **lens accommodation.**
   - a. When the ciliary muscle is relaxed, the ciliary body is positioned slightly posteriorly, farther away from the lens. This puts the zonule under tension, stretches the lens, and facilitates focus of objects that are farther away.
   - b. When the ciliary muscle is contracted, the ciliary body is drawn forward toward the lens, the zonular fibers are somewhat relaxed, the lens shortens, and focus on near objects is obtained.

D. Chambers. Three chambers are distinguished in the interior of the eye: the anterior, posterior, and vitreous chambers (see Figure 15–2).

1. The **anterior** and **posterior chambers** are demarcated by the iris and are intimately related.
   - a. The anterior chamber lies anterior to the iris, and the posterior chamber lies posterior to the lens.
   - b. These two chambers are in direct communication through the pupil and are filled with **aqueous humor.** The aqueous humor is continually produced by the ciliary part of the retina; it then flows into the posterior chamber, passes through the pupillary opening into the anterior chamber, and is resorbed by the scleral venous plexus in the iridocorneal angle.

Canine Clinical Correlation

Production of aqueous humor continues regardless of intraocular pressure. Even in severe cases of elevated intraocular pressure **(glaucoma),** production continues apace. Elevated intraocular pressure can lead to **retinal atrophy** and **blindness.**

2. The **vitreous chamber** accounts for approximately 80% of the volume of the globe.
   a. The **vitreous body,** a clear gel, fills the vitreous chamber.
      (1) The vitreous body is almost 98% water, with the remaining components being solids (e.g., proteins) and extremely fine fibers that support the structure of the body. The vitreous body is normally acellular.
      (2) Most borders are smooth, but the vitreous body is indented anteriorly by the lens (forming the hyaloid fossa), and also by the ciliary processes. The vitreous body is tightly adherent to the posterior lens capsule, the ciliary part of the retina, and the optic disk.

Canine Clinical Correlation

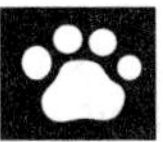

The adherence of the vitreous body to the lens capsule is so tight that attempted removal of the lens and its capsule (e.g., during cataract surgery) nearly always results in rupture of the vitreous body. Therefore, in dogs undergoing cataract surgery, the lens is removed from the capsule, which is left behind.

   b. The **hyaloid canal,** a remnant of the embryologic (primary) vitreous, passes through the vitreous body from the optic disc to the posterior lens capsule. The attachment of the hyaloid canal to the posterior lens capsule is sometimes visible on ophthalmoscopic examination.

III. ORBIT

A. The **bony orbit** is a deep bony cavity in the rostral surface of the skull that houses the globe and adnexa. The globe is situated in the orbit so that mainly only the limbal and corneal regions are visible, both in the intact state and with the eyelids dissected free. Normally only a small portion of the sclera is visible in the dog.

Canine Clinical Correlation

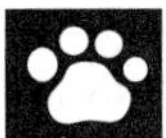

The bony orbit of brachycephalic breeds is considerably shallower than that of other breeds, resulting in marked protrusion of the globe from the orbit in brachycephalic breeds. These animals are predisposed to difficulties related to **inadequate closure of the lids over the globe** as well as **proptosis** (i.e., traumatic herniation of the eye from the orbit).

1. The **orbital rim** is bony around approximately 75% of its border; the lateral-most edge is completed by the orbital ligament (see also Chapter 8 II A 2 a).
2. The **medial wall** and much of the **roof** of the orbit are bony, but the remaining borders are formed by soft tissue. As one example, the **zygomatic salivary gland** forms the lateral two thirds of the orbital floor. Thus, appreciation of the complete orbit cannot be attained by studying the prepared skull.

B. The **orbital fasciae** invest the globe and adnexa. From superficial to deep, the orbital fasciae are the periorbita, the muscular fasciae, and the bulbar sheath.

1. The **periorbita** is the strongest and most readily visible fascial layer. It encloses the globe and all of its associated muscles, vessels, and nerves. This stout layer effectively delineates the floor of the orbital region.
   a. The periorbita is cone-shaped, with its apex in the region of the optic canal and its base

Canine Clinical Correlation

The incomplete nature of the bony orbit has several clinical ramifications:

- Several diseases not directly related to the eye can present with ocular signs. For example, involvement of the muscles of mastication in eosinophilic myositis can cause protrusion of the globe.
- Similarly, ocular processes can present with distant signs. For example, patients with a retrobulbar abscess may experience pain on opening the mouth when rostral movement of the coronoid process of the mandible compresses the abscess and causes pain.
- In some situations, the incomplete nature of the bony walls of the orbit renders obtaining surgical accesses to the orbital region less invasive, because it may not be necessary to cut bone.

at the orbital rim. Thus, this general area within the orbit (i.e., the caudal periorbita and associated structures) is referred to as the **orbital cone.** The nerves and vessels of the eye enter at the apex of the cone and pass rostrally under cover of the fascial layer.

b. The periorbita is attached to the skull near the optic foramen, where it is continuous with the periosteum of regional bone. At the margins of the optic canal and orbital fissure, it is also continuous with the dura mater of the nerves transmitted by these foramina [see Chapter 8 II A 2 b (3) (b)]. At the rostral extent of the periorbita (i.e., the orbital rim), the periorbita divides into two portions.

(1) One layer turns circumferentially around the orbital rim to become continuous with the periosteum of the facial bones.

(2) The other layer, the **orbital septum,** passes through each eyelid to form a fold in the free margin of each lid that is continuous with the tarsi (i.e., the thickened free margins of the lids that stiffen the free edge).

2. The **muscular fasciae** include the superficial, middle, and deep fasciae. These fasciae invest the extraocular muscles.

3. The **bulbar sheath** is a thin, fibrous capsule that enfolds the globe from the limbus to the optic nerve.

a. The **episcleral space** separates the bulbar sheath from the sclera. Fine **trabeculae** cross this space and anchor the bulbar sheath to the globe.

b. Near the equator, the bulbar sheath becomes continuous with the extraocular muscles that attach there.

C. The **orbital fat body (fat pad)** fills most of the free space within the orbit. This easily deformable body of fat **cushions** and **supports** the globe and adnexal structures and **facilitates rotation** and **retraction of the globe.** The fat body is divided into two portions, the:

1. **Intraperiorbital portion,** which surrounds the muscles, vessels, and nerves of the periorbita
2. **Extraperiorbital portion,** which consists of variably sized and variably continuous fat bodies placed between the periorbita and other orbital structures (e.g., the zygomatic salivary gland), as well as between the periorbita and the bony orbit

IV. ADNEXA

A. Conjunctiva. The conjunctiva is simply a mucous membrane that covers certain regions of the eye. The conjunctiva is attached to the globe by a loose layer of connective tissue containing abundant fibrocytes and inflammatory cells of several types (e.g., mast cells, lymphocytes, plasma cells, macrophages).

1. Regions

a. The **palpebral conjunctiva** lines the inner surface of the upper, lower, and third eyelids.

b. The **bulbar conjunctiva** covers the sclera and becomes continuous with the epithelium at the level of the limbus.
c. The **conjunctival fornix** is the point of reflection of the palpebral and bulbar conjunctiva. The two portions of the conjunctiva are continuous with each other (i.e., the palpebral conjunctiva reflects smoothly onto the surface of the globe to become the bulbar conjunctiva and vice versa).

2. **Vascularization.** The conjunctiva is well-vascularized by branches of several arteries, including the superior and inferior palpebral arteries, the malar artery, and the long ciliary arteries (see VII A).
   a. **Arteries.** Conjunctival vessels are visible on close inspection in health, and can become extremely prominent when inflamed. The vessels of the conjunctiva move when the loosely attached conjunctiva moves, thereby distinguishing them from the more deeply lying scleral vessels, which do not move.
   b. **Lymphatic nodules** are common throughout the conjunctiva, particularly on the bulbar surface of the third eyelid. These nodules respond emphatically to infection, and can become greatly enlarged. This is particularly true of those on the third eyelid which, when grossly enlarged during infection, may be confused with the gland of the third eyelid (see IV C 2).

B. **Eyelids (palpebrae).** The palpebrae are mobile skin folds, one upper and one lower, that close over the corneal surface to protect the cornea, exclude light, and spread the essential tear film over the corneal surface. The upper eyelid is larger and more mobile than the lower lid.

1. The eyelids are composed of an outer layer of **haired skin,** a middle **musculofibrous layer,** and an inner **palpebral conjunctiva,** which is simply a mucous membrane. The **conjunctival sac** is the space between the eyelid (upper or lower) and the globe. In life, this space normally contains tears and a small bit of mucus.
2. In the dog, only the superior eyelid possesses **eyelashes (cilia).**
3. The **medial** and **lateral commissures** are the points where the upper and lower lids meet. The **medial** and **lateral angles (canthi)** are the angles formed between the lids at the commissures. The **lacrimal caruncle** is an elevated area of skin in the medial canthus.
4. **Glands** of the eyelids include the:
   a. **Sebaceous glands,** which enter the follicles of the cilia (eyelashes)
   b. **Tarsal glands,** which are present on the free edges of both eyelids, are usually visible grossly on the everted lid margin as longitudinal yellow or white bars oriented perpendicular to the lid margin
5. **Ligaments.** The **palpebral ligaments** anchor the palpebral commissures to surrounding structures.
   a. The **lateral palpebral ligament,** which anchors the lateral commissure to the zygomatic arch, is relatively poorly developed.
   b. The **medial palpebral ligament,** which anchors the medial commissure to the frontal bone, is much better developed. This ligament serves for both the origin and insertion of the orbicularis oculi muscle.

C. **Third eyelid (semilunar fold).** The third eyelid originates as a fold of tissue in the ventromedial region of the medial canthus. The free edge of the fold conforms to the curvature of the globe, and has a conspicuous, darkly-pigmented free margin. A "T"-shaped plate of hyaline cartilage supports the third eyelid, with the upright of the "T" in the medial canthus and the crossbar of the "T" located at the free edge and molded to conform to the bulbar curvature.

1. **Movement.** The third eyelid is large and very mobile, and is capable of covering the entire corneal surface, although this feature is not apparent when the lid is at rest. Unlike movement of the upper and lower eyelids, motion of the third eyelid is **entirely passive.**
   a. When the eye is open, the third eyelid is withdrawn nearly completely into the medial canthus.
   b. When the globe is retracted into the orbit during closure of the eye, pressure is

placed on the base of the third eyelid by the retracted globe. The resultant pivot action displaces the base of the third eyelid forward.

c. As the globe returns to its resting position (as the eye opens), the pressure on the base of the third eyelid is relaxed, and the eyelid is passively retracted. Once retracted, smooth muscle cells derived from the periorbita assist in holding it in place.

Canine Clinical Correlation

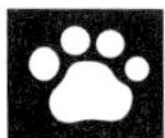

Clinical examination of the third eyelid (e.g., to search for a foreign body trapped between the third eyelid and the globe) is facilitated by applying gentle pressure on the sclera through the lid, which causes passive protrusion of the third eyelid.

2. **Gland.** The **superficial gland of the third eyelid** is a mixed seromucous gland that surrounds the base of the cartilage plate. Numerous ducts empty the secretion of the gland into the lower conjunctival fornix. These secretions form a substantial portion of the **tear film.** (The deep gland of the third eyelid is absent in dogs, but the "superficial" term is retained in the name to indicate its homology in other species.)

D. Lacrimal apparatus. The lacrimal apparatus is composed of the structures associated with the **production, dispersion,** and **disposal of tears.**

1. **Components of the lacrimal apparatus**
   a. **Tear-producing structures.** Structures involved with the production of the tear film are the lacrimal gland, the tarsal glands, the conjunctival goblet cells, and the gland of the third eyelid.
      (1) **Lacrimal gland.** The lacrimal gland lies under the periorbita on the dorsolateral aspect of the globe, separated from the adjacent extraocular muscle by a thin fascial sheet. Three to five ducts open from the lacrimal gland onto the adjacent conjunctival fornix. Surprisingly, removal of the lacrimal gland produces only a minor decrease in tear production, because the superficial gland of the third eyelid is able to markedly increase its tear production if necessary.
      (2) **Tarsal glands.** The tarsal glands are positioned in the free edge of the upper and lower eyelids, and also produce a characteristic part of the tear film.
      (3) **Conjunctival goblet cells** produce an essential part of the tear film.
      (4) **Superficial gland of the third eyelid.** This accessory lacrimal gland produces a major portion of the tear film.
   b. **Tear-dispersing structures**
      (1) The **eyelids** are the major structures involved in the dispersal of the tear film.
      (2) The **lacrimal lake** is a shallow depression in the region of the medial canthus between the lower palpebral conjunctiva and the third eyelid. Tears accumulate here prior to moving into the nasolacrimal duct system.
   c. **Tear-disposing structures.** Disposal of the tear film involves the **nasolacrimal duct system** (Figure 15–3).
      (1) The **lacrimal puncta** are located one on the inner surface of each lid margin at approximately the level of the lacrimal lake (i.e., very close to the medial commissure).
         (a) The puncta may be distinguished from the openings of the tarsal glands by their larger size, single occurrence on each lid, and positioning farther inward from the lid margin.
         (b) The puncta open into the lacrimal canaliculi.
      (2) The **lacrimal canaliculi** are tiny tubular pathways oriented with their long axes parallel with the lid margin. They travel medially to open into the lacrimal sac.

> **Canine Clinical Correlation**
>
> Introduction of contrast material into the nasolacrimal duct system is performed clinically to evaluate the integrity of the system. The canaliculi may be easily cannulated if the cannula is directed parallel with the lid margin (i.e., in the direction of the path of the canaliculi). Direction of the cannula in any other direction meets with considerable difficulty.

(3) The **lacrimal sac,** a dilatation at the junction of the canaliculi, represents the initial portion of the nasolacrimal duct itself. The lacrimal sac occupies a small fossa in the lacrimal bone.

(4) The **nasolacrimal duct** courses along the lateral border of the maxilla. It terminates by opening on the ventrolateral floor of the nasal vestibule, just ventral to the alar fold. (In order to see this opening in the living dog, it is necessary to use a speculum. In approximately 50% of the dog population, the opening is paired, with the second opening lying opposite the canine tooth.)

(a) The greatest part of the duct passes through the bony **lacrimal canal,** which first traverses part of the lacrimal bone and then the maxilla.

(b) The latter parts of the nasolacrimal duct run **deep to the nasal mucosa,** rather than within a bony canal.

2. **Composition of the tear film.** The tear film is **composed of three separate layers:**
   a. The **superficial oily layer** is produced by the tarsal glands (modified sebaceous glands).
   b. The **middle aqueous layer** is produced by the lacrimal gland and the gland of the third eyelid.
   c. The **deep mucous layer** is produced by the goblet cells of the conjunctiva.
3. **Functions of the tear film.** The normal tear film plays an absolutely essential role in

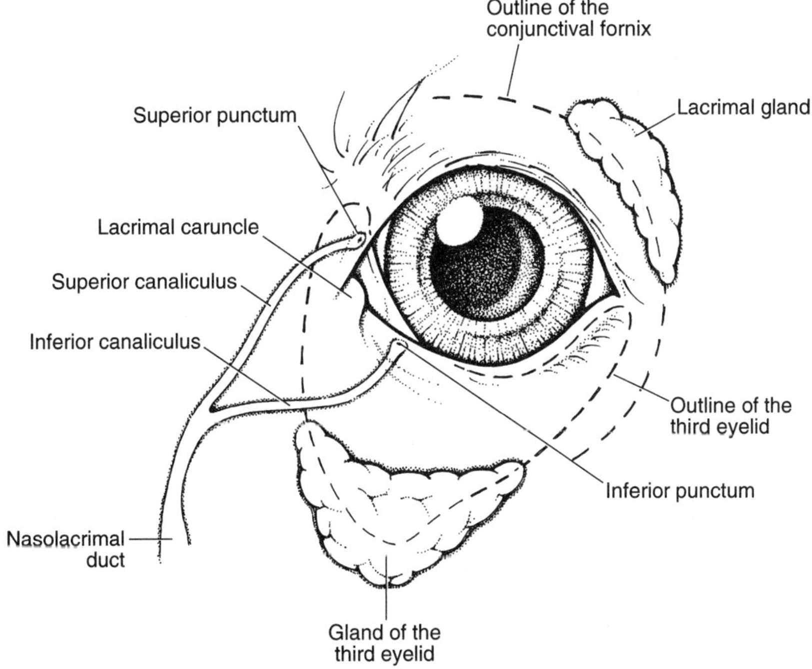

FIGURE 15–3. The lacrimal apparatus.

maintaining the health of the eye and the normal transparency of the cornea. The tear film:

a. Keeps the cells of the cornea moist
b. Washes foreign bodies away from the eye
c. Facilitates the diffusion of respiratory gases and nutrients to and from the avascular cornea
d. Contains antimicrobial substances and dissolved antibodies that help to protect against infection

V. MUSCULATURE.

MUSCULATURE. Recalling that the "eye" includes adnexal structures as well as the globe, three functional groups of muscles may be identified: the intraocular muscles ("intrinsic"), the extraocular muscles ("extrinsic"), and the muscles of the eyelids (palpebral muscles).

A. The **intraocular muscles** (i.e., the **ciliary muscle,** the **pupillary dilator,** and the **pupillary constrictor)** are all **smooth muscles** that lie entirely within the globe. These muscles are described in II B 2 b (3) and c (2).

B. The **extraocular muscles** are all **skeletal muscles.**

1. General considerations

a. All of the extraocular muscles, except for the ventral oblique muscle, originate in the pterygopalatine fossa near the group of foramina in its medial wall. The ventral oblique muscle arises from the palatine bone.
b. All of the extraocular muscles attach to the globe in the general equatorial region.
c. All of the extraocular muscles are enclosed within the periorbita.
d. All of the extraorbital muscles, except the retractor bulbi, become tendinous near their insertions. The retractor bulbi is muscular throughout its course.

2. Classification. There are seven extraorbital muscles. They can be classified as four rectus muscles, two oblique muscles, and one retractor muscle.

a. The **four rectus muscles** are named for the position of their insertion, just anterior to the global equator. They all course directly rostrally within the orbit in their respective positions.

(1) The **dorsal rectus muscle** courses on the dorsal surface of the globe. It acts to rotate the globe upward (dorsally) and is innervated by the oculomotor nerve (cranial nerve III).
(2) The **ventral rectus muscle** courses on the ventral surface of the globe. It acts to rotate the globe downward (ventrally) and is innervated by the oculomotor nerve (cranial nerve III).
(3) The **medial rectus muscle** courses on the medial surface of the globe. It acts to rotate the globe medially and is innervated by the oculomotor nerve (cranial nerve III).
(4) The **lateral rectus muscle** courses on the lateral surface of the globe. It acts to rotate the globe laterally and is innervated by the abducent nerve (cranial nerve VI). The innervation of the lateral rectus muscle by the abducent nerve makes sense in that lateral rotation of the eye can be considered a motion of abduction.

b. The **two oblique muscles** are named for their oblique course, as well as their orbital position.

(1) The **dorsal oblique muscle** courses rostrally in the orbit in a dorsomedial position, between the dorsal and medial recti. It sends its tendon medially around the **trochlea,** a small cartilaginous plate within the periorbita, which turns the tendon obliquely caudally, dorsally, and laterally to insert deep to the dorsal rectus muscle.

(a) The dorsal oblique muscle acts to rotate the dorsal surface of the globe medially.
(b) It is innervated by the trochlear nerve (cranial nerve IV).

(2) The **ventral oblique muscle** courses rostrally and laterally toward the anterior region of the globe, passing ventral to the ventral rectus before turning dorsally to reach its insertion points deep to the lateral rectus muscle and on the dorsolateral surface of the globe.

(a) The ventral oblique muscle acts to rotate the dorsal surface of the globe laterally.

(b) It is innervated by the oculomotor nerve (cranial nerve III).

c. The **one retractor muscle** is named for its action. The **retractor bulbi muscle** courses rostrally from its origin, progressively subdividing until nearly a complete cone of muscle is formed around the posterior surface of the eye. This muscular cone inserts along most of the equatorial surface. The retractor bulbi withdraws the globe deeper into the orbit and is innervated by the abducent nerve (cranial nerve VI).

C. The **palpebral muscles** [see also Chapter 11 I B 3 d (1); Table 11–1] move the eyelids to open or close the eye. They also adjust the eyelid position in response to positional changes of the globe. (For instance, when looking downward, the lower lid is depressed, and the upper lid follows the limbus down to keep the sclera from being exposed.)

1. The **orbicularis oculi** has an orbital part, surrounding the bony orbit, and a palpebral part, within the upper and lower eyelids. It acts almost like a sphincter to close the eye forcefully. The orbicularis oculi is innervated by the palpebral branches of the auriculopalpebral nerve of the facial nerve (cranial nerve VII).

2. The **levator palpebrae superioris** is the primary muscle acting to raise the upper eyelid.
   a. It originates deep within the orbit (in the general vicinity of the extraocular muscles) and passes rostrally within the periorbita (as do the other muscles with which it shares its site of origin) as the dorsal-most muscle within the orbit. It widens and flattens rostrally, and inserts by a broad aponeurosis into the substance of the upper eyelid.
   b. The levator palpebrae superioris is innervated by the oculomotor nerve (cranial nerve III).

3. The **retractor anguli oculi lateralis** is a small, superficial muscle that arises from the temporal fascia and inserts by blending with the palpebral part of the orbicularis oculi. It acts to draw the lateral canthus caudally and thereby assists in closure of the eye. It is innervated by the zygomatic branch of the auriculopalpebral branch of the facial nerve (cranial nerve VII).

4. The **palpebral part of the deep sphincter of the neck** consists of a few delicate fibers passing dorsally from the region of the ventral midline and inserting into the lower tarsus. The palpebral part of the deep sphincter of the neck depresses the lower lid, thus assisting in opening the eye, and is innervated by the buccal branches of the facial nerve (cranial nerve VII).

5. The **superior** and **inferior tarsal muscles** are muscular slips derived from the periorbita that insert into the eyelids and assist in holding them open. These muscles are innervated by sympathetic fibers, a feature that attains clinical significance in that the drooping lower lid encountered with brachial plexus avulsion (ptosis) is caused by loss of the sympathetic innervation to these muscles.

VI. INNERVATION.

The globe and its adnexa are innervated entirely by cranial nerves, these being the optic nerve (cranial nerve II), the oculomotor nerve (cranial nerve III), the trochlear nerve (cranial nerve IV), the trigeminal nerve (cranial nerve V), the abducent nerve (cranial nerve VI), and the facial nerve (cranial nerve VII). (Note that fully half of the cranial nerves have some participation in innervation of the globe and adnexa!) These nerves are discussed here only in their relation to the eye and their course external to the skull; a more complete description is provided in Chapter 11.

A. General considerations

1. Five of the six cranial nerves innervating the eye and ocular region are closely associated with each other as they leave the skull and pass rostrally into the orbit. These are the **optic nerve** (cranial nerve II), the **oculomotor nerve** (cranial nerve III), the **trochlear nerve** (cranial nerve IV), the **ophthalmic and maxillary divisions of the trigeminal nerve** (cranial nerve V_1 and V_2), and the **abducent nerve** (cranial nerve VI). Each of these nerves is associated solely or largely with innervation of the globe and adnexa, and thus has a **course exclusively or largely within the orbit.** In that intraorbital course, the nerves and their branches are **completely or largely contained within the periorbita.**
   a. The **optic nerve** (cranial nerve II) leaves the skull through its own private foramen (i.e., the **optic canal).**
   b. The **oculomotor nerve** (cranial nerve III), the **trochlear nerve** (cranial nerve IV), the **ophthalmic division of the trigeminal nerve** (cranial nerve V_1), and the **abducent nerve** (cranial nerve VI) leave the skull through the **orbital fissure.**
2. The **facial nerve** (cranial nerve VII) has a relatively small role in innervating the ocular adnexa—its primary function is innervating the muscles of facial expression. This nerve emerges from the skull at the **stylomastoid foramen,** and thus is not associated with the interior of the orbit.

B. Optic nerve (cranial nerve II). The optic nerve is **purely sensory,** functioning in the sense of **sight.**

1. **Identification with the central nervous system (CNS).** The optic nerve develops embryologically from an outgrowth of the retina, which itself develops from an outgrowth of the diencephalon. Therefore, the optic nerve is more similar structurally to the brain than to peripheral nerves.
   a. Myelination is achieved through CNS cells (oligodendrocytes) rather than through peripheral nervous system (PNS) cells (Schwann cells).
   b. The optic nerve is surrounded by an outer and an inner sheath, which are continuous with the dura mater and pia mater of the brain, respectively. The space between these layers (which is continuous with the same space in the brain) contains cerebrospinal fluid.
2. **Position.** The optic nerve lies within the cone formed by the extraocular muscles as they fan out from their origin to their insertion points. The space between the nerve and the muscular cone is filled by the substantial intraperiorbital fat pad.
3. **Course.** The optic nerve begins at the **optic disk** of the retina, and passes caudally (surrounded by the intraorbital fat pad and the extraocular muscles) to the **optic canal,** which it enters and traverses. After leaving the optic canal, the optic nerve enters the **middle cranial fossa,** passes through the **optic chiasm** (where approximately 75% of its fibers cross the midline), and continues as the **optic tract** into the brain (see Chapter 13, Figure 13–2).
   a. The length of the optic nerve exceeds the simple geometric distance between the posterior globe and the optic canal, so that there is sufficient "slack" for the nerve to follow the globe in its motions. The length of the optic nerve in the dog is sufficient that an animal can experience proptosis (herniation of the globe out of the orbit) without rupturing the nerve. Given the frequency of this event in brachycephalic breeds, this is a fortunate characteristic in that, assuming no damage to the globe itself, surgical replacement of the globe within the orbit is often followed by a return of normal ocular functioning.
   b. Certain fine vessels and nerves are closely applied to the surface of the optic nerve, which provides support and a pathway approaching the globe. These structures include the:
      (1) **Short ciliary nerves,** which carry postganglionic parasympathetic fibers
      (2) **Long ciliary nerves,** which carry mainly sensory but also postganglionic sympathetic fibers
      (3) **Long and short ciliary arteries,** which deliver blood to most structures of the globe

C. Oculomotor nerve (cranial nerve III)

1. The oculomotor nerve is **motor** to most of the extraocular muscles (i.e., the **dorsal rectus, lateral rectus, medial rectus, ventral oblique,** and **levator palpebrae superioris).** It emerges from the orbital fissure into the orbit, where it divides into a dorsal and a ventral branch.
   a. The smaller **dorsal branch** passes dorsally through the orbit *en route* to the dorsal rectus and levator palpebrae superioris.
   b. The smaller **ventral branch** also passes through the dorsal orbital region, but does so ventral to the dorsal rectus muscle. The ventral branch innervates the medial rectus, ventral rectus, and the ventral oblique muscles.
2. It also conducts **parasympathetic fibers.** The oculomotor nerve delivers preganglionic fibers to the **ciliary ganglion.** After synapsing in the ciliary ganglion, the postganglionic fibers pass as the **short ciliary nerves** along the surface of the optic nerve to the **pupillary constrictor** and the **ciliary muscle.**

Canine Clinical Correlation

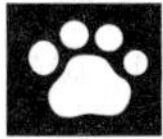

The pupillary dilatation (mydriasis) that is a common finding in conditions producing increased intracranial pressure results from compression of the ciliary ganglion against the bony orbit; the compression impairs the ciliary ganglion's ability to send messages to the pupillary constrictor.

Canine Clinical Correlation

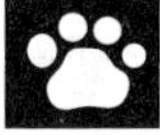

Lesions of the oculomotor nerve result in **pupillary dilation,** due to impairment of the pupillary sphincter, **ptosis** (drooping of the upper lid), due to impairment of the levator palpebrae superioris, **ventrolateral displacement of the globe** (due to the unopposed pull of the lateral rectus following paralysis of the other rectus muscles), and an **inability to retract the globe,** due to paralysis of the retractor bulbi.

D. Trochlear nerve (cranial nerve IV).

Trochlear nerve (cranial nerve IV). The trochlear nerve is **motor** to the **dorsal oblique muscle.** After passing out of the orbital fissure, the trochlear nerve attains the orbit and then passes along the dorsomedial orbital region to reach its target muscle.

E. Trigeminal nerve (cranial nerve V).

Trigeminal nerve (cranial nerve V). The trigeminal nerve plays a large role in innervating the globe and orbit.

1. **Ophthalmic division of the trigeminal nerve (cranial nerve V_1).** The **ophthalmic nerve** joins company with the oculomotor nerve (cranial nerve III), trochlear nerve (cranial nerve IV), and abducent nerve (cranial nerve VI) near the orbital fissure. After emerging from the orbital fissure, it divides into the frontal, lacrimal, and nasociliary nerves.
   a. The **frontal nerve,** a relatively small nerve, passes between the dorsal rectus and periorbita to the upper eyelid. It is **sensory** to most of the **upper eyelid** as well as to an area of skin passing medially from the upper eyelid to the dorsal midline.
   b. The **lacrimal nerve,** a very small nerve, passes along the dorsal rectus muscle toward the lacrimal gland. It carries (postganglionic) **sympathetic** fibers to the **lacrimal gland.**
   c. The **nasociliary nerve** is the largest branch of the ophthalmic nerve. This nerve itself has three branches:
      (1) The **long ciliary nerves** retain the position of the parent nerve adjacent to the optic nerve, follow the optic nerve rostrally into the orbit, arch onto the scleral surface by numerous branches, and pass anteriorly on the surface of the globe.

(a) These nerves provide rich sensory innervation to the **choroid, ciliary body, iris, cornea,** and **bulbar conjunctiva.**
(b) The (postganglionic) **sympathetic fibers to the pupillary dilator** travel with the long ciliary nerves.

(2) The **infratrochlear nerve** passes rostrally along the lateral rectus muscle ventral to the trochlea (as its name suggests) and provides numerous **sensory** branches to the **tissues and skin of the medial canthal region.**

(3) The **ethmoidal nerve** passes rostrally over the extraocular muscles, and then turns medially to depart from the orbit and reenter the skull via the ventral ethmoidal foramen, in company with the external ethmoidal artery. It is **sensory** to **part of the nasal mucosa** and **muzzle skin.**

2. **Maxillary division of the trigeminal nerve (cranial nerve V_2).** The **zygomatic nerve** enters the periorbital apex and divides into two branches.
   a. The **zygomaticotemporal nerve** passes rostrally on the lateral periorbital wall toward the orbital ligament, and from there sends branches into the upper eyelid and an area of skin over the temporal muscle reaching to the dorsal midline.
   b. The **zygomaticofacial nerve** courses rostrally parallel and ventral to the zygomaticotemporal nerve. Near the orbital margin, it turns ventrally and sends branches into the lower eyelid and the skin over the zygomatic arch.

F. Abducent nerve (cranial nerve VI).
Abducent nerve (cranial nerve VI). The abducent nerve provide **motor** innervation to the **lateral rectus** and **retractor bulbi muscles.**

G. Facial nerve (cranial nerve VII)

1. The facial nerve's primary role is to supply motor innervation to many of the muscles of facial expression and sensory innervation to the rostral two thirds of the tongue. Its involvement with the eye is limited to supplying **motor innervation** to certain **eyelid musculature** and **parasympathetic** (i.e., visceral motor) **innervation** to the **lacrimal gland.**
2. After passing through the stylomastoid foramen, the facial nerve gives off several motor branches to the side of the face, detaches the dorsal and ventral buccal branches, and then continues as the **auriculopalpebral nerve.** The auriculopalpebral nerve divides adjacent to the base of the zygomatic arch to form the:
   a. **Auricular branch**
   b. **Zygomatic branch,** which forms a plexus of nerves that then detaches the **palpebral branches,** providing **motor** innervation to the **orbicularis oculi** (both the upper and lower parts), **retractor anguli oculi lateralis,** and the **retractor anguli oculi medialis**

VII. VASCULATURE

A. Arteries.
Arteries. The main arterial supply to the globe and adnexa is complex and detailed. Most blood arrives through branches of the **external carotid artery** and the **external ophthalmic artery,** a branch of the **maxillary artery.**

1. **Arterial supply to the eyelids** arrives mainly from two arteries:
   a. The **superficial temporal artery,** one of the two terminal branches of the external carotid artery, terminates as the **superior** and **inferior lateral palpebral arteries,** which supply the lateral aspect of the conjunctiva as well as the eyelids.
   b. The **malar artery,** a branch of the infraorbital artery, supplies the:
      (1) **Superior** and **inferior medial palpebral arteries,** which supply the lateral aspect of the conjunctiva as well as the eyelids
      (2) **Branches to some adnexa,** including the third eyelid, ventral oblique muscle, and nasolacrimal duct
2. **Arterial supply to the globe** (Figure 15–4) arrives in largest part through branches of the external ophthalmic artery, a major branch of the maxillary artery. A small amount of blood also arrives from the internal ophthalmic artery (a branch of the rostral cerebral artery).

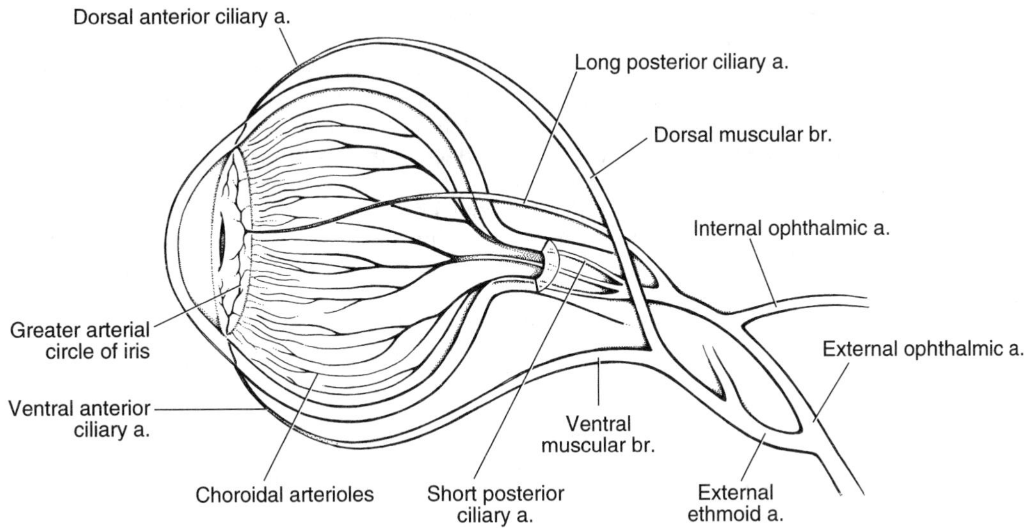

FIGURE 15–4. Schematized representation of the arterial supply to the globe.

a. The **external ophthalmic artery** arises from the maxillary artery almost immediately after the maxillary artery emerges from the alar canal. The external ophthalmic artery then almost immediately enters the periorbita, where it gives rise to two small anastomotic branches (which pass to the internal carotid and middle meningeal arteries) and the external ethmoid artery (see Chapter 9, Figure 9–2). After giving off the external ethmoidal artery, the external ophthalmic artery continues rostrally along the length of the optic nerve, where it anastomoses with the much smaller internal ophthalmic artery (see Figure 15–4).

(1) The **external ethmoid artery** leaves the external ophthalmic artery and usually provides the **dorsal** and **ventral muscular branches,** which are important in supplying the ocular adnexa. (Alternatively, these arteries may arise directly from the external ophthalmic artery.) Subsequently, the external ethmoidal artery enters the dorsal ethmoid foramen to assist the internal ethmoid artery in supplying the ethmoturbinates and nasal cavity. Adnexa supplied by the dorsal and ventral muscular branches include the:

- **(a) Extraocular muscles**
- **(b) Episcleral arteries**
- **(c) Bulbar conjunctiva**
- **(d) Lacrimal gland** (via the lacrimal artery)
- **(e) Gland of the third eyelid**

(2) The **dorsal** and **ventral anterior ciliary arteries** are the continuations of the dorsal and ventral muscular arteries, respectively. The dorsal anterior ciliary artery passes anteriorly from the equator to the limbal region (see Figure 15–4), where it pierces the sclera and divides into two branches, one directed medially and one laterally.

(a) Each of these branches continues ventrally through the sclera, parallel to the border of the iris, and eventually anastomoses with its ventral namesake, which has arrived by following a similar course. Thus, a complete circumferential arterial circle is formed within the sclera posterior to the iris.

(b) From this arterial circle, abundant arterioles pass to the capillary network of the limbal region. Fine arterioles also pass deeply to anastomose with the terminal branches of the posterior ciliary arteries (which supply the ciliary body).

b. The **internal ophthalmic artery** is almost rudimentary in domestic mammals, as compared with humans. This artery arises from the rostral cerebral artery within the cranial cavity and passes rostrally out of the cavity along with the optic nerve through the optic canal to anastomose with the external opthalmic artery (see Figure 15–4).

(1) The **long posterior ciliary arteries** arise from the anastomosis of the internal and external ophthalmic arteries on the surface of the optic nerve and supply the greatest part of blood to the anterior segment of the globe (see Figure 15–4). These arteries pass rostrally, still in contact with the optic nerve (placed mainly to its medial and lateral borders). On reaching the posterior surface of the globe, the long posterior ciliary arteries give rise to several short posterior ciliary arteries before continuing rostrally.

(2) The **short posterior ciliary arteries** branch to form a ring of several arteries that surround the optic nerve. These arteries participate in the formation of two arterial constructions.

(a) As they pass through the sclera adjacent to the area cribrosa, the short posterior ciliary arteries first give rise to the **retinal arteries.**

(i) These arteries pass to the interior of the globe in close apposition to the optic nerve and appear internally at the periphery of the optic disk.

(ii) At the optic disk, they branch in a radial pattern into 15–20 arterioles that course toward the retinal periphery. The retinal arterioles branch relatively uniformly throughout the retina, save for the region of the area centralis (i.e., that area of most acute vision) where the arterioles divert their path around its periphery.

Canine Clinical Correlation

Retinal arteries and veins can be easily distinguished from one another on ophthalmoscopic examination by the arteries' brighter color, smaller diameter, and more tortuous course.

(b) The short posterior ciliary arteries then pass on through the sclera and ramify in the choroid layer to form the **choroidal arterioles.** These arterioles pass anteriorly to reach the ciliary body and the ciliary margin of the iris, where they anastomose in a variable pattern with the anterior and long posterior ciliary arteries.

(3) Continuation of the long posterior ciliary arteries. After giving off the short posterior ciliary arteries at the posterior surface of the globe, the long posterior ciliary arteries continue rostrally along the medial and lateral borders of the globe.

(a) They are visible on the scleral surface as far as the equator. At this point, they pass deep to the sclera and continue in their anterior course.

(b) On reaching the ciliary margin of the iris, each long posterior ciliary artery divides into a **dorsal** and a **ventral branch,** which follow the caudal iridial border by coursing circumferentially around the globe. The circular arterial pattern thus formed is the **major arterial circle of the iris.** Fine branches leave the circle and pass either centrally toward the pupil (to supply the iris and its musculature) or the periphery (to anastomose with the arteries in the ciliary processes).

(4) Summary (Table 15–2). Consideration of where the three sets of ciliary arteries—the anterior, the long posterior, and the short posterior—enter the globe greatly simplifies their study, because the ciliary arteries are named for their site of entry into the globe:

(a) The **anterior ciliary arteries** enter the farthest anteriorly on the globe, in the region of the **limbus.** These arteries supply the **iris.**

(b) The **posterior ciliary arteries** enter more posteriorly, and are designated as long or short based on their entrance relative to the posterior surface of the globe:

TABLE 15–2. The Ciliary Arteries

Arteries	Source	Point of Entry Into the Globe	Structures Supplied
Anterior ciliary arteries	Dorsal muscular branch of the external ethmoid artery	Limbus	Iris, via the major arterial circle
Long posterior ciliary arteries	Anastomosis of external and internal ophthalmic arteries	Equator	Iris
Short posterior ciliary arteries	Long posterior ciliary artery	Surrounding optic nerve	Choroid, retina, parts of the iris

(i) The **short posterior ciliary arteries** enter the globe immediately adjacent to the exit of the optic nerve; hence their course is short compared with that of the long posterior ciliary arteries. These vessels supply the **choroid, retina,** and **parts of the iris.**

(ii) The **long posterior ciliary arteries** enter the globe at the equator; hence, their extraocular course is considerably longer than that of the short posterior ciliary arteries. These arteries also deliver blood to the **iris.**

B. Veins

1. **Drainage of the orbit.** Blood may leave the eye by one of three paths, all of which communicate with each other: via the angular vein (angularis oculi) to the facial vein, via the ophthalmic plexus to the cavernous sinus and maxillary vein, or via the anastomosis between the ventral external ophthalmic vein and the deep facial vein [see Chapter 9 II B 2 b (1), C 7 b].

   a. The **angular vein,** a superficial vein of the face that forms at the confluence of the dorsal nasal and facial veins, drains both superficial and deep structures.

      (1) The angular vein of the eye passes along the medial side of the orbit, and then turns deeply and enters the orbit just rostral to the zygomatic process of the temporal bone. Once in the orbit, the vein passes more deeply still by entering the periorbita at approximately the level of the equator of the globe. Here it flows into the dorsal external ophthalmic vein.

      (2) The angular vein of the eye lacks valves, and thus, depending on local factors, orbital blood may flow either by a superficial path into the facial vein, or by the deep path into the ophthalmic veins.

   b. The **dorsal external ophthalmic vein,** a deep vein lying within the orbit, is the largest of the individual veins associated with draining the eye.

      (1) The dorsal external ophthalmic vein receives the angular vein of the eye, and then courses caudoventrally within the orbit along its dorsomedial border. On reaching the posterior aspect of the globe, this vein sends a large anastomotic branch to the ventral external ophthalmic vein. The dorsal vorticose veins (which drain the vascular tunic; see VII B 2 b) usually enter the dorsal external ophthalmic vein near the exit of this anastomotic branch.

      (2) After the exchanges involving the anastomotic branch and the vorticose veins, the dorsal external ophthalmic vein dilates markedly and receives several small veins, including the external ethmoidal and lacrimal veins. The external ethmoidal vein undergoes marked dilatation and branching, forming the **ophthalmic plexus.** This plexus lies within the orbit near the orbital apex, and envelops the nervous and vascular structures entering the orbit.

      (3) The small **internal ophthalmic vein** leaves the plexus to pass through the optic canal along with the optic nerve and external ophthalmic artery.

c. The **ventral external ophthalmic vein** is another deep vein of the orbit, lying within the periorbita on the orbital floor.
   (1) At its rostral end, the ventral external opthalmic vein receives the large anastomotic branch from the dorsal external ophthalmic vein as well as the ventral vorticose veins from the vascular tunic of the eye.
   (2) At its caudal end, it receives numerous small branches from adjacent structures, and then enters the ophthalmic plexus formed by the dorsal external ophthalmic vein.
   (3) The ventral external ophthalmic vein **communicates with** the **deep facial vein** by a large anastomotic branch just caudal to the ventral orbital margin.

2. **Drainage of the globe**
   a. **Retina**
      (1) There are between three and five **retinal veins.** Their placement on the retina is fairly consistent, with the constant veins being directed dorsally, ventromedially, and ventrolaterally; a fourth vein directed straight ventrally is present in most dogs. The retinal veins anastomose in a circular pattern of variable completeness near the optic disk.
      (2) The retinal veins become confluent with each other as well as with the ciliary veins to form the **internal ophthalmic vein.**
   b. Vascular tunic. The iris, ciliary body, and choroid possess a unique drainage system that strictly follows its own course, and has no parallel arteries.
      (1) **Choroid**
         (a) **Choroidal venules** form within the substance of the choroid, and pass toward the sites of origin of the **vorticose veins.**
         (b) **Vorticose veins,** usually four in number, form from the confluence of the numerous choroidal venules. The vorticose veins provide the **major route of drainage from the choroid.** These veins pierce the sclera from the internal surface outward, and reach the superficial surface approximately at the equator.
            (i) The **dorsal pair** of vorticose veins drains into the **dorsal external ophthalmic vein.**
            (ii) The **ventral pair** of vorticose veins drains into the **ventral external ophthalmic vein.**
      (2) **Ciliary body.** The ciliary body is drained by the **ciliary veins,** which become confluent with each other as well as with the retinal veins to form the **internal ophthalmic vein.** Rather than being a single discrete vein, the internal opthalmic vein takes the form of several small veins coursing caudally in close association with the optic nerve. It joins in the formation of the ophthalmic plexus before passing into the optic canal with the optic nerve.

Chapter 16

Prominent Palpable and Visible Structures of the Head

I. PALPABLE STRUCTURES

A. Bony structures

1. **Mental foramina.** One or both of these foramina may be palpated in some individuals. The mental nerves, which are sensory, pass through these foramina; therefore, the examiner should be gentle.
2. **Mandible.** The **ventral mandibular border** is immediately subcutaneous; the **angular process** is slightly deeper, but still readily accessible.
3. **Teeth.** In addition to being readily visualized through the open mouth, the full length of both arcades of teeth is also palpable through the thin substance of the cheek.
4. **Infraorbital foramen.** This foramen is readily palpable on the maxilla a little less than halfway along the distance between the eye and external nose. When palpating for this structure, gentleness is again necessary because of the sensory nature of the infraorbital nerve, which passes through the foramen.
5. **Orbital rim.** The largely bony rim of the orbit is just subcutaneous, and thus readily accessible. Normally, little distinction can be felt between the bony part of the rim and the orbital ligament on its lateral edge.
6. **Zygomatic arch.** This heavy osseous arch is palpable along its full length, from the temporal region to where it blends with the maxilla at its rostral extent.
7. **Sagittal crest and external occipital protuberance.** The prominence of these structures varies, among breeds, between the sexes, and even among individuals. However, to some degree or another, the sagittal crest is normally palpable along the dorsal midline of the skull, and the external occipital protuberance is also normally accessible to the touch at the caudal end of the sagittal crest.
8. **Fontanelle.** In some individuals or toy breeds, the fontanelle on the dorsal surface of the skull does not entirely close, and can be detected as a yielding region of varying size along the dorsal midline of the skull.

B. Soft tissue structures

1. **Temporal and masseter muscle mass.** These heavy muscles of mastication are palpable directly beneath the skin, with the temporal muscle extending from the zygomatic arch dorsally to the dorsal midline, and the masseter muscle occupying the area on the lateral facial surface ventral to the zygomatic arch.
2. **Parotid duct.** This tubular structure is sometimes palpable as a cord-like structure beneath the skin as it passes in a caudorostral direction, about halfway down the expanse of the masseter muscle.
3. **Mandibular salivary gland.** The round, firm mass of this salivary gland is palpable on the ventrolateral neck, on the dorsal laryngeal border just caudal to the angle of the mandible.
4. **Mandibular lymph nodes.** These lymph nodes are palpable as a group of small, flattened structures just rostral to the mandibular salivary gland.
5. **External ear.** Several structures of the external ear are readily accessible to palpation:
   a. The full area of the **scapha** is visible and palpable, both over its flattened body as well as along its outer edges at the **helix.**
   b. The **cutaneous marginal pouch,** located at approximately the junction of the lateral helical margin and the head, is also readily visible and palpable.
   c. The **scutiform cartilage** may be palpable in the muscle mass rostral to the conchal opening.
   d. The **tragus** and **anthelix** are visible and palpable in the proximal part of the conchae.

e. Portions of the **external ear canal** are palpable through the musculature at the base of the ear.

6. **Basihyoid bone.** This bone is palpable in the base of the tongue just cranial to the larynx. This structure is delicate and should be palpated with caution.
7. **Larynx.** The **thyroid** and **cricoid cartilages** of the larynx are palpable caudal to the angle of the mandible in the cranial region of the neck. The larynx should also be palpated gently.

II. VISIBLE STRUCTURES

A. Oral cavity, oral vestibule, and oropharynx

1. The **frenulum** connects the body of the tongue to the floor of the oral cavity.
2. The paired **sublingual veins** are visible on the ventral surface of the tongue.
3. The **sublingual caruncles** are located just to each side of the midline ventral to the rostral region of the tongue. In some individuals, an elevation in the mucosa extending caudally from the sublingual caruncles indicates the submucosal position of the **ducts of the monostomatic sublingual** and **mandibular salivary glands.**
4. The **palatoglossal arches** can be seen extending from the base of the tongue dorsally to the soft palate.
5. The **opening of the parotid duct** can be seen in the vestibule adjacent to the upper carnassial tooth (fourth premolar).
6. The **palatine tonsil** can sometimes be seen within the palatine fossa in the lateral wall of the oropharynx, although it is usually partially hidden by the semilunar fold.

B. Eye

1. The **caruncle** is visible as a small, rounded elevation in the medial canthus.
2. The **punctae** are visible (if each lid is turned slightly outward) as small holes, one in each lid, just lateral to the medial edge of each eyelid. These openings to the lacrimal canaliculi are often present just at the junction of the pigmented and nonpigmented regions of the palpebral border.
3. The **third eyelid** is plain in the medial canthal region, where its darkly pigmented curved edge conforms to the curvature of the globe. The passive protrusion of the third lid may be demonstrated by applying gentle pressure through the eyelid on the scleral region of the globe: as the globe moves caudally, the third eyelid moves passively laterally over the corneal surface.

STUDY QUESTIONS

DIRECTIONS: Each of the numbered items or incomplete statements in this section is followed by answers or by completions of the statement. Select the ONE numbered answer or completion that is BEST in each case.

1. Which canine head form is most often associated with clinical difficulties?

(1) Brachycephalic
(2) Dolichocephalic
(3) Durocephalic
(4) Feracephalic
(5) Mesaticephalic

2. What is the temporal fossa?

(1) An excavation on the lateral surface of the skull from which the temporalis muscle originates
(2) A shallow groove in the middle cranial fossa through which the facial nerve runs
(3) The sinuous pathway of the temporal artery
(4) A convex region on the lateral surface of the skull from which the temporalis muscle originates

3. What is the region of the neurocranium where the mandible articulates with the remainder of the skull?

(1) Mandibular fossa
(2) Masseteric fossa
(3) Angular process
(4) Coronoid process
(5) Condylar process

4. What is the infraorbital foramen?

(1) The round opening on the bony floor of the orbit by which the optic nerve leaves the cranial cavity
(2) The elliptical opening on the lateral surface of the maxilla through which the infraorbital nerve passes
(3) An opening in the floor of the orbit that transmits a small group of sympathetic fibers
(4) A cleft in the ventrolateral orbital region through which a venous sinus passes

5. The caudolateral edge of the orbital rim is closed by the

(1) round ligament.
(2) orbital ligament.
(3) zygomatic process of the frontal bone.
(4) frontal process of the zygomatic bone.
(5) zygomatic process of the temporal bone.

6. Which one of the following statements regarding the pterygopalatine fossa is true?

(1) The pterygopalatine fossa is separated from the orbit by a stout horizontal shelf of bone.
(2) The pterygopalatine fossa is separated into two portions in the intact state by the body of the mandible.
(3) The pterygopalatine fossa is largely filled in the intact state by the temporalis muscle.
(4) The medial wall of the pterygopalatine fossa is the location of several foramina related to the eye and rostral facial region.
(5) The pterygopalatine fossa is bordered laterally by the pterygoid bone.

7. Which of the following adult teeth have three roots?

(1) Lateral incisors
(2) Central incisors
(3) Premolars 1 and 2
(4) Premolar 1 and molar 1
(5) Premolar 3 and molar 1

8. Which paranasal sinus or recess is most likely to be affected by a purulent sinusitis related to a tooth root abscess?

(1) Frontal sinus
(2) Sphenopalatine sinus
(3) Maxillary sinus
(4) Sphenoid sinus
(5) Maxillary recess

9. Which one of the following is located in the telencephalon?

(1) Lateral ventricles
(2) Hypothalamus
(3) Pyramids
(4) Optic chiasm

10. Which list correctly sequences the parts of the major white matter tract extending between the cerebral hemispheres and the spinal cord?

(1) Crus cerebri, pyramids, corona radiata, internal capsule
(2) Internal capsule, crus cerebri, transverse pontine fibers, pyramids
(3) Corona radiata, crus cerebri, pyramids, internal capsule
(4) Crus cerebri, longitudinal pontine fibers, pyramids

11. Which portion of the brain is involved in temperature regulation, visual reflexes, and auditory reflexes, and is also part of the visual path?

(1) Rhombencephalon
(2) Diencephalon
(3) Mesencephalon
(4) Brain stem

12. What is the correct sequence of cerebrospinal fluid flow through the ventricular system of the brain, from rostral to caudal?

(1) Lateral ventricles, third ventricle, mesencephalic aqueduct, fourth ventricle
(2) Third ventricle, fourth ventricle, lateral ventricles, mesencephalic aqueduct
(3) Mesencephalic aqueduct, lateral ventricles, third ventricle, fourth ventricle
(4) Lateral ventricles, third ventricle, fourth ventricle, mesencephalic aqueduct

13. Select the correct pairing of muscle and innervation.

(1) Buccinator—buccal nerve
(2) Temporal—auriculopalpebral nerve
(3) Orbicularis oris—dorsal buccal nerve
(4) Mentalis—mylohyoid nerve
(5) Levator palpebrae superioris—oculomotor nerve (cranial nerve III)

14. Which one of the following statements regarding the superficial facial region is true?

(1) The external nose is supported by paired and unpaired cartilages.
(2) The nasal plane is the vertical plane that divides the nasal region and muzzle into equal right and left halves.
(3) Vibrissae are specialized hairs designed to amplify sensory input that are distributed circumferentially around the margins of the lips.
(4) The scapha is the bony connection between the ear canal and the tympanic membrane.

15. Which one of the following statements regarding the parotid salivary gland is true?

(1) The parotid salivary gland closely embraces the base and ventral border of the orbit.
(2) The parotid salivary gland may have a small lymph node associated with its rostral border.
(3) The parotid duct of the parotid salivary gland courses rostrally over the deep surface of the masseter muscle.
(4) The parotid duct opens in the oral cavity near the last upper molar.

16. Which sequence correctly describes the course of sound waves through the inner ear?

(1) Vestibular window, cochlea, scala vestibuli, cochlear window
(2) Vestibular window, utricle, semicircular ducts, endolymphatic duct
(3) Cochlear window, cochlea, scala tympani, vestibule
(4) Cochlea, scala tympani, scala vestibuli, vestibule, semicircular canals

17. Which one of the following statements regarding the cochlear duct is true?

(1) It is filled with perilymph.
(2) It completes the division of the spiral canal into the scala tympani and scala vestibuli.
(3) It transfers mechanical impulses from the perilymph to the scala tympani, where they are transformed to electrical impulses.
(4) Crystals embedded in a gelatinous layer along its folds function in the perception of balance.

18. The nerves of the inner ear include the:

(1) chorda tympani, which innervates the tympanic membrane.
(2) cochlear nerve, which conducts impulses from the cochlea.
(3) spiral ganglion, which conducts impulses related to balance.
(4) vestibular nerve, which conducts impulses from the semicircular ducts.

19. Which one of the following statements regarding various structures of the eye is true?

(1) The ciliary body is located at the posterior extremity of the globe, where it produces vitreous humor.
(2) The tapetum lucidum is a feature of the fibrous tunic that serves to reflect light within the globe.
(3) Zonular fibers suspend the lens and play a role in changing its shape during accommodation.
(4) Pupillary dilatation is a parasympathetic response.

20. Which one of the following statements regarding the palpebrae is true?

(1) Cilia (eyelashes) are present on the free edges of both the upper and lower lids.
(2) The third eyelid has no intrinsic musculature.
(3) Tarsal glands are present in the free border of the upper lid only.
(4) The puncta open into the nasolacrimal duct system at the lateral canthal region.

21. Select the option below that correctly describes the sequence of tears through the nasolacrimal duct system.

(1) Lateral canthus, puncta, lacrimal sac, canaliculi, nasolacrimal duct proper
(2) Lateral canthus, canaliculi, puncta, lacrimal sac, nasolacrimal duct proper
(3) Medial canthus, nasolacrimal duct proper, lacrimal duct, canaliculi
(4) Medial canthus, puncta, canaliculi, nasolacrimal duct proper.

22. Which one of the following statements correctly describes the innervation of the eye?

(1) Sensory innervation to the globe arrives through the long ciliary nerves, branches of the ophthalmic nerve.
(2) Motor innervation to the pupil is provided by branches of the trochlear nerve.
(3) Much of the sensory innervation to the skin surrounding the orbit arrives through the facial nerve.
(4) Innervation to the levator of the upper lid and the orbicularis oculi are both provided by the oculomotor nerve.

23. Which one of the following statements correctly describes the arterial supply to the eye?

(1) The external ophthalmic artery is the direct parent of both the anterior and short posterior ciliary arteries.
(2) The long posterior ciliary arteries supply the iris.
(3) The internal ophthalmic artery supplies structures within the periorbita, and the external ophthalmic artery supplies structures outside the periorbita.
(4) Retinal arteries arise directly from the internal ophthalmic artery.

24. The external carotid artery typically terminates by dividing into the:

(1) deep temporal and maxillary arteries.
(2) superficial temporal and maxillary arteries.
(3) maxillary and infraorbital arteries.
(4) internal carotid and maxillary arteries.

25. Which one of the following statements regarding the infraorbital artery is true?

(1) It is the continuation of the sphenopalatine artery after it emerges from the intraorbital foramen.
(2) It supplies arterial branches to the lower arcade of teeth.
(3) It emerges from an elliptical foramen directly ventral to the orbit.
(4) It supplies the vibrissae.

26. Which one of the following statements regarding the maxillary vein is true?

(1) It drains the cranial cavity as well as the face.
(2) It originates in the medial part of the temporal fossa.
(3) It originates as the continuation of the infraorbital vein.
(4) It terminates in the maxillolinguofacial trunk.
(5) It receives no blood from the region of the ear.

27. Which non-cranial nerve supplies the most significant innervation to the head?

(1) Lesser auricular nerve
(2) Temporal nerve
(3) First cervical nerve
(4) Second cervical nerve

28. Which cranial nerve exits dorsally from the brain stem, innervates an extraocular muscle, and is the only cranial nerve to cross the brain entirely to innervate structures on the opposite side of its origin?

(1) Oculomotor nerve (cranial nerve III)
(2) Trochlear nerve (cranial nerve IV)
(3) Abducent nerve (cranial nerve VI)
(4) Glossopharyngeal nerve (cranial nerve IX)

29. Which group of cranial nerves exits the skull in the pterygopalatine fossa?

(1) III, VII, IX, and X
(2) II, III, IV, V, and VI
(3) IX, X, XI, and XII
(4) I, II, and VIII

30. Which component of the facial nerve (cranial nerve VII) carries parasympathetic fibers to the salivary and lacrimal glands?

(1) Genu
(2) Intermediate nerve
(3) Chorda tympani
(4) Medial ramus

31. Where are openings of the salivary glands found?

(1) In the oral cavity
(2) In the oral vestibule
(3) In the oral cavity and the oral vestibule
(4) Scattered along the walls of the oral cavity near the teeth

32. What structure does the sublingual fold cover?

(1) The sublingual artery
(2) The lyssa
(3) The ducts of the parotid and sublingual salivary glands
(4) The ducts of the mandibular and sublingual salivary glands

33. Which one of the following statements regarding the larynx is true?

(1) It receives both motor and sensory innervation from the vagus nerve (cranial nerve X).
(2) It is supported by paired bones and cartilages.
(3) It attaches directly to the occipital region of the skull by specialized ligaments.
(4) The arytenoid cartilage is its largest cartilage.

34. Which of the following structures is a prominently palpable feature on the lateral surface of the maxilla?

(1) The infraorbital foramen
(2) The rostral mental foramen
(3) The frenulum
(4) The anthelix

35. Which one of the following structures is normally palpable on the head?

(1) The ceratohyoid bone
(2) The arytenoid cartilage
(3) The angular process of the mandible
(4) The monostomatic sublingual salivary gland

36. Which two nerves are most extensively involved in the innervation of the pharynx?

(1) Vagus and hypoglossal nerves
(2) Vagus and glossopharyngeal nerves
(3) Glossopharyngeal and accessory nerves
(4) Hypoglossal and accessory nerves

37. Which muscle largely occupies the space dorsal to the zygomatic arch, inserts onto the coronoid process of the mandible, and is innervated by the mandibular division of the trigeminal nerve (cranial nerve V_3)?

(1) Temporalis muscle
(2) Medial pterygoid muscle
(3) Masseter muscle
(4) Lateral pterygoid muscle

DIRECTIONS: Each of the numbered items or incomplete statements in this section is negatively phrased, as indicated by a capitalized word such as NOT, LEAST, or EXCEPT. Select the ONE numbered answer or completion that is BEST in each case.

38. The walls of the neurocranium (braincase) are formed by contributions from all of the following bones EXCEPT the:

(1) zygomatic bone.
(2) frontal bone.
(3) parietal bone.
(4) temporal bone.

39. The zygomatic arch is formed by contributions from several bones. Which one of the following bones does NOT make a contribution to the zygomatic arch?

(1) Temporal bone
(2) Frontal bone
(3) Zygomatic bone
(4) Maxilla

40. Traumatic injury to the region surrounding the tympanic bulla would be LEAST likely to affect which one of the following cranial nerves?

(1) Glossopharyngeal nerve (cranial nerve IX)
(2) Vagus nerve (cranial nerve X)
(3) Facial nerve (cranial nerve VII)
(4) Mandibular nerve (cranial nerve V_3)

41. All of the following structures are prominent in the rostral view of the skull EXCEPT the

(1) zygomatic arch.
(2) incisor teeth.
(3) infraorbital foramen.
(4) alar canal.

42. Which of the following types of adult teeth do NOT have a deciduous precursor?

(1) All molars
(2) All premolars
(3) All premolars and molars
(4) The fourth premolars and the canines
(5) The third incisors and the molars

43. Which one of the following statements regarding the external ear is INCORRECT?

(1) The auricular cartilage is elastic in nature and supports the main portion of the erect or dependent portion of the ear.
(2) The external ear varies most in form among breeds in its more distal region.
(3) The external ear is characterized by a cutaneous marginal pouch along the medial margin of the ear.
(4) The external ear is characterized by an abrupt, almost 90-degree turn where the vertical portion joins the horizontal portion.

44. Which one of the following structures is NOT supplied by branches of the maxillary artery arising within the region of the deep face?

(1) Infraorbital area
(2) Temporal muscle
(3) Cranial cavity
(4) Periorbita

45. Which matching of ear part and function is INCORRECT?

(1) External ear—collects and transmits sound waves
(2) Middle ear—generates electrical impulses at the tympanic membrane
(3) Inner ear—functions in balance at the semicircular canals and maculae
(4) Inner ear—functions in hearing at the cochlear duct

46. Which one of the following descriptions INCORRECTLY describes the occipital artery?

(1) It is typically a branch of the internal carotid artery.
(2) It is associated with the medial retropharyngeal lymph node.
(3) It passes craniodorsally into the occipital region of the head.
(4) It supplies the caudal skull musculature and sends some branches into the meninges.

47. The lingual artery supplies all of the following structures EXCEPT the:

(1) tongue.
(2) hyoid apparatus.
(3) palatine tonsil.
(4) pharyngeal musculature.
(5) temporal muscle.

48. Which of the following veins does NOT accompany an artery of the same name?

(1) Superior labial
(2) Deep facial
(3) Superficial temporal
(4) Inferior alveolar

49. Which one of the following structures is NOT innervated by the trigeminal nerve (cranial nerve V)?

(1) Extraocular muscles
(2) Globe
(3) Tongue
(4) Skin on the lateral surface of the muzzle

50. Which one of the following structures is NOT innervated by the ophthalmic branch of the trigeminal nerve (cranial nerve V_1)?

(1) Lacrimal gland
(2) Nasal mucosa
(3) Cornea
(4) Levator palpebrae superioris

51. The eye (in the broad sense, including the globe and adnexa) receives innervation, either sensory or motor, from all of the following nerves EXCEPT the:

(1) facial nerve (cranial nerve VII).
(2) ophthalmic nerve.
(3) maxillary nerve.
(4) trochlear nerve (cranial nerve IV).
(5) pterygopalatine nerve.

52. Which one of the following statements describing the chorda tympani is INCORRECT?

(1) It is a branch of the facial nerve (cranial nerve VII).
(2) It carries taste fibers to the rostral two thirds of the tongue.
(3) It carries touch fibers from the tympanic membrane.
(4) It passes through the middle ear on its course.

53. All of the following cranial nerves contribute to the innervation of the teeth EXCEPT the:

(1) mandibular nerve.
(2) maxillary nerve.
(3) infraorbital nerve.
(4) facial nerve.

54. Which one of the following statements regarding the role of the tongue in taste is INCORRECT?

(1) The tongue is innervated by both cranial and cervical nerves.
(2) The rostral two thirds of the tongue is innervated for taste by different nerves from those that innervate the caudal third for taste.
(3) The rostral two thirds of the dorsal surface of the tongue is covered with filiform papillae, which are not gustatory in function.
(4) The tongue possesses two general types of papillae.

55. Select the INCORRECT statement describing the role of the pharyngeal musculature in alimentation. The pharyngeal muscles serve to:

(1) dilate the pharynx to receive the food bolus.
(2) close the pharynx over the food bolus.
(3) constrict the pharynx around the food bolus.
(4) elevate the pharynx over the larynx during liquid ingestion.

ANSWERS AND EXPLANATIONS

1. The answer is 1 [Chapter 7 II A 3 c]. Brachycephalic dogs are predisposed to several clinical conditions related directly to the shape of their heads. Brachycephalic dogs may experience complications related to mastication, breathing, and swallowing, as well as ocular problems, dermatologic disorders, and, in bitches, dystocia. (In fact, Caesarian deliveries are all but routine in some breeds, such as English bulldogs.) Mesaticephalic and dolichocephalic dogs typically have few difficulties related solely to head form. "Durocephalic" and "feracephalic" are fanciful terms.

2. The answer is 4 [Chapter 8 II A 3]. Despite its name, which implies a depression, the temporal fossa is convex in profile. The temporal fossa gives rise to the temporal muscle.

3. The answer is 1 [Chapter 8 II C 2 a, F]. The mandibular fossa, a transversely elongate projection of the squamous portion of the temporal bone, is where the mandible articulates with the rest of the skull. The condylar process, angular process, and the masseteric fossa are all named regions of the mandible itself.

4. The answer is 2 [Chapter 8 II A 1 (a) (2)]. The infraorbital foramen is a large ovoid foramen on the lateral surface of the maxilla through which the infraorbital nerve passes, as well as the infraorbital artery and vein. The other distractors are fanciful.

5. The answer is 2 [Chapter 8 II A 2 a (2)]. The caudal orbital rim, which is ligamentous rather than bony, is closed by the orbital ligament. The various round ligaments of the body are associated with the abdominal and pelvic viscera.

6. The answer is 4 [Chapter 8 II A 2 b (3) (b)]. The optic canal, the orbital fissure, and the rostral and caudal alar foramina are located in the medial wall of the pterygopalatine fossa. These foramina transmit structures related to the eye and the rostral facial region. The pterygopalatine fossa is directly continuous with the orbit. In the intact state, it is divided by the ramus (not the body) of the mandible and it is filled by the pterygoid muscles (not the temporal muscles).

7. The answer is 5 [Chapter 8 IV C 1]. Premolar 3 and molar 1 each have three roots. The number of roots is important to know when performing dental extractions. All incisors and canines have one root; the first two premolars have two roots, and the last premolar and both molars have three roots.

8. The answer is 5 [Chapter 8 II G 2 a]. The maxillary recess lies in close proximity to the roots of the upper molars and premolars, and the bone separating the teeth from the sinus is relatively thin. Therefore, tooth root abscesses can erode the bony partition and establish a purulent sinusitis within the maxillary recess. Drainage is best approached by removal of the carnassial tooth, allowing drainage into the mouth.

9. The answer is 1 [Chapter 13 I A 2 a; V A 1]. The lateral ventricles, the cerebrospinal fluid—filled spaces of the cerebral hemispheres, are part of the telencephalon. The telencephalon is the rostral derivative of the prosencephalon that develops into the cerebrum. The hypothalamus and optic chiasm are features of the diencephalon; the pyramids are features of the myelencephalon (medulla oblongata).

10. The answer is 4 [Chapter 13 IV A 2 c]. The longitudinal fibers of the pons are the continuation of the fibers from the crus cerebri (which in turn originated in the corona radiata of the cerebral hemispheres). Some longitudinal fibers synapse on the pontine nuclei, while others pass directly through to the pyramids of the medulla oblongata. Note that not all portions of the white matter tract are represented in the options.

11. The answer is 2 [Chapter 10 II B 2, 5 b]. The hypothalamus, part of the diencephalon, is involved in temperature regulation. The optic nerve begins development as an outgrowth from the diencephalon. The lateral and medial geniculate bodies (located in the metathalamus, which is also part of the diencephalon) are involved in visual and auditory function, respectively.

12. The answer is 1 [Chapter 13 V; Figure 13–6). Cerebrospinal fluid flows from the lateral ventricles, to the third ventricle, through the mesencephalic aqueduct, into the fourth ventricle, and from the fourth ventricle, either directly into the central canal of the spinal cord or through the lateral apertures into the subarachnoid space.

13. The answer is 5 [Table 11–1]. The levator palpebrae superioris, which raises the eyelid, is the only muscle of facial expression that is not innervated by a branch of the facial nerve (cranial nerve VII); the levator palpebrae superioris is innervated by the oculomotor nerve (cranial nerve III). The buccinator is innervated by the dorsal and ventral buccal branches of the facial nerve (CN VII), not the buccal nerve. The buccal nerve is a branch of the mandibular division of the trigeminal nerve (cranial nerve V_3), and is sensory rather than motor. Furthermore, there is no dorsal buccal nerve—rather, the dorsal and ventral buccal branches of the facial nerve innervate the orbicularis oris. The mentalis is innervated by the ventral buccal branch of the facial nerve (cranial nerve VII). [The mylohyoid nerve is a sensorimotor branch of the mandibular division of the trigeminal nerve (cranial nerve V_3).] The auriculopalpebral nerve innervates the muscles of the ear and eyelid. The temporal muscle is innervated by the temporal nerve.

14. The answer is 1 [Chapter 11 I]. The external nose is supported by paired and unpaired cartilages. The nasal plane is the region of thickened, hairless skin, commonly referred to as the "nose," that surrounds and extends beyond the borders of the nostrils. Vibrissae are specialized tactile hairs, but they do not circumferentially surround the lips (they are more restricted in their distribution). The scapha is the relatively flattened distal region of the auricular cartilage that begins at the area where the "scoop" of the conchal cavity is lost and the auricular cartilage becomes rather flat.

15. The answer is 2 [Chapter 11 I B 1 a, 2 b]. The parotid salivary gland may have a small lymph node associated with its rostral border. The parotid gland closely embraces the base of the ear, and sends its single duct rostrally over the superficial surface of the masseter muscle to open into the oral cavity near the last upper premolar.

16. The answer is 1 [Chapter 14 V C]. The first sequence—vestibular window, cochlea, scala vestibuli, cochlear window—correctly describes the course of sound waves through the inner ear. Although this sequence leaves out certain of the elements in the pathway, those represented are in correct order.

17. The answer is 2 [Chapter 14 IV C 4 c]. The membranous cochlear duct, along with the bony spiral lamina, partially bisects the spiral canal into two portions, the scala vestibuli and the scala tympani. The cochlear duct is filled with endolymph, and is the site where mechanical energy is transformed into electrical energy. The macules of the saccule and utriculus possess a gelatinous layer embedded with crystals, statoconia, which function in the perception of balance.

18. The answer is 4 [Chapter 14 IV E]. The vestibular nerve passes from the semicircular ducts and transmits information concerning balance. The chorda tympani is a branch of the facial nerve carrying taste fibers to the rostral two thirds of the tongue; it merely crosses over the tympanic membrane. Fibers from the spiral ganglion collect to form the cochlear nerve, which is involved with hearing. The cochlea is part of the bony labyrinth and thus generates no impulses at all (they come from the cochlear duct).

19. The answer is 3 [Chapter 15 II C 3]. Zonular fibers suspend the lens and function in changing its shape during accommodation. The ciliary body is positioned anteriorly in the globe and has no relation to the vitreous humor. The ciliary body is part of the choroid and is covered by the ciliary part of the retina: it is this portion of the retina, not the ciliary body itself, that produces aqueous humor. The tapetum lucidum is a feature of the choroid, not the fibrous tunic. Pupillary dilatation is a sympathetic response, not a parasympathetic response.

20. The answer is 2 [Chapter 15 IV B, C 1]. The third eyelid has no musculature at all—its movement is passive. The tarsal glands are found in both lids. The puncta open near the medial canthus. In dogs, cilia (eyelashes) are present on the free edge of the upper lid only.

21. The answer is 4 [Chapter 15 IV D 1 b (2), c]. After being produced and dispersed across the cornea, the tears accumulate in the lacrimal lake, which is a shallow depression in the medial canthus. From the lacrimal lake, the tears move into the puncta, which are located on the inner surface of each lid margin, very close to the lacrimal lake. The puncta open into the lacrimal canaliculi, which open into the nasolacrimal duct proper. The nasolacrimal duct terminates on the ventrolateral floor of the nasal vestibule.

22. The answer is 1 [Chapter 15 VI E 1 c (1)]. The long ciliary nerves, branches of the ophthalmic nerve (the opthalmic division of the trigeminal nerve, cranial nerve V), provide rich sensory innervation to the choroid, ciliary body, iris, cornea, and bulbar conjunctiva. The pupillary musculature is innervated by autonomic fibers. The facial nerve is motor to the orbicularis oculi, but not the levator palpebrae superioris. Sensory innervation to the periorbital skin is provided by the two divisions of the zygomatic nerve (the zygomatic nerve itself is a branch of the maxillary division of the trigeminal nerve, cranial nerve V).

23. The answer is 2 [Chapter 15 VII A 2 b (3); Table 15–2]. The long posterior ciliary arteries form the major arterial circle of the iris. The anterior ciliary arteries arise most directly from the external ethmoid artery (rather than the ophthalmic artery). The short posterior ciliary arteries arise most directly from the long posterior ciliary artery. Both the retinal and the external ophthalmic arteries supply structures within the periorbita. The retinal arteries arise from the short posterior ciliary arteries.

24. The answer is 2 [Chapter 9 I C 6]. The external carotid artery typically terminates by dividing into the superficial temporal and maxillary arteries.

25. The answer is 4 [Chapter 9 I D 2 a (2)]. The infraorbital artery is a continuation of the maxillary artery that emerges from the infraorbital foramen, which is situated a considerable distance rostral to the orbit. In addition to supplying the vibrissae, the infraorbital artery also supplies the teeth of the upper arcade.

26. The answer is 1 [Chapter 9 II C]. In addition to draining many structures of the face, the maxillary vein receives the temporomandibular articular vein, which drains a portion of the cranial cavity. The maxillary vein originates from the pterygoid plexus in the pterygopalatine fossa, receives the superficial temporal and caudal auricular arteries (both of which drain the auricular region), and terminates in the external jugular vein. The "maxillolinguofacial trunk" is a fanciful vessel.

27. The answer is 4 [Chapter 10 I B]. The second cervical nerve has three branches—the greater occipital, transverse cervical, and great auricular branches—and supplies the skin over the occipital, temporal, and caudal mandibular regions as well as over much of the pinna with sensory innervation. The "lesser auricular nerve" and "temporal nerve" are fanciful, and the first cervical nerve does not participate in innervation of the head region.

28. The answer is 2 [Chapter 10 II D 2]. The trochlear nerve is unique among the cranial nerves in three respects: it is the only cranial nerve to exit the dorsal brain stem surface, it is the only cranial nerve to cross the brain entirely to innervate the contralateral side, and it is the smallest cranial nerve.

29. The answer is 2 [Chapter 8 II A 2 b (3) (b)]. The optic nerve (cranial nerve II), oculomotor nerve (cranial nerve III), trochlear nerve (cranial nerve IV), ophthalmic and maxillary components of the trigeminal nerve (cranial nerve V_1 and V_2, respectively), and the abducent nerve (cranial nerve VI) exit the skull through a group of foramina on the caudoventral region of the pterygopalatine fossa (i.e., the optic canal, orbital fissure, and rostral alar foramen). The cranial nerves listed in the first option belong together because they all carry autonomic fibers. Those of the third option all exit the skull at the tympanooccipital fissure. Those of the fourth option are all purely sensory.

30. The answer is 2 [Chapter 10 II G 1 c (2)]. The intermediate nerve carries parasympathetic fibers to the salivary and lacrimal glands. The genu is simply a bend in the course of the facial nerve (cranial nerve VII) associated with a ganglion. The chorda tympani carries taste fibers to the rostral two thirds of the tongue. The "medial ramus" does not exist.

31. The answer is 3 [Chapter 12 I B 2, C 2 b]. The parotid and zygomatic salivary glands open into the oral vestibule near the upper carnassial tooth, and the major sublingual and mandibular salivary glands open in the oral cavity at the sublingual caruncle. No salivary gland openings are scattered along the walls of the oral cavity near the teeth.

32. The answer is 4 [Chapter 12 I C 2 a]. The sublingual fold covers the ducts of the mandibular and major sublingual salivary glands. The sublingual artery courses much more deeply within the substance of the tongue. The lyssa resides in the apex of the tongue. The parotid duct courses across the lateral surface of the masseter muscle.

33. The answer is 1 [Chapter 12 IV E]. The vagus nerve supplies all sensory and motor innervation to the larynx via the cranial and caudal laryngeal nerves. The larynx is composed of cartilage, not bone, and only one of the six cartilages is paired (the arytenoid cartilage). The thyroid cartilage is the largest of the six cartilages. The larynx attaches to the skull by way of the hyoid apparatus.

34. The answer is 1 [Chapter 16 I A 4]. The infraorbital foramen is the only structure listed that is located on the lateral surface of the maxilla: the mental foramina lie on the rostral lateral end of the mandible. The frenulum attaches the body of the tongue to the floor of the oral cavity. The anthelix is a portion of the ear.

35. The answer is 3 [Chapter 16 I A 2]. The angular process of the mandible is normally palpable. The basihyoid bone, not the ceratohyoid bone is also normally palpable. The cricoid and thyroid laryngeal cartilages, not the arytenoid cartilage, are normally palpable as well. The mandibular salivary gland, not the monostomatic sublingual salivary gland, is palpable.

36. The answer is 2 [Chapter 10 II I, K, L; Chapter 12 III A 3 d]. The vagus and glossopharyngeal nerves are most extensively involved in the innervation of the pharynx. The accessory nerve is motor only to various muscles of the ventral neck and the trapezius. The hypoglossal nerve is motor to only the tongue.

37. The answer is 1 [Chapter 11 II B 4 a (2)]. The temporal muscle extends from the bony wall of the temporal fossa to the coronoid process of the mandible. It occupies the space dorsal to the zygomatic arch and is innervated by the temporal branch of the mandibular nerve.

38. The answer is 1 [Chapter 8 I A 2 a (2)]. The zygomatic bone does not contribute to the neurocranium (braincase).

39. The answer is 2 [Chapter 8 II A 1 c]. Though the frontal bone contributes to the orbital rim by way of its zygomatic process, this process does not contribute to formation of the zygomatic arch.

40. The answer is 4 [Chapter 8 II C 2 b]. The glossopharyngeal nerve (cranial nerve IX) and the vagus nerve (cranial nerve X) both exit through the tympanooccipital fissure, and the facial nerve (cranial nerve VII) exits through the stylomastoid foramen. The tympanooccipital fissure and the stylomastoid foramen are directly adjacent to the tympanic bulla. The mandibular nerve (cranial nerve V_3) exits via the oval foramen, which is rostral to the area of the tympanic bulla. Furthermore, the mandibular nerve courses rostrally into the facial region rather than being distributed in the tympanic region.

41. The answer is 4 [Chapter 8 II A 2 b (4), E]. The alar canal is mainly visible from the lateral view. The appearance of the skull from the rostral aspect is marked plainly by the prominent nasal aperture, incisor and canine teeth, orbits, frontal region, and zygomatic arches.

42. The answer is 1 [Chapter 8 IV B 2]. There are no deciduous molars.

43. The answer is 3 [Chapter 11 I A 5 a (3)]. The cutaneous marginal pouch is a feature of the lateral margin of the ear, not the medial margin. The auricular cartilage is elastic in nature and supports the main portion of the erect or dependent portion of the ear. Variation in the form of the ear among breeds is most noticeable in the distal portion of the ear. The ear canal of the external ear has an "L"-shaped course, making a sharp 90-degree turn at the level of the external acoustic meatus.

44. The answer is 1 [Chapter 11 I B 4 a (4); II B 5 a]. Although the maxillary artery does ultimately carry blood to the infraorbital area, it does so by its continuation as the infraorbital artery, which is a feature of the superficial face. The temporalis muscle is supplied by the caudal deep temporal artery, the cranial cavity is supplied by the middle meningeal artery, and the periorbita is supplied by the external ophthalmic artery, all branches of the maxillary artery located in the deep face.

45. The answer is 2 [Chapter 14 V]. No nervous impulses are generated at the tympanic membrane—sound waves are simply transferred from the membrane to the chain of auditory ossicles. The external ear collects and transmits sound waves to the middle ear. The inner ear is involved in both hearing and balance; the cochlear duct is involved with hearing and the semicircular canals and maculae are involved with balance.

46. The answer is 1 [Chapter 9 I C 1]. The occipital artery is typically a branch of the external carotid artery, not the internal carotid artery. It passes craniodorsally into the occipital region of the head and supplies the skull musculature, as well as parts of the meninges. The occipital artery is associated with the medial retropharyngeal lymph node.

47. The answer is 5 [Chapter 9, Table 9–1]. The temporal muscle is not within the region supplied by the lingual artery. The lingual artery does supply the tongue, hyoid apparatus, palatine tonsil, and pharyngeal musculature.

48. The answer is 2 [Chapter 9 II B 2 b (4)]. The deep facial vein has no companion artery.

49. The answer is 1 [Chapter 10 II E 2]. The extraocular muscles are supplied by the oculomotor nerve (cranial nerve III) the trochlear nerve (cranial nerve IV), and the abducent nerve (cranial nerve VI). The trigeminal nerve (cranial nerve V) supplies the globe through its ophthalmic branch, the tongue through its mandibular branch, and the muzzle skin through its maxillary branch.

50. The answer is 4 [Chapter 10 II E 2 a]. The levator palpebrae superioris is innervated by the oculomotor nerve (cranial nerve III). Although it may seem unlikely that the nasal mucosa is innervated by the ophthalmic branch of the trigeminal nerve, it is—the ethmoidal nerve is a branch of the ophthalmic nerve.

51. The answer is 5 [Chapter 15 VI A–B]. The pterygopalatine nerve has no function related to the eye: it innervates the soft and hard palates, the nasal cavity, and the maxillary sinus. Fully half of the cranial nerves are involved in the innervation of the eye, including the trochlear nerve (cranial nerve IV), the maxillary and ophthalmic nerves (branches of cranial nerve V), and the facial nerve (cranial nerve VII).

52. The answer is 3 [Chapter 14 III B 2 c]. The chorda tympani is a branch of the facial nerve (cranial nerve VII) that carries taste fibers to the rostral two thirds of the tongue. The "tympani" in its name has to do with the nerve's physical proximity to the tympanic membrane on its course through the middle ear.

53. The answer is 4 [Chapter 10 II E 3 b (3), c, G 1]. The facial nerve has nothing to do with innervating the teeth. The maxillary nerve is a branch of the trigeminal nerve (cranial nerve V_2) and is sensory to the upper arcade. The mandibular nerve, also a branch of the trigeminal nerve (cranial nerve V_3) is sensory to the lower arcade via its branch, the inferior alveolar nerve.

54. The answer is 1 [Chapter 12 II F]. Only branches of cranial nerves (cranial nerves V, VII, IX, and XII) innervate the tongue. The chorda tympani, a branch of the facial nerve (cranial nerve VII), supplies taste innervation to the rostral two thirds of the tongue. The glossopharyngeal nerve (cranial nerve IX) supplies taste innervation to the caudal third of the tongue. The tongue possesses two general types of papillae, those with taste buds and those without. Filiform papillae, which lack taste buds, cover the rostral two thirds of the tongue's dorsum.

55. The answer is 4 [Chapter 12 VI A 2]. During deglutition, the pharyngeal dilator (stylopharyngeus muscle) widens the rostral part of the pharynx to receive the bolus of food. The pharyngeal shorteners/constrictors (the palatopharyngeus and pterygopharyngeus muscles) draw the pharynx onto and over the bolus. The middle and caudal pharyngeal constrictors (i.e., the hyopharyngeus, thyropharyngeus, and cricopharyngeus muscles) contract in a rostrocaudal direction, carrying solids over the laryngeal entrance and into the esophagus, and diverting fluids into the piriform recesses of the larynx.

PART III

NECK AND BACK

Chapter 17

Introduction to the Neck and Back

I. COMPONENTS

A. Vertebral column. The vertebral column, which forms the greatest part of the axial skeleton, is the central framework of the neck and back.

1. **Qualities.** The vertebral column is **firm yet flexible.** It consists of approximately 50 relatively small, separate bones that articulate with each other by synovial joints. Although for the most part, the mobility of each individual joint is relatively limited, the vertebral column as a unit is notably flexible, especially in the cervical and tail regions.
   a. The caudal area of the neck region is the most flexible of all. The mobility provided by joints in this region allow the dog to reach nearly all regions of its trunk with its mouth, although the interscapular region remains largely inaccessible (a fact seemingly well-known to fleas!)
   b. The considerable degree of flexion and extension characteristic of the late thoracic and all of the lumbar vertebrae is evidenced by the pronounced and dynamic motion of these regions of the column observed in the bounding gallop of a dog running at top speed. The column flexes so strongly that the hindfeet may be placed ahead of the forefeet at the start of each propulsion.
   c. The thoracolumbar region of the column is also capable of marked lateral extension and flexion, as demonstrated by the dog's ability to curl up into a "ball" when sleeping.
2. **Functions.** The bony vertebral column provides:
   a. Firm, yet flexible, central support for essentially the entire body
   b. A framework for the attachment of the ribs and sternum to the central body
   c. A framework for the attachment of the limbs to the body
   d. Protection for the spinal cord and spinal nerve roots

B. Muscles and ligaments. The musculature and ligaments of the neck and back serve a dual function. These structures:

1. Bind the numerous individual bones of the vertebral column into a cohesive unit sufficiently rigid to support the body
2. Impart significant mobility to the vertebral column, a quality that is essential to locomotion

II. EMBRYOLOGIC DEVELOPMENT.

The **somitic nature** of the embryo is clearly reflected in the final form of the neck and back.

A. The **vertebrae** are clear descendants of the ancestral regional somites (i.e., paired, block-like masses of mesoderm).

B. The **intrinsic musculature** of the back also retains clear connections to its somitic origin. The intrinsic muscles may cross one or multiple vertebral joints, but the segmental nature is retained in all cases.

C. The **innervation** pattern of the back musculature is traceable to the somitic origin of the muscles. As each muscle block develops, an adjacent spinal nerve grows outward into it. Regardless of where the muscle ultimately attaches, the original innervation is retained.

Chapter 18

The Vertebrae

I. INTRODUCTION

A. Terminology. The use of the terms "spine" and "spinal column" as synonyms for the vertebral column should be avoided. Although each vertebra is characterized by one or more spinous processes of varying prominence, use of the term "spine" (a term indicating merely a projection from some other, central structure) to describe the vertebral column as a whole is inaccurate.

B. Vertebral types and the vertebral formula

1. **Types.** Five named types of vertebrae are present in the vertebral column. Classification is based on the form of the vertebra and on its position within the chain of vertebrae comprising the column. From cranial to caudal, these types are the:
   - a. **Cervical vertebrae** (7 in the dog), found in the neck region
   - b. **Thoracic vertebrae** (13 in the dog), located in the chest region, each articulating with a pair of ribs
   - c. **Lumbar vertebrae** (7 in the dog), in the area of the loins (along the dorsal abdominal wall)
   - d. **Sacral vertebrae** (3 in the dog), in the area of the croup where the vertebral column articulates with the pelvis
   - e. **Caudal vertebrae** (approximately 20), found in the tail*
2. **Vertebral formula.** The vertebral formula may be written using a letter abbreviation to designate the region followed by the number of vertebrae within the region: therefore, in the dog, the vertebral formula is written as **C7, T13, L7, S3, Cd20–23.**

C. Alignment of the vertebral column. The position of the vertebral column within the body does not mirror the topline of the dog (see Figure 3–1).

1. **Cervical region.** In the cervical region, the column sweeps gently ventrally, so that in the midcervical region the bony column is positioned about midway down the dorsal to ventral depth of the neck.
2. **Thoracic, lumbar, and sacral regions**
   - a. In the **early thoracic region,** the main mass (i.e., the bodies) of the vertebrae are still positioned much deeper than the topline, although the long, dorsally projecting spinous processes extend to a subcutaneous position.
   - b. At the **midthoracic region,** the vertebral column begins to incline gently dorsally, so from this point caudally through the **lumbar** and **sacral regions,** the vertebral bodies are near the dorsal topline, and oriented essentially parallel with the ground.
   - c. In the **tail region,** the vertebral column occupies the middle of the tail, and lies very close to the surface from all aspects.

II. GENERAL VERTEBRAL MORPHOLOGY.

Except for the highly specialized vertebrae of the most cranial and caudal regions of the vertebral column, most vertebrae have basic

*The term "coccygeal" is sometimes used to described the caudal vertebrae. The coccyx is a structure found in humans that develops from the fusion of the first few caudal vertebrae. There is no homologous structure in domestic mammals; therefore, use of the term "coccygeal" to describe the individual and fully mobile vertebrae of the tail is discouraged in veterinary medicine.

structural features in common. Typically, vertebrae are formed from a body and an arch (composed of paired pedicles and laminae), from which project several types of processes: the dorsal or spinous, transverse, and articular in all vertebrae, and potentially the accessory and mamillary processes, as well.

A. Vertebral body. The vertebral body is the massive ventral portion of the vertebra (Figure 18–1).

1. The cranial surface of the vertebral body is slightly convex, while the caudal surface is slightly concave. This feature is related to the articulation of one vertebra with the next.
2. In the intact state, a fibrocartilaginous **intervertebral disc** is interposed between the articular surfaces of adjacent vertebral bodies. The intervertebral disc is composed of two parts:
   a. The **nucleus pulposus,** the central, gelatinous region, represents the sole remnant of the embryonic notochord in the definitive form.
   b. The **annulus fibrosus** is the tough outer fibrous area that encircles and retains the pulpy center.

B. Vertebral arch. The vertebral arch rises dorsally from the body (see Figure 18–1).

1. Paired **pedicles** project dorsally at essentially right angles for a short distance from the right and left sides of the vertebral body.
2. Paired **laminae,** again right and left, top the pedicles, each projecting medially from the

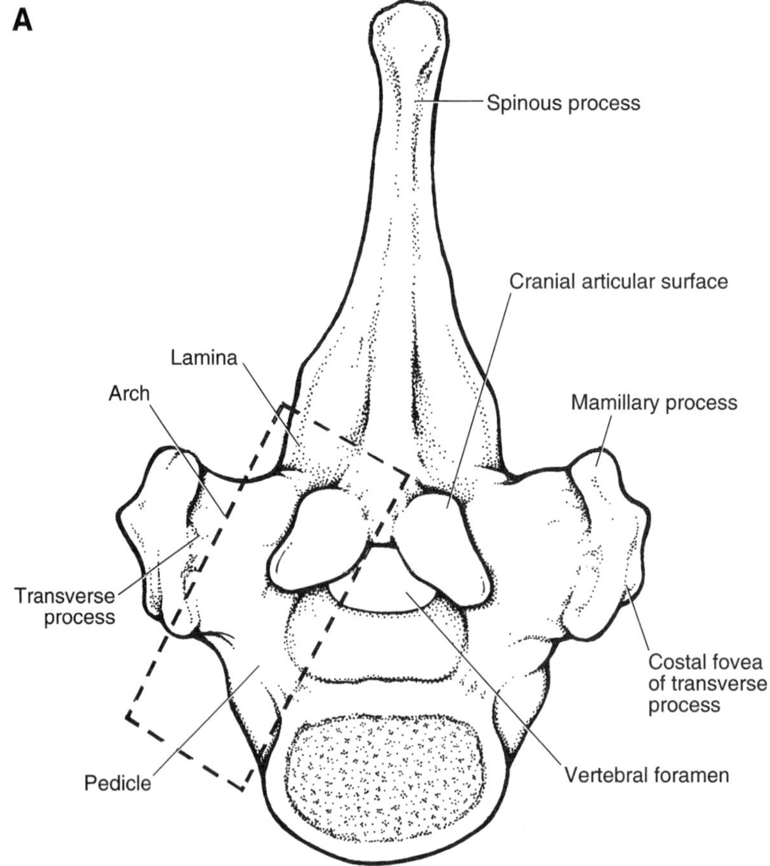

Figure 18–1. General morphologic form of the vertebrae. (*A*) Cranial view (thoracic vertebra). (*continued*)

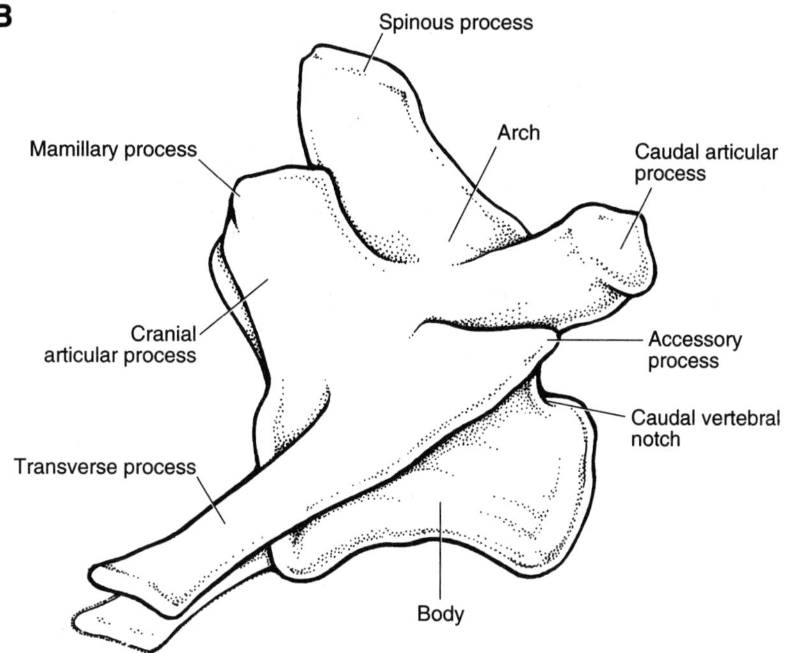

Figure 18–1—*continued* (*B*) Left lateral view (lumbar vertebrae).

Canine Clinical Correlation

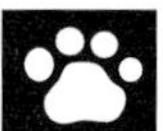

In the case of a **ruptured ("slipped") disc,** the annulus fibrosus ruptures, and the pulpy center of the disc protrudes outward from its normal confines. The protrusion of this material into the vertebral canal puts pressure on the associated nerve roots, spinal cord, or both, causing clinical signs that may range from moderate to incapacitating pain to loss of motor function of the affected nerves, depending on the direction of the rupture and the degree of impingement.

pedicle to meet its fellow on the midline. The base of each lamina bears a **cranial** and a **caudal vertebral notch.** When the vertebrae are articulated, the caudal notch from one vertebra adjoins the cranial notch of the preceding vertebra, forming the **intervertebral foramen** through which the spinal nerves and vessels pass.

C. **Vertebral foramen.** The vertebral foramen is the roundish hole described by the bony borders of the vertebral body ventrally, pedicles laterally, and laminae dorsally. The **vertebral canal,** formed by the juxtaposition of each succeeding vertebral foramen, houses and protects the spinal cord.

D. **Processes** (see Figure 18–1)

1. The unpaired **spinous process** (or dorsal spinous process) projects dorsally from the junction of the two laminae. The size of this process varies remarkably from one region of the vertebral column to another.
2. The paired **transverse processes** project laterally from the junction of the body and pedicles, dorsal to the intervertebral foramen. These processes are also highly variable in their degree of development and in their general form.
3. The **cranial** and **caudal articular processes,** both of which are paired (for a total of four on each vertebra), are located at the junction of the pedicle and the lamina. The cranial

articular process faces craniodorsally or medially, and the caudal one faces caudolaterally or ventrally. The articular processes are variable in the degree of their projection from the arch, being rather low in the cervical area and very prominent in the late thoracic and lumbar regions.

4. Paired **mamillary processes** are present from the second or third thoracic vertebra through the remainder of the column. These small protuberances project dorsally from the general area of the cranial articular process.
5. Paired **accessory processes** are present from the midthoracic vertebrae through the fifth or sixth lumbar vertebra. These relatively pointed, caudally directed processes arise from the caudal border of the pedicle, lateral to the caudal articular process. When well-developed (as in the lumbar vertebrae), the accessory processes embrace the lateral surface of the cranial articular process of the following vertebra. Table 18–1 summarizes the differences between the mamillary and accessory processes.

III. REGIONAL VERTEBRAL MORPHOLOGY.

The form of the vertebrae is distinct from region to region. Changes in identifying features typically take place in a gradual, progressive manner (passing cranially to caudally along the column). Thus, the vertebrae late in the series of a given region begin to resemble the cranial ones of the next series. (A few exceptions to this general rule include the unique first and second cervical vertebrae, the fused sacral vertebrae, and the small vertebrae of the tail.)

A. Cervical vertebrae

Cervical vertebrae (Figure 18–2A). The first two cervical vertebrae are highly specialized for articulation of the skull with the vertebral column, as well as for motion of the head on the neck. Therefore, these two vertebrae are individually named and require separate description. The remaining five cervical vertebrae are more similar in form, although C6 and

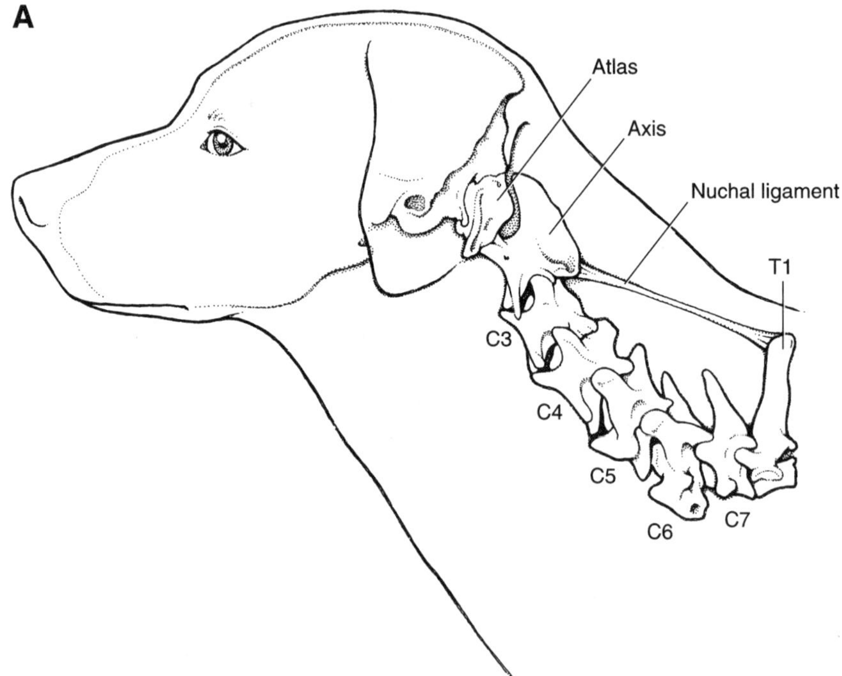

Figure 18–2. (*A*) Articulated cervical vertebrae and the nuchal ligament. Students who confuse the relation of the atlas (C1) to the axis (C2) may find it helpful to think of the head as the "Earth," which, in mythology, is borne on the shoulders of Atlas (the giant). (*continued*)

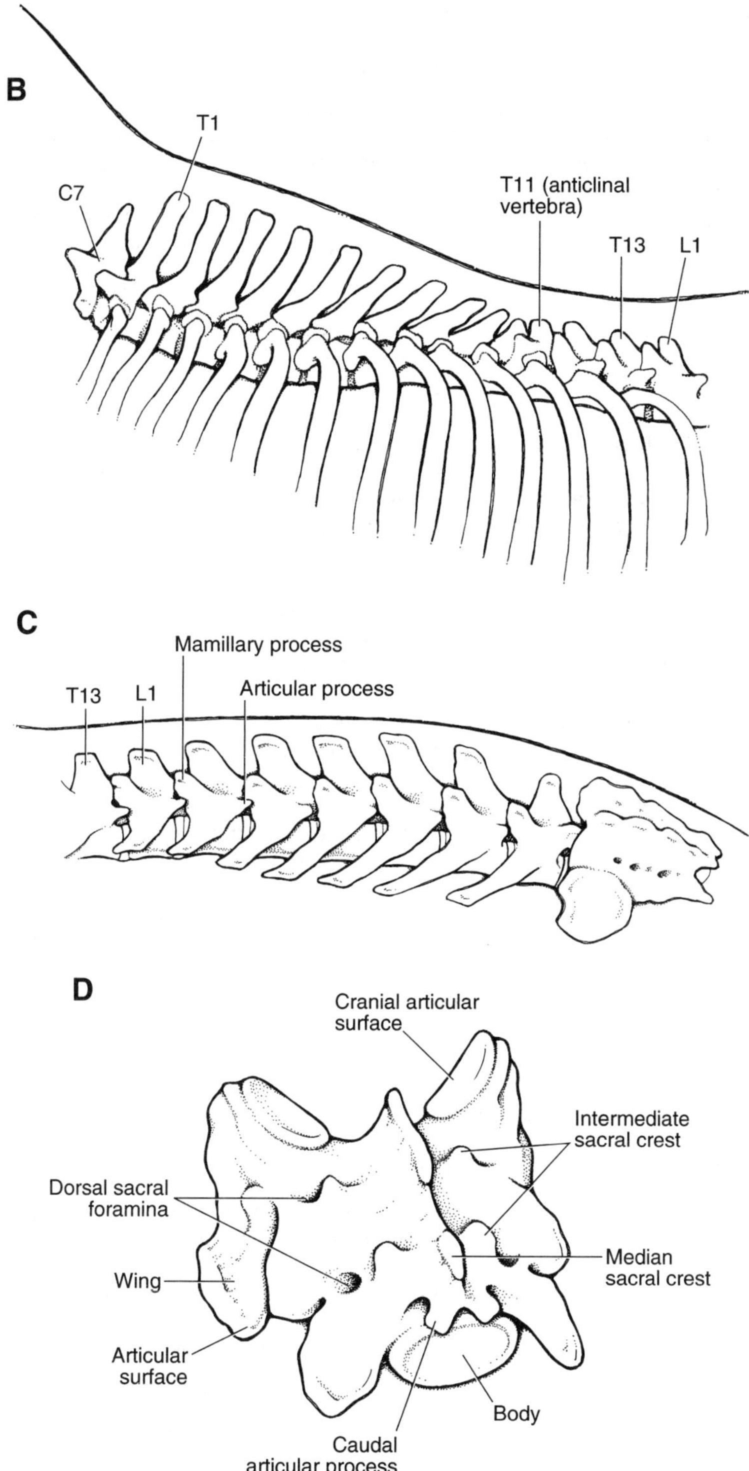

Figure 18–2—*continued* (*B*) Articulated thoracic vertebrae. (*C*) Articulated lumbar vertebrae. (*D*) Caudolateral view of the sacrum. (*D* Modified with permission from Evans HE, 1993, *Miller's Anatomy of the Dog,* 3e. Philadelphia, WB Saunders, p 177.)

C7 have features that allow them to be specifically identified. Despite these disparate features, the presence of **transverse foramina** distinguishes the cervical vertebrae as a group (with the exception of C7) from the other vertebrae of the vertebral column.

1. **Atlas (C1).** The atlas is unique in several respects.
   a. **Greatly reduced body.** The body of the atlas is so greatly reduced that it is sometimes referred to as the **ventral arch.** Therefore, the atlas is described as being composed of two large **lateral masses,** which are connected dorsally by the arch and ventrally by the reduced body (i.e., the ventral arch). Developmentally, a large part of the atlantal body comes free from the atlas and fuses to the succeeding vertebra, the axis.
   b. **Unique processes**
      (1) **No spinal process.** The atlas entirely lacks a spinous process.
      (2) **Modified transverse processes.** Paired **wings,** which are broad, flattened, shelf-like projections, extend laterally from each side of the atlantal body, and extend sufficiently caudally to overlap the atlantoaxial joint. Each wing bears two features of note:
         (a) The **transverse foramina** pass through the base of each wing near the junction of the wing with the lateral mass. The transverse foramina transmit the:
            (i) **Vertebral artery** *en route* to the cranial cavity
            (ii) **Vertebral vein** exiting the cranial cavity
            (iii) **Vertebral nerve**
         (b) The **alar notch** is a notch on the cranial border of the wing, again near the junction of the wing with the lateral mass. The alar notch transmits:
            (i) A branch of the vertebral vein
            (ii) The ventral branch of the first cervical nerve
   c. **Modified articular surfaces**
      (1) The **cranial surface** of the atlas is deep and cup-shaped for articulation with the large, rounded occipital condyles of the skull. The motion afforded by the **occipitoatlantal joint** is dorsoventral extension—flexion, such as occurs when a person nods "yes."
      (2) The **caudal surface** of the atlas bears paired, rather shallow **foveae** for articulation with the axis. The motion at the **atlantoaxial joint** is rotational from side to side, such as occurs when a person shakes his head "no."
      (3) The **dorsal surface** of the atlas bears the **fovea for the dens** (of the axis), a concave depression positioned between the caudal articular foveae that receives the dens.
   d. **Lateral vertebral foramen.** The lateral vertebral foramen passes obliquely, lateral to medial, through the cranial edge of the arch. The lateral vertebral foramen transmits the:
      (1) **Vertebral artery,** as it turns medially (after leaving the transverse foramen) *en route* to the cranial cavity
      (2) **First cervical nerve,** as it leaves the vertebral canal
   e. **Atlantooccipital membrane.** This membrane closes the relatively wide space between the foramen magnum and the dorsal arch of the atlas.

2. **Axis (C2).** The axis is the longest of the vertebrae in the column. The length of the axis, together with its heavy body and substantial arch, give it a notable robust appearance.
   a. **Dens.** The dens (odontoid process) of the axis, a stubby projection of bone extending cranially from the body of the axis, is actually a portion of the atlantal body that fuses with the axis during development.
      (1) In the intact state, the dens is positioned within the ventral part of the vertebral foramen of the atlas, resting on the floor of the foramen and bound in this position by the transverse ligament of the atlas.
      (2) The elongate, rounded contour of the dens forms the base for the side-to-side rotation that takes place at the atlantoaxial joint.
   b. **Vertebral processes**
      (1) The **spinous process** of the axis, like the bone itself, is markedly elongate, extending cranially and caudally slightly past those respective articular surfaces. The cranial edge of the spinous process extends as far cranially as the dens!

(2) The **transverse processes** are narrow and blade-like, and project caudolaterally from the body. The **transverse foramina** of the axis pass through the transverse processes very close to the pedicles.

3. **C3–C5.** Distinguishing cervical vertebrae C3–C5 from one another can be challenging. These vertebrae can be described as "typical" cervical vertebrae:
   a. **Body.** Progressing caudally from C2, the bodies of the cervical vertebrae become progressively shorter, and carry a ventral crest.
   b. **Articular surfaces.** The articular surfaces are oriented in essentially a dorsal plane, facing almost directly dorsally and ventrally.
   c. **Vertebral processes**
      (1) The **spinous processes** become more prominent and higher, and incline more strongly cranially, on succeedingly more caudal vertebrae. However, compared with the spinous processes of the thoracic vertebrae, the spinous process of the caudal cervical vertebrae are relatively short.
      (2) The **transverse processes** become larger and more complex, developing distinct cranial and caudal extensions called **tubercles.**
   d. **Transverse foramina** are present.

4. **C6–C7**
   a. **C6.** The **unique transverse process** of C6 allows it to be distinguished from the other cervical vertebrae.
      (1) The **caudal portion of the transverse process** is greatly expanded ventrally and laterally.
      (2) The **cranial portion of the transverse process** is reduced to a conical peg ventral and lateral to the transverse foramen.
   b. **C7** has the features typical of most cervical vertebrae, but also possesses individually identifying characteristics:
      (1) **No transverse foramina.** C7 is the only cervical vertebra that lacks transverse foramina.
      (2) **High spinous process.** The spinous process is the highest of all the cervical vertebrae, and is inclined strongly cranially.
      (3) **Costal foveae** may be present on the body ventral to the caudal vertebral notches, for articulation with the head of the first rib.

B. **Thoracic vertebrae** (Figure 18–2B). The **most characteristic features of the thoracic vertebrae** as a group are the **costal foveae** and the **transverse foveae,** both specializations for articulation with the ribs. As a group, thoracic vertebrae resemble each other fairly closely:

1. **Short body.** The vertebral bodies are notably short; they begin to increase in length from T10 on caudally (i.e., as the late thoracic vertebrae begin to adopt the form of the vertebrae of the lumbar segment of the vertebral column). The bodies of the thoracic vertebrae are so short that collectively, the length of the thoracic portion of the vertebral column is only approximately one third greater than that of the lumbar portion, although the thoracic vertebrae outnumber the lumbar vertebrae almost two to one.
2. **Costal foveae,** sites for articulation with the heads of the ribs, are located on the vertebral bodies of the thoracic vertebrae.
   a. **T1–T10.** The body of each vertebra possesses a **cranial** and **caudal costal fovea** or **demifacet** (i.e., "half" of an articulation site) at its cranial and caudal edges (i.e., there are four total sites on each body, two on each side). Therefore, through most of the length of the thoracic part of the column, the head of one rib articulates with the demifacets of two vertebral bodies.
   b. **T11** is variable, sometimes possessing both demifacets, and sometimes lacking the caudal set.
   c. **T12** and **T13** consistently present a single complete fovea on each side of the vertebral body.

3. **Short pedicles.** The thoracic vertebrae have notably short pedicles.
4. **Orientation of the articular surfaces**
   a. From T1 through about T10, the articular surfaces lie in a dorsal plane, like those of the cervical vertebrae. These joints thus permit mainly side-to-side lateral movement of the trunk.
   b. From approximately T10 on caudally, these surfaces are oriented in a sagittal plane, facing almost directly medially and laterally. These joints thus are designed for dorsal to ventral movement in the sagittal plane.
5. **Vertebral processes**
   a. The **spinous process** is well developed in the thoracic vertebrae.
      (1) **Length.** In the cranial six or seven thoracic vertebrae, the spinous process is particularly long and relatively massive. The processes begin to shorten at about T7 or T8, and become progressively shorter with each succeeding thoracic vertebra.
      (2) **Inclination**
         (a) **T1–T7.** The spinous processes of T1–T7 or T8 have a slightly caudal inclination.
         (b) **T8–T10.** The inclination becomes more strongly caudal from T8–T10.
         (c) **T11** is designated as the **anticlinal vertebra,** because its very short spinous process is classically described as projecting directly dorsally without inclination. (The prominence of this feature in actual skeletons is not always as plain as a textbook description might suggest, however.) Regardless of the prominence of the anticlinal nature of T11, it does represent a **transition point** along the vertebral column, in that all the spinous processes cranial to T11 are inclined caudally, whereas all those caudal to T11 are inclined cranially.
         (d) **T12–T13.** The spinous process of these vertebrae are inclined cranially.
   b. The **transverse processes** are **short and blunt.** Each presents a **transverse fovea** for articulation with the costal tubercle of the rib.
   c. The **mamillary processes** make their appearance, generally at T3.
      (1) **T3–T10.** The mamillary processes are small, short dorsal projections positioned on the cranial edge of the transverse processes.
      (2) **T11–T13.** The mamillary processes sit atop the cranial articular processes.
   d. The **accessory processes** first become visible in the midregion of the thoracic series, approximately at T6 or T7, and continue throughout the remaining thoracic vertebrae (and into the lumbar region, as well).

C. Lumbar vertebrae (Figure 18–2C). Like the thoracic vertebrae, the lumbar vertebrae resemble each other fairly closely. The most characteristic features of the lumbar vertebrae are their **massive vertebral bodies** and **distinctive transverse processes.**

1. **Body.** The vertebral bodies of the lumbar vertebrae are **massive, relatively long,** and **uniformly shaped,** particularly as compared with those of the thoracic region.
2. **Pedicles and laminae.** The pedicles and laminae are **longer** and **heavier** than those of the thoracic vertebrae.
3. **Orientation of articular surfaces.** The articular surfaces are oriented in the **sagittal plane** (facing medially and laterally). Therefore, the lumbar region of the vertebral column is mainly capable of flexion and extension in a dorsoventral direction, rather than from side-to-side.
4. **Vertebral processes**
   a. The **spinous processes** are **relatively short** and **wide** and they **incline cranially.**
   b. The **transverse processes** are **large, long, flattened dorsoventrally, directed at an angle ventrally from the body,** and **inclined cranially.**
   c. **Mamillary processes** are present on the cranial articular processes of all lumbar vertebrae.
   d. The **accessory processes** are consistently prominent from L1 to about L3 or L4 and absent on L5 and L6.

D. Sacral vertebrae. Three individual sacral vertebrae are present only in the fetus and young dog; by 12–18 months of age, the three vertebrae have fused together to form the **sacrum,** a four-sided, single mass of bone, slightly wider at its cranial end than at its caudal end (Figure 18–2D). The sacrum is **positioned between the iliac wings of the pelvis,** articulating with it very firmly and largely immovably in the normal situation. The sacrum forms the greatest part of the roof of the pelvic cavity.

1. The **sacral canal** is the continuation of the vertebral canal through the sacrum.
2. The **base** of the sacrum is its **cranial end.**
   a. The sacrum articulates with the seventh lumbar vertebra by its large **cranial articular processes** at the **sacrovertebral angle.**
   b. The **promontory,** a low, transverse ridge of bone on the cranioventral portion of the sacral base, helps to define the pelvic inlet (i.e., the entrance to the bony pelvic cavity).
3. The **sacral apex** is its **caudal end.** The sacral apex articulates with the first caudal vertebra by means of the small caudal articular processes.
4. The **wing** of the sacrum is its expanded lateral region. The **auricular surface** (named in humans for its vague resemblance in form to the human ear) is the roughed surface specialized for articulation with the wing of the ilium.
5. The **dorsal sacral surface** is rather complex, presenting several features reminiscent of the three original vertebrae that fused to form the sacrum.
   a. The **laminae** of the original sacral vertebra **do not fuse** on the dorsal midline in the region dorsal to the sacral canal. The bony incontinuity is closed by soft tissue.
   b. The **median sacral crest,** representing the fusion of the spinous processes, is a prominent ridge of bone passing down the dorsal sacral midline.
   c. The **intermediate sacral crest,** representing the fusion of the mamillary and articular processes, presents as a series of low "knobs" variably connected by an even lower bony crest.
   d. The **lateral sacral crest,** formed from the fusion of the transverse processes, runs along the lateral edge of the sacrum.
   e. The **dorsal sacral foramina,** present as two pairs, perforate the dorsal sacral surface just lateral to the fused vertebral bodies. These foramina transmit the dorsal branches of the sacral nerves and vessels.
6. The **pelvic (ventral) sacral surface** is **concave** (the degree varies among breeds and individuals).
   a. Two **transverse lines** mark the ventral sacral surface, representing the position of the intervertebral discs of the fetus and young dog.
   b. Two pairs of **ventral sacral foramina** perforate the ventral sacral surface in a position homologous to that of the dorsal sacral foramina (i.e., just lateral to the fused vertebral bodies). The ventral sacral foramina transmit the ventral branches of the sacral nerves and vessels.

E. Caudal vertebrae. The number of caudal vertebrae is highly variable among breeds, as well as among individuals within a breed.

1. **Progressive simplification.** The caudal vertebrae undergo a progressive decrease in size and a simplification in form from cranial to caudal. In general, the caudal vertebrae of the tail are longer, more narrow, and smoother than the cranial vertebrae of the tail.
   a. The first several caudal vertebrae are fairly regular in form, appearing much like lumbar vertebrae in miniature.
   b. Those of the midregion of the tail still present vestigial features recognizable as related to the defining features of the vertebral regions cranial to the tail.
      (1) The spinous processes are generally lost by the level of Cd7.
      (2) The cranial and caudal articular processes are generally lost by the level of Cd12.
      (3) The transverse processes are fairly typical through Cd4 or Cd5, after which they begin to regress, and are lost by Cd15.
   c. The caudal-most vertebrae are little more than elongate rods of bone.

2. **Hemal arches (vertebral arches)** are formed by the articulation of small, separate paired bones with the ventral surfaces of the vertebral bodies of Cd4, Cd5, and Cd6.
   a. The **"V"-** or **"Y"-shaped arches** are oriented with the point of the "V" or the stem of the "Y" projecting caudoventrally from the caudal end of the vertebra.
   b. The **median coccygeal artery** passes between the arms of the arch.

3. **Hemal processes** are similar in position to the hemal arches, but are formed from direct processes of the vertebra rather than from separate bones. The hemal processes persist the farthest caudally along the caudal vertebrae; they are still identifiable as far as Cd17 or Cd18.

Chapter 19

The Spinal Cord

I. INTRODUCTION.

INTRODUCTION. The spinal cord (see also Chapter 4 II A 2) is an elongate, cylindrical structure composed mainly of nervous tissue that is housed within the vertebral canal. Although the vertebral canal is filled throughout most of its length with nervous tissue, in adult dogs, the spinal cord is shorter than the vertebral canal.

II. SEGMENTATION

A. Identification and number of spinal cord segments. Attachment of the dorsal and ventral spinal nerve roots (see Chapter 4 II B 1) to the surface of the spinal cord is the means by which the spinal cord segments are identified: each cord segment extends between two sets of spinal roots. Spinal cord segments are identified in a manner similar to the way the vertebrae are identified (i.e., using a descriptive name based on location followed by a sequential number from cranial to caudal).

1. The **cervical spinal cord segments** number **8** (as opposed to 7 cervical vertebrae).
2. The **thoracic, lumbar** and **sacral spinal cord segments** number the same as the respective regions of the vertebral column (i.e., **13, 7,** and **3,** respectively).
3. The **caudal spinal cord segments** number only **5** (as opposed to approximately 20 caudal vertebrae).

B. Correlation of spinal cord segments and vertebrae. Clearly, not all spinal cord segments are directly related to the vertebrae to which they correspond in number.

1. **Factors contributing to disparity between the spinal cord segments and vertebrae**
   a. **Normal development.** The somitic nature of the early embryo is clearly reflected in the early development of the vertebral column and spinal cord: initially, the two are equal in length, and each segment of the cord is contained within the vertebral foramen of the vertebra with the same number as the spinal cord segment. As the animal grows, the rate of growth of the spinal cord and vertebral column do not keep similar pace; the column grows longer than the cord, resulting in discrepancies in the positioning of the spinal cord segments relative to the vertebrae.
   b. **Regional growth.** Differences in the regional growth of the cord and column also contribute to the discrepancy between the two. The spinal cord segments lengthen in the early cervical region, shorten in the midcervical to early thoracic regions, lengthen again through most of the thoracolumbar region, and finally shorten again in the caudal region.
2. **General description**
   a. From **most of the cervical region through the early thoracic region,** the segments lie approximately one half to one-and-a-half full vertebral body lengths cranial to their respective vertebrae, becoming closer to their respective vertebrae the farther caudally along the cord they lie. The **cervical spinal nerves** have a unique pattern of exit from the vertebral canal, because there are 8 cervical nerves but only 7 cervical vertebrae.
      (1) The **first cervical nerve** departs the vertebral canal through the lateral vertebral foramen of the atlas.
      (2) The **second, third, fourth, fifth, sixth,** and **seventh cervical nerves** leave the vertebral canal through the intervertebral foramen **cranial** to the vertebra of the same number. (For example, nerve C2 leaves cranial to vertebra C2.)
      (3) The **eighth cervical nerve** leaves the canal through the intervertebral foramen

caudal to vertebra C7, and thus establishes the pattern of exit for the remaining spinal nerves.

b. From the **late thoracic region** (T11 or T12) **through the early lumbar region** (approximately L3), the segments lie within the vertebra of the same number.

c. From the **midlumbar region through the remainder of the vertebral column,** the segments lie progressively cranial to their respective vertebrae, so that the cord typically ends at L6 (in medium and large breeds). In the small (toy) breeds, the cord segments may lie up to half a vertebral body caudal to the "typical" description, and may extend into the cranial sacral regions.

3. **Spinal nerve roots.** The spinal nerve roots always retain their original relation to the intervertebral foramina from which they depart. In other words, when the relative positions of the spinal cord segment and vertebral bodies change so that the segment is displaced cranial to the vertebra of the same number, the **spinal nerve roots must lengthen to retain their connection to the intervertebral foramen from which they exit.** Therefore, the spinal nerve roots are relatively:

a. **Short** in the initial cervical, thoracolumbar, and cranial lumbar regions (where the segments lie close to their respective vertebrae)

b. **Long** in the thoracic, midlumbar, sacral, and caudal regions (where the segments are displaced cranial to their respective vertebrae)

III. TRANSVERSE SECTIONAL FEATURES

A. The **central canal,** the remnant of the lumen of the embryonic neural tube, is filled with cerebrospinal fluid.

B. Grey matter

1. **Regions**. The gray matter is arranged in a pattern that resembles a butterfly (see Chapter 4 II A 2 c (1); Figure 4–4) and is positioned deep within the spinal cord.

a. The paired **dorsal horns** contain the cell bodies of **sensory (afferent) neurons**.

b. The paired **ventral horns** contain the cell bodies of **motor (efferent) neurons**.

c. The paired **intermediate horns** are located only in the **thoracolumbar region** of the spinal cord and contain the cell bodies of the **sympathetic nervous system.**

2. **Functional organization.** The grey matter is organized so that neurons having similar functions are grouped together. Two approaches have been developed to describe this functional organization:

a. **Nuclei or columns**

(1) **Dorsal horn nuclei** include the lateral cervical, marginal, thoracic, and proprius nuclei, as well as the substantia gelatinosa.

(2) **Intermediate substance nuclei** are mainly involved with autonomic nervous function. The nuclei here include the intermediomedial nucleus, the intermediolateral nucleus (the neurons of which form the lateral horn of the thoracolumbar spinal cord), and the sacral parasympathetic nucleus, which is concerned with parasympathetic innervation of the pelvic viscera.

(3) **Ventral horn nuclei** include the medial and lateral motor nuclei (which innervate the axial musculature) and the motor nucleus of the accessory nerve.

b. **Laminae.** Ten grey matter laminae have been identified, and are designated by Roman numerals. Functions have been described for each of the laminae, but are of mainly academic interest.

C. White matter is positioned superficially within the spinal cord and is composed of myelinated and nonmyelinated neuronal processes. The fatty myelinated nerve sheaths are responsible for the pale appearance of this region of the cord.

1. **Regions.** The white matter is divided into regions (funiculi) by the fissures and horns of the grey matter [see Chapter 4 II A 2 c (2); Figure 4–4].

a. A **funinculus** is a region of white matter that is grossly visible and readily identifiable on section.
b. A **fasciculus** is typically not visible grossly. Together, several fasciculi form a funiculus.

2. **Tracts.** The white matter pathways are often referred to as tracts.
   a. **Components.** White matter tracts potentially comprise:
      (1) **Afferent axons,** which bring sensory innervation into the cord via the dorsal roots
      (2) **Efferent axons,** which exit the spinal cord *en route* to their effectors via the ventral root
      (3) **Ascending** and **descending pathway axons,** which transmit information cranially and caudally (respectively) along the cord
   b. **Naming convention.** White matter tracts are named according to their course, with the origin named first, and the termination named last. Therefore, the name of a given tract not only gives information on what structures it connects, but also on the direction of impulse transmission within the tract: for example, the spinomedullary tract extends between the spinal cord and the brain stem, and carries information from the spinal cord to the medulla.
   c. **Specific white matter tracts**
      (1) **Fasciculus proprius.** This tract contains **intrinsic fibers** (i.e., fibers that both originate and terminate within the cord itself). The fasciculus proprius carries **intersegmental reflexes** that do not require higher input for execution, such as the reflex skin twitch of the cutaneous trunci.
      (2) **Ascending spinal tracts**
         (a) The **dorsal funiculus** is composed primarily of sensory fibers, some of which terminate in the spinal cord and others of which travel to the brain.
            (i) The **fasciculus cuneatus** transmits sensory fibers that function in discriminative touch, forelimb kinesthesia, and communication with the cerebellum from the thoracic limb and neck to the cuneate nuclei.
            (ii) The **fasciculus gracilis** carries sensory fibers from the caudal half of the body (especially the pelvis) to the nucleus gracilis, and also functions in discriminative touch.
         (b) The **lateral funiculus** is composed essentially of projection fibers. Tracts of the lateral funiculus are many, and conduct information related to nociceptive (painful), thermal, and tactile stimuli from the skin, muscles, joints, and viscera.
            (i) Perhaps the most noteworthy tract of the lateral funiculus is the **spinocervicothalamic tract,** the primary pathway conducting conscious pain perception in carnivores.
            (ii) Other tracts of the lateral funiculus include the **spinothalamic tract,** the dorsal, ventral, and cranial **spinocerebellar tracts,** the **spinomedullary tract,** and the **spinopontine tracts.**
         (c) The **ventral funiculus** is comprised mostly of fibers that receive information from both somatic and visceral sources. Tracts of the ventral funiculus include the **spinoreticular, spinovestibular, spinomesencephalic,** and **spino-olivary tracts.**
      (3) **Descending spinal tracts** convey motor information—they modify somatic and autonomic reflexes; control muscle tone, posture, and movement; and regulate impulses along ascending pathways. **Pyramidal systems** originate in the cerebral cortex and pass peripherally through the pyramids of the medulla *en route* to the spinal cord. **Extrapyramidal systems** originate in the brain stem nuclei and do not pass through the medullary pyramids.
         (a) **Descending tracts of forebrain origin** are **pyramidal.** The **lateral** and **ventral corticospinal tracts** originate in the motor cortex and terminate in the ventral horn. These tracts are concerned with voluntary skeletal muscle control.
         (b) **Descending tracts of midbrain origin** are **extrapyramidal.**
            (i) The **rubrospinal tract** is the **prime voluntary motor pathway** of the dog. This tract is distributed to all spinal cord segments.

(ii) Other tracts within this group include the **medial tectospinal** and **lateral tectotegmentospinal tracts,** which function in part in orientation of the head toward abrupt visual or auditory stimuli.

(c) **Descending tracts of hindbrain origin** are also **extrapyramidal.** Two tracts are of particular interest within this group:

(i) The **lateral vestibulospinal tract** carries neurons sensitive to **linear acceleration** of the head, as registered by the utricle and saccule of the inner ear. This tract contributes significantly to maintaining normal standing posture, and also in providing quick extension of the limbs to prevent the animal from stumbling and falling.

(ii) The **medial vestibulospinal tract** carries neurons sensitive to **angular acceleration** of the head, as registered by the semicircular canals of the inner ear. This tract helps maintain head position in response to information received from the external environment.

IV. VASCULATURE

A. Arterial supply.

Arterial supply. Three main arteries deliver blood to the spinal cord, each of which runs essentially the full length of the cord.

1. The **ventral spinal artery,** the largest of the three, lies along the ventral median fissure of the spinal cord.
   a. The ventral spinal artery is formed from the **ventral branches** of the **segmental spinal arteries.**
      (1) The segmental spinal arteries enter the spinal cord and divide into dorsal and ventral branches, the latter of which anastomose to form the unpaired ventral spinal artery.
      (2) The segmental spinal arteries arrive from regional vessels near the vertebral column. Within the neck, the pattern is consistent. However, more caudally, one branch at each intervertebral space is not always present. The following arteries give rise to the segmental spinal arteries in the neck, thoracic, lumbar, and sacral regions, respectively:
         (a) **Vertebral artery**
         (b) **Intercostal arteries**
         (c) **Lumbar arteries**
         (d) **Sacral artery**
   b. Structures supplied. The ventral spinal artery supplies the **grey matter** of the spinal cord and its **immediately adjacent white matter.**
2. The **dorsolateral spinal arteries** are smaller and pass longitudinally along the region where the dorsal roots enter the spinal cord.
   a. The dorsolateral spinal arteries are formed from the **dorsal branches** of the **segmental spinal arteries.** These arteries are plexiform in nature (rather than forming a continuous longitudinal channel).
   b. **Structures supplied.** The dorsolateral spinal arteries supply most of the **white matter** of the spinal cord.

B. Venous drainage.

Venous drainage. Veins drain into one of three sets of vertebral venous plexuses.

1. **Veins**
   a. The **spinal veins,** which are essentially tributaries of the spinal arteries, drain into the internal vertebral plexus.
   b. The **basivertebral veins,** which emerge from the vertebral bodies or the soft tissues ventral to them, also drain into the internal vertebral plexus.
   c. The **intervertebral veins** are found at each intervertebral foramen, and connect the internal vertebral plexus with veins and venous plexuses outside the vertebral column.

2. **Venous plexuses.** The venous plexuses of the spinal cord and vertebral column are multiple and complex, and they vary considerably in the degree of development from one region to another.
   a. The **internal vertebral venous plexus** extends the full length of the vertebral canal, although it is largest and best developed in the cervical region. It lies on the floor of the vertebral canal within the fat in the epidural space and takes the form of paired channels (i.e., the **right** and **left internal vertebral plexuses),** mostly positioned between consecutive intervertebral spaces. The channels from each side generally communicate with each other over each vertebral body by means of the **interarcuate branches**.
      (1) The plexus is formed from valveless, thin-walled veins; therefore, blood can pass in either direction along this plexus (a factor that plays a role in tumor metastasis).
      (2) The internal vertebral plexus drains the spinal cord as well as numerous additional structures, including the other structures housed within the vertebral canal, the vertebral bodies, and the regional musculature.
   b. The **dorsal external vertebral plexus,** which lies on the dorsal surface of the vertebral column, forms largely from anastomoses of succeeding intervertebral veins as they pass through the intervertebral foramina. This plexus is best-developed in the cervical and cranial thoracic regions.
   c. The **ventral external vertebral plexus** is not prominent in the dog. When recognizable, this plexus lies on the ventral surfaces of the vertebral bodies. It is formed from anastomoses of intervertebral veins (as is its dorsal fellow).

C. **Lymphatic system.** Lymph vessels and nodes are entirely lacking in central nervous tissue.

Chapter 20

The Ligaments, Muscles, and Fasciae of the Neck and Back

I. LIGAMENTS

A. Long ligaments of the vertebral column

1. The **nuchal ligament** (see Chapter 18, Figure 18–2A) assists in nonmuscular (and thereby nonfatiguing) support of the relatively heavy head.
   - **a.** The nuchal ligament is composed of paired longitudinal bundles of mainly elastic fibers.
   - **b.** The ligament originates from attachments along the dorsal extremities of the spinous processes of vertebrae T1–T10 and extends from the tip of the spinous process of T1 cranially (without contacting vertebrae C7–C3) to insert on the caudal broadened area of the spinous process of the axis (C2). Note that in dogs (as well as in cats) the nuchal ligament does not extend to the skull, as it does in larger animals.
2. The **supraspinous ligament** (Figure 20–1) is a greatly elongate structure, attaching along the dorsal tips of the vertebral spinous processes from T1–Cd3. This ligament helps prevent excessive spreading of the spinous processes when the vertebral column is flexed ventrally.
3. The **dorsal longitudinal ligament** (see Figure 20–1) lies directly on the dorsal surfaces of the vertebral bodies, and thus lies on the floor of the vertebral canal. This ligament extends from the axis to the caudal region.
4. The **ventral longitudinal ligament** (see Figure 20–1) lies directly on the ventral surfaces of the vertebral bodies and extends from the axis to the sacrum. This ligament is relatively poorly developed when compared with its dorsal counterpart, particularly in the regions cranial to the thorax.

B. Short ligaments of the vertebral column

1. The **interspinous ligaments** extend between adjacent vertebral spinous processes, thereby attaching them to each other (see Figure 20–1).
2. The **intertransverse ligaments** are present only in the lumbar region where, as their name suggests, they connect the transverse processes.
3. The **yellow ligaments (ligamentum flavum)** extend across the open spaces between the arches of adjacent vertebrae. The elastic fibers that form these ligaments give them their yellow color. These ligaments must be punctured when accessing the epidural or subarachnoid spaces.

II. MUSCLES. The attachments, innervation, and action of the muscles of the neck and back are summarized in Tables 20–1 through 20–6.

A. Musculature of the vertebral column as a whole. Both the neck and back are provided with a set of extrinsic muscles and a set of intrinsic muscles. Certain of these muscles also extend onto the tail.

1. **Extrinsic muscles** attach to the vertebral column as well as to other body areas (e.g., the thoracic or pelvic limb). Extrinsic muscles of the neck act mainly to turn the head and neck, and those of the back act mainly to move the head (relative to the rest of the vertebral column) or the limbs.
2. **Intrinsic muscles** both originate and insert on the vertebral column.
   - **a. Function.** These muscles primarily act to move one region of the vertebral column

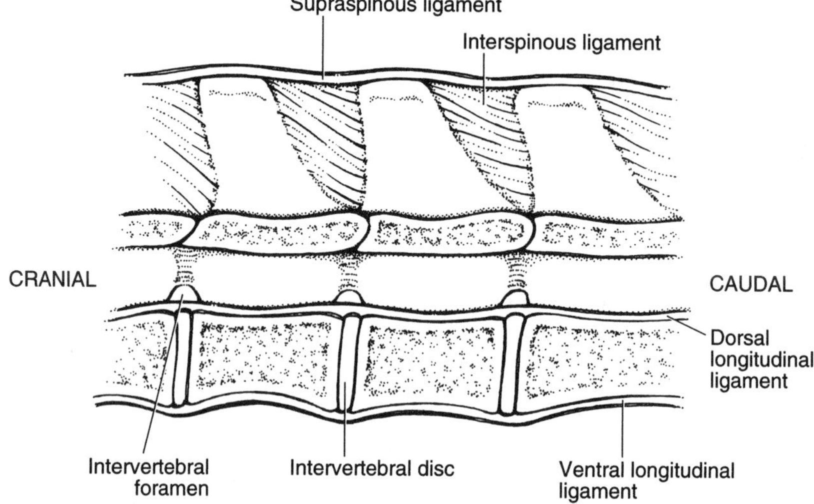

FIGURE 20–1. Ligaments of the vertebral column, left view of paramedian section.

TABLE 20–1. Attachments, Innervation, and Actions of the Intrinsic Vertebral Column Muscles

	Attachments	Innervation	Actions
Epaxial musculature	Generally attach to the bodies of the vertebrae (in the region of the articular or mamillary processes) or the iliac crest, and extend to various vertebral processes, or the skull	Generally by the dorsal branches of the regional spinal nerves	Extends the vertebral column dorsally (when both sides act together) Laterally flexes the column (when only one side contracts)
Hypaxial musculature	Generally attach to the bodies of the vertebrae and extend to the pelvis, proximal femur, or tail	Generally by the ventral branches of the regional spinal nerves	Ventrally flexes the vertebral column (when both sides act together) Laterally flexes the column (when only one side contracts)

relative to the other regions, and to hold the vertebral column firm against the pull of muscles from other areas.

b. Classification. The **intrinsic muscles** of the vertebral column are divided into two major groups, the **epaxial** and **hypaxial** muscles (Table 20–1). The axis of reference is the vertebral column itself, specifically, the level of its transverse processes. Both sets of muscles are generally oriented parallel to the long axis of the vertebral column in a caudal-to-cranial direction; hence, their positions and attachments are usually referred to in this manner as well.

(1) The **epaxial muscles** are positioned **dorsal** to the transverse processes of the vertebrae (*epi* = "upon"). They are well developed along the full length of the vertebral column, from the neck through tail, and are arranged in three adjacent longitudinal groups, medial to lateral (Figure 20–2). Each of these groups possesses regional segments related to the head, neck, or thoracolumbar (back) area.

(a) The **transversospinalis system,** the most medial system, lies directly adjacent to the vertebral bodies and the spinous processes.

(i) This system extends from the sacrum to the head and is composed of members that span one or multiple vertebrae.

(ii) The transversospinalis system is distinctly divided into one set of muscles associated with the neck, and one set of muscles associated with the back (which also continues onto the neck).

(b) The **longissimus system,** the intermediate system, is the longest and strongest of the three. It extends from the wing of the ilium to the skull and is composed of members that span several vertebrae in all cases.

(c) The **iliocostalis system,** the most lateral system, extends from the ilium to C7. This muscle group is composed of members that span several vertebrae, and is easily identified in most regions by the length of its flat, shiny tendons.

(2) The **hypaxial muscles** are positioned **ventral** to the transverse processes of the vertebrae (*hypo* = "under"). One region is distinctly associated with the neck, and the other is associated with the back. These two subdivisions have little relation to each other in terms of size and direction. The hypaxial muscles include the:

(a) Highly segmented muscles just ventral to the vertebrae in the cranial thoracic and cervical regions

(b) Poorly segmented muscles just ventral to the vertebrae in the lumbar region

(c) Segmented muscles of the ventral surface of the tail

(d) Muscles of the thoracic and abdominal walls (see Chapters 34 and 41, respectively)

B. Musculature of the neck

1. Muscles associated with the thoracic limb. The neck muscles associated with the thoracic limb (see also Chapter 28) are positioned relatively superficially on the neck. These muscles are derived from local condensations of mesenchyme associated with the limb bud, rather than from the somites associated with the vertebral column.

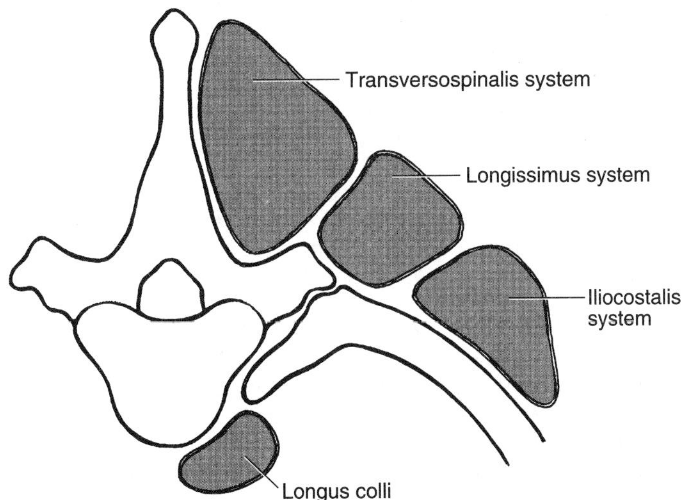

FIGURE 20–2. Diagrammatic representation of the positions of the epaxial and hypaxial muscles in the cranial thoracic region. The transversospinalis system is the most medial and the deepest of the three systems, lying adjacent to the vertebral bodies and spinous processes.

a. The **trapezius muscle** extends between the scapular spine and the dorsal midline of the neck.
b. The **cleidocephalicus portion** of the **brachiocephalicus muscle** itself has two portions, one that extends between the region of the shoulder and the mastoid bone (i.e., the **pars mastoideus)** and one that extends between the shoulder and the dorsal midline of the neck (i.e., the **pars cervicalis).**
c. The **rhomboideus cervicis** and **rhomboideus capitis** attach the medial surface of the scapula to the dorsal midline of the neck and the occiput, respectively.

2. **Muscles of the dorsal cervical surface.** This group includes muscles that are relatively large and superficially placed, as well as muscles that are tiny, delicate, and deeply placed.
   a. The **splenius** (Latin, *"bandage"*), a large, triangular, flat muscle of considerable substance, lies dorsolaterally on the neck and closely covers the several muscles deep to it. Through most of its extent, it is relatively superficial among the muscles of the neck, although it is covered by some of the muscles associated with the thoracic limb.
      (1) **Attachments and course.** The splenius **arises** from the distal portion of the spinous process of vertebra T1 (and sometimes T2), the nuchal ligament, and the median dorsal raphe of the neck. It **courses** cranioventrally toward the head and **inserts** by means of an aponeurotic tendon on the nuchal crest and mastoid process of the temporal bone.
      (2) **Innervation** is via regional cervical nerves.
      (3) **Actions.** The splenius:
         (a) **Extends and raises the neck and head** (when the paired muscles contract together)
         (b) **Moves the head to the side** (when only one muscle of the pair contracts)
   b. **Epaxial neck muscles** (Table 20–2; Figure 20–3)
      (1) **Transversospinalis system in the neck**
         (a) The **spinalis et semispinalis cervicis** originates along the thoracic vertebral bodies and inserts on the spinous processes of vertebrae C5–C2.
         (b) The **semispinalis capitis** lies adjacent to the nuchal ligament and has two parts:
            (i) The **biventer cervicis** is the more dorsal of the two. Four to five oblique tendinous insertions on the superficial surface of the biventer cervicis simplify identification of the muscle during dissection.
            (ii) The **complexus** is the more ventral of the two.
         (c) The **multifidus cervicis** is a series of small, deeply placed muscles. The bundles of the multifidus cervicis pass cranially from the midregion of one vertebra to the spinous process of the vertebra on which they insert. Generally, each muscle bundle crosses two vertebrae.
         (d) The **interspinales,** tiny muscles that extend between adjacent spinous processes, are distinct in the cervical region.
      (2) **Longissimus system in the neck**
         (a) The cervical part of the **longissimus cervicis** [a direct continuation of the thoracic portion of the muscle; see II C 2 a (2) (a)] is a muscle of considerable substance.
         (b) The **longissimus capitis** is a flattened yet relatively thick and strong muscle positioned fairly deeply. One to two tendinous intersections mark the muscle's course. At the cranial end, the muscle narrows and develops a broad, strong tendon.
         (c) The **longissimus atlantis** is an inconstant muscle, occurring in approximately 20% of dogs. When present, this muscle is a deep slip (i.e., elongate, narrow subdivision) of the longissimus capitis.
         (d) The **intertransversarius muscles** are a set of muscles derived from the deeper portions of the longissimus system. The **cervical intertransversarii,** rather robust muscles, are readily recognized.

TABLE 20–2. Epaxial Muscles of the Neck

Muscle	Action	Innervation	Course
Transversospinalis system			
Spinalis et semispinalis cervicis	Stabilize the vertebral column, assist in raising and extending neck	Dorsal branches of the cervical and thoracic spinal nerves	**Arises** along the thoracic vertebral bodies (as far caudally as T11) **Inserts** on the spinal processes of C5–C2
Semispinalis capitis	Elevates the head and neck, turns head and neck to the side	Dorsal branches of the cervical spinal nerves	
Biventer cervicis			**Arises** from the transverse processes of T4–T2 **Inserts** at the occipital skull region
Complexus			**Arises** from T1–C3 **Inserts** at the occipital skull region
Multifidus cervicis	Stabilizes the vertebral column	Dorsal branches of the cervical spinal nerves	**Arise** on T2 **Insert** at C2
Interspinales	Prevent excessive spreading of the spinous processes when the vertebral column is flexed ventrally	Dorsal branches of the cervical spinal nerves	**Extend** between adjacent spinous processes
Longissimus system			
Longissimus cervicis	Extends the neck, raises and draws the neck laterally	Dorsal branches of the cervical spinal nerves	**Arises** from the thoracic vertebrae **Inserts** on the transverse processes of C5–C3
Longissimus capitis	Extends the atlantooccipital joint, raises and draws the head laterally	Dorsal branches of the cervical spinal nerves	**Arises** from the transverse processes of T3–T1 and the bodies of C7–C4 or C3 **Inserts** on the mastoid region of the temporal bone
Longissimus atlantis (rare)	Extends the atlantooccipital joint, raises and draws the head laterally	Dorsal branches of the cervical spinal nerves	**Arises** along C7–C4 **Inserts** on the wing of the atlas
Cervical intertransversarii	Stabilize the neck, draw the neck slightly to one side	Dorsal branches of the cervical spinal nerves	**Extend** between the transverse processes of adjacent vertebrae

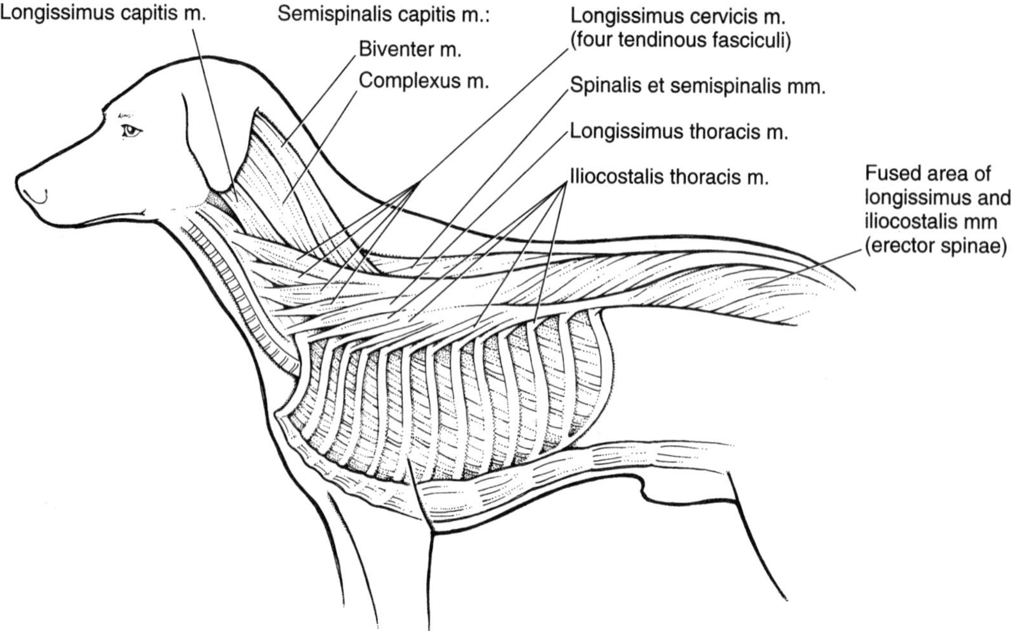

FIGURE 20–3. Epaxial musculature of the back and neck (superficial layer).

(3) **Iliocostalis system in the neck.** This system is minimally represented in the neck; only its cranial-most belly extends so far, and even then only to the transverse process of the last cervical vertebra (C7).

3. **Muscles of the ventral cervical surface**
   a. **Extrinsic muscles of the ventral neck**
      (1) The **sternocephalicus** flexes the neck and joints of the head and draws the head and neck laterally. The accessory nerve (cranial nerve XI) and the ventral branches of the cervical spinal nerves innervate the sternocephalicus. The two divisions of this muscle both **arise** from the sternum and **insert** on the head and neck. In their diverging paths, these two muscles embrace the ventral and lateral surfaces of the neck in the form of the letter "V."
         (a) The **sternomastoideus,** a muscle of considerable substance, is the more medial of the two divisions. It **inserts,** as its name suggests, on the mastoid process of the skull.
         (b) The **sternooccipitalis,** the more lateral division, is thinner and flatter than the sternomastoideus. It **inserts** along the dorsal midline of the neck from the midcervical region cranially to the skull, as well as along the nuchal crest.
      (2) The **sternohyoideus,** often referred to as one of the "strap" muscles of the neck, is a thin, flat muscle that draws the basihyoid bone (and thus the tongue) caudally.
         (a) **Course.** The sternohyoideus **arises** from the sternal manubrium, passes cranially along the ventral surface of the trachea (in close apposition to its fellow from the opposite side as well as the muscle just deep to it, the sternothyroideus), and **inserts** onto the basihyoid bone.
         (b) **Innervation** is via the ventral branches of the cervical spinal nerves.
      (3) The **sternothyroideus,** the other "strap" muscle of the neck, draws the larynx and tongue caudally.
         (a) **Course.** The sternothyroideus **arises** from the sternal manubrium and passes cranially along the ventral surface of the trachea, deep to the sternohyoideus through most of its course. It **inserts** onto the lateral surface of the thyroid cartilage of the larynx.

(i) The sternothyroideus is closely attached to the deep surface of the sternohyoideus in its proximal part.

(ii) Near its insertion, the sternothyroideus diverges laterally to some degree from deep to the sternohyoideus.

(b) **Innervation** is via ventral branches of the cervical spinal nerves.

(4) The **scalenus** flexes the neck ventrally and draws the neck laterally.

(a) **Course.** Separate bellies **arise** from the cranial ribs (1, 3, and/or 4, and 6–9, respectively) and **insert** on the caudal portion of the transverse processes of vertebrae C3–C7.

(b) **Innervation** is via ventral branches of the cervical spinal nerves.

b. Hypaxial neck muscles (Table 20–3) act as ventral flexors of the neck and occipitoatlantal joint.

(1) The **longus capitis,** an elongate, flattened muscle positioned on the ventrolateral surfaces of the cervical vertebrae is the lateral-most of the intrinsic neck muscles.

(2) The **longus colli** is composed of numerous segmental bundles located directly on

TABLE 20–3. Hypaxial Muscles of the Neck

Muscle	Action	Innervation	Course
Longus capitis	Flexes the atlantooccipital joint	Ventral branches of the cervical spinal nerves	**Arises** from the distinct caudal portion of the transverse processes of C2–C6 **Inserts** on the basioccipital bone between the tympanic bullae
Longus colli	Flexes the neck ventrally	Ventral branches of the cervical spinal nerves	
Thoracic portion			**Arises** on the ventral surfaces of the vertebral bodies of T6–T1 (i.e., medially) **Inserts** on the transverse processes of C7 and C6
Cervical portion			**Arises** on the transverse processes of C6–C3 (i.e., laterally) **Inserts** on the ventral surface of the vertebral body of the immediately preceding vertebra
Rectus capitus ventralis	Flexes the atlantooccipital joint	Ventral branches of the cervical spinal nerves	**Arises** from the ventral arch of the atlas and extends across the atlantooccipital joint **Inserts** on the basioccipital bone
Rectus capitus lateralis	Flexes the atlantooccipital joint	Ventral branches of the cervical spinal nerves	**Arises** on the ventral surface of the atlantal wing **Inserts** on the base of the jugular process of the occipital bone

the ventral surfaces of the vertebral bodies from C1 caudally as far as T6 (see Figure 20–2). Thus, the longus colli is divisible into cervical and thoracic portions.

Canine Clinical Correlation

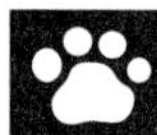

The bellies of the cervical portion of the longus colli form a set of overlapping "Vs," with the apices of the "Vs" (i.e., the points where the muscles attach to the vertebral body) directed cranially. These apices become convenient landmarks when performing surgery to correct a ruptured cervical disc because the attachment point lies directly cranial to the respective intervertebral joint. Thus, when myelographic studies have identified the site of rupture, the area of interest can be easily identified at surgery. Furthermore, the tendinous nature of the insertion area provides a relatively bloodless access point to the intervertebral space.

(3) The **rectus capitis ventralis** is a short yet strong muscle that flexes the atlantooccipital joint.

(4) The **rectus capitis lateralis** is a small muscle positioned immediately lateral to the rectus capitis ventralis.

4. **Specialized muscles.** Regional specializations have developed in the musculature dorsal and ventral to the atlas.

   a. The **rectus capitis dorsalis muscle** acts to extend the atlantooccipital joint and has three regions, designated as the rectus capitus dorsalis major, rectus capitus dorsalis intermedius, and rectus capitus dorsalis minor.

      (1) **Course.** This muscle **arises** from the spinous processes of the atlas and axis and **inserts** onto the occipital region of the skull.

      (2) **Innervation** is via the dorsal branch of the first cervical spinal nerve.

   b. The **obliquus capitus cranialis muscle** extends the atlantooccipital joint.

      (1) **Course.** This muscle **arises** mainly from the wing of the atlas and **inserts** on the mastoid portion of the temporal bone.

      (2) **Innervation** is via the dorsal branch of the first cervical spinal nerve.

   c. The **obliquus capitus caudalis muscle** is a rather robust muscle that stabilizes the atlantoaxial joint and rotates the atlas.

      (1) **Course.** This muscle **arises** along the full length of the spinous process of the axis and **inserts** on the cranial edge of the wing of the atlas, near the alar notch.

      (2) **Innervation** is via the dorsal branch of the first and second cervical spinal nerves.

C. Musculature of the back

1. **Extrinsic back muscles** are positioned superficially on the back and are derived from local condensations of mesenchyme associated with the limb bud rather than from the somites. These muscles include the:

   a. **Cutaneous trunci ("skin twitch") muscle,** which extends over most of the thoracolumbar area (see also Chapter 34 I D 1)

   b. **Trapezius,** which attaches the spine of the scapula to the neck and to the thorax (see also Chapter 28 I E)

   c. **Rhomboideus,** one part of which attaches the medial surface of the scapula to the dorsal midline of the thorax (see also Chapter 28 I F)

   d. **Latissimus dorsi,** which extends from the thoracolumbar fascia to the medial surface of the humerus (see also Chapter 28 I G)

2. **Intrinsic back muscles**

   a. **Epaxial muscles.** The epaxial muscles (Table 20–4) are entirely covered by the more superficial extrinsic back and limb muscles.

      (1) **Transversospinalis system in the back**

         (a) The **spinalis et semispinalis thoracis** divides into eight bundles with individual tendons that course cranially to insert on T6–C6 (one bundle for each vertebra).

TABLE 20–4. Epaxial Muscles of the Back

Muscle	Action	Innervation	Course
Transversospinalis system			
Spinalis et semispinalis thoracis	Stabilizes the thoracic portion of the vertebral column and extends the neck	Dorsal branches of the thoracic spinal nerves	**Arises** from the spinous processes of T11–T7 **Inserts** on the spinous processes of T6–C6
Multifidus thoracis et lumborum	Stabilizes the vertebral column	Dorsal branches of the thoracic and lumbar spinal nerves	
Multifidus thoracis			**Arises** from the mamillary or transverse processes of T11–T3 **Inserts** on the spinous processes of T8–C7
Multifidus lumborum			**Arises** from the processes of the sacrum and L7–T12 **Inserts** on the spinous processes of L6–T9
Rotatores	Stabilize the vertebral column Rotate the thoracic vertebral column around the longitudinal body axis	Dorsal branches of the thoracic and lumbar spinal nerves	**Arise** from the transverse processes of T10–T3 or T2 and cross over 1–2 intervertebral joints **Insert** on the spinous processes of the appropriate vertebrae
Interspinales	Prevent excessive separation of the spinous processes	Dorsal branches of the thoracic and lumbar spinal nerves	**Extend** between the spinous processes of adjacent vertebrae
Longissimus system			
Longissimus thoracis et lumborum	Extend the vertebral column	Dorsal branches of the thoracic and lumbar spinal nerves	
Longissimus thoracis			**Arises** from the iliac crest in its caudal portions, the lumbar vertebral bodies in its cranial portions, and from the spinous processes of the lumbar and thoracic vertebrae by way of an aponeurosis **Inserts** on the accessory processes of T13–T6 and the transverse processes of T5–T1 (caudal region), and on ribs 5–1 (cranial region)

continued

TABLE 20–4. Epaxial Muscles of the Back

Muscle	Action	Innervation	Course
Longissimus lumborum			**Arises** same as the longissimus thoracis **Inserts** on L7–L1
Intertransversarii lumborum et thoracis	Stabilize the thoracolumbar vertebral column	Dorsal branches of the thoracic and lumbar spinal nerves	**Extend** between the accessory or mamillary processes of L7–T9 and between the transverse processes of T12–T4
Iliocostalis system			
Iliocostalis thoracis et lumborum	Stabilize the vertebral column Flex the vertebral column laterally	Dorsal branches of the thoracic and lumbar spinal nerves	
Iliocostalis thoracis			**Arises** from ribs 2–12 **Inserts** on the costal angles of the ribs cranial to them (last segment inserts on the transverse process of C7)
Iliocostalis lumborum			**Arises** from the iliac wing and crest and the transverse processes of each lumbar vertebra **Inserts** on the transverse processes of the lumbar vertebrae and ribs 13–10 or 9

(b) **Multifidus thoracis et lumborum.** The multifidus lumborum is a strong muscle of considerable substance that is less distinctly divided into segments than the multifidus thoracis.

(c) The **rotatores muscles** are deeply placed, specialized subdivisions developed from the medial surface of the multifidus. They are located in the greater part of the cranial thoracic region, where the angle of the articular processes allows some degree of rotatory movement of the intervertebral joints. The rotatores are classified as long rotators or short rotators, depending on the number of intervertebral joints they cross.

(d) The **interspinales** in the thoracolumbar region, as elsewhere, are tiny muscles that extend between the spinous processes of adjacent vertebrae.

(2) **Longissimus system in the back.** The longissimus thoracis et lumborum forms a thick and wide expanse of muscle in the area between the ilium and the last ribs. Together with the iliocostalis lumborum [see II C 2 a (3) (b)], the longissimus thoracis et lumborum forms the **erector spinae,** the large muscle mass that acts as a powerful extensor of the vertebral column. The origins of the thoracic and lumbar

portions of the longissimus thoracis et lumborum are largely fused, although the insertions of each portion are clearly separate.

(a) **Longissimus thoracis.** Each subdivision of the longissimus thoracis extends cranially over several vertebral segments and inserts via a separate tendon. The insertion points of the individual bellies form a progression, with the most caudal bellies inserting relatively dorsally on the vertebrae, the middle bellies inserting more laterally on the vertebrae, and the most cranial bellies inserting further laterally and slightly ventrally on the proximal part of the ribs.

(i) The **caudal region** of the longissimus thoracis **inserts** by way of a **two-pronged tendon** onto vertebrae T13–T1 and the proximal portion of ribs 13–6.

(ii) The **cranial region** of the longissimus thoracis **inserts** by way of an undivided tendon in its attenuated cranial segments, passing to the proximal portion of ribs 5–1.

(b) The **longissimus lumborum** extends craniolaterally, passing over multiple vertebral segments.

(c) The **intertransversarii lumborum et thoracis** is divided into two groups:

(i) One group extends between the accessory or mamillary processes of vertebrae L7–T9.

(ii) One group extends between the transverse processes of vertebrae T12–T4.

(3) **Iliocostalis system in the back.** The thoracic region of the iliocostalis system is a long, narrow muscle group. The individual segments fuse in their midportion before separating again. These terminal segments end in long, thin, prominent tendons that are superficially placed.

(a) **Iliocostalis thoracis muscle** (see Figure 20–3). The fascicles of the iliocostalis thoracis extend craniolaterally (passing over one or more ribs) to insert (more proximally than the level at which they arose) on the ribs cranial to them or, in the case of the most cranial segment, on the transverse process of C7.

(b) **Iliocostalis lumborum.** The iliocostalis lumborum is more robust than its thoracic counterpart. The more caudal region of the muscle forms a muscle mass of considerable substance distinct from that of the longissimus system. Together with the longissimus thoracis et lumborum, the iliocostalis lumborum forms the more lateral part of the **erector spinae.**

b. Hypaxial (sublumbar) muscles. The hypaxial muscles of the back (Table 20–5) extend between the vertebral column and os coxae ("hip bone") or femur and are arranged in layers dorsally to ventrally.

(1) The **psoas minor** is a long, thin, flat muscle that is largely tendinous over approximately 75% of its caudal portion. The tendon is long, flat, thin, and glistening white, even in embalmed specimens.

(2) The **iliopsoas muscle** is a compound muscle formed from the **psoas major** and the **iliacus.**

(a) The **iliacus portion** of the iliopsoas muscle passes caudally and laterally from the ilium and joins with the fibers of the psoas major.

(b) The **psoas major portion** of the iliopsoas muscle originates via a relatively narrow and tendinous region that attaches directly to the ventral surfaces of L2 and L3, and also by aponeuroses to L4 through L7. This muscle passes caudally and very slightly laterally, ventral to the ilium, where it becomes more substantial and receives the fibers of the iliacus muscle.

(3) The **quadratus lumborum muscle** lies directly on the ventral surfaces of vertebrae T11–L7.

3. Muscles of the tail (Table 20–6)

a. General considerations

(1) The tail muscles arise on the lumbar vertebrae, sacrum, and caudal vertebrae, and insert exclusively on the tail. They are relatively fleshy cranially (where they enclose the majority of the substance of the caudal vertebrae), but passing cau-

TABLE 20–5. Hypaxial Muscles of the Back

Muscle	Action	Innervation	Course
Psoas minor	Flexes the lumbar portion of the vertebral column	Ventral branches of the lumbar spinal nerves	**Arises** from the ventral surfaces of the last thoracic and first four or five lumbar vertebrae, as well as from a fascial attachment to the quadratus lumborum **Inserts** on the cranial surface of the pelvis near the junction of the ilium and the pubis
Iliopsoas	Flexes the hip and draws the femur cranially (when limb is free); ventrally flexes the vertebral column (when limb is weight-bearing)	Ventral branches of the lumbar spinal nerves	
Iliacus portion			**Arises** from the ventral surface of the body of the ilium **Inserts** on the lesser trochanter of the femur
Psoas major portion			**Arises** from the ventral surfaces of L2–L4 **Inserts** on the lesser trochanter of the femur
Quadratus lumborum	Stabilizes the lumbar vertebral column	Ventral branches of the lumbar spinal nerves	
Thoracic portion			**Arises** along the bodies of T11–T13 and the transverse process of all seven lumbar vertebrae **Inserts** on the ventromedial surface of the iliac wing
Lumbar portion			**Arises** along the lateral and ventral edges of the lumbar transverse processes **Inserts** on the ventromedial surface of the iliac wing

TABLE 20–6. Muscles of the Tail

Muscle	Action	Innervation
Dorsal group		
Sacrocaudalis dorsalis medialis (short tail levator)	Raises the tail, assists in lateral flexion	Branches of the dorsal caudal trunk
Sacrocaudalis dorsalis lateralis (long tail levator)	Raise the tail, assists in lateral flexion	Branches of the dorsal caudal trunk
Intertransversarius dorsalis caudalis	Lateral flexion	Branches of the ventral caudal trunk
Ventral group		
Sacrocaudalis ventralis medialis (short tail depressor)	Ventral flexion, assists in lateral flexion	Branches of the ventral caudal trunk
Sacrocaudalis ventralis lateralis (long tail depressor)	Ventral flexion, assists in lateral flexion	Branches of the ventral caudal trunk
Intertransversarius ventralis caudalis	Lateral flexion	Branches of the ventral caudal trunk

dally, they decrease progressively in size, so that in the caudal-most regions of the tail, only tendons are present.

(2) The tail musculature may be conceptualized as **two major paired groups,** one **dorsal** and one **ventral,** each largely an inverse image of the other. The dorsal and ventral groups each contain a **medial member** (which is relatively short, a **lateral member** (which is relatively long), and an **intertransverse member** (which extends between the transverse processes). Thus, longitudinal muscle groups of varying length on the tail are positioned as follows:

- **(a) Dorsomedial layer**
- **(b) Dorsolateral layer**
- **(c) Dorsal intertransverse layer**
- **(d) Ventral intertransverse layer**
- **(e) Ventrolateral layer**
- **(f) Ventromedial layer**

(3) The **dorsal tail muscles** are direct **continuations of the epaxial trunk musculature** and are relatively well developed; the **ventral tail muscles** are similar in position to the **hypaxial musculature,** and as is the case in the more cranial body regions, are less complex than their dorsal counterparts.

b. Dorsal group. These muscles are presented from medial to lateral.

(1) The **sacrocaudalis dorsalis medialis (short tail levator)** is the continuation of the **multifidus system** onto the tail. The short tail levator **arises** on the spinous processes of L7, the sacrum, and most of the caudal vertebrae, and extends caudally as far as the last caudal vertebra. It **inserts** by two tendons per belly:

(a) The **deep tendon** ends on the processes or tubercles of the dorsal vertebral body of the vertebra at the caudal end of the tendon's extent.

(b) The **superficial tendon** ends in common with an adjacent tendon of the sacrocaudalis dorsalis lateralis [see II C 3 b (2)].

(2) The **sacrocaudalis dorsalis lateralis (long tail levator)** represents the continuation of the **longissimus system** onto the tail. The substance is distinctly fleshy through approximately the level of Cd14. The muscle **arises** from the aponeurosis of the longissimus and from various processes of the lumbar vertebrae, sacrum, and first several caudal vertebrae. It **inserts** by means of approximately fourteen long, distinct tendons to each caudal vertebra from approximately Cd5 to the end of the tail.

(3) The **intertransversarius dorsalis caudalis** has two distinct portions:

(a) The **cranial portion arises** from the dorsal sacroiliac ligament and vertebra S3, forms a long tendon that receives other small muscular strands of the muscle originating on the transverse processes of adjacent vertebrae, and **inserts** on the transverse process of Cd5 or Cd6. The **abductor caudae dorsalis** is a subdivision of this muscle marked by broad, flat tendons that insert separately on the transverse processes of Cd6–Cd7 or 8.

(b) The **caudal portion arises** from the caudal edge of the transverse process of a tail vertebra, extends across only a single joint, and **inserts** on the cranial edge of the following transverse process.

c. **Ventral group.** These muscles are presented from medial to lateral.

(1) The **sacrocaudalis ventralis medialis (short tail depressor)** forms a segmented column close to the midline along the ventral surfaces of the vertebral bodies. The short tail depressor **arises** from the last sacral vertebra and the ventral surfaces of the succeeding caudal vertebrae. It forms individual flat tendons, which **insert** by blending with the tendon of the adjacent segment of the sacrocaudalis ventralis lateralis (long tail depressor) and then passing to the hemal process of the next succeeding vertebra.

(2) The **sacrocaudalis ventralis lateralis (long tail depressor)** closely parallels its dorsal counterpart in form. This muscle **arises** from the ventral surface of L7 and the sacrum for its first segment, and from the ventral surfaces and transverse processes of succeeding caudal vertebrae for the more caudal segments. The long tail depressor then passes caudally over several segments, forming long, prominent tendons that **insert** on the ventral surfaces of the caudal vertebrae from Cd6 through the last vertebra. Just prior to insertion, each tendon of the long tail depressor receives the small tendon of the adjacent segment of the short tail depressor.

(3) The **intertransversarius ventralis caudalis** commences at the third caudal vertebra and continues in a readily recognizable form throughout the length of the tail. It **arises** on the caudal edge of the transverse process of a given caudal vertebra, passes caudally across one segment, and **inserts** on the cranial edge of the succeeding vertebra.

III. FASCIAE

A. Fasciae of the neck

1. The **superficial cervical fascia** is a delicate layer immediately underlying the skin that sheathes essentially the entire length of the neck. The cutaneous cervical muscles are contained within this fascial layer, and the superficial cervical muscles are covered by it. The superficial cervical fascia has no specialized attachment to deeper structures along the dorsal midline; therefore, the skin is not held tightly to the dorsal midline of the neck.

Canine Clinical Correlation

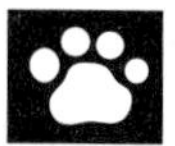

The looseness of the superficial fascial attachment in the neck allows the skin to be readily grasped and elevated, providing a convenient site for the administration of subcutaneous injections.

2. The **deep cervical fascia** is a more substantive layer that envelops the deeper musculature as well as the cervical viscera (e.g., the trachea, esophagus, thyroid glands). The **prevertebral portion** of the deep cervical fascia passes as deeply as the vertebral bodies (the longus colli muscle lies on this fascial layer).

B. Fasciae of the trunk and tail. As is the case throughout the body, the fasciae of the trunk and tail have a superficial and a deep layer. Additionally, the thorax, abdomen, and pelvis also contain cavities that are lined by a fascial layer. Thus, on the trunk (though obviously not the tail), the fascial layers are usually specified as either "external" or "internal." External fascial layers of the trunk and the fascia of the tail include the following:

1. The **superficial truncal fascia** covers the thorax and abdomen on essentially all sides. This layer is continuous cranially with the superficial fascia of the neck and thoracic limb, and caudally with the fascia of the gluteal region and pelvic limb.
   a. The superficial fascia is largely areolar (loosely arranged) in nature.
   b. As in the cervical region, the fascia is not attached to the vertebral spinous processes, and thus is quite mobile over nearly all of the thoracolumbar and abdominal regions. The subcutaneous tissues provide a significant area for fat storage.

Canine Clinical Correlation

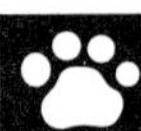

The mobility of the superficial fascia over the thoracolumbar area provides a convenient opportunity for the administration of parenteral fluids. Considerable volumes of replacement fluids can be administered and will be slowly absorbed at a fairly constant rate. This technique facilitates rehydration in cases of moderate dehydration by providing a constant and steady fluid source without requiring placement and management of an intravenous catheter. Suitable sites include over the shoulders, back, and much of the thorax.

   c. The superficial fascia sends significant supporting leaves to the mammary gland.

2. The **deep truncal (thoracolumbar) fascia** is well developed, taking the form in certain areas of a thick, almost tendinous layer with a shiny appearance, even in the embalmed animal. The thick substance of this layer renders it suitable for holding sutures.
   a. Unlike the superficial fasciae of the neck and back, this deeper fascial layer is attached to the spinous processes of the vertebrae via its attachment to the supraspinous ligament. The thoracolumbar fascia extends from its attachment at the dorsal midline over the dorsal, lateral, and ventral surfaces of the trunk to meet its fellow along the linea alba, a longitudinal tendinous band on the ventral midline that extends from the sternum to the pubis.
   b. The **aponeurosis of the longissimus and iliocostalis muscles** in the thoracolumbar region is a particularly well-developed deeper leaf of the thoracolumbar fascia that is separate from the remainder of the thoracolumbar fascia. This layer provides direct and substantive attachment for many fibers of these epaxial muscles.
   c. Parts of the **external** and **internal abdominal oblique muscles** arise directly from the thoracolumbar fascia.
   d. The deep truncal fascia is continuous with the deeper fasciae of other parts of the body.
      (1) Cranially, the connection to the cervical fascia is fairly plain.
      (2) Caudally, the thoracolumbar fascia continues as the **deep gluteal fascia** (which itself is comprised of superficial and deep layers).

3. The **spinotransversalis fascia** is a fascial layer in the deep shoulder region and across the thorax that is largely separate from the thoracolumbar fascia. This fascial layer also has superficial and deep layers. Muscles arising from various parts of the spinotransversalis fascia include the **serratus dorsalis cranialis,** the **serratus dorsalis caudalis** (see Chapter 34 I D 2–3), and the **splenius** (see II B 2 a).
4. The **superficial fascia of the tail** arises from the superficial layer of the gluteal fascia and is relatively thin and weak, serving mainly in the attachment of the skin to the tail.
5. The **deep fascia of the tail** is thick and almost tendinous in places. This layer closely invests the various caudal muscle groups and their terminal tendons.

Chapter 21

Vasculature of the Neck, Back, and Tail

I. VASCULATURE OF THE NECK

A. Arterial supply

1. The **common carotid artery** is the largest vessel in the neck, coursing along the full cervical length from the thoracic inlet to the base of the skull (see also Chapter 9 I B). The vagosympathetic trunk and internal jugular vein are closely associated with the common carotid artery through the greatest length of the neck.
   a. **Course.** The common carotid artery arises from the brachiocephalic trunk just cranial to the heart, and courses cranially within the carotid sheath on the lateral surface of the trachea. It terminates by dividing into the internal and external carotid arteries at approximately the angle of the mandible.
   b. **Branches.** The common carotid artery branches minimally in the neck, because it serves mainly as a conduit to the head. In the neck, the common carotid artery has **one inconstant** and **one constant branch.**
      (1) The **caudal thyroid artery** is highly variable in its origin, usually arising from a common trunk off the brachiocephalic artery.
      (2) The **cranial thyroid artery** (see also Chapter 9 I B 1) is the only constant cervical branch of the common carotid artery, and it is also the largest.
         (a) It has several **named branches,** which supply various cervical structures. From caudal to cranial, these branches are the:
            (i) **Thyroid branches,** which supply the thyroid gland and provide esophageal and tracheal branches
            (ii) **Pharyngeal branch,** the smallest branch, which travels to the pharynx and also supplies many adjacent structures (e.g., the larynx and esophagus)
            (iii) **Cricothyroid branch,** which supplies the same-named muscle but also provides numerous branches to the adjacent musculature and the larynx
            (iv) **Muscular branches,** which supply a small amount of blood to the sternocephalicus and cleidomastoideus muscles
         (b) Several **unnamed branches** also supply the submandibular and medial retropharyngeal lymph nodes, the capsule of the mandibular salivary gland, and the longus capitis and longus colli muscles.
2. The **vertebral artery** serves as a primary conduit of blood to the brain, but is also extremely important to the arterial supply of the skin and musculature of the neck.
   a. **Course.** The vertebral artery leaves the subclavian artery within the bony thorax and ascends cranially, passing through the **transverse canal** of the vertebral column. The vertebral artery enters the transverse foramen of the atlas, passes ventral to the atlantal wing for a short distance, and then emerges dorsally via the **alar notch** in the cranial edge of the wing. The artery then turns medially to enter the vertebral canal via the **lateral vertebral foramen** of the atlas and turns cranially, dividing into branches.
      (1) Caudally, the branches anastomose with the **ventral spinal artery** (see Chapter 19 IV A 1).
      (2) Cranially, the branches anastomose to form the **basilar artery** (see Chapter 13 VI A 1 a).
   b. **Branches**
      (1) A small **unnamed branch** arises near the thoracic inlet and passes to the longus capitis.

(2) The **muscular branches** arise at each intervertebral space and pass outward into the surrounding musculature and regional skin.
   (a) The **dorsal branches** extend into the scalenus, cervical intertransversarii, serratus ventralis cranialis, and omotransversarius muscles. Terminal twigs from these branches pierce the muscles to supply the skin.
   (b) The **ventral branches** extend mainly to the longus capitis and longus colli muscles.

(3) The **spinal branches** arise at each intervertebral space and pass medially to enter the vertebral canal. These branches contribute to the formation of the ventral spinal artery and supply some other spinal cord structures on their own (see Chapter 19 IV A 1 a, 2).

B. **Veinous drainage.** The neck is characterized by a large superficial vein not directly associated with an artery, as well as a deep set of veins that are (for the most part) satellites of named arteries.

1. The **external jugular vein,** the largest vein in the neck, is superficial in position and subcutaneous along the greatest part of the length of the neck. Because of its prominence, the external jugular vein is often referred to as simply the "jugular vein."

Canine Clinical Correlation

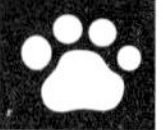

The size and accessibility of the external jugular vein make it an excellent site for the collection of large amounts of blood. The length of its course through the neck permits the novice to access multiple sites if necessary. Interestingly, physicians do not have this advantage—in humans, the external jugular is the small vein, whereas the internal jugular is the large one!

   a. The external jugular vein forms cranially at the confluence of the maxillary and linguofacial veins near the angle of the mandible. It courses caudally along the lateral surface of the sternocephalicus muscle and receives the omobrachial and cephalic veins just cranial to the shoulder before passing into the thoracic inlet.
   b. It terminates within the thorax by becoming confluent with the **subclavian vein** to form the **brachiocephalic vein,** which in turn becomes confluent with its fellow to form the **cranial vena cava.**

2. The minuscule **internal jugular vein** forms cranially at the confluence of various veins of the cranial cavity (usually the vertebral vein and sigmoid sinus). The vein courses within the carotid sheath, where it receives the cranial thyroid vein. Usually, the vein terminates by entering the external jugular vein (occasionally, it enters the brachiocephalic vein instead).
3. The **vertebral vein** is a satellite of the same-named artery, passing caudally through the transverse canal and receiving spinal veins at each intervertebral foramen.
4. The **internal** and **external vertebral plexuses** lie on the dorsal and ventral surfaces of the vertebral bodies. These plexuses are discussed more fully in Chapter 19 IV B 2.

C. **Lymphatic system**

1. **Lymph nodes**
   a. The **medial retropharyngeal lymph node** is discussed in Chapter 11 II B 3 a.
   b. The **lateral retropharyngeal lymph node** is discussed in Chapter 11 II B 3.
   c. The **superficial cervical lymph nodes** are positioned near the shoulder and are often palpable. They drain the skin of the neck, shoulder, and forelimbs.
   d. The **deep cervical lymph nodes** are positioned along the ventral and lateral surfaces of the trachea. These lymph nodes drain the deepest structures of the neck.

2. **Lymphatic trunk.** In addition to the many small afferent and efferent lymphatic vessels in

the neck, a single large lymphatic trunk is present, the **tracheal trunk.** The tracheal trunk originates as the efferent vessels from the medial retropharyngeal lymph node and is positioned deeply (within the carotid sheath). Termination varies:

a. The **left tracheal duct** enters the thoracic duct.

b. The **right tracheal duct** enters the great vessels cranial to the heart, usually near the junction of the right external jugular and subclavian veins.

II. VASCULATURE OF THE BACK

A. Arterial supply. The back is largely supplied by paired segmental arteries. Most of these are direct branches of the aorta and are referred to collectively as **"parietal" branches,** because they supply the body wall rather than the body cavity viscera.

1. The **dorsal intercostal arteries** are paired arteries numbering **twelve** on each side.
   - **a. Origin**
     - **(1) Intercostal arteries 1–3 or 4** arise from the **thoracic vertebral artery,** which is a branch of the costocervical trunk. (The thoracic vertebral artery is not the same as the vertebral artery.)
     - **(2) Intercostal arteries 4 or 5–12** arise from the dorsal surface of the **thoracic aorta.**
   - **b. Course**
     - **(1)** The dorsal intercostal arteries pass a short distance dorsally around the body of the corresponding vertebra, giving off a:
       - **(a) Nutrient artery,** which supplies the adjacent vertebral body
       - **(b) Spinal branch,** which enters the vertebral canal to contribute to the arterial supply of the spinal cord (see Chapter 19 IV A 2 a)
       - **(c) Dorsal branch,** which passes dorsally between the epaxial muscles (supplying them *en route*), crosses the vertebral spinous process, and continues dorsally to become cutaneous, supplying more adjacent epaxial muscles and the regional skin (Figure 21–1)

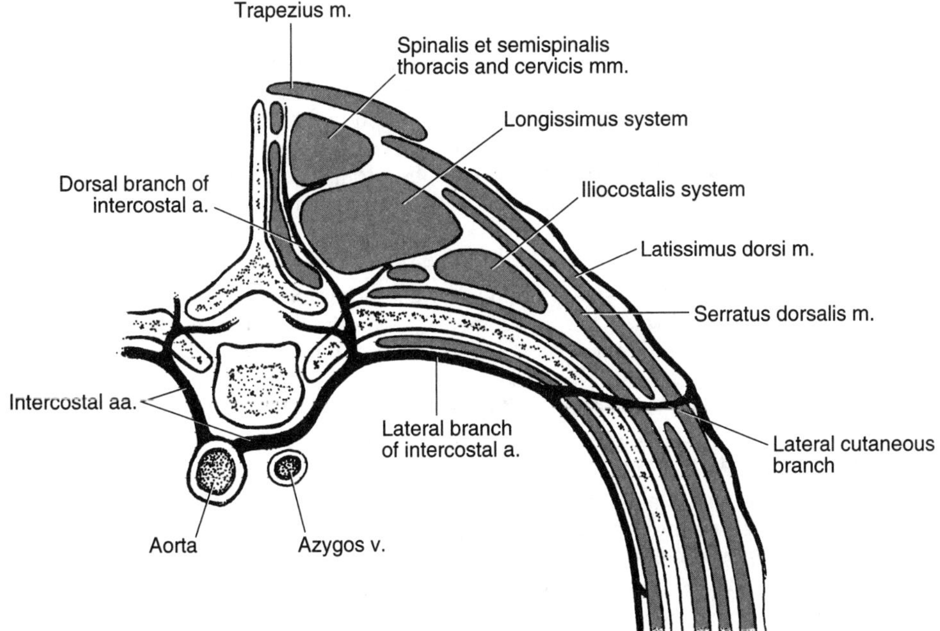

FIGURE 21–1. Branching of an intercostal artery as related to the epaxial musculature.

(2) After giving off these branches, the dorsal intercostal arteries continue laterally to contribute to the arterial supply of the thorax. The **lateral cutaneous branches** leave the dorsal intercostal arteries, one near the ventral edge of the epaxial musculature, and the second slightly less than halfway down the lateral thoracic wall. These arteries supply the skin over much of the dorsolateral and lateral thoracic wall.

2. The **dorsal costoabdominal artery** is also a branch of the thoracic aorta. This artery courses and branches similarly to the intercostal arteries, but is located caudal to the last rib; therefore, it cannot be termed an "inter"-costal artery, and takes an appropriately descriptive name instead.
3. The **lumbar arteries** are paired arteries numbering **seven** on each side. Their course and branching in the back is essentially like that of the dorsal intercostal and costoabdominal arteries, because these arteries are all segmental in nature.
   a. **Origin**
      (1) **Lumbar arteries 1–2** arise from the **thoracic aorta.**
      (2) **Lumbar arteries 3–7** arise from the **abdominal aorta.** (The last two often arise from a common trunk.)
   b. **Course**
      (1) The **first six pairs** of lumbar arteries have a course similar to that of the intercostal arteries.
         (a) These vessels arise from the aorta, pass dorsally around the body of the adjacent vertebra, and give off a **spinal branch** (which supplies the spinal cord) and a **dorsal branch,** which, in addition to supplying the adjacent epaxial muscles and regional skin, gives off small branches that run on the ventral surface of the lumbar transverse processes. These branches send out twigs that supply the adjacent regions of the internal abdominal oblique and transverse abdominal muscles.
         (b) The first six pairs of lumbar arteries continue laterally to participate in the arterial supply of the abdominal wall (see Chapter 41 V A 1).
      (2) The **last pair of lumbar arteries** differs slightly in origin and distribution from the more cranial pairs.
         (a) These arteries may arise separately or from a common trunk, either from the abdominal aorta or the median sacral artery (i.e., the direct continuation of the aorta after the origin of the internal iliac arteries).
         (b) The seventh pair of lumbar arteries divides into a:
            (i) **Dorsal branch,** similar in distribution to the other lumbar (as well as the dorsal intercostal and dorsal costoabdominal) arteries
            (ii) **Caudal branch,** which continues into the pelvis and supplies the sympathetic trunk and the ventral sacrocaudal muscles

B. Veinous drainage. Satellite veins follow the intercostal, costoabdominal, and lumbar arteries.

1. The **dorsal intercostal veins** vary slightly in their termination.
   a. **Dorsal intercostal veins 1–3 or 4** generally enter the thoracic vertebral vein (a satellite of the artery of the same name that gives rise to the first few dorsal intercostal arteries).
   b. **Dorsal intercostal veins 4 or 5–12** enter the azygous vein (on the right) or the inconstant hemiazygos vein (on the left). When the hemiazygos vein is absent, these dorsal intercostal arteries simply enter the azygous vein.
2. The **dorsal costoabdominal vein** enters the azygous (or hemiazygos) vein.
3. The **lumbar veins** are diverse in their terminations.
   a. **Lumbar veins 1–2** enter the azygous vein.
   b. **Lumbar veins 3–4** approach each other on the midline and **join to form the azygous vein.**
   c. **Lumbar veins 5–6** anastomose with each other, and the trunks thus formed enter the caudal vena cava.
   d. **Lumbar vein 7** empties into the common iliac vein.

III. VASCULATURE OF THE TAIL

A. Arterial supply. The tail has an irregularly arranged, ladder-like pattern of arteries. Many members of this ladder are small, inconstant, or both.

1. The paired **lateral caudal arteries** are two of only three arteries that extend entirely to the tip of the tail. These arteries supply the skin and fascia of the caudal gluteal region as they pass to the end of the tail.
   a. **Origin.** Each lateral caudal artery arises from the **cranial gluteal artery.**
   b. **Course.** Each lateral caudal artery courses along the dorsolateral surface of the tail all the way to its end and terminates by anastomosing with its fellow from the other side as well as with the median caudal artery at the tip of the tail.
   c. **Branches and anastomoses.** The lateral caudal arteries send branches from both their dorsal and ventral surfaces at irregular intervals. In addition, they anastomose in an irregular manner with adjacent caudal arteries along the length of the tail.

2. The single **median caudal artery** is the other artery that extends entirely to the tip of the tail. The median caudal artery supplies the tail along its length by means of segmental branches to the bone and muscle as well as dorsal branches to the skin.
   a. **Origin.** The median caudal artery is the **direct continuation of the median sacral artery.**
   b. **Course.** The median caudal artery courses along the ventral midline of the tail, passing first through the **hemal arches** and then through the **hemal processes** of the vertebrae possessing these structures (usually Cd4–6). The median caudal artery becomes **plexiform** near its caudal extremity as it anastomoses with the two lateral caudal arteries.

3. The paired **ventral caudal artery** is inconstant. When present, the ventral caudal artery arises as the first branch of the median caudal artery and typically rejoins the median caudal artery after exiting the pelvis. The ventral caudal artery supplies the adjacent vertebrae and soft tissue.
4. The paired **dorsolateral caudal artery** is a tiny artery that courses along the dorsal surfaces of the transverse processes of the caudal vertebrae. The dorsolateral caudal artery anastomoses with the segmental branches of other tail arteries at each vertebra. It decreases in size caudally and is usually lost at approximately the level of Cd9.
5. The paired **ventrolateral caudal artery** is similar to the dorsolateral caudal artery, except that it courses along the ventral surfaces of the transverse processes and is not as straight and regular as its dorsal counterpart.
6. The **caudal branch of the seventh lumbar artery** also participates in supplying the tail (its branches enter the ventral sacrocaudal muscles).

B. Veinous drainage. Only the left and right **lateral caudal veins** are recognizable as veins on the surface of the tail. These veins largely parallel the arteries of the same name.

Chapter 22

Innervation of the Neck and Back

I. VERTEBRAL NERVE.

I. VERTEBRAL NERVE. The vertebral nerve is the portion of the autonomic nervous system (ANS) that carries **sympathetic fibers to the head and neck.**

A. The vertebral nerve originates in the thorax at the level of the first intercostal space and is associated with the **cervicothoracic ganglion.**

B. The vertebral nerve enters the transverse foramen of vertebra C6 and, as a small plexiform nerve, ascends the neck through the vertebral canal in company with the vertebral artery and vein.

II. CERVICAL NERVES

A. Overview

1. **Eight pairs** of cervical spinal nerves are present. Each pair of nerves arises from the same-numbered spinal cord segment.
2. **Cervical plexus.** Many of the cervical spinal nerves form a plexus before forming the named nerves of the neck. Members of the plexus are variable among individuals, but many, most, or all of the cervical nerves may contribute to the plexus.
3. **Branching pattern.** The fundamental branching pattern of most cervical nerves is similar, although the first two cervical nerves depart considerably from the pattern. Generally, the cervical nerve leaves the vertebral column and divides almost immediately into a dorsal and ventral branch.
   a. **Dorsal branch.** The dorsal branch has a medial and lateral division.
      (1) The **medial (cutaneous) division** of the dorsal branch is purely **sensory** in nature. The cutaneous branch supplies the skin on the dorsal and lateral surfaces of the neck.
      (2) The **lateral (motor) division** of the dorsal branch supplies the regional cervical musculature.
   b. **Ventral branch.** The ventral branch has a medial and ventral division.
      (1) The **medial (motor) division** of the ventral branch supplies the regional cervical musculature, including the longissimus capitis, longus colli, intertransversarius, omotransversarius, and brachiocephalicus muscles.
      (2) The **ventral (cutaneous) division** of the ventral branch supplies large areas of skin over the ventrolateral surfaces of the neck.

B. Nerve C1. The first cervical nerve departs considerably from the pattern outlined in II A 3. The first cervical nerve emerges from the lateral vertebral foramen of the atlas and sends out a dorsal and a ventral branch.

1. The **dorsal branch of C1 (suboccipital nerve)** is **entirely motor** and supplies regions of the cranial cervical musculature (i.e., the obliquus capitis cranialis, obliquus capitis caudalis, rectus capitis dorsalis, and the cranial portions of the semispinalis and splenius muscles).

2. The **ventral branch of C1,** which gains the ventral side of the body by passing through the **alar notch,** is also **entirely motor.** It usually participates in forming the **cervical loop,** a loop of nervous tissue that receives fibers from the hypoglossal nerve and some cervical nerves, depending on the individual. The cervical loop supplies several branches to the sternohyoid and sternothyroid muscles.

C. **Nerve C2.** The second cervical nerve also departs considerably from the basic branching pattern. It emerges from the intervertebral foramen cranial to the axis (vertebra C2) and sends out a dorsal and a ventral branch, which ultimately fuse.

1. The **dorsal branch of C2 (greater occipital nerve)** is **motor** to the semispinalis capitis and splenius muscles and **sensory** to a large area of the skin over the temporal muscle and convex surface of the pinna. The sensory component is the largest of all the cervical or thoracic nerves.
2. The **ventral branch of C2** divides into two large **sensory** nerves.
   a. The **transverse cervical nerve** supplies the skin over the mandibular space as well as the lateral and ventral surfaces of the neck as far caudally as the first tracheal ring.
   b. The **great auricular nerve** divides into at least two branches, which supply both surfaces of the pinna.

D. **Nerves C3–C8** emerge through the intervertebral foramen, cranial to the vertebra of the same number for nerves C3–C7, and caudal to vertebra C7 for nerve C8. They generally follow the fundamental pattern of branching described in II A 3.

1. The **dorsal branches** of **nerves C3–C8** progressively decrease in size (moving cranially to caudally), with the seventh being only a twig, and the eighth sometimes being absent. Each dorsal branch sends a few fibers to the multifidus muscle shortly after leaving the vertebral canal.
   a. The **medial (cutaneous) division** of the dorsal branch is **absent** from **nerves C7–C8.**
   b. The **lateral (motor) division** supplies the regional cervical muscles, including the biventer and complexus portions of the semispinalis muscle and the splenius muscle.
2. **Ventral branches** of **nerves C3–C8**
   a. The ventral branches of nerves C3–C5 decrease in size progressing in a cranial-to-caudal direction.
      (1) The ventral branches of nerves C3 and C4 (as well as nerve C2) intermix with the accessory nerve.
      (2) The field of distribution of the ventral (cutaneous) division of the ventral branch of nerve C5 is particularly large, including a large portion of the skin over the brachium.
   b. The ventral branches of nerves C6–C8 contribute (along with nerves T1 and T2) to the formation of the **brachial plexus,** the large network of nerves that is the source of the motor and sensory innervation of the thoracic limb (see Chapter 30 I). For this reason, the latter cervical nerves are not consistently represented in the typical branching pattern.

III. THORACIC NERVES.

Thirteen pairs of thoracic nerves are present, each of which exits the intervertebral foramen caudal to the vertebra of the same number as the nerve. On leaving the intervertebral foramen, each thoracic nerve divides into a **dorsal branch** and a **ventral branch.**

A. The **dorsal branches** of the thoracic nerves are important when considering the innervation of structures intrinsic to the back. The dorsal branch itself divides into medial and lateral branches.

1. The **medial branch** of the dorsal branch passes caudodorsally across the spinous process of the associated vertebra and is **motor only.** It supplies all of the **regional epaxial musculature** except the iliocostalis muscle. Specifically, it supplies the:
   a. **Rotatores**
   b. **Interspinales thoracis**
   c. **Multifidus thoracis**
   d. **Longissimus thoracis**
   e. **Spinalis et semispinalis thoracis et cervicis**

2. The **lateral branch** of the dorsal branch is **motor** and **sensory.**
   a. It passes caudolaterally between the longissimus and iliocostalis muscles and turns ventrally to gain a position where it can reach and supply the **iliocostalis thoracis,** the most ventral thoracic epaxial muscle group.
   b. The lateral branch then turns directly laterally to **perforate the skin,** becoming the **dorsal cutaneous branches.** The dorsal cutaneous branches divide into two branches that supply the **skin over the dorsal third of the thorax.**

B. The **ventral branches** of certain thoracic nerves contribute to the innervation of some of the muscles on the back, such as the extrinsic muscles of the thoracic limb. These branches are discussed in more detail in Chapter 30.

IV. LUMBAR NERVES.

Seven pairs of lumbar nerves are present, each of which exits the intervertebral foramen caudal to the vertebra of the same number as the nerve. On leaving the intervertebral foramen, each lumbar nerve divides into a **dorsal branch and a ventral branch.**

A. The **dorsal branches** are important when considering the innervation of structures intrinsic to the back.

1. **Nerves L1–L3 or L4.** The dorsal branch of nerves L1–L3 or L4 divides into medial and lateral branches.
   a. The **medial branch** of the dorsal branch is **motor only.** It passes caudodorsally across the spinous process of the associated vertebra, supplying the **regional epaxial musculature:**
      (1) **Multifidus lumborum**
      (2) **Interspinales lumborum**
      (3) **Longissimus lumborum**
   b. The **lateral branch** of the dorsal branch is both **motor** and **sensory.**
      (1) It passes caudolaterally between the longissimus and iliocostalis muscles, and turns ventrally to gain a position where it can reach and supply the **abdominal wall** and the **iliocostalis lumborum,** the most ventral lumbar epaxial muscle group.
      (2) This branch then turns directly laterally to perforate the skin, becoming the **dorsal cutaneous branches (cranial cluneal nerves).** The dorsal cutaneous branches supply the **skin over the dorsal third of the abdominal wall.**
2. **Nerves L4 or L5–L7.** In these nerves, the dorsal branch typically does not divide into medial and lateral branches. Therefore, the dorsal branches of lumbar nerves L4 or L5–L7 lack dorsal cutaneous branches and terminate by arborizing in the regional epaxial musculature.

B. The **ventral branches** of the lumbar nerves are described with the abdominal wall and pelvic limb (see Chapter 43 II C). They do not participate in innervation of the back.

V. SACRAL NERVES.

Three pairs of sacral nerves emerge from the dorsal sacral foramina and contribute to the formation of the **dorsal sacral trunk or plexus,** a small nerve plexus on the dorsal surface of the sacrum. They then divide into **dorsal and ventral branches.**

A. **The** dorsal branch of each sacral nerve is important to the innervation of the back and tail. The dorsal branch divides into a:

1. **Medial branch,** which is **motor** to the **lateral and medial dorsal sacrocaudal muscles**
2. **Lateral branch,** which terminates as the **dorsal cutaneous branch (middle cluneal nerves)** and is **sensory** to the **regional skin**

B. The **ventral branch** is important in the innervation of the pelvic limb and other structures and is discussed in Chapter 61.

VI. CAUDAL NERVES.
The caudal nerves are variable in number, ranging between four and seven pairs.

A. The **dorsal branches** of the caudal nerves communicate with each other and also receive fibers from the last sacral nerve (S3) to form the **dorsal caudal trunk,** which is positioned immediately dorsal to the transverse processes of the caudal vertebrae. Delicate **motor** branches leave the dorsal caudal trunk to supply the tail musculature dorsal to the transverse processes of the caudal vertebrae (i.e., the **lateral and medial dorsal sacrocaudal muscles).**

B. The **ventral branches** of the caudal nerves play an important role in the innervation of the regional musculature of the vertebral column. A **ventral caudal trunk** is formed from the ventral branches of the caudal nerves together with contributions from the last sacral nerve (S3). The ventral caudal nerve trunk is larger than its dorsal counterpart, because it supplies an extra set of muscles as well as the skin. It lies immediately ventral to the transverse processes of the caudal vertebrae.

1. **Motor branches** leave both the dorsal and ventral surfaces of the ventral caudal trunk to supply the tail musculature ventral to the transverse processes of the caudal vertebrae (i.e., the **lateral and medial ventral sacrocaudal muscles),** as well as both parts of the **intertransverse tail muscles.**
2. **Cutaneous branches** may be associated with the first seven to nine ventral branches of the ventral caudal trunk.

Chapter 23

Soft Tissue Structures of the Neck

I. INTRODUCTION. The **visceral compartment of the neck** is bounded by muscle:

A. **Deeply** (i.e., against the vertebral bodies)—the longus capitis and longus colli muscles

B. **Superficially** (i.e., closer to the skin)—the sternohyoideus and sternothyroideus muscles

II. TRACHEA. The trachea conducts air from the pharynx to the lungs.

A. **Position.** The trachea extends through the full length of the neck from the larynx to the thoracic inlet. Its course runs deeply, close along the ventral cervical midline and adjacent to the longus colli muscle over the ventral surfaces of the cervical vertebral bodies.

B. **Structure.** The trachea is a semirigid, tubular organ composed of **tracheal rings** of hyaline cartilage, which are separated by narrow membranous regions, the **annular tracheal ligaments.** The tracheal rings are incomplete dorsally, where the gap is bridged by the **trachealis muscle.** The form of the trachea renders it both noncollapsible (to maintain a permanently open airway) and flexible (to permit motion of the head and neck).

C. **Vascularization.** Arterial supply arrives to the trachea mainly from the **cranial** and **caudal thyroid arteries,** as well as from the **bronchoesophageal artery.**

D. **Innervation** of the trachea is essentially autonomic. Parasympathetic fibers arrive through the **pararecurrent laryngeal nerves.**

III. ESOPHAGUS. The esophagus is the muscular tube that connects the pharynx with the stomach.

A. **Position.** The esophagus undergoes positional changes relative to other organs as it courses cranially to caudally through the neck.

1. In the cranial cervical regions, the esophagus lies dorsal to the trachea.
2. In the midcervical region, the esophagus moves to the left of the midline and trachea, and holds this position as far caudally as the thoracic inlet. Therefore, throughout most of the cervical length, both the esophagus and trachea are in contact with the longus colli muscle.

B. **Vascularization**

1. The **cervical portion** of the esophagus is supplied mainly by the **cranial** and **caudal thyroid arteries,** and drained by their satellite veins.
2. The **thoracic portion** of the esophagus is supplied mainly by the **bronchoesophageal** or **dorsal intercostal arteries,** or both. The **left gastric artery** supplies the caudal-most part of the esophagus (i.e., the part adjacent to the cardia of the stomach).

C. **Innervation**

1. **Motor innervation**
   a. The **cervical region** receives motor innervation through two sets of paired nerves, the **pharyngoesophageal nerve** (from the vagus) and the **pararecurrent laryngeal nerve** (also from the vagus, but via the recurrent laryngeal nerve).
   b. The **cranial thoracic region** receives motor innervation via the **pararecurrent laryngeal nerves.**

c. The **caudal thoracic region** receives motor innervation via the **dorsal** and **ventral vagal branches** and the **dorsal** and **ventral vagal trunks.**

2. **Sensory innervation** to the esophagus essentially mirrors the motor innervation, except that the pharyngoesophageal nerve does not participate.

IV. CAROTID SHEATH. The carotid sheath, formed from the **deep cervical fascia,** surrounds and supports several vascular and nervous structures as they traverse the length of the neck.

A. Position. The carotid sheath is located in the angle between the longus colli muscle and the trachea; on the left, it is also related to the esophagus.

B. Structures contained. The carotid sheath contains the:

1. **Common carotid artery,** as it ascends the neck *en route* to the head and brain
2. **Internal jugular vein,** as it passes caudally to enter the external jugular vein
3. **Vagosympathetic trunk,** as it carries sympathetic input to the head and parasympathetic input to the thorax and abdomen
4. **Recurrent laryngeal nerve,** as it ascends the neck *en route* to the larynx
5. **Tracheal lymphatic duct,** as it carries lymph from the deep structures of the head to the great vessels cranial to the heart

V. THYROID GLANDS. The thyroid glands (see also Chapter 6 II C) are positioned on the ventrolateral surfaces of the first several tracheal rings.

A. Vascularization

1. **Arterial supply**
   a. The **cranial thyroid artery** [see Chapter 21 I A 1 b (2)] sends numerous tiny branches that enter the gland around its perimeter.
   b. The **caudal thyroid artery** is variable in origin, but usually arises as a branch of the brachiocephalic artery within the thorax. This artery ascends along the trachea to supply the gland.

2. **Venous drainage** occurs through the **cranial and caudal thyroid veins,** which enter the internal jugular vein.

B. Innervation of the thyroid gland arrives through the **thyroid nerve,** which is formed by contributions from the **cranial cervical ganglion** (sympathetic) and **cranial laryngeal nerve** (parasympathetic).

VI. PARATHYROID GLANDS (see also Chapter 6 II D)

A. Position

1. The **external parathyroid glands** are located on the lateral surface of the cranial pole of the thyroid gland.
2. The **internal parathyroid glands** are located on the medial surface of the caudal pole of the thyroid gland.

B. Vascularization

1. **Arterial supply** to the parathyroid glands is essentially the same as that of the thyroid glands.
   a. The **external parathyroid glands,** the more cranial of the glands, receive their supply from the cranial thyroid artery.
   b. The **internal parathyroid glands** receive branches from the thyroid parenchyma.

2. **Venous drainage** of the parathyroid glands is similar to that of the thyroid glands.

C. Innervation of the parathyroid glands is also similar to that of the thyroid glands.

Chapter 24

Prominent Palpable Features of the Neck and Back

I. BONY STRUCTURES

A. The **atlantal wings** are located directly under the skin in the dorsolateral region of the neck, caudal and slightly ventral to the level of the junction of the pinna and the head. In smooth-haired dogs with a short coat (e.g., Doberman pinschers), the edges of the wings are often visible.

B. The **spinous processes** of the thoracic and lumbar vertebrae (i.e., from the axis caudally) are easily palpated by applying moderate pressure along the dorsal midline. Those of the thoracic region are most prominent.

C. The **transverse processes** of the cervical and lumbar vertebrae may be appreciated in many normal dogs as a general, unyielding firmness along the lateral surface of the neck and back. However, because the transverse processes are covered by substantial muscle mass, they are not as prominent as the spinous processes and may not be palpable at all in dogs with particularly thick neck or back musculature. Conversely, in emaciated animals, the transverse processes become more prominent.

D. The **caudal vertebral column** can be appreciated as a general firmness within the substance of the tail, although the bony features of individual caudal vertebrae cannot be detected.

II. SOFT TISSUE STRUCTURES

A. The **epaxial musculature** can be appreciated as the dorsally positioned, symmetrical, rounded mass of soft tissue on each side of the dorsal midline.

B. The **thyroid gland** is readily palpable in dogs only when it is enlarged.

C. The **trachea** is felt as a firm, tubular structure extending throughout much of the cervical length on the ventral surface of the neck near the midline. The cartilaginous nature of the trachea allows it to be grasped between the fingers. With careful, moderate pressure, the flattened dorsal surface where the incomplete cartilage rings are bridged by the trachealis muscle may sometimes be appreciated.

> **Canine Clinical Correlation**
>
> The freely palpable nature of the trachea allows **diagnostic elicitation of a cough during physical examination.** Placing light digital pressure on the trachea should evoke a light, brief, single cough that is not repeated. When performing this test, it is important to remember the importance of maintaining an open lumen in the cartilaginous trachea; only light pressure should be used!

D. The **esophagus** is more difficult to palpate because it is composed entirely of soft tissue and is normally collapsed (unless a bolus is passing through it). However, the esophagus can sometimes be appreciated as a pliant, elongate structure positioned to the left of and dorsal to the trachea.

STUDY QUESTIONS

DIRECTIONS: Each of the numbered items or incomplete statements in this section is followed by answers or by completions of the statement. Select the ONE numbered answer or completion that is BEST in each case.

1. Which of the following descriptions would identify a vertebra as being any one from the sequence C3–C7?

(1) A longitudinal crest along the dorsal surface of the body
(2) A transverse foramen in the transverse process
(3) A relatively short spinous process
(4) Cranial articular facets that face ventrally

2. What is the correct canine vertebral formula?

(1) C8, T12, L7, Cd25–30
(2) C7, T12, L6, Cd15–20
(3) C7, T13, L7, Cd20–23
(4) C7, T13, L7, S3, Cd20–23
(5) C8, T13, L7, S3, Cd20–30

3. Consider this description of vertebrae from a particular region: massive body, long transverse processes projecting cranially, relatively long and heavy pedicles and laminae, mamillary and accessory processes. This description applies to vertebrae of the:

(1) cervical region.
(2) thoracic region.
(3) lumbar region.
(4) caudal region.

4. The region of the vertebral column that departs most significantly from the dorsal topline of the intact dog is the:

(1) cervical region.
(2) thoracic region.
(3) lumbar region.
(4) caudal region.

5. Which one of the following statements regarding the vertebral bodies is true?

(1) They are most massive in the thoracic region.
(2) They are perforated by the transverse foramina in the cervical region.
(3) They are positioned dorsal to the transverse processes.
(4) They form the floor of the vertebral canal.
(5) They incline caudally cranial to T11 and cranially from that point on.

6. Identify the correct pairing of vertebral foramen and structures passing through it.

(1) Intervertebral foramen—ventral branch of spinal nerves
(2) Lateral vertebral foramen—ventral branch of the first cervical nerve
(3) Transverse foramen—vertebral nerve
(4) Alar notch—dorsal branch of the first cervical nerve

7. Select the descriptor most applicable to thoracic vertebrae as a group.

(1) Small vertebral bodies
(2) Tall pedicles
(3) Absent transverse processes
(4) Absent spinous processes

8. The orientation of the surfaces of the articular facets of the lumbar vertebrae:

(1) facilitates lateral flexion.
(2) facilitates dorsoventral flexion—extension.
(3) prevents dorsoventral flexion—extension.
(4) is essentially similar to that of the more cranial vertebrae.

9. Which pairing of sacral structures with structures of individual vertebrae is correct?

(1) Sacral canal—transverse canal
(2) Median sacral crest—mamillary processes
(3) Lateral sacral crest—transverse processes
(4) Intermediate sacral crest—accessory processes

10. It is necessary for a veterinarian to obtain a cerebrospinal fluid sample for analysis. One area where the vertebral canal is accessible to needle puncture is the:

(1) thoracolumbar junction.
(2) intervertebral space T10–T11, at the anticlinal vertebra.
(3) ventral surface of the lumbosacral junction.
(4) atlantooccipital junction.

11. What is the general pattern of exit of spinal nerves from the vertebral canal, relative to the vertebrae?

(1) All spinal nerves exit cranial to the vertebra of the same number.
(2) All spinal nerves exit caudal to the vertebra of the same number.
(3) The first seven cervical nerves exit cranial to the vertebra of the same number, and the remaining spinal nerves exit caudal to the vertebra of the same number.
(4) The first seven cervical nerves exit caudal to the vertebra of the same number, and the remaining spinal nerves exit cranial to the vertebra of the same number.

12. The discrepancy between the location of spinal cord segments and vertebral bodies of the same number is caused by:

(1) the different number of neurons in various segments.
(2) different rates of growth for the spinal cord and vertebral column.
(3) different patterns in blood supply of the cord and column.
(4) different dural attachments in the cranial and caudal cord segments.

13. A funiculus is distinguished from a fasciculus by:

(1) size.
(2) position.
(3) blood supply.
(4) direction of impulse conduction.

14. Which one of the following statements regarding descending white matter tracts is true?

(1) They carry sensory impulses.
(2) They carry motor impulses.
(3) They are located deep to the central grey matter surrounding the central canal.
(4) They are located within the dorsal funiculus.

15. Injury to which one of the following structures would affect sensory function?

(1) Dorsal funiculus
(2) Descending tracts
(3) Ventral horn of the spinal cord
(4) Ventral root of the spinal cord

16. The main channel flow of arterial blood along the spinal cord:

(1) runs in the dorsal median sulcus.
(2) runs along the ventral midline.
(3) takes the form of paired arteries on the dorsolateral cord surface.
(4) is an unpaired artery running just ventral to the central canal.

17. The grey matter of the spinal cord receives most of its arterial supply from the:

(1) ventral spinal artery.
(2) dorsal spinal artery.
(3) dorsolateral spinal arteries.
(4) basilar artery.

18. Which one of the following statements regarding the lymphatic drainage of the spinal cord is true?

(1) It is best-developed in the white matter tracts.
(2) It follows the ventral spinal but not the dorsolateral spinal arteries.
(3) It drains into tiny paired lymph nodes at each intervertebral foramen.
(4) It is absent.

19. The venous plexuses associated with the spinal cord and vertebral canal:

(1) have prominent valves to ensure strictly cranial flow of blood within the plexuses.
(2) drain the cord as well as the surrounding structures.
(3) are contained within the epidural space.
(4) are absent in the regions of the cervical and lumbar intumescences.

20. The nuchal ligament may be regarded as a specialization of the:

(1) supraspinous ligament.
(2) yellow ligament.
(3) intertransverse ligament.
(4) dorsal longitudinal ligament.

21. Which one of the following statements regarding the extrinsic muscles of the neck is true?

(1) The extrinsic neck muscles have attachments that extend from one side of the back to the other, across the dorsal midline.
(2) The extrinsic neck muscles extend the vertebral column dorsally.
(3) The extrinsic neck muscles are innervated by cranial nerves.
(4) The extrinsic neck muscles are attached to the thoracic limb.

22. Which system of epaxial muscles generally extends from the ilium to the ribs, is positioned most laterally among the muscle groups, and is characterized by muscles that span multiple vertebrae in all cases?

(1) Longissimus system
(2) Transversospinalis system
(3) Longus thoracolumbalis system
(4) Iliocostalis system
(5) Psoas major system

23. The truncal fascia that supports the mammary gland is the:

(1) superficial external fascia.
(2) superficial leaf of the deep external fascia.
(3) deep leaf of the deep external fascia.
(4) thoracolumbar fascia.

24. The broad, flattened neck muscle that is most superficial among the intrinsic neck musculature and wraps the deeper muscles in a manner reminiscent of a bandage is the:

(1) semispinalis capitis, complexus portion.
(2) semispinalis capitis, biventer portion.
(3) splenius.
(4) longissimus atlantis.

25. Which neck muscle of the transversospinalis system acts to elevate the head and is innervated by dorsal branches of the cervical spinal nerves?

(1) Semispinalis et spinalis cervicis
(2) Semispinalis capitis
(3) Longissimus capitis
(4) Longissimus atlantis
(5) Rhomboideus capitis

26. Which one of the following neck muscles has a general action that is different from that of the other listed muscles?

(1) Longissimus cervicis
(2) Longus colli, thoracic portion
(3) Semispinalis et spinalis cervicis
(4) Semispinalis capitis

27. Which one of the following pairs represents members of the transversospinalis system of the back?

(1) Interspinales and intertransversarii muscles
(2) Multifidus and rotatores muscles
(3) Multifidus and intertransversarii muscles
(4) Iliocostalis and spinalis et semispinalis thoracis muscles

28. Which epaxial muscle acts mainly to stabilize the vertebral column?

(1) Iliocostalis thoracis
(2) Sacrocaudalis dorsalis lateralis
(3) Interspinales
(4) Multifidus
(5) Longissimus thoracic et lumborum

29. The epaxial muscle systems whose caudal regions fuse together into the large, relatively unsegmented mass of muscle covering the dorsal lumbar region are the:

(1) transversospinalis and iliocostalis systems.
(2) transversospinalis and longissimus systems.
(3) iliocostalis and longissimus systems.
(4) multifidus and longissimus systems.

30. Which group of tail muscles is most involved in lateral movement of the tail?

(1) Sacrocaudalis dorsalis lateralis
(2) Sacrocaudalis ventralis lateralis
(3) Sacrocaudalis lateralis
(4) Intertransversarius dorsalis caudalis

31. Which one of the following is a typical branch of the common carotid artery in the neck?

(1) Medial thyroid artery
(2) Cranial thyroid artery
(3) Ascending pharyngeal artery
(4) Vertebral artery

32. Place the following structures in correct caudal-to-cranial sequence to describe the course of the vertebral artery.

(1) Transverse foramen of C7, transverse canal, dorsal surface of atlantal wing, alar notch, lateral vertebral foramen, vertebral canal
(2) Transverse foramen of C7, transverse canal, ventral surface of atlantal wing, lateral vertebral foramen, alar notch, vertebral canal
(3) Transverse canal, alar notch, lateral vertebral foramen, vertebral canal
(4) Transverse canal, lateral vertebral foramen, alar notch, vertebral canal

33. Place the following letters in the correct order to describe the typical branching pattern of a dorsal intercostal artery after it has arisen from the parent artery.

A—Nutrient artery to vertebral body
B—Spinal branch to ventral spinal artery
C—Dorsal branch to epaxial musculature and skin
D—Lateral branch to body wall

(1) A, B, C, D
(2) A, B, D, C
(3) B, A, C, D
(4) C, A, B, D

34. Which one of the following statements regarding the main arteries of the tail is true?

(1) They take the form of paired dorsal and ventral channels along the respective surfaces of the tail.
(2) They become discontinuous in the caudal fourth of the tail, with regions caudal to that level being supplied by arteriovenous sinuses.
(3) They arise from the median sacral and cranial gluteal arteries.
(4) They are present as a single dorsal and a single ventral midline channel extending the full length of the tail.

35. The dorsal branches of the thoracic and lumbar spinal nerves divide into medial and lateral branches. Which one of the following statements regarding these second branchings is true?

(1) The medial branch is motor to the epaxial muscles.
(2) The medial branch is motor to the hypaxial muscles.
(3) The lateral branch is motor to the hypaxial muscles.
(4) The lateral branch is sensory to the skin over the ventral abdominal wall.

36. Which group of spinal nerves fits the following description: divides into dorsal and ventral branches on exiting the intervertebral foramen; dorsal branch is sensory and motor; medial branch of the dorsal branch is sensory; lateral branch of the dorsal branch is motor.

(1) Cervical spinal nerves
(2) Thoracic spinal nerves
(3) Lumbar spinal nerves
(4) Sacral spinal nerves

37. Which statement regarding the caudal spinal nerves or nerve trunks is true?

(1) The ventral caudal nerves supply their musculature directly, but the dorsal caudal nerves first form a trunk from which nerves to the dorsal tail region arise.
(2) The caudal nerves correspond to each caudal vertebral segment, although they become progressively smaller from cranial to caudal.
(3) Cutaneous branches of the ventral caudal trunk are associated with the first several ventral branches.
(4) The dorsal caudal nerve trunk is positioned dorsal to the spinous processes of the caudal vertebrae.

38. Which one of the following features is normally readily palpable in the cranial cervical region?

(1) Atlantal wing
(2) Spinous process of the atlas
(3) Lateral vertebral foramen of the axis
(4) Dens of the axis
(5) Transverse processes of vertebra C3

DIRECTIONS: Each of the numbered items or incomplete statements in this section is negatively phrased, as indicated by a capitalized word such as NOT, LEAST, or EXCEPT. Select the ONE numbered answer or completion that is BEST in each case.

39. Which statement regarding the muscles of the tail is INCORRECT?

(1) The tail muscles are arranged in paired dorsal and ventral groups, each of which contains a lateral, a medial, and an intertransverse member.
(2) The tail muscles have lateral members that are relatively short and medial members that are relatively long.
(3) The tail muscles are supplied by branches of the dorsal and ventral caudal plexuses.
(4) The dorsal group of tail muscles raise the tail and the ventral group of tail muscles lower the tail.

40. Contraction of which one of the following would NOT induce movement of the head?

(1) The epaxial muscle system deepest and closest to the midline
(2) The transversospinalis system
(3) The longissimus system
(4) The iliocostalis system

41. Which feature of the final body form in the neck and back area is LEAST traceable to the somitic nature of the early embryo?

(1) Vascularization
(2) Innervation
(3) Bony form
(4) Musculature

42. Which one of the following arteries does NOT contribute significantly to the main channel flow of arterial supply to the spinal cord?

(1) Vertebral artery
(2) Intercostal artery
(3) Lumbar artery
(4) Sacral artery
(5) Caudal artery

43. Which one of the following structures is NOT typically supplied directly by the vertebral artery?

(1) Epaxial musculature
(2) Hypaxial musculature
(3) Spinal cord
(4) Cervical skin

44. Which one of the following statements regarding the external jugular vein is INCORRECT?

(1) The external jugular vein is a large vein superficial in position throughout most of the cervical length.
(2) The external jugular vein forms at the confluence of the superficial temporal and maxillary veins.
(3) The external jugular vein receives the omobrachial and cephalic veins.
(4) The external jugular vein terminates in the thorax at the brachiocephalic vein.

45. Which statement regarding the thoracic and lumbar spinal nerves is INCORRECT?

(1) They have dorsal branches important in the innervation of the intrinsic muscles of the back.
(2) They have ventral branches important in the innervation of the extrinsic back muscles.
(3) They have ventral branches important in the innervation of the intrinsic back muscles.
(4) They have ventral branches important in the innervation of the thoracic, but not the pelvic, limbs.

46. Which statement regarding the cervical viscera is INCORRECT?

(1) The carotid sheath passes along the tracheal surface.
(2) The esophagus lies dorsal to the trachea in the cranial cervical region, but eventually lies to the right of the midline and trachea.
(3) The incomplete tracheal rings are closed dorsally by the trachealis muscle.
(4) The cervical viscera lie in contact with the longus colli and longus capitus muscles dorsally.

47. Soft tissue structures normally palpable in the neck and back include all of the following EXCEPT the:

(1) trachea.
(2) larynx.
(3) thyroid glands.
(4) epaxial muscle mass in the lumbar region.

ANSWERS AND EXPLANATIONS

1. The answer is 3 [Chapter 18 III A 3–4; Figure 18–2]. Vertebrae C3–C7 are distinguished by relatively short spinous processes (when compared with the spinous processes of the thoracic vertebrae). The longitudinal crest characteristic of the cervical vertebrae runs along the ventral, not the dorsal, surface of the body. Vertebra C7 lacks a transverse foramen. The cranial articular facets do not face ventrally in any vertebra.

2. The answer is 4 [Chapter 18 I B 2]. The correct vertebral formula for the dog is C7, T13, L7, S3, Cd20–23.

3. The answer is 3 [Chapter 18 III C]. The vertebrae of the lumbar region are generally characterized by a massive vertebral body, long transverse processes that project cranially, relatively long and heavy pedicles and laminae, and the presence of mamillary and accessory processes.

4. The answer is 1 [Chapter 18 I C; Figure 3–1]. Much of the cervical portion of the vertebral column is located far ventral to the topline of the dog's neck, with no portion of the vertebrae extending to a subcutaneous position. Although the thoracic vertebral bodies are also somewhat removed from the topline, their spinous processes are nonetheless subcutaneous.

5. The answer is 4 [Chapter 18 II C, D 2; III A 4 b (1), B 5 a (2) (c), C]. The vertebral bodies form the floor of the vertebral canal. The vertebral bodies are most massive in the lumbar area, and in all cases lie ventral to the transverse processes. The transverse processes (not the vertebral bodies) of C1–C6 are perforated by transverse foramina, but C7 lacks transverse foramina. The spinous processes, not the vertebral bodies, incline caudally cranial to T11 and cranially thereafter. The lumbar vertebrae, not the thoracic vertebrae, are known for their massive vertebral bodies.

6. The answer is 3 [Chapter 18 II B 2, III A 1 b (2) (a), d; Chapter 22 I B]. The transverse foramen transmits the vertebral nerve, along with the vertebral artery and vein. The intervertebral foramen transmits the entire spinal nerve before it branches. The lateral vertebral foramen transmits the entirety of the first cervical nerve. The alar notch transmits the ventral, not the dorsal, branch of the first cervical nerve.

7. The answer is 1 [Chapter 18 III B]. Thoracic vertebrae possess both spinous and transverse processes (although the latter are short and blunt), but their pedicles are short and their bodies are small.

8. The answer is 2 [Chapter 18 III C 3]. The articular surfaces of the lumbar region are oriented in a sagittal plane, which is different from the orientation of the vertebral articular surfaces in the thoracic area. The orientation in the sagittal plane facilitates dorsoventral flexion–extension (e.g., the type of movement seen when a dog arches its back while running at top speed).

9. The answer is 3 [Chapter 18 III D 1, 5 b–d]. The lateral sacral crest is formed by the fusion of the transverse processes of the original vertebrae. The sacral canal is the continuation of the vertebral canal, not the transverse canal. The median sacral crest forms from the fusion of the original spinous processes. The intermediate sacral crest forms from the fusion of the mamillary and articular processes.

10. The answer is 4 [Chapter 18 I A 1 e; III D 5 a]. The atlantooccipital membrane may be punctured with a needle to access the cerebellomedullary cistern beneath it. Although this is the correct answer to this question, accessing the cerebellomedullary cistern to obtain a cerebrospinal fluid sample or introduce contrast material carries a greater risk than obtaining access at the dorsal (not the ventral) lumbosacral junction. The dorsal lumbosacral junction is safer because in this more caudal region, only the nerve roots (i.e., the cauda equina) are present, rather than the spinal cord itself. The nerve roots are mobile and can evade the needle. Even if damage to a nerve root should occur, the results will likely be far less devastating to the patient than a cord injury in the cervical region.

11. The answer is 3 [Chapter 19 II B 2 a]. The first seven cervical nerves exit cranial to the vertebra of the same number, and the remaining spinal nerves exit caudal to the vertebra of the same number. This pattern is formed because there are eight cervical nerves and seven cervical vertebrae. The first cervical nerve exits the lateral vertebral foramen of the atlas, nerves C2–C7 exit the intervertebral foramen cranial to the vertebra of the same number, nerve C8 exits caudal to vertebra C7, and the remaining nerves exit caudal to the vertebra of the same number.

12. The answer is 2 [Chapter 19 II B 1]. The spinal cord and vertebral column are initially the same length, but after birth, the cord grows more slowly than the column, causing the column to become longer than the cord.

13. The answer is 1 [Chapter 19 III C 2 c (2)]. A funiculus is a grossly visible white matter tract, whereas a fasciculus is a smaller, subgross tract, several of which compose a funiculus.

14. The answer is 2 [Chapter 19 III C 2 c (3)]. Descending tracts carry motor commands caudally from higher centers ("down"); ascending tracts carry sensory information cranially ("up"). White matter tracts are all located superficially on the cord. The dorsal funiculus is largely sensory.

15. The answer is 1 [Chapter 19 III C 2 c (2) (a)]. The dorsal funiculus is a major sensory tract ascending to the brain. Descending tracts, the ventral horn, and the ventral root are all motor in nature.

16. The answer is 2 [Chapter 19 IV A 1]. The unpaired ventral spinal artery is the main arterial channel of the spinal cord, and is positioned superficially along the plane of the ventral median fissure. The paired dorsolateral spinal arteries are much smaller and more discontinuous than the ventral spinal artery.

17. The answer is 1 [Chapter 19 IV A 1 b]. The grey matter of the spinal cord is supplied mainly by the ventral spinal artery. The dorsolateral spinal arteries supply the majority of the white matter of the spinal cord and the basilar artery supplies the brain. A "dorsal spinal artery" is a fictitious structure.

18. The answer is 4 [Chapter 19 IV C]. Part of the central nervous system (CNS), the spinal cord has no lymphatic channels.

19. The answer is 2 [Chapter 19 IV B]. The venous plexuses drain the spinal cord as well as the surrounding structures housed within the vertebral canal. The venous sinuses are valveless, are present both within and outside of the vertebral canal, and are present in the area of the cervical and lumbar intumescences.

20. The answer is 1 [Chapter 20 I A 1–2]. The nuchal ligament extends cranially along the dorsal midline in essentially the same plane as the supraspinous ligament.

21. The answer is 4 [Chapter 20 II A 1, B 1]. By definition, the extrinsic musculature of any region has attachments both in that region as well as external to it. The extrinsic neck muscles attach to the head and thoracic limb. They do not cross the dorsal midline. They are innervated by cervical spinal nerves and act mainly to turn the head and neck.

22. The answer is 4 [Chapter 20 II A 2 b (1) (c)]. The iliocostalis system extends from the ilium to C7. Its members span multiple vertebrae in all cases, and are positioned most laterally among the three epaxial muscle systems. The longissimus system extends from the ilium to the head and is intermediate in position among the three epaxial groups. The transversospinalis system extends onto the head and occupies the intermediate position. The psoas major is a member of the hypaxial muscle group. The "longus thoracolumbalis" is a whimsical group of muscles.

23. The answer is 1 [Chapter 20 III B 1 c]. The superficial external fascia sends significant supporting leaves to the mammary gland. All portions of the deep fascia are too deep to support the mammary gland, which is essentially a cutaneous structure. The thoracolumbar fascia is a subdivision of the deep external fascia, and is too far dorsal to support the mammary gland.

24. The answer is 3 [Chapter 20 II B 2 a]. The splenius is the most superficial of the intrinsic neck musculature (although it lies deep to the extrinsic limb muscles). The semispinalis capitis and longissimus atlantis are both deeper than the splenius.

25. The answer is 2 [Table 20–2]. The semispinalis capitis attaches to the occipital skull region and acts to elevate the head. The semispinalis et spinalis cervicis is not attached to the head, and functions primarily to stabilize the vertebral column. The longissimus capitis and the longissimus atlantis are part of the longissimus system. The rhomboideus capitis is an extrinsic limb muscle.

26. The answer is 2 [Tables 20–2 and 20–3]. The longus colli is a hypaxial muscle that flexes the neck ventrally. The longissimus cervicis, semispinalis et spinalis cervicis, and semispinalis capitis are all epaxial muscles that act in extension.

27. The answer is 2 [Table 20–4]. The multifidus muscles and the rotatores muscles are members of the transversospinalis system of the epaxial back musculature. The spinalis et semispinalis thoracis and the interspinales muscles are also members of the transversospinalis system on the back, but the intertransversarii are members of the longissimus group, and the iliocostalis forms its own group separate from the transversospinalis system.

28. The answer is 4 [Table 20–4]. The multifidus thoracis et lumborum acts primarily to stabilize the vertebral column. The iliocostalis thoracis and longissimus thoracis et lumborum are members of the group of muscles that extends the vertebral column. The sacrocaudalis muscles give mobility to the tail. The interspinales prevent excessive separation of the spinous processes.

29. The answer is 3 [Chapter 20 II C 2 a (3) (b)]. The caudal regions of the iliocostalis and longissimus systems fuse together to form a large muscle mass that covers the dorsal lumbar region. "Erector spinae" is a term used to describe the longissimus thoracis et lumborum together with the iliocostalis lumborum. The large mass of these combined muscles forms a powerful extensor of the vertebral column.

30. The answer is 4 [Table 20–6]. The intertransversarius dorsalis caudalis muscles, along with the intertransversarius ventralis caudalis muscles, are responsible for lateral flexion of the tail. The dorsal sacrocaudal muscles elevate the tail and the ventral sacrocaudal muscles lower it. There is no "sacrocaudalis lateralis" muscle.

31. The answer is 2 [Chapter 21 I A 1 b (2)]. The cranial thyroid artery is the only constant cervical branch of the common carotid artery. There is no such thing as a "medial thyroid artery." The ascending pharyngeal artery typically is a branch of the external carotid artery. The vertebral artery normally arises from the subclavian artery.

32. The answer is 3 [Chapter 21 I A 2 a]. The vertebral artery leaves the subclavian artery and ascends cranially, passing through the transverse canal of the vertebral column. The vertebral artery enters the transverse foramen of the atlas, passes ventral to the atlantal wing, and then emerges dorsally via the alar notch in the cranial edge of the wing. The artery then turns medially to enter the vertebral canal via the lateral vertebral foramen of the atlas and turns cranially, dividing into branches. Vertebra C7 has no transverse foramen.

33. The answer is 1 [Chapter 21 I II A 1 b; Figure 21–1]. The segmented dorsal intercostal arteries arise from the parent artery (either the thoracic vertebral artery or the thoracic aorta) and pass dorsally around the body of the corresponding vertebra. They then give off a nutrient artery (which supplies the vertebral body), a spinal branch (which contributes to the arterial supply of the spinal cord), and a dorsal branch (which supplies the adjacent epaxial musculature and the regional skin). After branching, the dorsal intercostal arteries continue laterally to supply the body wall (the thorax, in this case).

34. The answer is 3 [Chapter 21 III A 1 a, 2 a]. The three large, constant arteries of the tail, which extend the entire length of the tail, are the paired lateral caudal arteries and the median caudal artery. The lateral caudal arteries arise from the cranial gluteal artery, and the median caudal artery is the direct continuation of the median sacral artery. Several smaller (and often inconstant) arteries are present on the tail as well. No arteriovenous sinuses are formed.

35. The answer is 1 [Chapter 22 III A 1; IV A 1 a]. The medial divisions of the dorsal branches of the thoracic and lumbar spinal nerves are motor to the regional epaxial muscles (i.e., the rotatores, interspinalis thoracis, multifidus thoracis, longissimus thoracis, spinalis et semispinalis thoracis et cervicis, multifidus lumborum, interspinales lumborum, and longissimus lumborum). Hypaxial muscles are innervated by ventral branches of the spinal nerves. The lateral branch of the dorsal branch does have a large sensory component, but to the dorsal, rather than the ventral, body region.

36. The answer is 1 [Chapter 22 II A 3]. The cervical spinal nerves typically divide into dorsal and ventral branches on exiting the intervertebral foramen. The dorsal branch is sensory and motor: the medial branch of the dorsal branch is sensory and the lateral branch of the dorsal branch is motor. Having a sensory medial division of the dorsal branch is characteristic only of the cervical spinal nerves; that branch in the remaining spinal nerves is motor only.

37. The answer is 3 [Chapter 22 VI]. Cutaneous branches may be associated with the first seven to nine ventral branches of the ventral caudal trunk. Only five pairs of caudal nerves are present, corresponding to the five caudal segments of the spinal cord. Both the dorsal and ventral branches of caudal nerves form nerve trunks. The dorsal caudal nerve trunk lies dorsal to the transverse processes of the caudal vertebrae, and the ventral trunk lies ventral to the transverse processes of the caudal vertebrae.

38. The answer is 1 [Chapter 24 I A]. The atlantal wings are readily palpated and may actually be visible in dogs with short, smooth coats. The atlas lacks a spinous process. The lateral vertebral foramen of the axis, the dens of the axis, and the transverse processes of vertebra C3 are too deep to be palpated.

39. The answer is 2 [Chapter 20 II B 3 a (2)]. The tail musculature may be conceptualized as consisting of two major paired groups, one dorsal and one ventral, each largely an inverse image of the other. The dorsal and ventral groups each contain a medial member (which is relatively short), a lateral member (which is relatively long), and an intertransverse member (which extends between the transverse processes). The dorsal group of tail muscles raises the tail and the ventral group of tail muscles lowers the tail. Dorsal and ventral arterial plexuses supply the tail musculature.

40. The answer is 4 [Chapter 20 II A 2 b (1) (c)]. The iliocostalis system extends from the ilium to C7; therefore, it is not involved in movement of the head. The longissimus and transversospinalis systems both attach to the head. The transversospinalis system is the epaxial muscle system deepest and closest to the midline.

41. The answer is 1 [Chapter 17 II]. The innervation, bony form, and musculature of the neck and back retain their relation to the original segmentation of the embryo, but the vasculature is more malleable and changes with development, losing the original segmental relation.

42. The answer is 5 [Chapter 19 IV A 1 a (2)]. The caudal artery takes part only in supplying the tail. The vertebral, intercostal, lumbar, and sacral arteries directly feed into the main channel flow on the ventral surface of the spinal cord, according to region.

43. The answer is 4 [Chapter 21 I A 2 b]. The cervical skin and parts of the cervical viscera are supplied only after the vertebral artery has divided into its dorsal and ventral branches. The vertebral artery supplies the longus colli muscle (a hypaxial muscle) and the longissimus capitus (an epaxial muscle), as well as the spinal cord.

44. The answer is 2 [Chapter 20 I B 1 a]. The external jugular vein forms at the confluence of the maxillary and lingual veins, not at the confluence of the superficial temporal and maxillary veins. It is superficial in position throughout most of the cervical length. It receives the omobrachial and cephalic veins before terminating in the thorax, where it becomes confluent with the brachiocephalic vein.

45. The answer is 3 [Chapter 22 III B; IV B]. The ventral branches of the thoracic and lumbar spinal nerves are not important when considering the innervation of the intrinsic back muscles—they play a more important role in the innervation of the extrinsic back muscles. Both the pelvic and thoracic limbs receive innervation from ventral branches of the lumbar and thoracic nerves, respectively. The dorsal branches of the thoracic and lumbar spinal nerves innervate the epaxial muscles, which are intrinsic back muscles.

46. The answer is 2 [Chapter 23 III A]. The esophagus attains a position to the left, not the right, of the midline and trachea throughout most of the neck. The carotid sheath is located in the angle between the longus colli muscle and the trachea; therefore, it does pass along the tracheal surface. The incomplete tracheal rings are closed dorsally by the trachealis muscle. The longus colli and longus capitus muscles form the deep wall of the visceral compartment of the neck; therefore, the cervical viscera lie in contact with these muscles dorsally.

47. The answer is 3 [Chapter 24 II B]. The thyroid glands are normally not palpable unless they are enlarged. The trachea, larynx, and epaxial muscle mass in the lumbar region are normally palpable.

PART IV

THORACIC LIMB

Chapter 25

Introduction to the Thoracic Limb

I. ATTACHMENTS. Dogs and other domestic mammals differ significantly from primates as well as climbing quadrupeds (e.g., rats) because the attachment of the limb to the body is entirely muscular.

A. The **serratus ventralis** provides the major attachment of the thoracic limb to the body.

B. Numerous **other muscles** extending between the limb and the trunk also contribute to this attachment, but their major role is movement of the limb or associated structures, rather than the provision of a substantive connection between the limb and the body. These muscles include the **rhomboideus, trapezius, omotransversarius,** and **latissimus dorsi** muscles.

II. REGIONS. The thoracic limb can be thought of as having five regions (Figure 25–1).

A. The **scapular region** occupies the lateral surface of the trunk, roughly at the junction of the neck and thorax.

1. **Bones.** The bone of the scapular region is the **scapula.**
2. **Muscles.** The scapula (except for its spine) is clothed in thick muscular layers along its full extent, both medially and laterally.

B. The **brachium (arm)** is the region of the thoracic limb extending between the shoulder and the elbow.

1. **Bones.** The bone of the brachium is the **humerus.**
2. **Muscles.** Most of the humerus is thickly clothed in muscle along its full length.

C. The **antebrachium (forearm)** is the region of the thoracic limb extending between the elbow and the carpus (wrist).

1. **Bones.** The antebrachium contains two bones, the **radius** and the **ulna**. The radius, the weight-bearing bone of the antebrachium, is stouter than the ulna.
2. **Muscles.** The antebrachial region is variably ensheathed in muscle:
   a. Proximally, the muscle bellies are large, and the muscular layers are thick around all surfaces of the antebrachium.
   b. Distally, the muscular "coat" tapers to mainly tendons, making the bones more prominent; indeed, much of the distal radial shaft as well as the caudal border of the ulna are subcutaneous.

D. The **carpus (wrist)** is the region of the thoracic limb extending between the antebrachium (forearm) and the manus (forepaw).

1. **Bones**
   a. **Large bones.** There are seven large bones of the carpus, arranged in two rows, one proximal and one distal.
      (1) **Proximal row.** From medial to lateral, the bones of the proximal row are the **intermedioradial (radial), ulnar,** and **accessory carpal bones.**
      (2) **Distal row.** From medial to lateral, the bones of the distal row are numbered **I–IV.**
   b. The **sesamoid bone of the abductor pollicis longus muscle** is a tiny bone located in the tendon of insertion of this muscle. Although tiny, this bone is consistently present and visible on many radiographs.

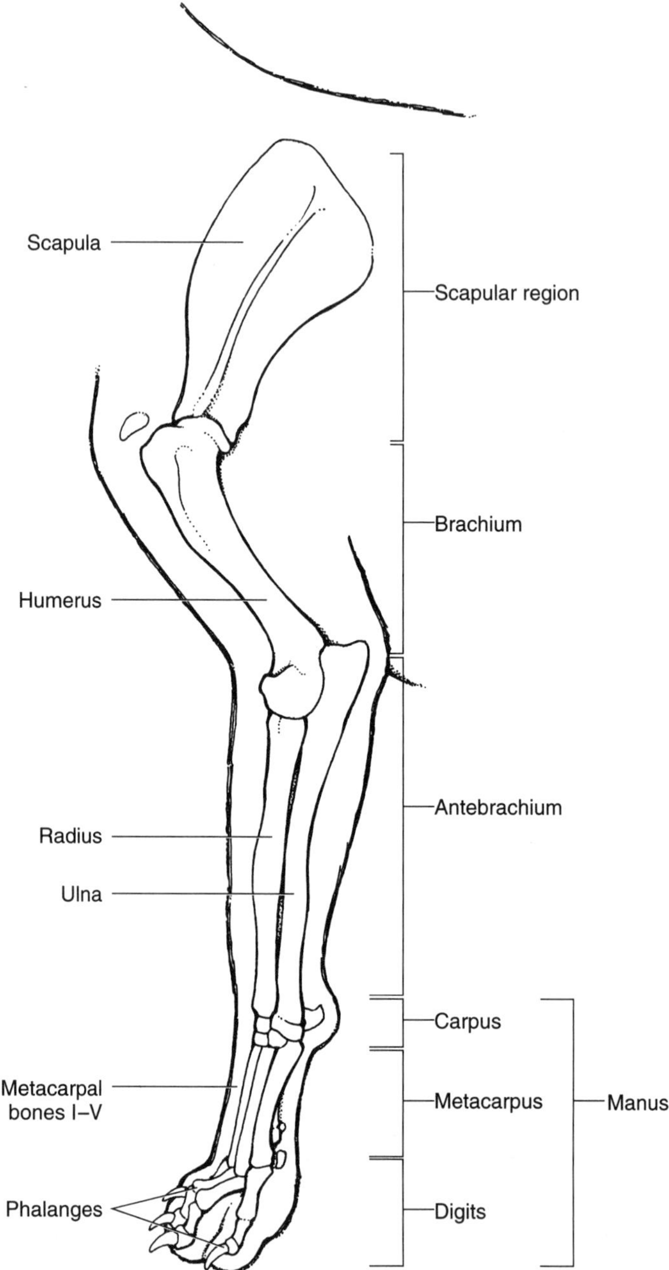

Figure 25–1. Regions of the thoracic limb.

2. **Joints.** The numerous **intercarpal joints** are designated according to the bones between which they extend (e.g., the intermedioradial-ulnar joint). Motion at the intercarpal joints is restricted to a small degree of sliding between the various carpal elements.

E. The **manus (forepaw)** is the region of the thoracic limb extending between the carpus and the ground.

1. **Bones.** There are 19 bones in the manus.
   a. Five **metacarpal bones** are present in the region corresponding to the palm of the human hand (i.e., between the wrist and the digits). These bones are designated **I–V,** from medial to lateral.
   b. **Phalanges** are the small bones that compose the five **digits,** which, like the metacarpal bones, are designated I–V from medial to lateral.
      (1) Digit I consists of two phalanges.
      (2) Digits II through IV are each composed of three phalanges.

Canine Clinical Correlation

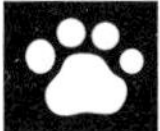

The first digit (digit I) is often referred to as the "dewclaw," and is treated variably. In many instances, this digit is removed shortly after birth for cosmetic reasons or to prevent trauma to the digit, which is non–weight-bearing. In some breeds, the digit must be present for the individual to be entered into the breed registry.

2. **Joints.** The joints of the manus are usually referred to colloquially as the "knuckles." Two bones contribute to the formation of each joint. The joints are saddle joints, a modification of a ginglymus (hinge) type.
   a. The **metacarpophalangeal joints** are present at the articulation of the metacarpal and proximal phalangeal bones.
   b. The **interphalangeal joints** connect the bones of the digits.
      (1) **Digit I.** The interphalangeal joint is located between the proximal and distal phalanges.
      (2) **Digits II–V**
         (a) The **proximal interphalangeal joints** are present between the proximal and middle phalanges of digits II–V.
         (b) The **distal interphalangeal joints** are present between the middle and distal phalanges of digits II–V.

III. JOINTS.

The joints of the thoracic limb are named anatomically for the regions of the limb contributing to the joint from proximal to distal (thus, "antebrachiocarpal," rather than "carpoantebrachial").

A. The **glenohumeral (shoulder) joint** is the region where the thoracic limb joins the trunk. The shoulder joint is formed by the articulation of the **scapula** and the **humerus.**

B. The **brachioantebrachial (elbow, cubital) joint** is the articulation between the brachium and the antebrachium. The **humerus, radius,** and **ulna** contribute to the formation of the elbow joint.

C. The **antebrachiocarpal joint** is the articulation between the antebrachium and the carpus. This entire area, which is composed of several subjoints, is colloquially referred to as the **wrist**. Five bones contribute to the antebrachiocarpal joint—the **radius, ulna,** and the **proximal row of carpal bones** (i.e., the intermedioradial, ulnar, and accessory carpal bones).

D. The **carpometacarpal joint** is the joint between the carpus and the manus. Ten bones form this joint: the four members of the **distal row of carpal bones,** the five **metacarpal bones,** and the **ulnar carpal bone.**

Chapter 26

Bones of the Thoracic Limb

I. PECTORAL GIRDLE. The pectoral girdle, consisting of the clavicle and the scapula, is classically described as the set of bones attaching the thoracic limb to the trunk. In domestic quadrupeds (including dogs), this definition must be modified slightly, because the clavicle does not articulate with the axial skeleton.

A. Clavicle. In dogs (and many other quadrupeds), the clavicle is reduced to the **clavicular remnant,** a small bit of bone or a tendinous thickening in the substance of the brachiocephalicus (an extrinsic muscle of the limb). When ossified (as it is in many dogs), the clavicular remnant is usually positioned at the **clavicular intersection,** within the substance of the cleidobrachialis muscle cranial to the shoulder joint. The major importance of the clavicle in canine medicine is awareness of its presence, lest its inconstant appearance on radiographs be misinterpreted as a bone fragment.

B. Scapula. The scapula is a large, flat bone positioned against the lateral surface of the trunk at the junction of the neck and the ribs.

1. The **medial (costal) surface** of the scapula is quite flat.
   a. The **dorsal border** of the medial scapular surface provides attachment for the **rhomboideus muscles.**
   b. The **facies serrata,** a roughened region representing approximately the dorsal third of the craniomedial scapular surface, provides attachment for the **serratus ventralis muscle.**
   c. The greatest part of the medial scapular surface bears the **subscapular fossa,** a slightly scooped region that is the attachment site for the **subscapularis muscle.**
2. The **lateral surface** is marked by the prominent **scapular spine,** a tall ridge of bone that extends essentially the full length of the bone and divides it into nearly equal regions, the **supraspinous fossa** and the **infraspinous fossa.** The **acromion** is a knob-like thickening on the distal end of the spine where part of the deltoideus muscle attaches.
3. The **ventral angle** of the scapula is the expanded ventral portion of the scapula, where the bone is specialized for articulation with the humerus.
   a. The **neck** of the scapula is a slightly constricted area where the major part of the bone meets the ventral angle.
   b. The **scapular notch** is a marked inward curve at the cranial side of the scapular neck, around which the suprascapular nerve passes from medial to lateral.
   c. The **glenoid cavity** is a shallow depression that receives the head of the humerus. The glenoid cavity is so shallow that most of the stability of the shoulder joint is afforded by the heavy musculature surrounding it on all sides, rather than by its bony form.
   d. The **supraglenoid tubercle** is a thickened elevation on the cranial surface of the ventral angle, just over the glenoid cavity, where the biceps brachii muscle originates. The **coracoid process,** a tiny elevation that projects medially from the supraglenoid tubercle, is specialized for attachment of the diminutive coracobrachialis muscle.
   e. The **infraglenoid tubercle** is an elevation on the caudal scapular border positioned just proximal to the glenoid cavity, where the teres minor and part of the triceps brachii muscles originate.

II. BRACHIUM. The **humerus** is the bone of the brachium.

A. Proximal humerus

1. The **head** is the almost hemispherical portion that faces caudally and articulates with the glenoid cavity of the scapula.
2. The **greater tubercle,** an elaboration on the lateral side of the proximal humerus, is specialized for attachment of the lateral scapular musculature.
3. The **lesser tubercle,** a smaller elaboration on the medial side of the proximal humerus, is specialized for attachment of the medial scapular musculature.
4. The **intertubercular groove** lies between the greater and lesser tubercles and provides passage (but not attachment) for the tendon of origin of the biceps brachii.
5. The **neck** is a relatively indistinct constriction at the junction of the proximal humerus and the shaft of the humerus.

B. Humeral shaft. Prominent features are found mainly on the lateral surface.

1. The **deltoid tuberosity** is a large elevation on the lateral humeral surface located roughly halfway down the humeral shaft. The deltoideus muscle inserts here.
2. The **tricipital line** extends along the lateral humeral surface between the humeral head and the deltoid tuberosity and is the site of attachment for the triceps brachii muscle.
3. The **brachialis (musculospiral) groove** is a smooth, spiraling path (rather than a distinct groove) that extends from the caudolateral to the craniolateral surface of the humeral shaft. The brachialis muscle passes along this path.
4. The **teres major tuberosity** is a small elevation positioned a short distance distal to the lesser tubercle on the medial side of the humeral shaft. The teres major and latissimus dorsi muscles insert here.
5. The **medial epicondyle** is an enlarged region on the distomedial humerus just proximal to the trochlea (see II C 1). Flexors of the carpus and digits originate here.
6. The **lateral epicondyle** is an enlargement situated in a similar position on the lateral side of the condyle, just proximal to the capitulum (see II C 1). This is the region of origin of the extensors of the carpus and digits.

C. Distal humerus (humeral condyle)

1. The **trochlea** (medially) and **capitulum** (laterally) are regions that articulate with the radius and ulna jointly, and the radius alone, respectively.
2. The **olecranon fossa** is a deep hollow on the caudal aspect of the humeral condyle that receives the anconeal process of the ulna when the elbow is fully extended.
3. The **radial fossa** is a small excavation located on the cranial aspect of the condyle that receives the radial head on full elbow flexion.
4. The **supratrochlear foramen** is a hole in the thinned bone of the central region of the distal condyle that connects the olecranon and radial fossae. Nothing passes through this foramen.

III. ANTEBRACHIUM. The **radius** and **ulna** are the bones of the antebrachium. In the normal standing position, the radius and ulna cross each other obliquely in the midantebrachial region. The radius is considerably shorter than the ulna; in the articulated state, the radius does not meet either the proximal or distal extremity of the ulna.

A. Radius

1. **General form and position**
   a. The radius is noticeably flattened craniocaudally, so that its width is broader than its depth throughout its length.
   b. The proximal radius is positioned laterally at the elbow. The radial body inclines medially as it passes distally and obliquely crosses the ulna, so that it is positioned along

the craniomedial antebrachial region. The distal radius is positioned medially at the carpus.

2. **Notable features**
   a. The **proximal radius** is composed of the head and neck.
      (1) The **head** is the irregularly oval, proximal-most region that faces directly dorsally and articulates with the humerus and ulna at the elbow.
         (a) The **fovea capitis** is the depression on the cranial extremity of the bone that articulates with the humerus and provides its weight-bearing surface.
         (b) The **articular circumference** is a flattened, smooth, ring-like area just distal to the fovea capitis that encircles the greater part of the radial head. It is incomplete laterally. This region articulates with the ulna and allows limited rotation at the elbow.
      (2) The **neck** is a slight constriction at the junction of the head and body.
   b. The **radial body** continues smoothly from the neck, and presents:
      (1) The **radial tuberosity,** a small, variably developed elevation on the medial radial border just distal to the neck that is the lesser insertion site for the biceps brachii
      (2) A **roughened caudal surface,** a site for ligamentous attachment to the ulna
   c. The **distal radius** is broader and wider than the other parts of the bone, and is sometimes referred to as the trochlea. Features of note on the distal radius include the:
      (1) **Articular surface,** which is concave, faces directly ventrally, and articulates with the carpal bones
      (2) **Ulnar notch,** a small and indistinct facet for articulation with the ulna
      (3) **Medial styloid process,** a sharp, beak-like projection on the medial end of the distal extremity that extends distal to the ventral border of the remainder of the bone

B. Ulna. The ulna, the longest bone of the body, bears no weight. Nonetheless, the ulna is essential to normal function of the limb in that its articulation with the humerus provides all of the hinge action at the elbow, and its body provides essential surface area for muscular attachment.

1. **General form and position**
   a. The ulna has an irregular form—it is noticeably elaborate proximally, and greatly simplified distally. Distal to the marked specializations for articulation with the humerus, the ulna narrows to an unspecialized shaft of bone that gently tapers to a nondescript termination at the carpus.
   b. The proximal ulna is positioned medially in the region of the elbow. The ulnar body is positioned along the caudal antebrachial region, and it inclines laterally so that it obliquely crosses the radius and its distal end is positioned laterally at the carpus.

2. **Notable features**
   a. **Proximal ulna (olecranon)**
      (1) The **olecranon tuber ("point of the elbow")** is the most proximal extent of the bone. This stout, elongate, rounded projection proximal to the elbow joint is the insertion site for the elbow extensors.
      (2) The **trochlear notch** is a deep, half-moon–shaped concavity that faces cranially and articulates with the trochlea of the humerus. This articulation allows the hinge action of the elbow joint.
         (a) The **anconeal process** is a sharp, beak-like process on the proximal end of the trochlear notch that, in full extension, is seated within the olecranon fossa of the humerus.
         (b) The **medial** and **lateral coronoid processes** are pointed extensions at respective sides of the distal end of the trochlear notch.
            (i) The medial coronoid process is considerably larger than the lateral one.
            (ii) The two coronoid processes are positioned on each side of a concavity referred to as the **radial notch.** These two processes together with the radial notch form a rounded "scoop" that receives and cradles the articular circumference of the radius.

Canine Clinical Correlation

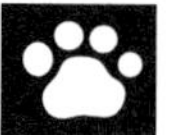

The anconeal process develops from a separate ossification center than the rest of the ulna. In many large breeds, faulty fusion of this process with the olecranon occurs. The resulting **un-united anconeal process** causes a painful lameness. If left untreated, the condition causes severe and debilitating degeneration of the elbow joint. Treatment consists of surgical removal of the bone fragment.

b. **Ulnar body.** The ulnar body tapers as it continues distally from the neck. In lateral or medial view, the ulnar body is distinctly bowed cranially.
   (1) The **ulnar tuberosity** is a small elevation on the medial surface of the proximal ulnar body, just distal to the medial coronoid process. The biceps brachii and brachialis have their major insertions here.
   (2) The **interosseous border** of the ulna is the border extending distally from the area of the radial notch, where a tight ligamentous attachment to the radius is formed.

c. **Distal ulna.** Two features are described on the distal extremity of the ulna.
   (1) The **articular circumference** is a small, smooth spot that articulates with the ulnar notch of the radius.
   (2) The **lateral styloid process** is a prominent, pointed projection on the distal ulnar extremity. (In human anatomy, the styloid process is the "bump" visible on the lateral edge of the proximal wrist when the hand is placed in a palm-down position.)

C. **Interosseous space.** The interosseus space is a roughly rectangular space that separates the radius and ulna through the greatest part of their length.

1. The **antebrachial interosseous membrane** is a thin, membranous sheet extending across the antebrachial interosseous space through most of the length of the forearm.
2. The **antebrachial interosseous ligament** is a short, heavy ligament extending between the radius and ulna, beginning about a third of the way distally down the radius, and ending just proximal to the midpoint of the bone. The interosseous ligament of the antebrachium can be viewed as a thickened region of the interosseous membrane, which extends both proximal and distal to it.
3. The **antebrachial interosseous muscle** also bridges the interosseous space, assisting in retaining the normal positions of the antebrachial bones.

IV. MANUS.

The bones of the forepaw include the bones of the carpus, metacarpus, and digits, as well as several sesamoid bones (Figure 26–1).

A. Carpus

1. **Proximal row**
   a. The **intermedioradial (radial) carpal bone,** the largest of the carpal bones, forms from the fetal fusion of the radial, intermediate, and central carpal bones. The radial carpal bone is positioned most medially in the proximal row and articulates with nearly the entire distal surface of the radius proximally, and with the full distal row of carpal bones (I–IV) distally.
   b. The **ulnar carpal bone** is positioned on the lateral side of the carpus, where it articulates with the ulna and radius proximally, and with carpal bone IV and metacarpal bone V distally.
   c. The **accessory carpal bone** is positioned laterally on the carpus and projects distinctly palmarly ("caudally") from the plane of the other carpal bones. The accessory carpal bone articulates with the lateral styloid process proximally and the ulnar carpal bone distally.

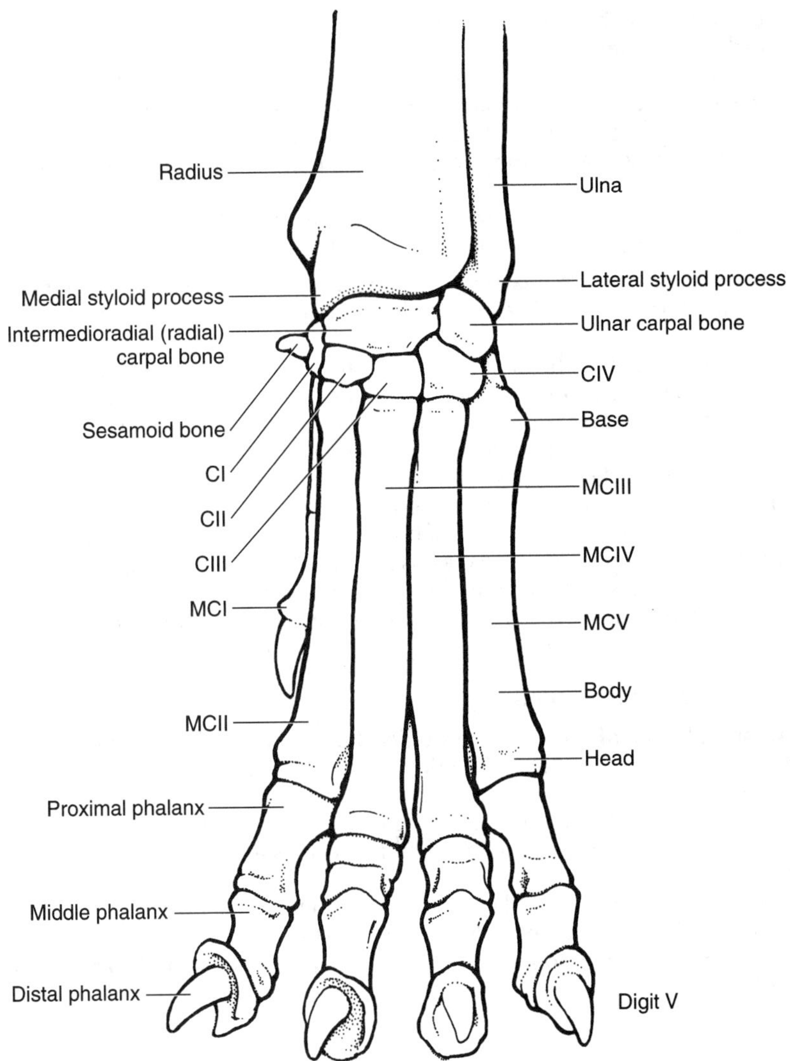

Figure 26–1. Bones of the left distal antebrachium and manus, dorsal view. *CI, CII, CIII, CIV*—carpal bones I–IV; *MCI, MCII, MCIII, MCIV, MCV*—metacarpal bones I–V.

2. **Distal row.** Each of the four carpal bones in the distal row has several distinguishing features that permit positive and fairly ready identification of each individual bone. However, these features are generally of academic interest, and will not be discussed here.
   a. The bones of the distal row increase in size from medial to lateral, so that carpal bone I is the smallest and carpal bone IV is the largest.
   b. Carpal bones I–IV articulate proximally with the radial and ulnar carpal bones, distally with the metacarpal bones, and medially or laterally with each other.

B. Metacarpus. The metacarpal bones (designated I–V) are small, elongate, rod-shaped bones that have specializations at each end for articulation with neighboring bones. Metacarpal bone I differs from metacarpal bones II–V in that it is shorter and non–weight-bearing.

1. The **base** is the **proximal end,** which articulates proximally with the distal row of carpal bones and distally with the corresponding digit.

2. The **body (shaft)** of the bone is relatively long.
3. The **head** is the **distal end.**
4. **Interosseous space.** The **interosseous spaces** of the metacarpal bones are developed distal to the **interosseous metacarpal ligament,** which connects the proximal-most portions of the metacarpal bones. The interosseous spaces permit the bones to splay slightly to afford space for muscle attachment, as well as to better support the weight of the dog.

C. Digits. The digits ("toes"), designated I–V, are composed of the **phalanges.** The phalanges progressively shorten in length from proximal to distal.

1. The **proximal** and **middle phalanges** have a **base** (proximally), **body,** and **head** (distally), like the metacarpal bones. The proximal phalanges are about one third longer than the middle ones.
2. The **distal phalanges** are highly modified in shape. Many of these features are important in terms of radiographic examination and some surgical techniques.
   a. The **extensor process** is a rounded proximal projection on the dorsal surface where the tendon of the common digital extensor inserts.
   b. The **flexor tubercle** is a small elevation on the proximal palmar surface where the tendon of the deep digital flexor inserts.
   c. The **unguicular crest** is a "shelf" of bone that completely surrounds the proximal portion of the distal phalanx. The crest is separated from the phalanx by a space. The bed of the claw is embedded in this space under the bony shelf.
   d. The **unguicular process** is the claw-shaped distal extremity of the distal phalanx. In the intact state, this process is closely covered by the claw itself.

D. Sesamoid elements of the manus

1. The **sesamoid bone of the abductor pollicis longus muscle** is positioned medially, against the distal edge of the intermedioradial carpal bone or proximal end of the first metacarpal bone.
2. The four (unpaired) **dorsal sesamoid bones** are positioned dorsal to **metacarpophalangeal joints II–V** and are contained within the substance of the common digital extensor tendons.
3. The four **dorsal sesamoid cartilages** are similar to the dorsal sesamoid bones, but they are positioned at the **distal interphalangeal joints.**
4. Two **proximal sesamoid bones** are positioned palmar to each **metacarpophalangeal joint (II–V)** and are contained within the substance of the tendons of the interosseous muscles.

Chapter 27

Joints and Ligaments of the Thoracic Limb

I. GLENOHUMERAL (SHOULDER) JOINT

A. Motion. The shoulder joint is a **ball-and-socket joint,** which allows movement in essentially every direction. In quadrupeds, however, most of the motion takes place in a direct cranial-to-caudal plane, resulting in mainly extension and flexion of the joint.

B. Structure

1. **Bones** contributing to formation of the shoulder joint are proximally, the **scapula** (by the **glenoid cavity)** and distally, the **humerus** (by its **head).**
2. **Joint capsule.** The shoulder joint capsule consists of a single cavity that extends between the scapula and humerus. A subdivision of the joint capsule surrounds the tendon of origin of the biceps brachii muscle, and travels with it through the intertubercular groove as the tendon's synovial sheath.
3. **Ligaments**
   a. The **medial** and **lateral glenohumeral ligaments** are thickenings of the respective surfaces of the joint capsule. These ligaments are weak; it is the strength of the heavy musculature surrounding the joint that maintains the joint integrity.

Canine Clinical Correlation

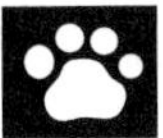

Because of the thickness of the musculature surrounding the shoulder joint and the relatively limited range of motion of quadrupeds, subluxations and luxations of the shoulder are extremely rare in veterinary medicine.

   b. The **transverse humeral ligament** is a thick band of ligamentous tissue that bridges the intertubercular groove (located between the greater and lesser tubercles). The tendon of the biceps brachii and its synovial sheath are retained in the intertubercular groove by this ligament.

II. BRACHIOANTEBRACHIAL (ELBOW, CUBITAL) JOINT

A. Motion. The elbow joint is a **ginglymus (hinge) joint.** Typical of ginglymus joints, the main motion is flexion–extension, together with a small gliding component. A small amount of rotation is also possible (e.g., allowing the dog to supinate the paw to remove a burr from between the pads).

B. Structure

1. **Bones.** The elbow is a complex joint formed by contributions from the humerus, the radius, and the ulna. Three separate subjoints are thus identified, each of which plays an essential role in the normal function of the joint.
   a. The **humeroulnar joint** is formed proximally by the **humeral trochlea** and distally by the **trochlear notch of the ulna.** This articulation affords the main **flexion–extension** motion of the elbow.
   b. The **humeroradial joint** is formed proximally by the **humeral capitulum** and distally

by the **radial head.** This articulation provides the major **weight-bearing** function of the elbow.

c. The **proximal radioulnar joint** is formed by the **articular circumference of the radius** and the **radial notch of the ulna.** This articulation contributes to the **rotary** motion of the elbow.

2. **Joint capsule.** A **single cavity** comprises the elbow joint capsule, serving all three subjoints.
3. **Ligaments**
   a. The **medial** and **lateral collateral ligaments** are stout thickenings of the joint capsule formed on the respective sides of the joint. Each of these two ligamentous bands steadies the joint against excessive transverse motion toward the opposite side of the limb.
      (1) The medial collateral ligament attaches proximally (to the medial humeral epicondyle) and divides distally into two branches to afford separate attachment to both the radius and ulna.
      (2) The lateral collateral ligament attaches proximally (to the lateral humeral epicondyle) and divides distally into two branches to attach to each antebrachial bone.
   b. The **annular ligament of the radius** is a thin ligamentous band that passes transversely around the articular circumference of the radius (deep to the collateral ligaments), essentially surrounding the bone and maintaining its position against the ulna when the radius rotates.
   c. The **oblique ligament** is a relatively minor ligament on the cranial (flexor) surface of the joint. This ligament begins on the lateral side of the humerus dorsal to the supratrochlear foramen, crosses obliquely, and terminates on the medial side of the radius. Hypothetically, this ligament assists in prevention of hyperextension.
   d. The **olecranon ligament** is a short band that extends between the lateral side of the olecranon and the medial side of the lateral humeral condyle. This ligament assists in retaining the proximity of the olecranon and the humerus.

III. RADIOULNAR JOINTS. The radius and ulna articulate directly in two regions.

A. Motion. The radioulnar joints contribute to the limited degree of rotation characteristic of the thoracic limb in dogs.

B. Structure

1. The **proximal radioulnar joint** is considered with the elbow (see II B 1 c).
2. The **distal radioulnar joint** is formed by the **articular circumference of the ulna** and the **ulnar notch of the radius.**

IV. CARPAL JOINTS

A. Overview. The three main joints of the carpus are the:

1. **Antebrachiocarpal joint,** between the radius and ulna proximally and the proximal row of carpal bones distally
2. **Middle carpal joint,** between the proximal and distal row of carpal bones
3. **Carpometacarpal joints,** between the distal row of carpal bones and the metacarpal bones

B. Motion. The many individual joints of the carpus act together as a **ginglymus** joint, thus permitting mainly extension–flexion, and a limited amount of gliding (i.e., lateral) movement.

1. The antebrachiocarpal and middle carpal joints are the most mobile in the carpus. These joints "open" widely when the joint is fully flexed.

Canine Clinical Correlation

The wide separation of the proximal two carpal subjoints renders these joints readily accessible to needle puncture.

2. Very limited movement occurs at the carpometacarpal and intercarpal joints (i.e., the joints formed between individual carpal bones).

C. Structure

1. **Bones.** The bones that form the carpal joints are enumerated in IV A.
2. **Joint capsule.** The joint capsule extends like a sheath across the entire carpal area, but it has **cavities** (consisting of three separate compartments).
   a. The **antebrachiocarpal compartment** does not communicate with the compartment of the two distal joints.
   b. The **middle carpal** and **carpometacarpal compartments** communicate with each other, but not with the antebrachiocarpal compartment.

Canine Clinical Correlation

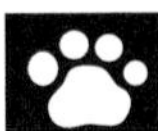

Knowledge of the compartments of the carpal joint capsule becomes important when obtaining diagnostic fluid from a portion of the joint is necessary. For example, analysis of fluid obtained from the antebrachiocarpal compartment will not provide information on the status of the more distal subjoints. Communications between the compartments can also be used to the veterinarian's advantage: although the carpometacarpal joint does not open significantly when the joint is strongly flexed, the middle carpal joint does, and thus is readily accessible to needle puncture; because these two joint cavities communicate, information can be obtained on the status of the difficult-to-access carpometacarpal joint simply by obtaining fluid from the easy-to-access middle carpal joint.

3. **Ligaments**
   a. The **extensor retinaculum,** a significant thickening over the midregion of the joint capsule's dorsal surface, serves to bind down the tendons of the extensor muscles of the carpus and digits and to maintain the integrity of the joint.
   b. The **flexor retinaculum** is a restricted thickening of the carpal fascia on the palmar surface of the joint. Laterally, the flexor retinaculum attaches to the **accessory carpal bone.** Medially, it attaches to the **styloid process of the ulna** and to the **medial-most carpal bones of both rows** (i.e., the radial carpal bone and carpal bone I).
   c. The **palmar carpal fibrocartilage** ("ligament") is an extremely thick layer of fibrocartilaginous tissue applied intimately to the palmar surface of the carpal bones. This fibrocartilage has several important functions:
      (1) Preventing collapse of the carpus when the limb is weight-bearing
      (2) Smoothing the irregular palmar surface of the carpal bones into an even surface for passage of the digital flexor tendons through the carpal canal
      (3) Providing the origin site for most of the small digital muscles
   d. The **special ligaments of the carpus** are tiny individually named ligaments that extend between the individual carpal bones.

V. METACARPAL JOINTS

A. Intermetacarpal joints. The intermetacarpal joints lie between adjacent metacarpal bones at their proximal ends. Motion is limited.

B. Metacarpophalangeal joints

1. **Motion.** The metacarpophalangeal joints are **ginglymus joints;** thus, motion at these joints is mainly extension–flexion.
2. **Structure**
   a. **Bones**
      (1) The metacarpophalangeal joints are formed proximally by the **head** (i.e., distal end) **of the metacarpal bones** and distally by the **base** (i.e., proximal end) **of the proximal phalanges.**
      (2) The tiny **dorsal sesamoid bones** are present on the dorsal surface of the joint.
      (3) The large, paired **proximal sesamoid bones** lie on the palmar surface of metacarpophalangeal joints II–V (i.e., the weight-bearing digits).
   b. **Joint capsule.** Each metacarpophalangeal joint has its own, separate synovial joint capsule.
   c. **Ligaments**
      (1) **Medial** and **lateral collateral ligaments** are present at each metacarpophalangeal joint, as with most ginglymus joints.
      (2) **Sesamoidean ligaments** are present at the joint, both dorsally and palmarly.

VI. INTERPHALANGEAL JOINTS.

The proximal and distal interphalangeal joints are similar to each other in terms of articulations and support, and are discussed together here. (Keep in mind, however, that for digit I, there is only a single interphalangeal joint, because this digit is comprised of two, rather than three, phalanges.)

A. Motion.

The joints are **saddle joints** (modified ginglymus joints), allowing mainly flexion–extension.

B. Structure

1. **Bones.** The interphalangeal joints are formed by the articulation of the **head** (distal end) **of the more proximal phalanx** and the **base** (proximal end) of the **more distal phalanx.**
2. **Joint capsule.** The interphalangeal joints have individual joint capsules.
3. **Ligaments**
   a. The interphalangeal joints are supported by **medial** and **lateral collateral ligaments.**
   b. In addition, the **distal interphalangeal joints** have **dorsal ligaments,** paired elastic ligaments that pass over the dorsal surface of the joint and serve to hold the claw in passive semiretraction.

Chapter 28

Muscles of the Thoracic Limb

I. EXTRINSIC MUSCLES (Table 28–1, Figure 28–1) have one attachment on the limb and the other attachment on another portion of the body. **Limb attachment sites** include either the scapula or humerus, and **non-limb attachment sites** include the sternum, scapula, head, neck, and back. All extrinsic muscles are paired.

A. The **superficial pectoral** is a powerful muscle that extends between the sternum and the humerus. It is subcutaneous over most of its extent, and covers the most proximal regions of the deep pectoral muscle. Each superficial pectoral muscle is divided into two portions:

1. The **descending pectoral** is the most superficial, smallest portion.
2. The **transverse pectoral** is the deeper, larger portion.

B. The **deep pectoral (pectoralis profundus, ascending pectoral)** also extends between the sternum and humerus, but is larger and longer than the superficial pectoral muscle, and is thereby extremely powerful. The most cranial region of the deep pectoral is covered by the superficial pectoral, but most of its surface is subcutaneous.

C. The **brachiocephalicus** extends between the brachium and the head. This muscle lies on the cranial surface of the brachium and shoulder, and sweeps proximally along the lateral surface of the neck. It is subcutaneous through essentially all of its course. The brachiocephalicus is a **compound muscle,** consisting of two parts, one of which is subdivided:

1. The **cleidobrachialis** originates at the clavicular intersection, courses distally along the cranial brachial surface, and inserts on the distal, cranial humerus.
2. The **cleidocephalicus** is composed of two parts extending between the clavicular intersection and the head.
   a. **Cervical part (pars cervicalis).** This thinner portion attaches to the dorsal midline (cervical raphe) of the cranial two-thirds of the neck.
   b. **Mastoid part (pars mastoideus).** This thicker portion attaches to the mastoid process of the skull.

D. The **omotransversarius** is an elongate, strap-like muscle that extends between the distal scapular spine and the wing (transverse process) of the atlas. The omotransversarius passes deep to the cleidocephalicus shortly after leaving its origin. The superficial cervical lymph nodes are located deep to the omotransversarius, just cranial to its scapular attachment.

E. The **trapezius** is a thin, flat, triangular sheet of muscle extending between the scapular spine and the dorsal midline. It is divided into two parts, both of which are subcutaneous through most or all of their extent.

1. The **cervical part** is the larger, more cranial portion.
2. The **thoracic part** is the smaller, more caudal portion.

F. The **rhomboideus** is composed of triple parts. All parts of the rhomboideus lie deep to the trapezius muscle and insert mainly on the medial dorsal border of the scapula.

1. The **rhomboideus capitis** is a long, thin, strap-like muscle that **originates** on the **occipital bone.**
2. The **rhomboideus cervicis** is somewhat more substantive than its capital part, but is also strap-like. The rhomboideus cervicis **originates** on the **cervical raphe.**
3. The **rhomboideus thoracis** is a short, thick expanse of muscle of considerable substance. It **originates** on the **spinous processes of vertebrae T4–T7.**

TABLE 28–1. Extrinsic Muscles of the Thoracic Limb

Muscle	Action	Innervation	Course
Superficial pectoral	Holds limb against body wall (fixed); adducts the limb (free)*	Cranial pectoral nerves of the brachial plexus	
Descending pectoral			**Arises** on the cranial-most sternebra **Courses** obliquely caudolaterally over the transverse pectoral **Inserts** on the crest of the greater tubercle of the humerus
Transverse pectoral			**Arises** on the cranial two or three sternebrae **Courses** directly laterally **Inserts** on the crest of the greater tubercle of the humerus
Deep pectoral	Extends the shoulder and pulls the body cranially (fixed); adducts the limb (free)	Caudal pectoral nerves of the brachial plexus	**Arises** along the length of the sternum **Courses** craniolaterally toward the proximal humerus **Inserts** on the lesser tubercle of the humerus and on the greater tubercle of the humerus (by means of a tendinous extension)
Brachiocephalicus	Extends the shoulder and draws the head laterally (fixed); draws the limb cranially (free)	Cranial nerve XI (accessory nerve) and ventral branches of the cervical spinal nerves	**Arises** at clavicular intersection **Courses** distally toward limb or proximally toward head and neck **Inserts:**
Cleidobrachialis			distal-cranial humerus
Cleidocephalicus			
Pars cervicalis			dorsal cervical midline
Pars mastoideus			mastoid process of skull
Omotransversarius	Flexes the neck laterally (fixed); draws the limb cranially (free)	Cranial nerve XI (accessory nerve)	**Arises** from the distal end of the scapular spine just proximal to the acromion **Courses** cranially and dorsally **Inserts** on the wing of the atlas

continued

TABLE 28–1. Extrinsic Muscles of the Thoracic Limb

Muscle	Action	Innervation	Course
Trapezius	Elevates and adducts the limb (fixed or free)	Cranial nerve XI (accessory nerve)	
Cervical part	Draws the limb cranially (free)		**Arises** from the cervical raphe from vertebrae C3–C7 **Courses** caudoventrally **Inserts** on the greatest length of the scapular spine
Thoracic part	Draws the limb caudally (free)		**Arises** from the dorsal midline of the back (from vertebra T1–T9) **Courses** cranioventrally **Inserts** on the greatest length of the scapular spine
Rhomboideus	Adducts the scapula against the body (fixed); elevates the limb (free)	Ventral branches of the cervical and thoracic spinal nerves	
Rhomboideus capitis			**Arises** on the nuchal crest of the occipital bone **Inserts** on the dorsal border of the scapula
Rhomboideus cervicis			**Arises** on the cervical raphe from vertebrae C1–C7 **Inserts** on the dorsal border of the scapula
Rhomboideus thoracis			**Arises** on the spinous processes of vertebrae T4–T7 **Inserts** on the dorsal border of the scapula
Latissimus dorsi	Flexes the shoulder joint (fixed); flexes the shoulder and draws the brachium caudally (free)	Thoracodorsal nerve of the brachial plexus	**Arises** from the thoracolumbar fascia and spinous processes of T6 or T7 and all of the lumbar vertebrae (aponeurotic origin), as well as from ribs 11 or 12 through 13 (muscular origin)

continued

TABLE 28–1. Extrinsic Muscles of the Thoracic Limb

Muscle	Action	Innervation	Course
			Courses cranioventrally toward the humerus **Inserts** on the teres major tuberosity on the medial humeral shaft
Serratus ventralis Cervical portion	Supports the trunk (fixed); draws the limb cranially (free)	Ventral branches of the cervical spinal nerves	**Arises** on the transverse processes of vertebrae C3–C7 **Courses** caudodorsally toward the scapula **Inserts** on the serrated face of the scapula
Thoracic portion	Supports the trunk (fixed); draws the limb caudally (free)	Long thoracic nerve of the brachial plexus	**Arises** on ribs 1–7 or 8, just ventral to their midpoints **Courses** craniodorsally toward the scapula **Inserts** on the serrated face of the scapula

*"Fixed" = weight-bearing limb; "free" = non–weight-bearing limb.

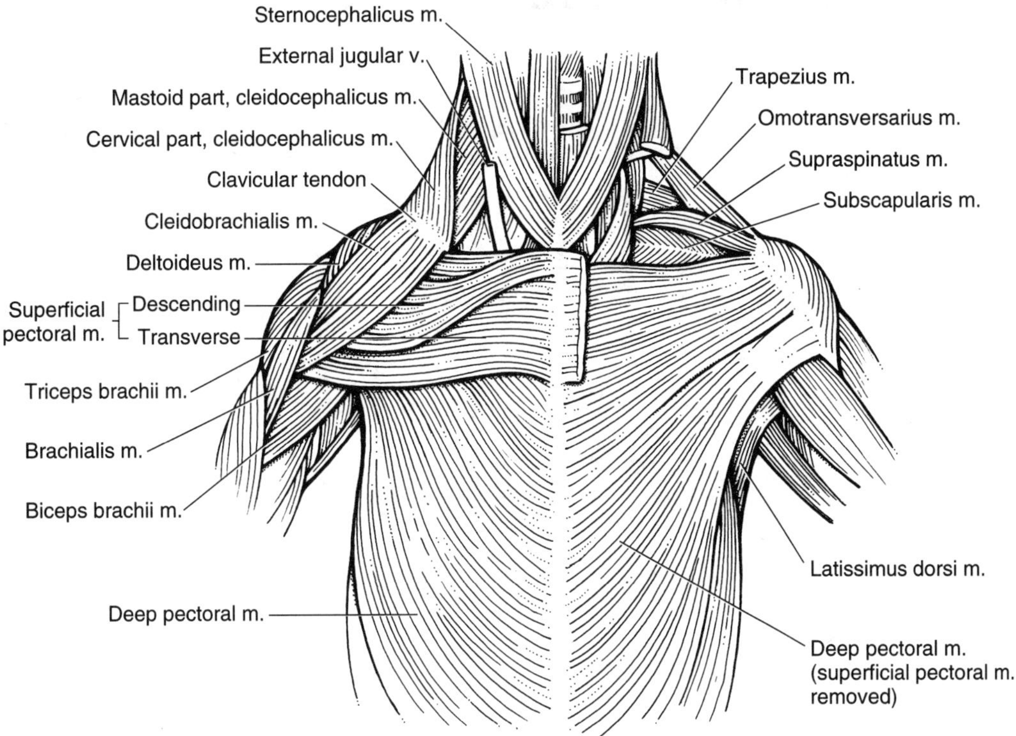

FIGURE 28–1. Extrinsic muscles of the thoracic limb, ventral view. Portions of some intrinsic muscles (i.e., the deltoideus, supraspinatus, and subscapularis muscles) are also shown. (Modified with permission from Evans HE, 1993, *Miller's Anatomy of the Dog,* 3e. Philadelphia, WB Saunders, P 325.)

G. The **latissimus dorsi** is a broad, flat sheet of muscle that extends between the dorsal midline and the brachium. This muscle is roughly triangular in shape, filling the space between the dorsal midline and the area caudal to the scapula. The latissimus dorsi covers most of the dorsal as well as parts of the lateral body wall, and is thus subcutaneous over most of its area. This muscle is sometimes referred to as the "digging dog" or "swimming dog" muscle, because it is responsible for the powerful caudal stroke of the brachium required for both motions.

H. The **serratus ventralis** is a deeply placed, expansive, thick, fan-shaped muscle that covers the caudal half of the lateral neck and the cranial half of the lateral thorax. Together with its fellow from the opposite side, the serratus ventralis forms a **muscular sling that suspends the trunk between the thoracic limbs** and **provides the major attachment of the thoracic limb to the trunk.** The serratus ventralis is divided into two portions, based on the origin of the muscle fibers:

1. The **cervical portion**
2. The **thoracic portion**

II. INTRINSIC MUSCLES

INTRINSIC MUSCLES (Table 28–2, Figure 28–2) arise and insert on the thoracic limb. All intrinsic muscles are paired and essentially surround the thoracic limb on all sides in most places.

TABLE 28–2. Intrinsic Muscles of the Thoracic Limb

Muscle	Action	Innervation	Course
Shoulder muscles			
Subscapularis	Adducts, extends, and stabilizes the shoulder joint	Subscapular nerve	**Arises** from the subscapular fossa **Courses** craniodistally **Inserts** via a stout tendon on the lesser tubercle of the humerus
Teres major	Flexes the shoulder and slightly rotates the brachium medially	Axillary nerve	**Arises** from the caudal scapula **Courses** craniodistally on the caudal surface of the shoulder joint **Inserts** by blending its tendon with that of the latissimus dorsi and attaching to the teres major tuberosity on the medial humeral shaft
Deltoideus	Flexes the shoulder	Axillary nerve	**Courses** distally **Inserts** on the deltoid tuberosity of the lateral humerus
Scapular part			**Arises** from an aponeurosis that attaches to most of the length of the scapular spine
Acromial part			**Arises** from the acromion
Supraspinatus	Extends and stabilizes the shoulder	Suprascapular nerve	**Arises** from the supraspinous fossa **Courses** craniodistally (cranial to the shoulder joint) **Inserts** on the greater tubercle of the humerus via a stout tendon
Infraspinatus	Flexes, extends, and stabilizes the shoulder; rotates the brachium laterally	Suprascapular nerve	**Arises** from the infraspinous fossa **Courses** craniodistally (caudal to the shoulder joint) **Inserts** on the greater tubercle of the humerus via a stout tendon (distal to the insertion of the supraspinatus)
Teres minor	Flexes the shoulder and slightly rotates the brachium medially	Axillary nerve	**Arises** from the infraglenoid tubercle **Courses** craniodistally (caudal to the shoulder joint)

continued

TABLE 28–2. Intrinsic Muscles of the Thoracic Limb

Muscle	Action	Innervation	Course
			Inserts on the teres minor tuberosity of the medial humeral shaft
Arm muscles			
Biceps brachii	Extends the shoulder, flexes the elbow, and supinates the paw (to a limited degree)	Musculocutaneous nerve	**Arises** via a long tendon from the supraglenoid tubercle **Courses** distally **Inserts** on the radial and ulnar tuberosities
Brachialis	Flexes the elbow	Musculocutaneous nerve	**Arises** from the proximal lateral humerus **Courses** along the caudolateral humeral shaft and then turns medially and crosses the elbow **Inserts** on the ulnar tuberosity
Coracobrachialis	Adducts and extends the shoulder joint	Musculocutaneous nerve	**Arises** via a tendon from the coracoid process **Courses** obliquely (medially and caudodistally) **Inserts** via a tendon on the crest of the lesser humeral tubercle
Triceps brachii	Extends the elbow; long head also flexes the shoulder	Radial nerve	**Courses** distally toward elbow **Inserts** via a tendon on the olecranon tuber
Tensor fasciae antebrachii	Tenses the antebrachial fascia; extends the elbow	Radial nerve	**Arises** from the fascia of the latissimus dorsi **Courses** distally **Inserts** on the olecranon tuber
Anconeus	Extends the elbow; assists in tensing the antebrachia fascia	Radial nerve	**Arises** from the supracondylar crest and the medial and lateral epicondyles **Courses** distally over the cavity of the olecracon fossa **Inserts** on the olecranon tuber
Forearm muscles			
Brachioradialis	Flexes elbow; rotates radius laterally	Radial nerve	**Arises** on lateral humeral epicondyle **Courses** obliquely distomedially

continued

TABLE 28–2. Intrinsic Muscles of the Thoracic Limb

Muscle	Action	Innervation	Course
			Inserts on radial periosteum approximately three fourths of the way distally
Extensor carpi radialis	Extends the carpus; flexes the elbow	Radial nerve	**Arises** from the lateral epicondyle and the epicondylar crest of the humerus **Courses** distally on the craniolateral radial surface **Inserts** via separate tendons on the proximal ends of metacarpal bones II and III
Common digital extensor	Extends the carpus and the digital joints	Radial nerve	**Arises** on the lateral humeral epicondyle **Courses** distally on the cranial radial surface **Inserts** via separate tendons on the extensor processes of the distal phalanges of digits II–IV
Lateral digital extensor	Extends the carpus and the digital joints	Radial nerve	**Arises** on the lateral humeral epicondyle **Courses** distally **Inserts** via separate tendons on the proximal and middle phalanges of digits III–V
Ulnaris lateralis	Flexes the carpus	Radial nerve	**Arises** from the lateral humeral epicondyle **Courses** distally on the lateral radial surface **Inserts** via separate tendons on the proximal end of metacarpal bone V and on the accessory carpal bone
Supinator	Rotates the antebrachium laterally so that the palmar surface of the paw turns dorsally ("up")	Radial nerve	**Arises** from the lateral humeral epicondyle **Courses** obliquely medially toward the radial shaft **Inserts** on the proximal, cranial fourth of the radial shaft
Abductor pollicis longus	Abducts digit I; extends the carpus	Radial nerve	**Arises** from the craniolateral radial and ulnar shafts **Courses** obliquely from lateral to medial

continued

TABLE 28–2. Intrinsic Muscles of the Thoracic Limb

Muscle	Action	Innervation	Course
			Inserts on the proximal end of metacarpal bone I
Pronator teres	Rotates the antebrachium medially so that the palmar surface of the paw turns palmarly ("down"); flexes the elbow	Median nerve	**Arises** from the medial humeral epicondyle **Courses** obliquely laterally toward the radial shaft **Inserts** on the radial shaft
Flexor carpi radialis	Flexes the carpus	Median nerve	**Arises** from the medial humeral epicondyle and the adjacent radial shaft **Courses** distally **Inserts** on metacarpal bones II and III proximally on the palmar sides
Superficial digital flexor	Flexes the carpus, metacarpophalangeal joints, and proximal interphalangeal joints	Median nerve	**Arises** from the medial humeral epicondyle and the adjacent radial shaft **Courses** directly distally **Inserts** on the middle phalanges of digits II–V proximally on the palmar sides
Flexor carpi ulnaris	Flexes the carpus	Ulnar nerve	**Courses** distally **Inserts** on the accessory carpal bone
Ulnar head			**Arises** on the proximal caudal ulna
Humeral head			**Arises** on the medial humeral epicondyle
Deep digital flexor	Flexes the carpus and all digital joints		**Courses** distally **Inserts** on the distal phalanges of digits I–V proximally on the palmar sides
Radial head		Median nerve	**Arises** along the proximal medial radius
Humeral head		Median and ulnar nerves	**Arises** on the medial humeral epicondyle
Ulnar head		Ulnar nerve	**Arises** on the caudal ulnar border over most of its length

continued

TABLE 28–2. Intrinsic Muscles of the Thoracic Limb

Muscle	Action	Innervation	Course
Pronator quadratus	Rotates the antebrachium medially so that the palmar surface of the paw turns palmarly ("down")	Median nerve	**Arises** and **inserts** along the opposed edges of the radius and ulna
Forepaw muscles			
Interossei	Flex the metacarpophalangeal joints; maintain the joint angle when the dog is standing	Ulnar nerve	**Arise** on the proximal ends of the metacarpal bones **Course** distally **Insert** via two tendons on the proximal ends of the associated proximal phalanges

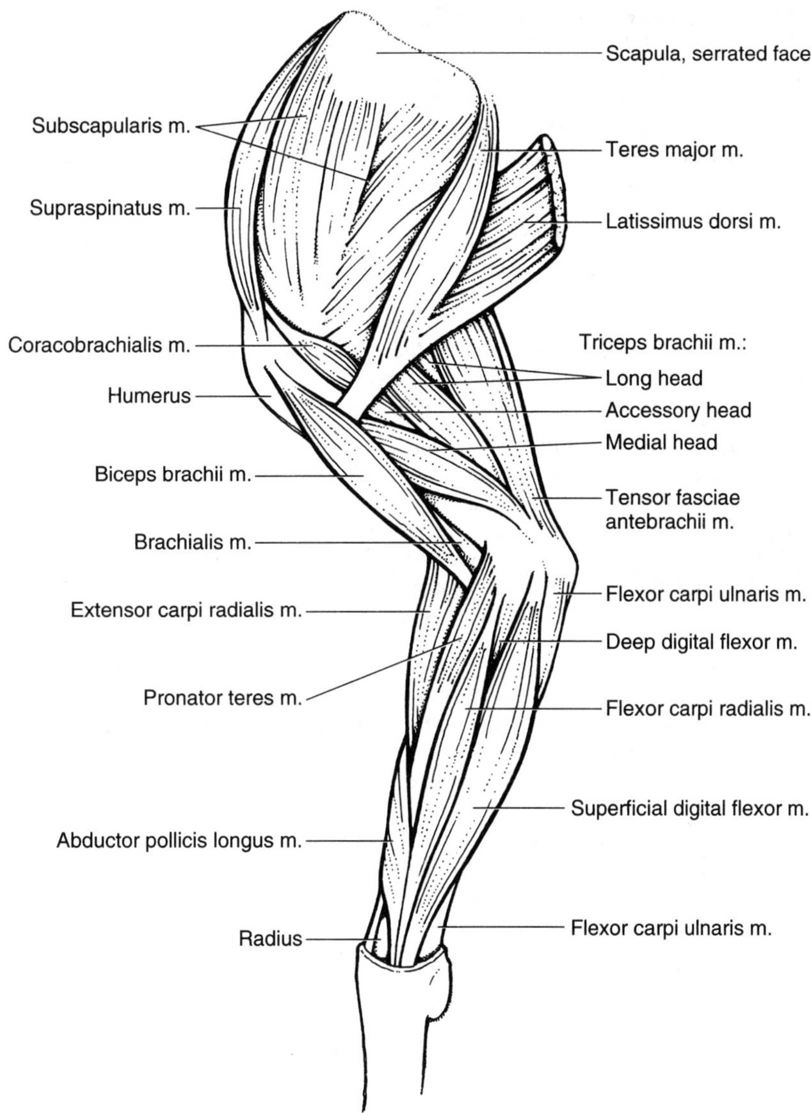

FIGURE 28–2. Intrinsic muscles of the left thoracic limb, medial view.

A. Muscles of the shoulder

1. **Medial shoulder musculature.** The **subscapularis** is a large, thick muscle that occupies essentially the entire subscapular fossa (i.e., nearly all of the medial scapular surface).
2. **Caudal shoulder musculature.** The **teres major** is positioned directly caudal to the subscapularis, and is sometimes grouped with it as a medial shoulder muscle. This large, thick, quadrilateral muscle extends between the caudal scapula and the humerus.
3. **Lateral shoulder musculature.** From superficial to deep, the lateral shoulder muscles are the deltoideus, the supraspinatus, the infraspinatus, and the teres minor.
   a. The **deltoideus,** which extends between the scapula and the proximal–lateral humerus, is subcutaneous over the lateral shoulder surface, where it covers the infraspinatus. It has two parts, which fuse before they insert and act together as a single unit.

(1) The **scapular part** is thin and sheet-like.
(2) The **acromial part** is thicker and is fusiform in shape.

b. The **supraspinatus** is a robust muscle that lies dorsal to the scapular spine and entirely fills the supraspinous fossa. Its lateral surface is largely covered by the cervical trapezius and the omotransversarius.

c. The **infraspinatus** is a thick muscle that entirely fills the infraspinous fossa and is largely covered by the spinous part of the deltoideus.

d. The **teres minor** is a small muscle positioned relatively deeply on the lateral scapular surface. It lies just caudal to and in approximately the same plane as the infraspinatus. In the intact state, it is entirely covered by the spinous part of the deltoideus, the infraspinatus, and the triceps brachii.

B. Muscles of the brachium (arm). For study purposes, the brachial muscles are generally described as "cranial" or "caudal." This distinction is based on the muscles' distal attachments, rather than on their position on the humerus.

1. **Cranial brachial musculature.** These muscles generally flex the elbow.

a. The **brachioradialis** is an inconstant muscle that extends between the lateral humeral epicondyle and the distal radius. When present, this thin slip of muscle is interposed between the superficial and deep layers of the antebrachial fascia; therefore, it is physically removed from the remaining antebrachial muscles.

b. The **biceps brachii** is a fusiform muscle of considerable substance and strength. A distinct, heavy tendinous band that is readily visible on cut section runs through the center of the muscle, adding to its strength.

(1) The biceps brachii, which belies its name by having only **one head,** covers some of the cranial and most of the medial humeral surface. It is **unusual among the brachial musculature in that it bridges the full length of the humerus but has no attachment to it.**

(2) The biceps brachii extends proximally past the shoulder joint and distally past the elbow joint. Of the brachial musculature, only the long head of the triceps brachii also **passes two joints** [see III B 2 a (1)].

c. The **brachialis** is grouped with the cranial brachial musculature, but a large part of its substance lies on the lateral shaft of the bone. The brachialis is long and rather flat, and courses along the brachial groove of the humerus. The long head of the triceps brachii largely covers the brachialis laterally.

d. The **coracobrachialis** is a small muscle that courses craniomedially so that its greatest bulk lies on the medial surface of the shoulder joint. This muscle is unique in that it originates and inserts via long tendons. The substance of the muscle belly forms once the tendon of origin gains the medial shoulder surface, so that much of the muscle's fleshy portion lies over the medial surface of the shoulder joint capsule.

2. **Caudal brachial musculature.** These muscles generally **extend the elbow.**

a. The **triceps brachii** is a large, powerful muscle covering most of the medial, caudal, and lateral brachial surface. The **four heads** of the triceps brachii each have a unique origin, but share a common insertion.

(1) The **long head** originates along the **caudal scapular border** and **bridges the full length of the humerus,** extending proximally past the shoulder joint and distally past the elbow joint. This head is roughly triangular and is the largest of the four. Two (sometimes three) bellies are present, and can convincingly look like separate muscles.

(2) The **lateral head** originates along the **tricipital line** on the lateral humeral surface. A roughly rectangular muscle of considerable substance, the lateral head can be difficult to distinguish from the long head.

(3) The **medial head** is spindle-shaped and originates from the **crest of the lesser tubercle** on the medial humerus. This head is relatively small, and not particularly thick.

(4) The **accessory head,** roughly rectangular in shape, originates on the **caudal part of the humeral neck** and generally maintains a position caudal to the humerus

through its course. The accessory head is the smallest and deepest of the heads, and is almost completely covered in the intact state by the other tricipital heads.

b. The **tensor fasciae antebrachii** is a thin, flat, narrow sheet of muscle on the medial surface of the brachium that covers the caudal portion of the medial surface of the triceps brachii.

c. The **anconeus** is small, thin muscle of irregular shape positioned caudally over the elbow. The anconeus essentially covers the olecranon fossa and is almost entirely covered in the intact state by the surrounding musculature.

C. **Muscles of the antebrachium (forearm).** Antebrachial muscles, especially those of the craniolateral group, tend to be fleshy in their proximal regions but taper to long flat tendons in their distal regions. Therefore, although the proximal antebrachium is surrounded by muscle on essentially all sides, the distal radial shaft and the distal caudal border of the ulna are subcutaneous.

1. **Craniolateral antebrachial musculature** (Figure 28–3A). These muscles extend the carpus, the digits, or both, and can be grouped into a continuous superficial layer, and a noncontinuous deeper layer.
   a. **Superficial layer.** From cranial to caudal, these muscles are the extensor carpi radialis, the common digital extensor, the lateral digital extensor, and the ulnaris lateralis.
      (1) The **extensor carpi radialis** is the largest member of the craniolateral antebrachial muscle group. This muscle lies subcutaneously on the cranial radial surface.
      (2) The **common digital extensor** also lies subcutaneously on the cranial radial surface and has considerable substance, although it is somewhat smaller than the extensor carpi radialis.
      (3) The **lateral digital extensor** is the smallest of the superficial craniolateral antebrachial muscle group. Its belly is hardly larger than its tendon. The lateral digital extensor lies subcutaneously on the cranial radial surface.
      (4) The **ulnaris lateralis,** a muscle of considerable substance, lies subcutaneously on the lateral radial surface. Unlike most other members of its group, the ulnaris lateralis is fleshy throughout much of its length.
   b. **Deep layer.** This layer consists of the supinator and the abductor pollicis longus.
      (1) The **supinator,** a short, broad, flat muscle that lies directly on the radius, is positioned deep to the extensor carpi radialis and common digital extensor muscles.
      (2) The **abductor pollicis longus** is a flat, triangular sheet of muscle that largely occupies the groove between the radius and ulna and is covered by the superficial layer of cranial antebrachial muscles. The muscle is directly applied to the surfaces of the antebrachial bones and covers the tendon of the extensor carpi radialis. The abductor pollicis longus forms a prominent tendon that runs down the cranial edge of most of the muscle's length.
2. **Caudomedial antebrachial musculature** (Figure 28–3B). These muscles flex the carpus, digits, or both, and can be grouped into a continuous superficial layer, a deep layer, and an extremely deep layer.
   a. **Superficial layer.** From cranial to caudal, these muscles are the pronator teres, the flexor carpi radialis, the superficial digital flexor, and the flexor carpi ulnaris.
      (1) The **pronator teres** lies obliquely on the radial shaft and is sort of a "mirror image" of the supinator.
      (2) The **flexor carpi radialis** is small in terms of overall size, but its short belly is of considerable thickness. The muscle belly extends only approximately one third of the way down the antebrachium, after which it is replaced by a thin, flat, strong tendon.
      (3) The **superficial digital flexor** is a large, flat muscle that is fleshy almost to the carpus. Its subcutaneous belly covers a large part of the caudal antebrachial surface.
      (4) The **flexor carpi ulnaris,** the lateral-most of the muscles in this group, consists of two parts that originate separately, and remain separate throughout their length.
         (a) The **ulnar head** is the more superficial of the two parts, and lies directly over the deeper and larger humeral head. The ulnar head of the flexor carpi ulnaris

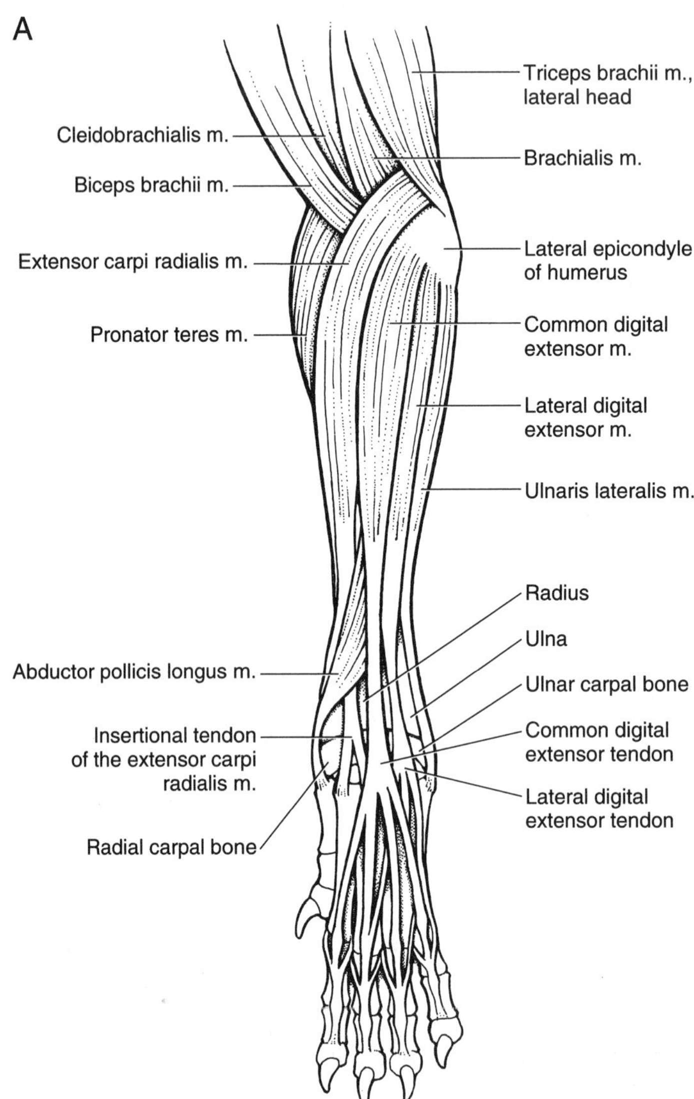

FIGURE 28–3. Superficial view of left antebrachial muscles. (*A*) Cranial surface. (*continued*)

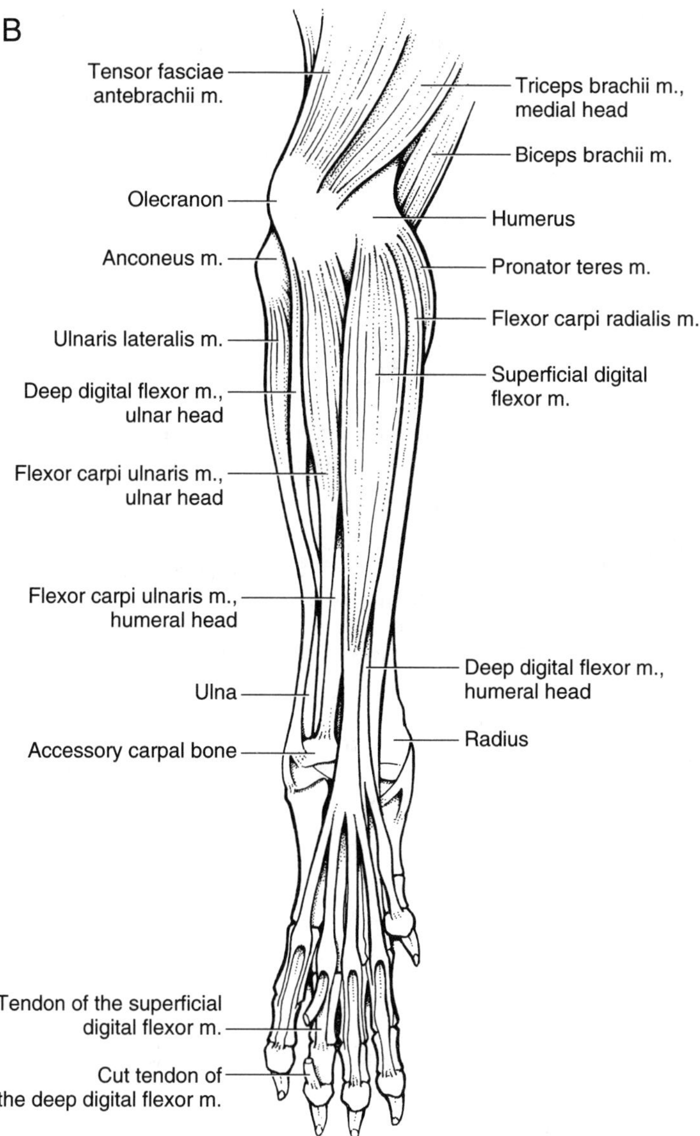
B
Tensor fasciae antebrachii m.
Triceps brachii m., medial head
Biceps brachii m.
Olecranon
Humerus
Anconeus m.
Pronator teres m.
Flexor carpi radialis m.
Ulnaris lateralis m.
Superficial digital flexor m.
Deep digital flexor m., ulnar head
Flexor carpi ulnaris m., ulnar head
Flexor carpi ulnaris m., humeral head
Deep digital flexor m., humeral head
Ulna
Radius
Accessory carpal bone
Tendon of the superficial digital flexor m.
Cut tendon of the deep digital flexor m.

FIGURE 28–3—*continued* (*B*) Caudal surface.

is thin and flat, and muscular only through the proximal third of its length. A thin, flat, strong tendon forms on its medial side and continues to the carpus.

(b) The **humeral head** is the deeper of the two parts, and lies directly over the deep digital flexor. The humeral head of the flexor carpi ulnaris is thick and fleshy, and remains fleshy through most of its length. It forms a short, thick tendon just proximal to its insertion.

b. Deep layer. The deep layer of caudomedial antebrachial muscles is composed of the bellies and heads of the **deep digital flexor,** which are positioned between the superficial layer of caudomedial antebrachial muscles superficially and the pronator quadratus deeply. The deep digital flexor consists of **three heads** of disparate size and character.

(1) The **humeral head,** the largest of the three heads, is composed of several (unnamed) bellies. The humeral head of the deep digital flexor remains fleshy through most of its length. It forms a short, thick tendon just proximal to the carpus.

(2) The **radial head** is hardly more than a wisp of muscular tissue attached to the radius. A tendon along its free surface joins the tendon of the humeral head at the carpus.

(3) The **ulnar head** is thin and elongate, and like the radial head, forms a tendon along much of its free edge. The tendon of the ulnar head joins the tendon of the humeral head at the carpus.

c. Deepest layer. The deepest layer is composed of the **pronator quadratus,** which essentially fills the interosseous space between the radius and ulna.

D. Muscles of the manus (forepaw). Approximately one dozen highly specialized muscles are present in the paw, some homologous to those of the thenar and hypothenar regions of the human hand. Most of these muscles are of academic interest only. Only one group of paw muscles warrants discussion here, the **interosseous muscles.** The four interosseous muscles are similar in size, shape, position, and attachments. The interossei lie deep to the deep digital flexor and cover the palmar surfaces of the metacarpal bones.

III. MUSCLE ACTION.

Consideration of a muscle's attachments relative to the flexor/extensor angles of the joints across which the muscle passes permits intuitive comprehension of the major action of the muscle. The **flexor surfaces** of the thoracic limb joints **alternate** from the **caudal** to the **cranial surface** of the limb from the shoulder through the carpus, and then remain on the palmar surface of the limb from the carpus distally (Figure 28–4). Therefore, a muscle's function alternates according to the surface of the limb on which it is found.

A. Glenohumeral (shoulder) joint. The flexor surface is on the caudal limb surface.

1. Muscles on the **cranial side** of the shoulder are **shoulder extensors** (the supraspinatus and coracobrachialis).
2. Muscles on the **caudal side** of the shoulder are **shoulder flexors** (the infraspinatus, deltoideus, teres minor, and teres major).

B. Brachioantebrachial (elbow) joint. The flexor surface is on the cranial limb surface.

1. Muscles on the **cranial side** of the elbow are **elbow flexors** (the biceps brachii, brachialis, supinator, and pronator teres).
2. Muscles on the **caudal side** of the elbow are **elbow extensors** [the tensor fasciae antebrachii, triceps brachii (all heads), and anconeus].

C. Antebrachiocarpal joint (carpus). The flexor surface is on the caudal limb surface.

1. Muscles on the **cranial side** of the carpus are **carpal extensors** (the extensor carpi radialis, common digital extensor, and lateral digital extensor).
2. Muscles on the **caudal side** of the carpus are **carpal flexors** (the ulnaris lateralis, flexor

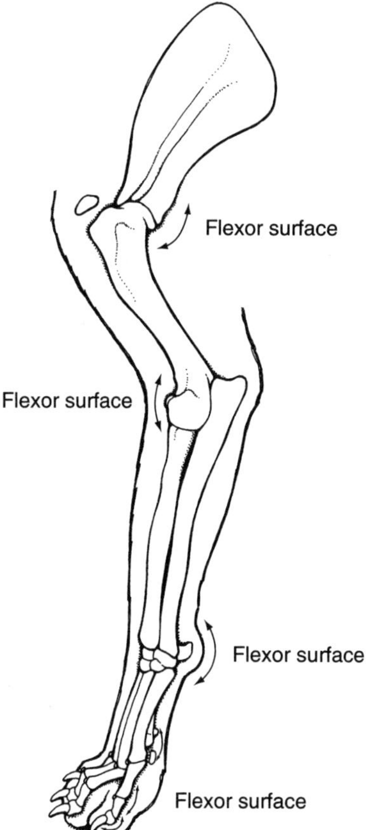

FIGURE 28–4. Flexor surfaces of the joints of the thoracic limb.

carpi radialis, superficial digital flexor, and deep digital flexor). Although the ulnaris lateralis shares its origin site with the carpal and digital extensors, its insertion is so far lateral that the action of the muscle changes from extension to flexion of the carpal joint.

D. **Metacarpophalangeal joints.** The flexor surface is on the palmar limb surface.

1. Muscles on the **cranial side** of the metacarpus are **metacarpal extensors** (the common digital extensor and lateral digital extensor). The extensor carpi radialis is not included in this list because it does not extend past the carpus.
2. Muscles on the **caudal side** of the metacarpus are **metacarpal flexors** (the superficial digital flexor and deep digital flexor). The flexor carpi ulnaris and flexor carpi radialis are not included in this group, because they do not extend past the carpus.

E. **Interdigital joints.** The flexor surface is on the caudal limb surface.

1. Muscles on the **cranial side** of the digits are **digital extensors** (the common digital extensor and lateral digital extensor).
2. Muscles on the **caudal side** of the digits are **digital flexors** (the superficial digital flexor and deep digital flexor).

Chapter 29

Vasculature of the Thoracic Limb

I. ARTERIES OF THE THORACIC LIMB (Figure 29–1, Table 29–1). The typical branching pattern is described in this section; the reader must keep in mind that variations are relatively common, and that **arteries are named for the structures they supply, rather than for the source from which they branch.**

A. Introduction

1. **Position.** Most arteries of the limbs are positioned on the medial side of the limb and deeply among muscles (which protects against surface trauma) and on the flexor surface of joints (which minimizes stretching of the artery during limb motion).
2. **Flow of arterial blood to the thoracic limb.** Arterial flow to and through the thoracic limb is proximal to distal via a central continuous channel, from which smaller branches periodically arise to deliver blood to regional structures. The **main arterial channel** to and through the thoracic limb takes the following sequence:
   a. **Subclavian artery**
   b. **Axillary artery**
   c. **Brachial artery**
   d. **Median artery**
   e. **Palmar common digital arteries**
   f. **Palmar proper digital arteries**

B. Arteries of the shoulder

1. **Superficial cervical artery**
   a. **Origin.** The superficial cervical artery originates inside the thorax from the cranial surface of the **subclavian artery.**
   b. **Course.** The superficial cervical artery courses through the region between the neck and shoulder and extends from the area of the first rib as far dorsally as the trapezius muscle.
   c. **Branches.** The superficial cervical artery has **five named branches** that provide at least partial supply to much of the musculature in the shoulder and cranial cervical regions.
      (1) The **suprascapular artery** courses around the cranial side of the scapular neck to reach the lateral scapular surface. It supplies the **supraspinatus, infraspinatus,** and **teres minor** muscles, the **scapula,** and the **shoulder joint.**
      (2) The **supraspinous artery** courses around the cranial side of the mid-dorsal border of the scapula and primarily supplies the **supraspinatus** muscle.
      (3) The **deltoid branch** passes ventrally and laterally to supply the **pectoral** and **brachiocephalicus** muscles.
      (4) The **ascending cervical artery** courses dorally to supply numerous muscles of the cervical region (e.g., the **sternocephalicus, brachiocephalicus, rhomboideus, omotransversarius,** and **scalenus** muscles).
      (5) The **prescapular artery** supplies the **trapezius** muscle.
2. **Axillary artery.** The axillary artery is the first segment of the main arterial channel of the thoracic limb proper.
   a. **Origin.** The axillary artery is the continuation of the subclavian artery lateral to the first rib; therefore, it is the major pathway for blood from the interior of the thoracic cavity to the thoracic limb.
   b. **Course.** Throughout its course, the axillary artery is buried deeply among the muscles medial to the scapula in the axillary region. The axillary artery extends from the point

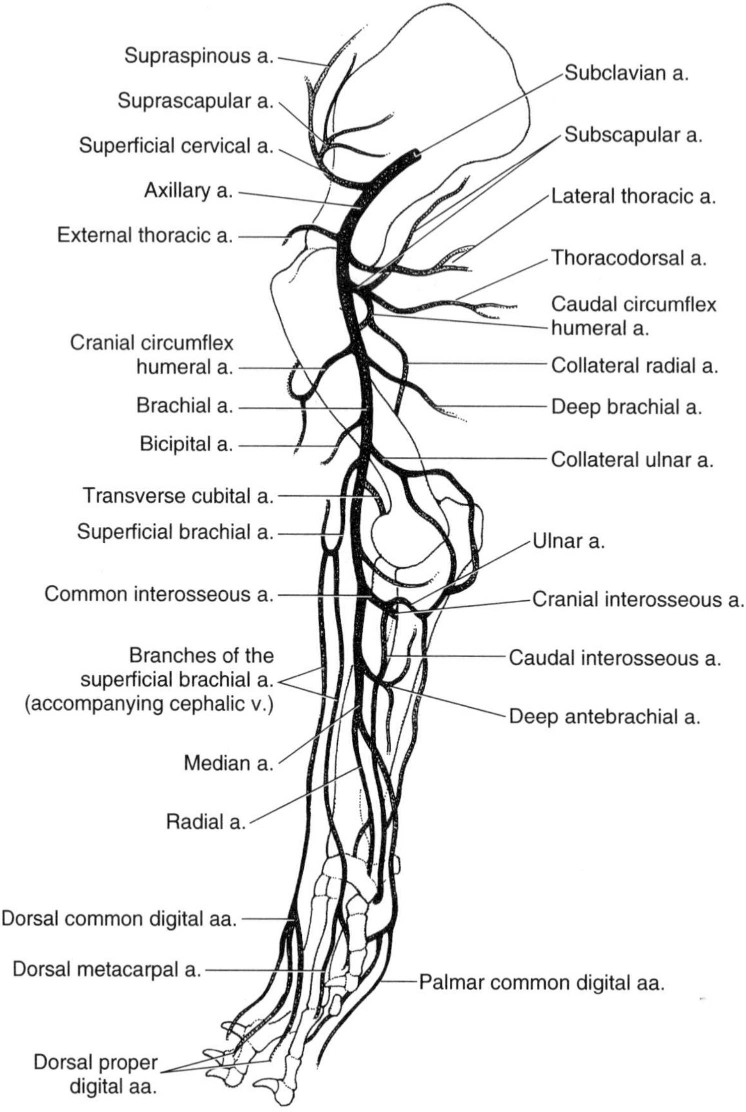

FIGURE 29–1. Arteries of the right thoracic limb, medial view.

where the subclavian artery turns lateral to the first rib, as far as the conjoined tendon of the teres major and latissimus dorsi muscles.

c. **Branches.** Typically, **four major branches** arise from the axillary artery.
   (1) The **external thoracic artery** usually arises from the cranial surface of the axillary artery and courses cranially around the cranial border of the deep pectoral muscle to supply the **superficial pectoral muscle.**
   (2) The **lateral thoracic artery** usually arises from the caudal surface of the axillary artery.
      (a) **Course.** The lateral thoracic artery courses caudally through the axilla, across the axillary lymph node, and along the lateral border of the deep pectoral muscle.
      (b) **Structures supplied** include (but are not limited to) the **deep pectoral muscle,** the **axillary lymph node,** and the **mammary glands.**

TABLE 29–1. Main Arterial Supply of the Major Thoracic Limb Muscles

Muscle	Main Arterial Supply	Parent Artery
Extrinsic muscles		
Superficial pectoral	External thoracic	Axillary
Deep pectoral	Lateral thoracic	Axillary
Brachiocephalicus	Superficial cervical	Subclavian
Omotransversarius	Superficial cervical	Subclavian
Trapezius	Superficial cervical	Subclavian
Rhomboideus	Superficial cervical	Subclavian
Latissimus dorsi	Thoracodorsal	Subscapular (axillary)
Serratus ventralis	Thoracodorsal	Subscapular
Shoulder muscles		
Subscapularis	Subscapular	Axillary
Supraspinatus	Suprascapular and supraspinous	Superficial cervical (subclavian)
Infraspinatus	Suprascapular	Superficial cervical (subclavian)
Teres major	Subscapular and thoracodorsal	Axillary
Deltoideus	Caudal circumflex humeral	Subscapular (axillary)
Teres minor	Suprascapular	Superficial cervical (subclavian)
Brachial muscles		
Cranial muscles		
Biceps brachii	Cranial circumflex humeral	Axillary or subscapular
	Bicipital	Brachial
Brachialis	Collateral radial	Caudal circumflex humeral
	Transverse cubital	Brachial
Coracobrachialis	Caudal circumflex humeral	Subscapular
Caudal muscles		
Triceps brachii	Caudal circumflex humeral	Subscapular (axillary)
	Deep brachial and collateral ulnar	Brachial
Tensor fasciae antebrachii	Collateral ulnar	Brachial
Anconeus	Collateral ulnar	Brachial
Antebrachial muscles		
Craniolateral muscles		
Extensor carpi radialis	Transverse cubital	Brachial
	Cranial interosseous	Common interosseus
Common digital extensor	Cranial interosseous	Common interosseous (brachial)
Lateral digital extensor	Cranial interosseous	Common interosseous (brachial)
Ulnaris lateralis	Cranial interosseous	Common interosseous (brachial)
Supinator	Cranial interosseous	Common interosseous (brachial)
	Transverse cubital	Brachial

continued

TABLE 29–1. Main Arterial Supply of the Major Thoracic Limb Muscles

Muscle	Main Arterial Supply	Parent Artery
Abductor pollicis longus	Cranial interosseous	Cranial interosseous
Caudomedial muscles		
Pronator teres	Common interosseous	Brachial
Flexor carpi radialis	Collateral ulnar	Brachial
	Deep antebrachial	Median
Superficial digital flexor	Common interosseous	Brachial
	Deep antebrachial	Median
Flexor carpi ulnaris	Collateral ulnar	Brachial
	Deep antebrachial	Median
Deep digital flexor	Collateral ulnar	Brachial
	Deep antebrachial	Median
	Ulnar artery	Common interosseus (brachial)
Pronator quadratus	Common interosseous	Brachial
Interossei	Deep palmar arch	Caudal interosseous (brachial)
		Radial (median)

(3) The **subscapular artery,** a major branch of the axillary artery, may actually be larger than the continuation of the axillary artery itself.

(a) Course. The subscapular artery usually arises from the caudal surface of the axillary artery and courses dorsocaudally between the subscapularis and teres major muscles. For most of its course, the artery lies deeply, but its terminal branches become subcutaneous caudal to the dorsal scapula.

(b) Branches and structures supplied. The subscapular artery has several branches of its own, including the:

(i) Thoracodorsal artery, a large artery that usually arises from the caudal surface of the subscapular artery close to its origin and supplies most of the **latissimus dorsi,** and usually a part of the **teres major**

(ii) Caudal circumflex humeral artery, which usually arises from the lateral surface of the subscapular artery near the thoracodorsal artery and courses deeply (between the humeral head and the teres major muscle) to supply the **triceps brachii** and a large portion of the **deltoideus,** as well as providing small twigs to nearby muscles

(4) The **cranial circumflex humeral artery** usually arises from the medial surface of the axillary artery, but is frequently a branch of the subscapular artery instead.

(a) Course. This small artery courses cranially around the humeral neck, deep to the tendon of origin of the biceps brachii muscle.

(b) Structures supplied. The cranial circumflex humeral artery supplies part of the **biceps brachii,** as well as the **coracobrachialis.**

C. Arteries of the brachium. The **brachial artery** is the main artery of the brachium.

1. **Origin.** The brachial artery is the direct continuation of the axillary artery.
2. **Course.** The brachial artery descends the medial surface of the brachium in a relatively straight path, extending from the conjoined tendon of the teres major and latissimus dorsi muscles through the origin of the common interosseous artery. Because the com-

mon interosseous artery arises distal to the elbow, the brachial artery continues a short distance into the antebrachium.

3. **Relations.** The brachial artery consistently demonstrates a positional relation to the neurovascular and muscular structures of the brachium. It lies:
   a. Caudal to the biceps brachii muscle and the musculocutaneous nerve
   b. Cranial to the combined median and ulnar nerves and the brachial vein
   c. On the medial surface of the medial head of the triceps brachii

4. **Branches and structures supplied**
   a. The **deep brachial artery** is a moderately large artery that usually arises from the caudal surface of the brachial artery in the proximal third or half of the brachium. This artery immediately plunges into the substance of the **triceps brachii** muscle to supply its **medial** and **long heads.**
   b. The **bicipital artery** is a small artery that usually arises from the cranial surface of the brachial artery about a third of the way distally along the arm. It courses craniodistally to enter and supply the **biceps brachii** at its distal end.
   c. The **collateral ulnar artery** is a fairly large artery that usually arises from the caudal surface of the brachial artery in the distal third of the brachium and has several small, unnamed branches of its own.
      (1) **Course.** The major part of the artery courses caudodistally toward the elbow, providing small branches to muscles and deeper structures as it goes.
      (2) **Structures supplied.** The main part of the artery enters the **antebrachial flexor muscle mass.** In addition, the artery supplies the **elbow joint capsule, anconeus,** and parts of the **triceps brachii.**
   d. The **superficial brachial artery** is a small artery that usually arises from the cranial surface of the brachial artery just proximal to the elbow.
      (1) **Course.** The superficial brachial artery courses obliquely craniodistally toward the flexor surface of the elbow, where it becomes subcutaneous and **gives off a medial branch.** It then **continues** as the **cranial superficial antebrachial artery.** The medial branch and the cranial superficial antebrachial artery continue on either side of the cephalic vein to the level of the paw.
      (2) **Structures supplied.** The superficial brachial artery sends twigs to the **skin** (*en route* to the paw) and contributes to the **dorsal carpal rete** (i.e., a vascular network on the dorsal surface of the carpus).
   e. The **transverse cubital artery** is a small artery that usually arises from the lateral surface of the brachial artery just proximal to where the brachial artery passes deep to the pronator teres muscle. It courses distally and slightly caudally (deep to the biceps brachii) to reach and supply the **extensor carpi radialis.**

D. Arteries of the antebrachium

1. **Common interosseous artery**
   a. **Origin.** The common interosseous artery is a large but short branch that usually arises from the lateral surface of the **brachial artery** just distal to the elbow. (Recall that the brachial artery retains its name a short distance into the antebrachium.)
   b. **Course.** The common interosseous artery courses cranially and slightly ventrally, providing a few twigs to adjacent muscles. The artery then immediately plunges into the interosseous space between the radius and ulna, where it **terminates by trifurcating into three arteries.**
      (1) The **ulnar artery** courses distally to and travels the length of the antebrachium, deep to the ulnar head of the flexor carpi ulnaris. It supplies both heads of the **flexor carpi ulnaris** and the **humeral** and **ulnar heads** of the **deep digital flexor.** In addition, the ulnar artery contributes to the supply of the **paw.**
      (2) The **caudal interosseous artery** courses directly distally in the interosseous space, deep to the pronator quadratus muscle. The artery supplies at least seven **adjacent muscles** of the **extensor and flexor groups,** the **radius** and **ulna,** and some structures of the **paw.**
      (3) The **cranial interosseous artery** courses cranially through the interosseous space,

then emerges from the space and turns proximally just distal to the lateral humeral epicondyle. At this level it enters the **extensor muscle group** on the craniolateral antebrachium, supplying those muscles as well as the **adjacent muscles,** the **flexor carpi radialis,** and the **elbow joint capsule.**

2. **Median artery.** The median artery is the largest artery of the antebrachium.
   a. **Origin.** The median artery is the **direct continuation of the brachial artery;** therefore, it forms the third segment of the main arterial channel of the thoracic limb.
   b. **Course.** The median artery, which begins after the origin of the common interosseous artery, descends the caudomedial surface of the antebrachium in a fairly straight path and continues to the proximal metacarpus. Here, it turns transverse to the long axis of the limb to form the predominant part of the superficial palmar arch, the principal arterial supply to the paw.
   c. **Branches**
      (1) The **deep antebrachial artery** is a rather large artery that usually arises from the caudal surface of the median artery not far distal to the common interosseous artery.
         (a) **Course.** The deep antebrachial artery courses distally, passing into the substance of the deep digital flexor and continuing through the length of the antebrachium. During its course, the artery anastomoses with regional arteries. The artery then continues as a small vessel through the carpal canal.
         (b) **Structures supplied** include the **flexors carpi radialis** and **ulnaris** and the **superficial** and **deep digital flexors.**
      (2) The **radial artery** is a small artery that usually arises from the median artery approximately one third to halfway distally along the antebrachium.
         (a) **Course.** The radial artery courses distally along the caudomedial border of the radius, dividing into dorsal and palmar branches approximately at the carpus.
         (b) **Structures supplied**
            (i) The **dorsal branch** contributes to the **dorsal carpal rete.**
            (ii) The **palmar branch** makes a tiny contribution to the **deep palmar arch,** which supplies the digits.

E. Arteries of the manus (see Chapter 30, Figure 30–2)

1. **General pattern of arterial supply.** A description of the paw's general pattern of arterial supply assists understanding of the regional vasculature. The arterial supply is best considered in two general regions: the **metacarpal region** and the **digital region.**
   a. **Metacarpal region.** By using a set of **three descriptors (surface, depth, position)** in a consistent sequence, each of the arteries in the metacarpal region can be identified.
      (1) **Surface.** The surface of the paw is identified as either **dorsal** or **palmar.**
      (2) **Depth.** Two separate sets of arteries, one **superficial** and one **deep,** are present on each surface. Four arteries are usually present in each set (i.e.,the superficial dorsal set, deep dorsal set, superficial palmar set, and deep palmar set). The **depth of the artery** is identified as either:
         (a) **Common digital,** for the more **superficial set** on both the dorsal and palmar surfaces.
            (i) Dorsally, the common digital arteries are superficial to the digital extensor tendons.
            (ii) Palmarly, the common digital arteries are placed between the superficial and deep digital flexors.
         (b) **Metacarpal** for the **deeper set** on both the dorsal and palmar surfaces (located on the surfaces of the metacarpal bones deep to the extensor or flexor tendons)
      (3) **Position.** The arteries take a course relative to a position between adjacent metacarpal bones and are **numbered to correspond to the lower-numbered metacarpal bone** (i.e., the arteries are numbered from medial to lateral, beginning with I, as are the digits—although the numbering stops at IV because there are only four interosseous spaces).

b. Digital region. Like the metacarpal region, the digital region is supplied with arterial blood on both its **dorsal** and **palmar** surfaces. However, unlike the metacarpal region, there is only one vessel on each surface of each digit.

2. Arteries of the metacarpal region

a. Dorsal surface

(1) Dorsal common digital arteries I–IV arise from the superficial brachial artery (via the trifurcation of the **cranial superficial antebrachial artery** and the continuation of the **medial branch of the superficial brachial artery).**

(2) Dorsal metacarpal arteries I–IV are very small. These arteries arise from the **dorsal carpal rete,** the fine arterial network on the dorsum of the carpus formed by contributions from the **radial, caudal interosseous,** and **ulnar arteries.**

b. Palmar surface. The arteries of the palmar surface of the metacarpus arise from the **palmar arches,** one superficial and one deep.

(1) Palmar common digital arteries I–IV are quite large, and **supply most of the arterial blood to the paw.** They arise from the **superficial palmar arch,** a structure of varying prominence formed mainly from the **median artery,** together with a small contribution from the **caudal interosseous artery.** The contribution from the caudal interosseous artery is so small that the palmar common digital arteries sometimes appear to simply arise as direct branches of the median artery.

(2) Palmar metacarpal arteries I–IV are much smaller, and arise from the **deep palmar arch,** a structure that is consistently recognizable as an arch and is formed by the anastomosis of the palmar branch of the **radial artery** and the termination of the **caudal interosseous artery.**

3. Arteries of the digital region. The **dorsal** and **palmar proper digital arteries** are the arteries that supply arterial blood to the individual digits.

a. Formation (Figure 29–2). The proper digital arteries are formed in the following manner:

(1) Near the distal end of the metacarpus, **each dorsal (or palmar) metacarpal artery anastomoses with the dorsal (or palmar) common digital artery of the same number.** The common digital artery then continues for a short distance until it reaches the level of the metacarpophalangeal joint, where the toes begin to diverge from the metacarpal region.

(2) At the metacarpophalangeal joint, each common digital artery **bifurcates into two arteries,** each of which courses down the adjacent surfaces of adjacent digits. These arteries supply blood to one side (medial or lateral) of one surface (dorsal or palmar) of one digit proper ("proper" = "only") and are called the proper digital arteries.

(a) The proper digital arteries **take the number of the digit on which they are located.**

(b) By virtue of the bifurcation of adjacent common digital arteries, each toe is provided with an artery passing down its medial and lateral surface. In order to distinguish these two arteries, one final set of descriptive terms is introduced: **axial** and **abaxial.** This terminology refers to the conventional designation of the **axis of the digits,** which **passes between digits III** and **IV.**

(i) The **axial surface** of the digit **faces the axis.**

(ii) The **abaxial surface** faces **away from the axis.**

b. Identification

(1) General example. Dorsal common digital artery I, running in the space between metacarpal bones I and II, terminates by bifurcating into the arteries on facing surfaces of digits I and II (i.e., the **axial dorsal proper digital artery I** and the **abaxial dorsal proper digital artery II).**

(2) Digits separated by digital axis. Because the digital axis passes between digits III and IV, the arteries on the adjacent surfaces of these two digits both face the axis, and thus dorsal (or palmar) digital artery III bifurcates into two axial arteries, rather than one axial and one abaxial artery.

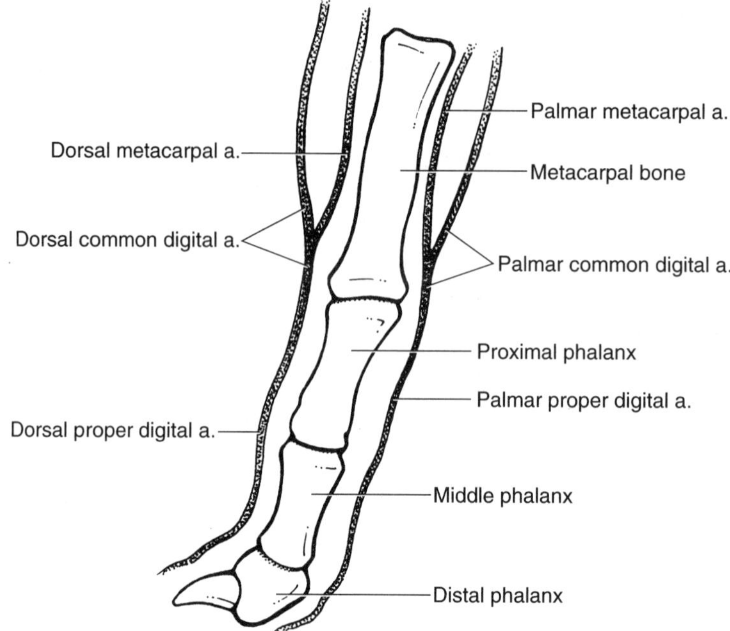

FIGURE 29–2. Formation of the proper digital arteries, dorsal and palmar, from the respective common digital and metacarpal arteries (highly schematized).

II. VEINS OF THE THORACIC LIMB.

II. VEINS OF THE THORACIC LIMB. Two sets of veins are present in the limbs, a deep set that parallels the arteries, and a superficial set that has no relation to the arteries.

A. The **deep veins** are largely **satellite veins** of the named arteries. At times, the satellite veins may be doubled, in which case the two veins simply share the same name with each other as well as with the companion artery. Nearly all of the arteries detailed in I are accompanied by satellite veins.

B. The **superficial veins** are subcutaneous. The distal members of this group are often accessible to venipuncture. These veins are best considered in the direction of their blood flow (i.e., from distal to proximal).

1. The **dorsal common digital veins** flow together to form the **accessory cephalic vein,** which leaves the dorsal surface of the metacarpal region and ascends across the carpus and into the antebrachium to join the **cephalic vein** in the distal antebrachial region.
2. The **cephalic vein,** the major superficial vein of the paw and antebrachium, originates from the **superficial palmar venous arch** [i.e., the satellite of the deep palmar (arterial) arch], courses proximally on the palmar surface of the paw, and then inclines medially to gain the dorsum of the carpus. The vein then continues proximally along the craniomedial antebrachial surface as the **antebrachial part of the cephalic vein** to the elbow, and then continues proximally as the **brachial part of the cephalic vein.**
   a. The **antebrachial part of the cephalic vein** receives tributaries draining both superficial and deep structures. The **cranial superficial antebrachial artery** and the **medial branch of the superficial brachial artery** accompany this part of the vein, as do the **medial and lateral branches of the superficial radial nerve.**
   b. The **brachial part of the cephalic vein** passes deep to the cleidobrachialis muscle about a third of the way proximal along the antebrachium, continues proximally, and then **terminates by entering the external jugular vein.**

Canine Clinical Correlation

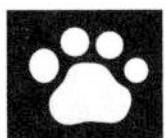

The antebrachial part of the cephalic vein is the most commonly accessed vein for venipuncture in dogs. Accidental placement of the needle into one of the sensory branches of the radial nerve is often what prompts a vigorous escape attempt by the dog undergoing venipuncture!

3. The **median cubital vein** is a prominent vein that lies obliquely across the flexor surface of the elbow, joining the antebrachial part of the cephalic and the median veins.
4. The **axillobrachial vein** appears to be a direct continuation of the brachial part of the cephalic vein. From the site where the cephalic vein turns cranially deep to the cleidobrachialis muscle, the axillobrachial vein continues directly proximally over the lateral head of the triceps (receiving tributaries from this muscle). It passes deep to the deltoideus muscle and caudal to the humerus, becomes confluent with the subscapular vein, and **terminates by entering the axillary vein.**
5. The **omobrachial vein** passes over the surface of the proximal shoulder and arm. This vein branches from the axillobrachial vein (just before that vein passes deep to the deltoideus muscle), passes subcutaneously across the deltoideus, inclines cranially, passes over the brachiocephalicus, and **terminates by entering the external jugular vein.**

III. LYMPHATIC VESSELS OF THE THORACIC LIMB.

Two lymphocenters are present consistently.

A. Superficial cervical lymphocenter

1. **Lymph nodes.** The **superficial cervical lymph nodes** are positioned cranial to the supraspinatus muscle, deep to the cervical part of the brachiocephalicus, the omotransversarius, and the cervical part of the trapezius.
2. **Lymphatics**
   a. **Afferent lymphatics** arrive from almost the entire thoracic limb, as well as the head and neck.
   b. **Efferent lymphatics** terminate in the respective lymphatic ducts, right or left.

B. Axillary lymphocenter

1. **Lymph nodes**
   a. The **axillary lymph node,** a constant lymph node, is large, roundish, and flattened in form. This node is positioned on the medial surface of the shoulder, caudal to the shoulder joint. **The axillary lymph nodes of the right and left sides communicate with each other** by means of connections between the efferent lymphatics from each node. This communication takes place across the cranial ventral thoracic region.
   b. The **accessory axillary lymph node,** rarely present, lies caudal to the axillary node and is considerably smaller in size.
2. **Lymphatics**
   a. **Afferent lymphatics** arrive from the deep structures of the thoracic limb, much of the mammary gland chain, and the thoracic wall.
   b. **Efferent lymphatics** terminate in the thoracic duct, tracheal trunks, external jugular vein, or any combination of these on a given side.

Canine Clinical Correlation

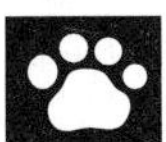

The communication across the midline between the two axillary lymph nodes provides a potential route of metastasis for mammary adenocarcinoma.

Chapter 30

Innervation of the Thoracic Limb

I. BRACHIAL PLEXUS

A. Definition. The brachial plexus is the network of nerves that supplies most structures of the thoracic limb with both sensory and motor innervation.* (Note that "sensory" includes cutaneous information, as well as sensory information from the muscle spindle fibers, periosteum, and joint capsule.)

B. Formation (Figure 30–1)

1. **Roots.** The **ventral branches of cervical nerves 6, 7,** and **8 (C6, C7, C8)** and **thoracic nerves 1** and **2 (T1, T2)** form the brachial plexus in most dogs [occasionally cervical nerve 5 (C5) contributes; the contribution of T2 is then reduced or absent]. These nerves are referred to as the **roots of the brachial plexus.**
   a. The ventral branches of the contributing spinal nerves cross the scalenus muscle, extending into and traversing the **axilla** (i.e., the triangular space between the medial shoulder region and the lateral body wall).
   b. As the ventral branches of the contributing spinal nerves traverse the axillary space, they **intercommunicate extensively** to form the brachial plexus.
2. **Derivatives.** From the network that is the brachial plexus, fibers from multiple nerve roots coalesce to form the **named nerves** of the plexus. These named nerves pass into the thoracic limb along constant routes.

II. NERVES OF THE BRACHIAL PLEXUS IN THE SHOULDER, BRACHIUM, AND ANTEBRACHIUM.

Consideration of the nerves of the brachial plexus is most convenient according to their level of origin from the brachial plexus, from cranial to caudal.

A. The **brachiocephalic nerve** is formed from the ventral branches of **C7** and **C8.**

1. The brachiocephalic nerve **courses** directly laterally into the brachiocephalicus muscle at the level of the shoulder joint.
2. It provides **motor branches** to the **brachiocephalicus muscle,** and **sensory branches** to the **skin of the craniolateral, cranial,** and **craniomedial brachial regions**

B. The **subscapular nerve** is formed from the ventral branches of **C6** and **C7** and may be doubled.

1. The subscapular nerve **courses** directly from its origin into the musculature on the medial scapular surface.
2. It provides **motor fibers** to the **subscapularis muscle.**

C. The **suprascapular nerve** is formed from the ventral branches of **C6** and **C7.**

1. The suprascapular nerve **courses** between the subscapularis and supraspinatus muscles (in company with the artery and vein of the same name), and then passes around the cranial surface of the neck of the scapula to gain the lateral surface of the scapula.

*Thoracic limb structures not supplied by the brachial plexus include the trapezius, omotransversarius, part of the brachiocephalicus, the rhomboideus, and the cervical part of the serratus ventralis, as well as the skin of the proximal shoulder region.

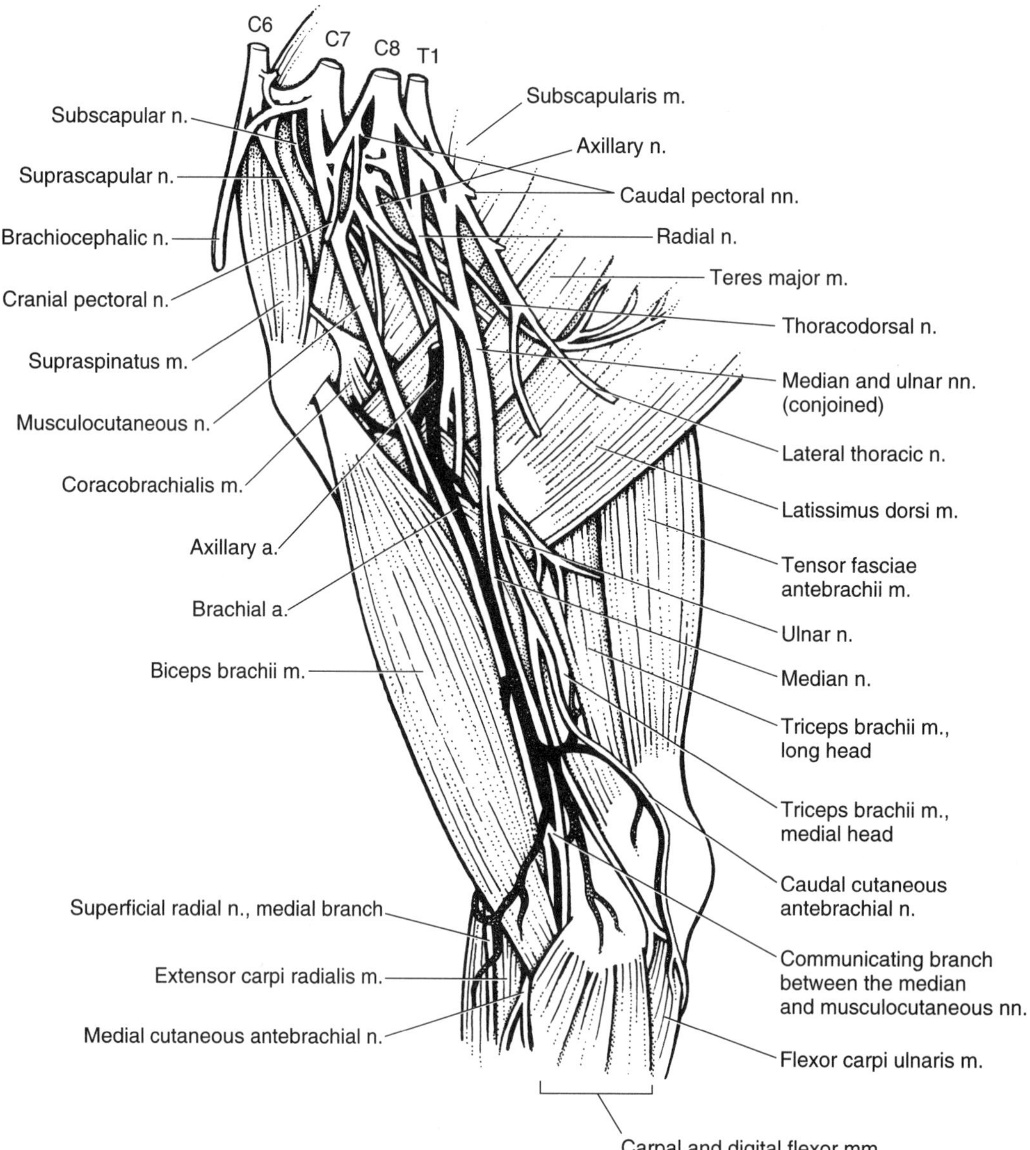

FIGURE 30–1. Formation of the brachial plexus and nerves of the right shoulder and brachium, medial view. (Modified with permission from Evans HE, 1993, *Miller's Anatomy of the Dog,* 3e. Philadelphia, WB Saunders, p 842.)

2. It provides **motor innervation** to the **supraspinatus** and **infraspinatus muscles** and **sensory fibers** to the **shoulder joint capsule.**

D. The **cranial pectoral nerves** are formed from the ventral roots of **C6, C7,** and **C8.**

1. These nerves **course** medially into the pectoral region, in company with the external thoracic artery.
2. The cranial pectoral nerves provide **motor fibers** to the **superficial pectoral muscles.**

E. The **caudal pectoral nerves,** formed from the ventral branches of **C8, T1,** and **T2,** are considered here despite their more caudal origin, for the sake of conceptual grouping with the cranial pectoral nerves.

1. These nerves **course** medially from the brachial plexus, in company with the lateral thoracic artery.
2. They provide **motor innervation** to the **deep pectoral muscles.**

F. The **long thoracic nerve** is formed from the ventral branches of **C7.**

1. This nerve **courses** caudally and horizontally along the superficial surface of the serratus ventralis muscle.
2. It provides **motor fibers** to the **thoracic part of the serratus ventralis muscle.**

G. The **musculocutaneous nerve** is formed from the ventral branches of **C6, C7,** and **C8.**

1. The musculocutaneous nerve **courses** distally through the brachium in a constant position (i.e., **caudal** to the **biceps brachii muscle** and **cranial** to the **brachial artery).** In the distal third of the antebrachium, a **communicating branch** of the musculocutaneous nerve forms a loop and joins with the **median nerve,** delivering motor and sensory fibers to this nerve.
2. **Branches.** The musculocutaneous nerve is responsible for much of the supply to the cranial brachial muscles and has an important sensory component.
   a. **Motor.** The musculocutaneous nerve supplies **motor innervation** to the **biceps brachii** (via a branch into the proximal part of the muscle), the **brachialis** (via a branch into the distal part of the muscle), and the **coracobrachialis.**
   b. **Sensory.** After its last muscular branch, the musculocutaneous nerve continues as the **medial cutaneous antebrachial nerve,** which enters the antebrachium from the flexor surface of the elbow and supplies a branch to the **elbow joint capsule** and an area of **skin on the craniomedial antebrachium.**

H. The **axillary nerve** is formed from the ventral branches of **C7** and **C8.**

1. The axillary nerve **courses** laterally to gain the lateral shoulder region by passing **between the subscapularis** and **teres major muscles.**
2. **Branches**
   a. **Motor.** Branches of the axillary nerve supply the **subscapularis, teres major, teres minor,** and the **deltoideus** (both the spinous and acromial parts).
   b. **Sensory**
      (1) The axillary nerve sends a sensory branch to the **shoulder joint capsule.**
      (2) The **cranial-lateral cutaneous brachial nerve** arises from the axillary nerve as the axillary nerve enters the deltoideus muscle. This branch supplies the **skin over the lateral brachial surface;** this nerve continues into the antebrachium as the **cranial cutaneous antebrachial nerve,** which supplies **skin over the cranial antebrachial surface.**

I. The **thoracodorsal (dorsal thoracic) nerve** is formed from the ventral branches of **C7, C8,** and **T1.**

1. The thoracodorsal nerve **courses** caudally and horizontally along the deep surface of the latissimus dorsi muscle, adjacent to the vessels of the same name.
2. It provides **motor branches** to the **latissimus dorsi muscle.**

J. The **lateral thoracic nerve** is formed from the ventral branches of **C8** and **T1.**

1. The lateral thoracic nerve **courses** caudally in a horizontal position, between the borders of the latissimus dorsi and deep pectoral muscles.
2. It provides **motor innervation** to the **cutaneous trunci muscle** and the **deep pectoral muscles.**

K. The **radial nerve** is formed from the ventral branches of **C7, C8, T1,** and **T2.** The **largest nerve** of the brachial plexus, the radial nerve is often described as the **key nerve of the thoracic limb.**

1. The radial nerve **courses** laterally from the brachial plexus, passing **between the medial and long heads of the triceps brachii,** providing muscular branches *en route.* When it reaches the level of the brachialis muscle, it **follows the brachialis through the musculospiral groove of the humerus** and **divides** into **deep** and **superficial branches** at the level of the lateral head of the triceps.

Canine Clinical Correlation

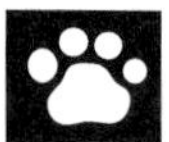

At the level of the division into the deep and superficial branches, the radial nerve lies on the surface of the humerus; therefore, here, it is susceptible to both traumatic and iatrogenic injury.

a. The **deep branch of the radial nerve** passes deep to the extensor carpi radialis.
b. The **superficial branch of the radial nerve** becomes subcutaneous just distal to the lateral head of the triceps, and then **divides** into **medial** and **lateral branches,** which pass distally along the lateral and medial branches of the superficial brachial artery, which courses adjacent to the cephalic vein.
(1) The lateral of the two branches gives rise to the **lateral cutaneous antebrachial nerve.**
(2) Both the medial and lateral cutaneous branches continue distally to the paw.

2. **Branches.** The radial nerve innervates a tremendous amount of muscle mass, including the extensors of the elbow, carpus, and digits. Additionally, the radial nerve has a significant cutaneous component.
a. **Motor**
(1) Before it divides, the **radial nerve** supplies motor innervation to the **extensors of the elbow** (i.e., all heads of the triceps brachii, the tensor fasciae antebrachii, and the anconeus). Intact functioning of the portions of the nerve innervating the triceps brachii is obligatory for weight-bearing of the limb.
(2) The **deep branch of the radial nerve** supplies motor innervation to the **extensors of the carpus and digits** (i.e., the extensor carpi radialis, common digital extensor, lateral digital extensor, and abductor pollicis longus), as well as the **supinator** and **ulnaris lateralis.**
b. **Sensory**
(1) The **superficial branch of the radial nerve** supplies the **skin of the cranial antebrachial surface,** as well as the **skin of the dorsum of the paw.**
(2) The **lateral branch of the superficial branch of the radial nerve** supplies the **skin over the lateral humeral epicondyle.**

L. The **median nerve** is formed from the ventral branches of **C8, T1, T2,** and a **common trunk with the ulnar nerve.**

1. It **courses** through the brachium, without giving off any muscular or sensory branches, and into the antebrachium.
a. **Brachial region.** The median nerve remains **caudal to the brachial artery and vein** throughout its brachial course.
(1) **Proximal brachial region.** The median nerve is **loosely bound with and positioned cranial to the ulnar nerve;** the two diverge approximately halfway distally along the brachium.
(2) **Distal brachial region.** The median nerve detaches a **communicating branch** to the **musculocutaneous nerve.**
b. **Antebrachial region.** At the level of the elbow, the median nerve passes **deep to the pronator teres,** where it provides numerous muscular branches to the muscles on the caudomedial antebrachial surface. It then continues distally into the antebrachium, where it is first **associated with the median artery,** and then with the **ulnar artery.**

2. **Branches**
   a. **Motor.** The median nerve provides motor innervation to **most flexors of the carpus and digits** (i.e., the flexor carpi radialis, superficial digital flexor, and the radial and ulnar heads of the deep digital flexor), the **pronator teres,** and the **pronator quadratus.** The median nerve also contributes minor motor innervation to the **paw.**
   b. **Sensory.** The median nerve provides a twig to the **elbow joint capsule** and plays an important role in the cutaneous innervation of the **paw.**

M. The **ulnar nerve** is formed from the ventral branches of **C8, T1, T2,** and a **common trunk with the median nerve.**

1. The ulnar nerve **courses** through the brachium and into the antebrachium.
   a. **Brachial region.** The ulnar nerve remains **caudal to the brachial artery and vein** throughout its brachial course.
      (1) **Proximal brachial region.** The ulnar nerve is **loosely bound with and positioned caudal to the median nerve** in the proximal brachial region, where the two run together.
      (2) **Distal brachial region.** After diverging from the median nerve, the ulnar nerve passes along the **cranial border of the medial head of the triceps brachii.** At about this level, the **caudal cutaneous antebrachial nerve** leaves the ulnar nerve and passes over the medial surface of the olecranon process and into the antebrachium. The caudal cutaneous antebrachial nerve accompanies the collateral ulnar artery and vein throughout its distal brachial course.
   b. **Antebrachial region.** After detaching its antebrachial cutaneous branch, the ulnar nerve crosses the medial humeral epicondyle, passes deep to the ulnar head of the flexor carpi ulnaris, and then passes between the humeral heads of the flexor carpi ulnaris and deep digital flexor, where it courses the remainder of the length of the antebrachium. At about midantebrachium, the ulnar nerve **divides** into a **dorsal part** (mostly sensory to the skin) and a **palmar part** (sensory to the skin and motor to the paw muscles).

2. **Branches**
   a. **Motor**
      (1) **Antebrachium.** The ulnar nerve provides motor innervation to **some flexors of the carpus and digits** (i.e., the flexor carpi ulnaris and the ulnar and humeral heads of the deep digital flexor).
      (2) **Paw.** The ulnar nerve is motor to the **interosseus** and **other muscles of the paw.**
   b. Sensory. By means of its primary course and also via ascending branches, the **caudal cutaneous antebrachial nerve** supplies the **skin of the distal brachial** and **caudolateral antebrachial regions.** The terminal parts of the ulnar nerve are also essential to the cutaneous innervation of the **paw.**

III. NERVES OF THE BRACHIAL PLEXUS IN THE MANUS. The **radial, median,** and **ulnar nerves** provide motor and sensory innervation of the manus (Table 30–1, Figure 30–2).

A. **General pattern of innervation.** As is the case with the arterial supply, the nerves of the manus are best considered in two general regions: the metacarpal region and the digital region.

1. **Metacarpal region.** By using three descriptors (surface, depth, position), the nerves in the metacarpal region can be identified (see also Chapter 29 I E 1).
   a. **Surface.** As with the arteries of the manus, the **nerves of the manus** are divided into **dorsal** and **palmar sets.**
   b. **Depth**
      (1) **Dorsal set (dorsal common digital nerves).** The dorsal set consists only of a **superficial** set of nerves. The nerves are superficial to the extensor tendons and parallel the common digital arteries.

TABLE 30–1. Summary of the Contributions of the Radial, Median, and Ulnar Nerves to the Innervation of the Manus

Nerve	Sensory Innervation	Motor Innervation
Radial nerve	Skin on the dorsum of the paw (except for the lateral-most surface of digit V); skin over the first metacarpal bone and the first digit on the palmar surface of the paw	None
Median nerve	Skin on the palmar surface of the paw over metacarpal bones II–IV, the metacarpal pad, and most of the palmar surfaces of digits II–V	Interflexorius muscle
Ulnar nerve	Skin on the palmar edge of the paw, over metacarpal bone IV, the abaxial surface of digit IV, and both surfaces of digit V	Most muscles of the paw

(2) **Palmar set.** The palmar nerves comprise both a **superficial** and a **deep set,** which parallel the adjacent arteries.

(a) The **palmar common digital nerves** are the **superficial set,** placed between the superficial and deep digital flexor tendons.

(b) The **palmar metacarpal nerves** are the **deep set,** placed directly on the palmar surfaces of the metacarpal bones.

c. **Position.** Like the arteries, the common digital and metacarpal nerves are numbered I–IV, from medial to lateral.

2. **Digital region.** The digital region is innervated on both its **dorsal** and **palmar** surfaces.

a. **Formation.** Like the arteries, the metacarpal and common digital nerves join together at the metacarpophalangeal region, and then each common digital nerve bifurcates into two nerves, which pass distally on the adjacent sides of adjacent digits. These nerves parallel the proper digital arteries and are called the **proper digital nerves.**

b. **Identification.** The proper digital nerves are **identified by number,** according to the digit on which they are located, and because each digit has two proper digital nerves, the terms **abaxial** and **axial** are used to differentiate the two.

B. Sensory innervation

1. **Metacarpal region**

a. **Dorsal surface.** Dorsal digital nerve I and the dorsal common digital nerves II–IV **arise from the terminal branches of the radial nerve.**

b. **Palmar surface**

(1) **Palmar common digital nerves**

(a) **I–III** arise from the terminal branches of the **median nerve.**

(b) **IV** arises from the **dorsal branch of the ulnar nerve.**

(2) **Palmar metacarpal nerves I–IV** arise from the **palmar branch of the ulnar nerve.** Occasionally, the **median nerve** contributes to the first two palmar metacarpal nerves.

2. **Digital region**

a. **Dorsal surface.** The **dorsal proper digital nerves,** all save one, arise from the terminal branches of the **radial nerve** via the dorsal common digital nerves. **Abaxial dorsal proper digital nerve V** is the continuation of the dorsal branch of the **ulnar nerve.**

b. **Palmar surface**

(1) **Axial and abaxial palmar proper digital nerves I–III** and **axial palmar proper digital nerve IV** arise from the terminal branches of the **median nerve.**

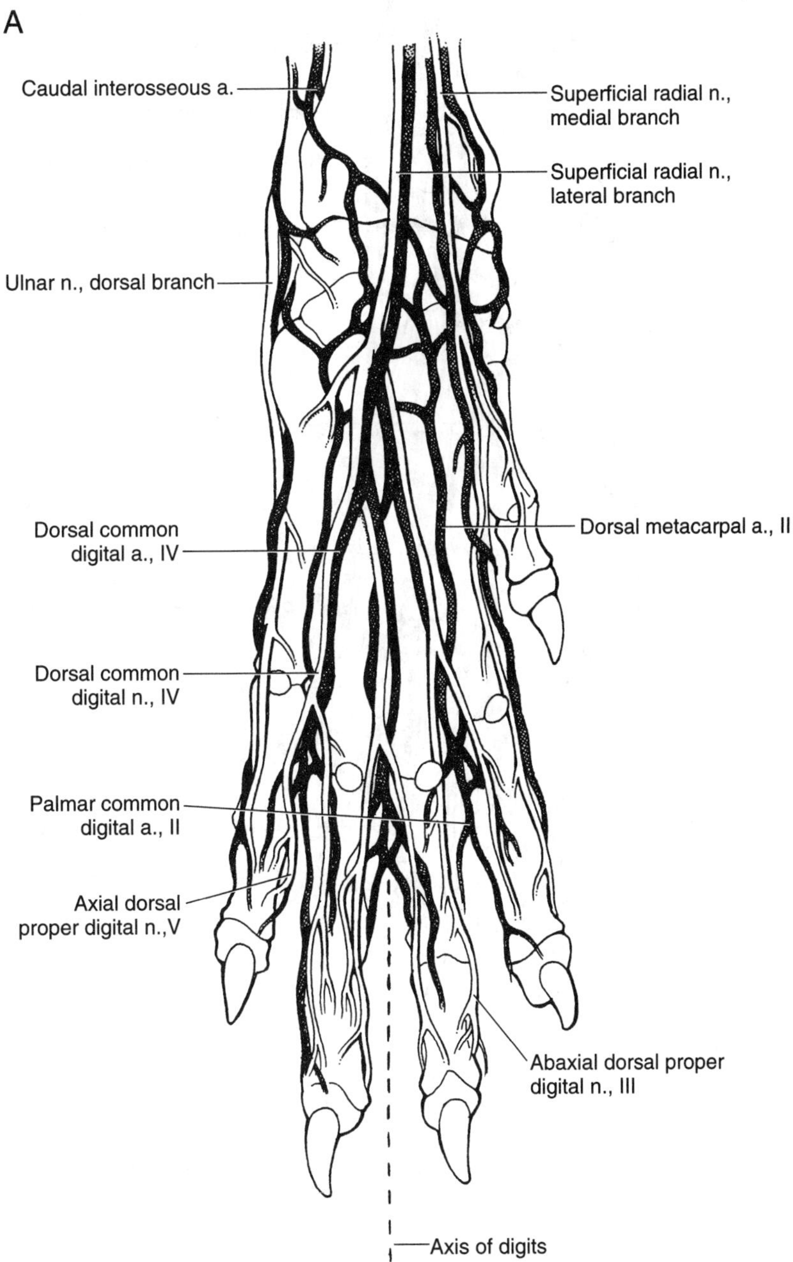

FIGURE 30–2. Nerves and arteries of the right manus. (*A*) Dorsal view. (*continued*)

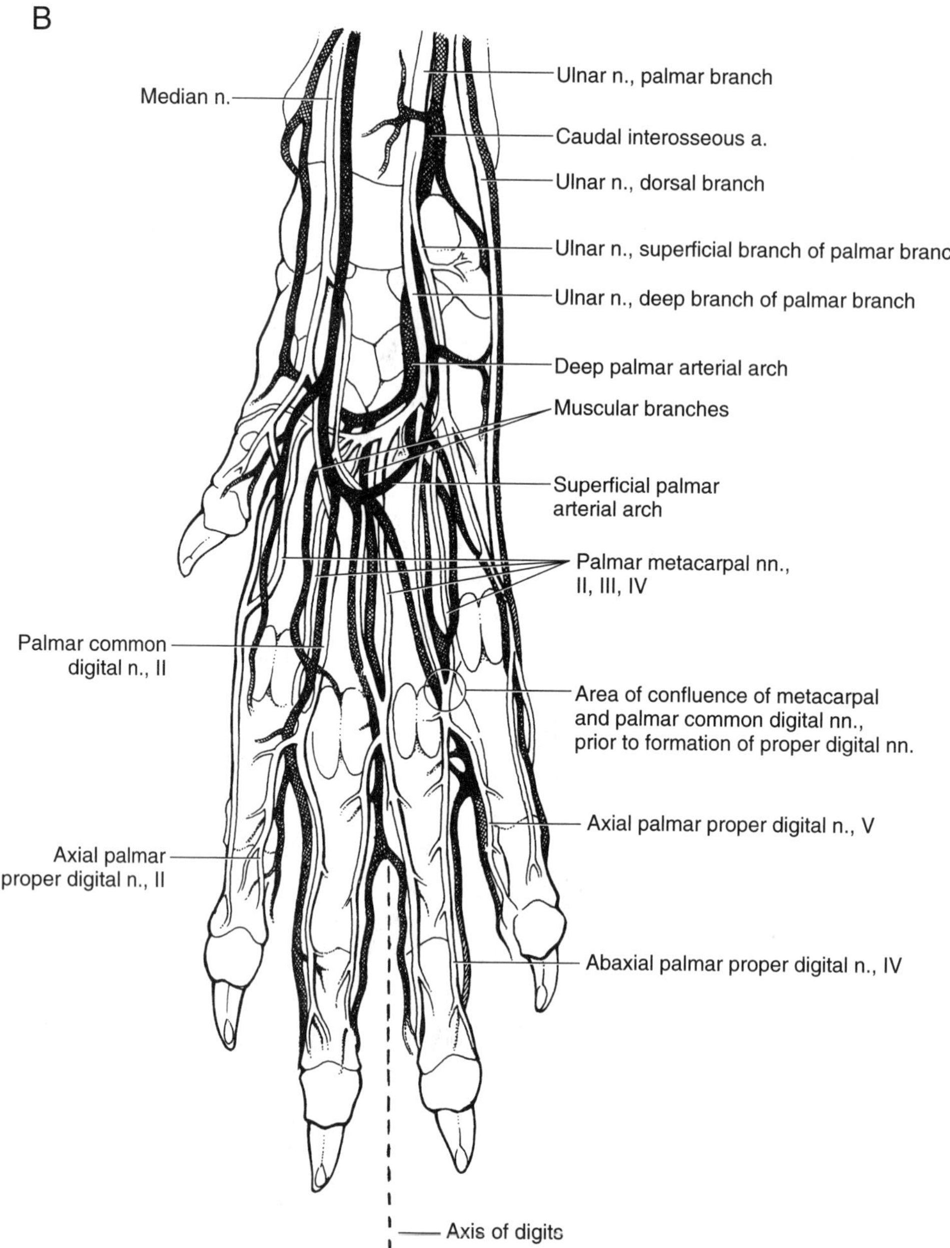

FIGURE 30–2—*continued* (*B*) Palmar view. (Modified with permission from Evans HE, 1993, *Miller's Anatomy of the Dog,* 3e. Philadelphia, WB Saunders, pp 855, 856.)

(2) **Abaxial palmar proper digital nerve IV** and **axial and abaxial palmar proper digital nerves V** arise from the terminal branches of the **ulnar nerve.**

C. **Motor innervation.** Most motor nerves of the manus, which pass to the interosseous muscles and the minute specialized digital muscles, arise from the **ulnar nerve,** either directly from its deep branch or from the palmar metacarpal nerves.

Chapter 31

Prominent Palpable Features of the Thoracic Limb

I. BONY STRUCTURES

A. Shoulder region

1. The **scapula** presents several palpable features.
   a. **Dorsal border**—prominent over nearly the full length of the scapula
   b. **Cranial border**—palpable over the proximal half
   c. **Cranial** and **caudal angles**—readily recognizable
   d. **Supraglenoid tubercle**—can be appreciated deep on the cranial end of the ventral angle
   e. **Spine**—prominent essentially throughout its length
   f. **Acromion**—readily recognizable at the distal end of the spine
2. The **shoulder joint** can be appreciated by placing the flat part of the fingers a bit distal to the acromion and flexing and extending the shoulder by moving the humerus.

B. Brachial region. Several features of the **humerus** are palpable:

1. The **greater tubercle** is prominent on the lateral proximal surface of the humerus, as is its **crest** passing distally from it.
2. The **cranial humeral border** is palpable through much of its length, between the lateral and medial muscle masses.
3. The **deltoid tuberosity** is prominent on the lateral humeral shaft approximately one third of the way distally along the bone.

C. Elbow region

1. The **medial** and **lateral humeral epicondyles** are prominent as distinctly elevated structures on the proximal part of the humeral condyle, on the respective sides of the elbow.
2. The **medial** and **lateral surfaces of the humeral condyle** continue distally from the epicondyles. The rounded contours of each side of the condyle can be felt all the way around, beginning in the area of the olecranon and continuing cranially.
3. The **olecranon tuberosity** is immediately recognizable as a large, almost rectangular bar projecting proximal to the caudal surface of the elbow joint. The tuberosity projects to the medial side of the joint.
4. The **radial head** is palpable deeply on the medial surface of the elbow joint. Placing a thumb over the surface of the radial head and then passing the elbow through its limited rotational range of motion often causes the radial head to turn appreciably under the thumb.
5. The **flexion** and **extension of the elbow joint** is best appreciated by placing the thumb and fingers just cranial to the humeral condyles while moving the joint.
6. The limited **rotation of the elbow joint** is best appreciated by cupping the caudal surface of the proximal ulna in the fingers, placing the thumb over the radial head, and passing the joint through its rotatory motion.

D. Antebrachial region

1. **Radius**
   a. The **radial head** is easily discerned (see I C 4).
   b. The **radial shaft** is palpable subcutaneously over much of the distomedial third of the antebrachium, where it becomes prominent after the muscle bellies of the extensors and flexors of the carpus and digits have narrowed to tendons.

c. The **medial styloid process** is palpable subcutaneously at the distal extremity of the radius, just proximal to the carpus.

2. **Ulna**

a. The **olecranon tuberosity** can be palpated as described in I C 3.

b. The **ulnar shaft** is palpable subcutaneously over almost the full length of the caudal antebrachium.

c. The **lateral styloid process** is palpable subcutaneously at the distal extremity of the ulna, just proximal to the carpus. The caudal border of the ulna can be palpated all the way to the lateral styloid process.

E. Carpal region

1. The **carpal bones** can be appreciated distal to the distal ends of the antebrachial bones. Only the **accessory carpal bone** can be individually identified, because it projects so far caudally from the remaining carpal bones.
2. The **antebrachiocarpal joint** can be recognized as a soft area between the rows of bones when the joint in flexed.

F. Metacarpal region

1. The **metacarpal bones** are palpable both as a group (proximally) and individually (distally, where they diverge to meet the proximal phalanges of their respective digits). The bony substance of the metacarpal bones is best appreciated from the dorsal surface, because palmarly they are largely covered by the substantive interosseous muscles.
2. The **metacarpophalangeal joints** are largely inaccessible to palpation, because those within the antebrachial region are largely immobile, and those within the proximal phalanges are covered by the metacarpal pad.

G. Digital region.

Digital region. In this region, structures are largely reduced to bones, tendons, and tiny vessels and nerves. Essentially the sole structures that can be appreciated by palpation are the **proximal interdigital joints,** because the distal interdigital joints are largely obscured by the digital pads.

II. SOFT TISSUE STRUCTURES

A. Shoulder region

1. The **borders of the axilla** can be palpated softly with the hands if the forelimb is gently abducted from the body wall. The borders are the:

a. Pectoral muscles (cranially)

b. Teres major muscle (caudally)

c. Thoracic wall (medially)

d. Subscapularis muscle on the medial surface of the scapula (laterally)

d. Skin (ventrally)

2. The **supraspinatus muscle** fills the supraspinous fossa dorsocranial to the scapular spine, where it is readily palpable.
3. The **infraspinatus muscle** is palpable in the infraspinous fossa ventrocaudal to the scapular spine; here it is covered by the thin substance of the **spinous part of the deltoideus muscle.**

B. Brachial region

1. The **superficial** and **deep pectoral muscles** are palpable as they approach the humeral tubercles. These muscles are best appreciated in the standing dog by placing the hands over the back and reaching in cranial to the thoracic limb (to palpate the superficial pectoral muscles) and reaching in caudal to the thoracic limb (to palpate the deep pectoral muscles).

2. The **latissimus dorsi muscle** is palpable on the caudomedial proximal humerus as it nears its insertion point. The **teres major** is also present in this vicinity, though it cannot be appreciated as a separate entity.
3. The **deltoideus muscle** is palpable proximal to the deltoid tuberosity as it approaches this elevation for insertion.
4. The **biceps brachii muscle** is readily palpable on the craniomedial humeral region along the distal two-thirds of the humerus, distal to the insertion of the pectoral muscles.
5. The **brachialis muscle** is readily accessible on the distal lateral humeral shaft as it passes distally from under cover of the lateral head of the triceps brachii.
6. The **triceps brachii muscle** is palpable over much of the caudomedial and caudolateral brachial region. The **long, lateral,** and **medial heads** essentially fill the triangular space between the caudal scapular border and the humeral shaft; together, they form the huge muscular mass that can be grasped between the thumb and fingers from the caudal humeral surface.

C. Carpal region

1. The **tendons of the extensor carpi radialis** (medially, just as the muscle belly lies at the proximal end of the antebrachium) and the **common digital extensor** are palpable as they cross the antebrachiocarpal joint.
2. The **insertions of the flexor carpi ulnaris** and the **ulnaris lateralis on the accessory carpal bone** are readily appreciable.

D. Metacarpal region

1. The **tendons of the digital extensors** are palpable as they cross the dorsal surface of the metacarpal bones. Rolling the tendons against the metacarpal bones beneath them may allow appreciation of the tendons passing to individual digits.
2. The **tendons of the digital flexors** are palpable as a soft mass as they cross the palmar surface of the metacarpal bones. However, they are not distinguishable individually, partly because of the position of the interosseous muscles deep to them.
3. The **interosseous muscles** can be appreciated as a yielding soft tissue mass on the palmar surface of the metacarpus.

STUDY QUESTIONS

DIRECTIONS: Each of the numbered items or incomplete statements in this section is followed by answers or by completions of the statement. Select the ONE numbered answer or completion that is BEST in each case.

1. Which of the following joints has the greatest number of bones involved in forming the joint?

(1) Glenohumeral joint
(2) Brachioantebrachial joint
(3) Antebrachiocarpal joint
(4) Carpometacarpal joint

2. Which one of the following statements regarding the digits of the manus is true?

(1) They are composed of phalanges.
(2) They articulate with the proximal manus at the metacarpodigital joints.
(3) They are numbered 1–5 from lateral to medial.
(4) Their distal bony elements are rounded nubbins that seat the claw.

3. Which one of the following statements regarding the canine clavicle is true?

(1) It is generally ossified.
(2) It is embedded in the substance of the major pectoral muscle.
(3) It is unimportant clinically because of its small size and variable ossification.
(4) It provides the major supportive attachment for the musculature in the area of the clavicular intersection.

4. Which one of the following statements regarding the scapula is true?

(1) It is marked by a prominent longitudinal spine on its medial surface.
(2) It presents a deep glenoid fossa that contributes to the ball-and-socket form of the shoulder joint.
(3) It provides attachment for muscles extending between the body and limb, as well as among areas of the limb itself.
(4) It presents the coracoid process, a prominent, medially directed elevation providing attachment for the coracobrachialis muscle.

5. Where does the deltoideus muscle attach to the scapula?

(1) Supraglenoid tubercle
(2) Acromion
(3) Deltoid tuberosity
(4) Coracoid process

6. The humerus is characterized by:

(1) greater and lesser condyles at its distal end.
(2) a hemispherical head that faces laterally and articulates with the scapula.
(3) the large and prominent deltoid tuberosity on the medial side of the humeral shaft.
(4) a relatively indistinct neck at the junction of the head and the shaft.

7. Which one of the following statements regarding the bones of the antebrachium is true?

(1) The ulna is the major weight-bearing bone.
(2) The radius and ulna share weight-bearing approximately equally.
(3) The ulna courses largely parallel to the radius but extends beyond it both proximally and distally.
(4) The radius articulates with the lateral side of the distal humerus, and the ulna articulates with the medial side of the distal humerus.

8. The ulnar notch of the radius:

(1) articulates with the anconeal process of the ulna.
(2) articulates with the distal end of the ulna.
(3) is an indentation midway down the shaft of the radius where the two bones contact each other.
(4) provides an articulation site for the radius with the styloid process of the ulna.

9. Which one of the following statements regarding the carpal bones is true?

(1) The ulnar carpal bone is the most lateral bone in the proximal-most row.
(2) The first carpal bone is the most lateral in the distal-most row.
(3) There are four carpal bones in the proximal row and three carpal bones in the distal row.
(4) The rows of carpal bones contribute to three different joints.

10. Which one of the following statements regarding the metacarpal bones is true?

(1) They number five and are identified by Roman numeral from medial to lateral.
(2) They number four and are identified by Roman numeral from medial to lateral.
(3) They articulate with the distal row of carpal bones by their heads.
(4) They articulate with the proximal phalanges by their bases.

11. Which one of the following accurately characterizes the glenohumeral (shoulder) joint?

(1) Formed by the scapula, the humerus, and a sesamoid bone
(2) Robust thickenings in the medial and lateral surfaces of the joint capsule
(3) Single cavity of the joint capsule
(4) Wide range of motion

12. Which joint is characterized by the following features: single joint capsule, two bones contributing to the joint, no collateral ligaments, transverse humeral ligament?

(1) Glenohumeral joint
(2) Brachioantebrachial joint
(3) Humeroradial subjoint
(4) Humeroulnar subjoint

13. Which subjoint affords the limited range of rotation characteristic of the brachioantebrachial joint in the dog?

(1) Humeroradial
(2) Humeroulnar
(3) Proximal radioulnar
(4) Distal radioulnar

14. In the manus, the dorsal ligament characterizes the:

(1) metacarpophalangeal joint.
(2) proximal interphalangeal joint.
(3) middle interphalangeal joint.
(4) distal interphalangeal joint.

15. Which muscle is the smallest muscle in the superficial layer of antebrachial muscles?

(1) Extensor carpi radialis
(2) Common digital extensor
(3) Lateral digital extensor
(4) Ulnaris lateralis

16. Which flexor muscle is innervated by the radial nerve?

(1) Pronator quadratus
(2) Flexor carpi radialis
(3) Ulnaris lateralis
(4) Deep digital flexor

17. Which extrinsic thoracic limb muscle originates on the sternum, passes across the ventral body surface, inserts on the humerus, and is innervated by the cranial pectoral nerves?

(1) Superficial pectoral
(2) Deep pectoral
(3) Serratus ventralis
(4) Pectoralis profundus

18. All of the following muscles are shoulder flexors. Which member of the group does not belong with the others, based on the nature of the attachments of the muscles?

(1) Teres major
(2) Latissimus dorsi
(3) Teres minor
(4) Long head of the triceps brachii

19. Which one of the following muscles follows a convoluted course from its attachment site (the proximal caudolateral humeral surface) to its insertion site (the distal craniomedial humeral surface)?

(1) Brachialis
(2) Biceps brachii
(3) Coracobrachialis
(4) Long head of the triceps

20. Which thoracic limb muscle extends across the medial surface of the shoulder joint, is innervated by the musculocutaneous nerve, and possesses uniquely elongate tendons both at its origin and insertion point?

(1) Supraspinatus
(2) Subscapularis
(3) Coracobrachialis
(4) Lateral head of the triceps

21. Which caudal antebrachial muscle is characterized by innervation by two nerves?

(1) Flexor carpi radialis
(2) Flexor carpi ulnaris
(3) Pronator quadratus
(4) Deep digital flexor

22. The interosseous muscles of the paw:

(1) arise from the metacarpal bones.
(2) are powerful flexors of the interphalangeal joints.
(3) lie deep to the superficial digital flexor tendons.
(4) are characterized by paired sesamoid bones in the tendons of the dorsal set.

23. Although most of the thoracic limb musculature is supplied by arterial branches arising from the axillary artery external to the thoracic cavity, some thoracic limb muscles receive their major arterial supply from an artery arising inside the thorax. What is this artery?

(1) Deep cervical artery
(2) Infraclavian artery
(3) Superficial cervical artery
(4) Brachiocephalic artery

24. It is necessary to amputate the left thoracic limb of a German shepherd that has been hit by a car. The veterinarian wishes to preserve the scapula and its associated musculature. Where should ligation of the arterial supply to the thoracic limb take place?

(1) At the origin of the axillary artery
(2) Distal to the origin of the axillary artery, but proximal to the origin of the subscapular artery
(3) Just proximal to the origin of the deep brachial artery
(4) Distal to the origin of the subscapular artery but proximal to the origin of the cranial circumflex humeral artery

25. Essentially complete compromise of the arterial flow to the biceps brachii muscle would result from occlusion of which two of the following arteries?

(1) Bicipital and deep brachial arteries
(2) Bicipital and cranial circumflex humeral arteries
(3) Bicipital and caudal circumflex humeral arteries
(4) Deep brachial and cranial circumflex humeral arteries
(5) Cranial and caudal circumflex humeral arteries

26. Which thoracic limb artery is unusual in that it extends beyond the anatomic region for which it is named?

(1) Median artery
(2) Brachial artery
(3) Deep brachial artery
(4) Deep antebrachial artery

27. Which branch of the brachial artery is most important in the blood supply to the dorsal part of the forepaw?

(1) Median artery
(2) Collateral ulnar artery
(3) Deep antebrachial artery
(4) Superficial brachial artery

28. Which artery occupies the space between metacarpal bones II and III on the palmar surface of the paw?

(1) Palmar metacarpal artery II
(2) Palmar metacarpal artery III
(3) Palmar common digital artery II
(4) Palmar common digital artery III

29. Which vein is most commonly accessed for venipuncture in the dog?

(1) Antebrachial part of the cephalic vein
(2) Cranial antebrachial vein
(3) Satellite vein of the median artery
(4) External jugular vein

30. A veterinarian is performing shoulder surgery on a dog, necessitating reflection of the distal part of the deltoideus muscle. What major vein passing just under this muscle must he watch for in this approach?

(1) Axillary vein
(2) Cephalic vein
(3) Omobrachial vein
(4) Axillobrachial vein

31. Trauma to the medial epicondyle of the humerus affects muscles innervated by the:

(1) radial nerve.
(2) median nerve.
(3) ulnar nerve.
(4) median and ulnar nerves.

32. A dog sustains a fracture to the neck of the scapula. What action is most likely to be impaired as a result of concomitant nerve injury?

(1) Extension of the shoulder
(2) Flexion of the shoulder
(3) Adduction of the shoulder
(4) Extension and flexion of the shoulder

33. Which one of the following nerves has a cutaneous component in both the brachium and antebrachium?

(1) Long thoracic nerve
(2) Axillary nerve
(3) Median nerve
(4) Ulnar nerve

34. Compromise of the ulnar nerve would most directly affect:

(1) the ability of the limb to bear weight.
(2) extension of the carpus and digits.
(3) cutaneous sensation over the medial antebrachium.
(4) maintenance of proper joint angle in the carpal region.

35. A dog is brought to the veterinarian because he is limping. He carries the shoulder and elbow in active flexion (i.e., by active muscle contraction) and the carpus in passive flexion (i.e., limply, without muscular effort). The dorsum of the paw is turned toward the ground. Which nerve has most likely been injured?

(1) Axillary nerve
(2) Radial nerve
(3) Median nerve
(4) Musculocutaneous nerve

36. Which nerve passes on the dorsal surface of the paw and is related to the space between the third and fourth metacarpal bones?

(1) Dorsal common digital nerve III
(2) Dorsal metacarpal nerve III
(3) Dorsal common digital nerve IV
(4) Dorsal metacarpal nerve IV

37. Which nerve passes along the lateral side of the palmar surface of digit IV?

(1) Abaxial palmar common digital nerve IV
(2) Axial palmar common digital nerve IV
(3) Abaxial palmar digital nerve IV
(4) Axial palmar digital nerve IV

38. Which carpal bone can be individually palpated?

(1) Radial carpal
(2) Ulnar carpal
(3) Accessory carpal
(4) Intermedioradial carpal

DIRECTIONS: Each of the numbered items or incomplete statements in this section is negatively phrased, as indicated by a capitalized word such as NOT, LEAST, or EXCEPT. Select the ONE numbered answer or completion that is BEST in each case.

39. Which of the following descriptors is NOT a feature of the common digital extensor?

(1) It extends the carpus.
(2) It is innervated by the same nerve as the supinator.
(3) It originates from the medial humeral epicondyle.
(4) It crosses six joints.

40. Which one of the following is NOT an action of the biceps brachii?

(1) Shoulder extension
(2) Shoulder flexion
(3) Elbow rotation
(4) Elbow flexion

41. Fracture of the lateral epicondyle of the humerus could potentially affect all of the following motions. Which one would be LEAST affected?

(1) Elbow flexion
(2) Carpal joint extension
(3) Rotation of the paw inward
(4) Interphalangeal joint extension

42. Venous blood returning to the heart from the thoracic limb could reach the central venous flow by entering any of the following veins EXCEPT the:

(1) omobrachial vein.
(2) axillobrachial vein.
(3) internal jugular vein.
(4) external jugular vein.

ANSWERS AND EXPLANATIONS

1. The answer is 4 [Chapter 25 III]. Ten bones contribute to the carpometacarpal joint, which is the joint between the carpus (wrist) and the manus (paw). These ten bones are the five metacarpals, the four bones of the distal carpal row, and the accessory carpal bone. The glenohumeral (shoulder) joint is formed by the articulation of the scapula and humerus. The brachioantebrachial (elbow) joint is formed from the humerus, radius, and ulna. The antebrachiocarpal joint, which is the joint between the arm and the wrist, is contributed to by five bones (the radius, ulna, and the proximal row of carpal bones).

2. The answer is 1 [Chapter 25 II E 1 b; Chapter 26 IV C]. The digits are composed of small bones called the phalanges and are numbered I–V from medial to lateral. The digits articulate with the manus at the metacarpophalangeal joints. Their distal bony elements are modified into a curved elongate shape similar to the claw itself.

3. The answer is 1 [Chapter 26 I A]. The canine clavicle is ossified in approximately 80% of dogs. The clavicle lies within the cleidobrachialis muscle, but affords little substantive attachment for the muscle. Attachment for the muscle is actually provided by the thick, fibrous substance of the clavicular intersection itself. The clavicle is clinically important because its appearance on a radiograph may be misinterpreted as an anomaly.

4. The answer is 3 [Chapter 26 I B]. The scapula provides attachment for muscles extending between the body and the limb, as well as among areas of the limb itself. The prominent scapular spine is a feature of the lateral, not the medial, surface of the bone. The glenoid fossa is markedly shallow. The coracoid process is a small medial eminence.

5. The answer is 2 [Chapter 26 I B 2]. The acromion is a knob-like thickening on the distal end of the spine of the scapula where part of the deltoideus muscle attaches. The supraglenoid tubercle of the scapula provides attachment for the biceps brachii muscle, while its coracoid process provides attachment for the coracobrachialis muscle. The deltoid tuberosity does provide attachment for the deltoideus muscle, but the deltoid tuberosity is a feature of the humerus, rather than the scapula.

6. The answer is 4 [Chapter 26 II A 5]. The humerus is characterized by a relatively indistinct neck at the junction of the head and the shaft. "Greater" and "lesser" refer to the tubercles of the humerus. The hemispherical humeral head faces caudally. The deltoid tuberosity is located on the lateral surface of the humeral body.

7. The answer is 4 [Chapter 26 III A 1 b, B 1 b]. Rather than paralleling each other, the ulna and radius cross each other obliquely on their course through the antebrachium. The proximal radius is positioned laterally, and the proximal ulna is positioned medially. The ulna bears no weight whatsoever.

8. The answer is 2 [Chapter 26 III A 2 c (2)]. The ulnar notch is a small, indistinct facet for articulation with the ulna located on the distal radius. Neither the anconeal nor the styloid processes of the ulna articulate with the radius. The radius and ulna are separated from each other along most of their shafts, including the midregion, by the interosseous space.

9. The answer is 4 [Chapter 25 II D 1; III C–D]. The two rows of carpal bones contribute to the antebrachiocarpal, intercarpal, and carpometacarpal joints. The proximal carpal bones are, from medial to lateral, the intermedioradial carpal bone, the ulnar carpal bone, and the accessory carpal bone. The distal carpal bones are, from medial to lateral, I–V.

10. The answer is 1 [Chapter 25 II E 1 a; Chapter 26 IV B]. There are five metacarpal bones, designated I–V from medial to lateral. The orientation of the metacarpal bones (and phalanges) may seem backwards, but these bones are described as oriented with their bases proximally and their heads distally.

11. The answer is 3 [Chapter 27 I]. The shoulder joint capsule consists of a single cavity that extends between the scapula and the humerus. No sesamoid bones are associated with the shoulder. The medial and lateral glenohumeral ligaments are quite thin and weak. Although the glenohumeral joint is a ball-and-socket joint, in dogs, the practical range of motion is mainly extension and flexion.

12. The answer is 1 [Chapter 27 I B]. The lack of collateral ligaments and the presence of the transverse humeral ligament positively identify the joint as the glenohumeral (shoulder) joint.

13. The answer is 3 [Chapter 27 II B 1 c]. The proximal radioulnar subjoint of the brachioantebrachial joint contributes to the limited rotatory motion of the elbow. The nestling of the articular circumference of the radius into the radial notch of the ulna provides the surface for the elbow's rotatory movements. The motion at the humeroulnar and humeroradial joints is mainly extension–flexion. The distal radioulnar joint is found in the carpal region.

14. The answer is 4 [Chapter 27 VI B 3 b]. The dorsal ligament holds the claw in passive retraction, and thus is found at the distal interphalangeal joint. (Note that no "middle" interphalangeal joint is present in the manus.)

15. The answer is 3 [Chapter 28 II C 1 a (3)]. The lateral digital extensor is the smallest of the four muscles in the craniolateral antebrachial muscle group. This muscle extends the carpus and the digital joints.

16. The answer is 3 [Table 28–2]. The ulnaris lateralis, which flexes the carpus, is innervated by the radial nerve. This muscle developmentally groups with the extensor muscles of the carpus and digits, but in the final form attaches sufficiently caudally that it becomes a functional flexor of the joint. The pronator teres rotates the antebrachial bones and is innervated by the median nerve. Like the ulnaris lateralis, the flexor carpi radialis flexes the carpus, but this muscle is innervated by the median nerve. The deep digital flexor flexes the carpus and the digital joints, but is innervated by the median and ulnar nerves.

17. The answer is 1 [Chapter 28 I A; Table 28–1]. Both the superficial and deep pectoral muscles originate on the sternum, pass across the ventral body surface, and insert on the crest of the greater tubercle of the humerus. However, the deep pectoral muscle (pectoralis profundus) is innervated by the caudal pectoral nerves, whereas the superficial pectoral muscle is innervated by the cranial pectoral nerves. Therefore, the description given in the question most aptly applies to the superficial pectoral muscle.

18. The answer is 2 [Chapter 28 I G; Table 28–1; Table 28–2]. The latissimus dorsi is an extrinsic limb muscle that originates from the thoracolumbar fascia. The teres major, teres minor, and long head of the triceps brachii are intrinsic to the limb (i.e., they arise and insert on the limb).

19. The answer is 1 [Table 28–2]. The brachialis muscle arises from the proximal lateral humerus, and then courses along the caudolateral humeral shaft, turning medially to cross the elbow. The brachialis then inserts on the distal craniomedial humeral surface. The biceps brachii, coracobrachialis, and lateral head of the triceps do not have their proximal attachments on the humerus. The biceps brachii courses medially to insert on the radial and ulnar tuberosities; the coracobrachialis takes a direct course from the scapula to the proximal (not distal) humerus, and the long head of the triceps, placed caudally on the brachium, has no humeral attachment at all.

20. The answer is 3 [Table 28–2]. The coracobrachialis extends across the medial surface of the shoulder joint, is innervated by the musculocutaneous nerve, and possesses tendons at both its origin and insertion points.

21. The answer is 4 [Table 28–2]. The deep digital flexor is innervated by both the median and ulnar nerves—the radial head of the deep digital flexor is supplied by the median nerve, the ulnar head is supplied by the ulnar nerve, and the humeral head (because of its large size) is supplied by both the median and ulnar nerves. The flexor carpi radialis and pronator quadratus are innervated by the median nerve, and the flexor carpi ulnaris is innervated by the ulnar nerve.

22. The answer is 1 [Chapter 27 V B 2 a (2)–(3); Chapter 28 II D; Table 28–1]. The interossei arise from the metacarpal bones and lie directly on the palmar surface of the metacarpal bones; therefore, they are deep to the deep digital flexor tendons, not the superficial digital flexor tendons. These muscles are flexors of the metacarpophalangeal joints, not the interphalangeal joints. There is no dorsal set of interosseous muscles, although paired sesamoid bones are present in the muscles at the metacarpophalangeal joints.

23. The answer is 3 [Chapter 29 I B 1 a, c (1)–(2)]. The superficial cervical artery supplies muscles of the shoulder and caudal neck region associated with the limb, such as (but not limited to) the supraspinatus, infraspinatus, and brachiocephalicus muscles. It originates inside the thorax.

24. The answer is 4 [Chapter 29 I B 2 (c) (3), (4)]. In order to preserve the scapula and its associated musculature, the axillary artery should be ligated distal to the origin of the subscapular artery but proximal to the origin of the cranial circumflex humeral artery. Ligation of the axillary at its origin (i.e., at the level of the first rib) or proximal to the subscapular artery would interrupt flow to the subscapular artery, which supplies a large amount of arterial blood to the scapular and dorsal regions, including (but not limited to) the subscapularis and latissimus dorsi. Ligation just proximal to the deep brachial artery is at a mid-brachial level; therefore, this would be too far distal.

25. The answer is 2 [Table 29–1]. The biceps brachii receives most of its blood supply from the bicipital and cranial circumflex humeral arteries. The deep brachial and caudal circumflex arteries supply mainly the triceps brachii muscle.

26. The answer is 2 [Chapter 29 I C 2]. The brachial artery passes distal to the elbow, but does not change its name until it gives off the common interosseous artery at the level of the proximal part of the interosseous space (i.e., the space between the radius and ulna in the antebrachium).

27. The answer is 4 [Chapter 29 I E 2 a]. The superficial brachial artery contributes to the dorsal carpal rete, the fine network of vessels on the dorsal carpal surface. The median artery is not a branch of the brachial artery; it is a continuation of the brachial artery. Furthermore, it supplies mainly the palmar surface of the manus. The deep antebrachial and collateral ulnar arteries have nothing to do with the dorsal part of the limb.

28. The answer is 1 [Chapter 29 I E 1 a]. The artery that occupies the space between metacarpal bones II and III on the palmar surface of the paw is the palmar metacarpal artery II. The arteries of the paw are identified according to surface (palmar or dorsal), depth [metacarpal (deep) or common digital (superficial)], and position (I–IV). By convention, the metacarpal and common digital arteries take the name of the lower-numbered of the two metacarpal bones between which they run.

29. The answer is 1 [Chapter 29 II B 2 a]. The antebrachial part of the cephalic vein is the most commonly accessed site for venipuncture in dogs.

30. The answer is 4 [Chapter 29 II B 4]. The axillobrachial vein passes deep to the deltoideus muscle *en route* to the axillary vein.

31. The answer is 4 [Chapter 26 II B 5; Table 28–2]. The flexors of the carpus and digits, which include muscles innervated by both the median and ulnar nerves, arise from the medial humeral epicondyle.

32. The answer is 4 [Table 28–2; Chapter 30 II C]. The suprascapular nerve, which innervates the supraspinatus and infraspinatus muscles, passes around the cranial surface of the neck of the scapula and would most likely be the injured nerve. The supraspinatus is a shoulder extensor and the infraspinatus can either flex or extend the shoulder, depending on the position of the limb when the muscle contracts. Therefore, extension and flexion of the shoulder are most likely to be impaired with a scapular fracture that involves the neck of the scapula.

33. The answer is 2 [Chapter 30 II H 2 b (2)]. The axillary nerve continues after its last motor branch, first as the cranial-lateral cutaneous brachial nerve, and then, distal to the elbow, as the cranial cutaneous antebrachial nerve. The long thoracic nerve does not pass to the brachium or antebrachium, nor does it have a cutaneous component. The median and ulnar nerves have no cutaneous branches in the brachium.

34. The answer is 4 [Table 28–2; Chapter 30 II M 2]. The interosseous muscles, innervated by the ulnar nerve, are responsible for maintenance of proper joint angle in the carpal region. The ulnar nerve innervates the carpal and digital flexors (not extensors), and supplies the skin of the caudolateral (not the medial) antebrachium. The radial nerve is responsible for extending the elbow and allowing the limb to bear weight.

35. The answer is 2 [Chapter 30 II K 2]. The gait of this dog indicates inability to extend the elbow, carpus, and digits, which is suggestive of a radial nerve injury.

36. The answer is 1 [Chapter 30 III A 1]. Dorsal common digital nerve III passes on the dorsal surface of the paw and is related to the space between the third and fourth metacarpal bones. The nerves of the paw, by convention, take the lower number of the metacarpal bones with which they are associated. No dorsal metacarpal nerves are present on the manus; therefore, the nerve must be a common digital nerve.

37. The answer is 3 [Chapter 30 III A 2]. Abaxial palmar proper digital nerve IV passes along the lateral side of the palmar surface of digit IV. Lying on a single digit, the nerve is a proper digital nerve, and the lateral surface of the fourth digit faces away from this axis, thus the nerve is designated abaxial.

38. The answer is 3 [Chapter 31 I E 1]. The accessory carpal bone projects caudally from the remaining carpal bones, and can therefore be individually identified.

39. The answer is 3 [Table 28–2]. The common digital extensor originates from the lateral, not the medial, humeral epicondyle, along with the other carpal and digital extensors. Both the common digital extensor and the supinator are innervated by the radial nerve. The six joints crossed by the common digital extensor are, in order, the elbow, the antebrachiocarpal joint, the middle carpal joint, the carpometacarpal joint, the proximal interdigital joint, and the distal interdigital joints.

40. The answer is 2 [Table 28–2]. The biceps brachii does not pass over the caudal surface of the shoulder joint; therefore, it cannot flex the shoulder. The biceps brachii's origin from the supraglenoid tubercle and passage over the cranial surface of the shoulder joint allows it to extend the shoulder. The same muscle rotates (supinates) the elbow via its attachment to the radial tuberosity and flexes the elbow via its attachment to the ulnar and radial tuberosities.

41. The answer is 1 [Table 28–2]. Although the extensor carpi radialis originates from the lateral epicondyle and epicondylar crest of the humerus and acts to flex the elbow, its action here is minor, and would easily be compensated for by the action of the biceps brachii and brachialis muscles. The extensor carpi radialis, common digital extensor, lateral digital extensor, and ulnaris lateralis muscles, which originate from the lateral epicondyle of the humerus, are the sole extensors of the carpus and digits; therefore, those actions would be greatly affected. The supinator, the major inward rotator of the paw, also arises from the lateral epicondyle and its action would be severely compromised in the event of fracture of the lateral epicondyle of the humerus.

42. The answer is 3 [Chapter 29 II]. The cephalic vein, the main channel of venous flow back to the heart from the thoracic limb, terminates by entering the external jugular vein. The omobrachial vein also enters the external jugular vein, and the axillobrachial vein is directly confluent with the cephalic vein *en route* to the head.

PART V

THORACIC REGION

Chapter 32

Introduction to the Thoracic Region

I. DEFINITIONS. When considering the thoracic region, one must consider the **thoracic cage** and the **thoracic cavity.**

A. The **thoracic cage (bony thorax)** surrounds the thoracic cavity, as well as other structures. It **houses and protects** several major organs, and **provides a rigid framework** for ventilatory movements.

1. **Boundaries** (Figure 32–1). The thoracic cage is bounded:
   a. **Cranially,** by the **thoracic inlet** (i.e., the space between the first pair of ribs, the body of vertebra T1, and the manubrium)
   b. **Caudally,** by the **thoracic outlet** (i.e., the space between the last pair of ribs and the costal arch, the body of vertebra T12, and the xiphoid process)
   c. **Dorsally,** by the **bodies of the thoracic vertebrae** and the **proximal regions of the ribs**
   d. **Ventrally,** by the **sternum,** the **distal regions of the ribs,** and the **cranial parts of the abdominal muscles**
   e. **Laterally,** by **ribs 1–12** and the **intercostal muscles**
2. **Contents** of the thoracic cage include the:
   a. **Contents of the thoracic cavity** (see I B 2)
   b. **Diaphragm**
   c. **Spleen**
   d. **Liver** and **gall bladder** (normally, little to none of the liver projects outside the bony cage of the ribs)
   e. **Stomach**
   f. **Transverse colon**
   g. **Jejunum** (variable number of loops)
   h. **Right kidney** and **adrenal gland**
   g. **Abdominal aorta** and **caudal vena cava** (in part)
   h. **Abdominal sympathetic chain** (in part)

B. The **thoracic cavity** is described in relation to both soft and bony tissue. The thoracic cavity is contained within the thoracic cage.

1. **Boundaries.** The **thoracic cavity** is limited by the **same boundaries as the bony thorax, except caudally,** its boundary is the **diaphragm.**
   a. The diaphragm, a muscle of inspiration, forms the **musculotendinous boundary** between the thoracic and abdominal cavities.
      (1) The diaphragm's **thoracic (cranial) surface** is covered by the endothoracic fascia, which is covered by the pleura.
      (2) The diaphragm's **abdominal (caudal) surface** is covered by the transversalis fascia, which is covered more deeply by the peritoneum.
      (3) **Openings** in the diaphragm are provided for structures that must pass between the thoracic and abdominal cavities (see Chapter 34, Figure 34–2).
         (a) **Caval foramen.** The **caudal vena cava** passes through the caval foramen of the diaphragm.
         (b) **Esophageal hiatus.** The **esophagus** and **dorsal** and **ventral vagal trunks** pass through the esophageal hiatus.
         (c) **Aortic hiatus.** The **aorta, azygos vein** (and the hemiazygos vein, when it is present), and the **thoracic duct** pass through the aortic hiatus.
   b. The diaphragm is positioned within the bony thorax so that it is **convex cranially,** and extends into the thoracic cavity in a domed fashion. In effect, this orientation results

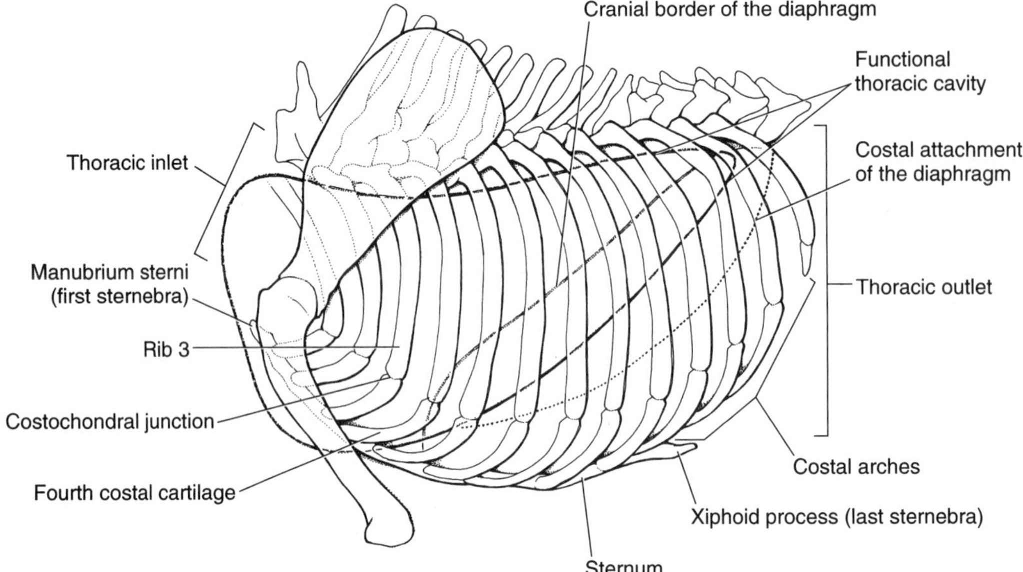

FIGURE 32–1. The thoracic skeleton with relation to the thoracic limb. The thoracic cage comprises the full expanse of the ribs and the costal arches. However, the doming of the diaphragm into the thoracic cage and the costal attachments of the diaphragm decrease the size of the functional thoracic cavity.

in the thoracic cavity being restricted to the more cranial part of the bony thorax. Consequently, the abdominal viscera project a considerable distance into the bony thorax, so that the most caudoventral portions of the last several ribs lie over digestive rather than cardiopulmonary viscera.

Canine Clinical Correlation

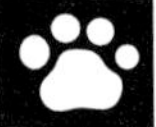

The positioning of the diaphragm and the cranial placement of some of the digestive viscera enable the clinician to hear digestive sounds over a considerable region of the caudoventral bony thorax during auscultation. This fact must be remembered when performing physical examination, lest an erroneous diagnosis of diaphragmatic hernia or another similar mistake be made!

2. **Contents**
   a. **Structures contained entirely within the thoracic cavity** include the:
      (1) **Heart** and **great vessels** (i.e., aortic arch, cranial vena cava)
      (2) **Lungs**
      (3) **Pleurae** and **pleural cavities**
      (4) **Thymus**
      (5) **Some lymph nodes** (e.g., the cranial mediastinal and tracheobronchial nodes)
      (6) **Some sympathetic ganglia** (e.g., the cervicothoracic and middle cervical ganglia)
      (7) **Mediastinum**
   b. **Structures contained partially within the thoracic cavity** include the:
      (1) **Trachea**
      (2) **Esophagus**
      (3) **Aorta**
      (4) **Caudal vena cava**

(5) **Phrenic nerves**
(6) **Sympathetic chain**
(7) **Vagus nerves, branches,** and **trunks**

II. BONY THORAX MORPHOLOGY

A. Internal morphology. The bony thorax is roughly **cone-shaped,** with the apex of the cone directed cranially and the base directed caudally. Two anatomic features account for the conical shape of the bony thorax:

1. The **vertebral column and sternum diverge** progressing cranially to caudally, increasing the dorsal to ventral dimensions of the bony thorax.
2. The **arch of the ribs increases** progressing cranially to caudally, increasing the medial to lateral dimensions of the bony thorax.

Canine Clinical Correlation

The space at the thoracic inlet is small: only 4–5 centimeters wide and 6–7 centimeters high in a 20-kg dog. Therefore, the inlet is a potential site for obstruction (e.g., in dogs that bolt their food or attempt to swallow unyielding objects, such as pieces of bone, toys, or wood).

B. External morphology. The thorax of quadruped mammals is compressed laterally (in contrast with the dorsoventrally flattened thorax of bipeds and reptiles). The lateral compression causes the limbs to fall in a straight line from the shoulder, greatly facilitating motion of both the thoracic and pelvic limbs. In contrast, the rather rounded thorax of quadruped amphibians and reptiles causes the brachium to project almost horizontally from the shoulder (turning ventrally at the elbow), resulting in laborious, slow motion. Although the thoracic cage is generally laterally compressed in all breeds, selective breeding has resulted in a wide range within the limit.

1. A **deep, narrow thorax** is characteristic in greyhounds, boxers, and Doberman pinschers. Many (although not all) of these breeds have been bred for speed, endurance, or both.
2. A **wide, barrel-shaped thorax** is characteristic in English bulldogs, dachshunds, and basset hounds. Most barrel-chested dogs are also chondrodystrophic (i.e., they have short legs).

Chapter 33

Bones, Joints, and Ligaments of the Thoracic Region

I. BONES

A. Thoracic vertebrae. The thoracic vertebrae form the narrow midline strip of the dorsal bony wall of the thorax. These bones are discussed in Chapter 18 I B 1 b; III B.

B. Sternum. The sternum forms part of the floor of the thoracic cage. **Eight bones (sternebrae)** and their intervening **intersternebral cartilages** compose the sternum.

1. **Bones of the sternum**
   a. The **manubrium,** the **first sternebra,** is specialized in form: largely cylindrical, the manubrium is longer than sternebrae 2–7, and slightly flared at its cranial end.
   b. **Sternebrae 2–7** are short, cylindrical bones, slightly constricted in their middles, that in many respects resemble the vertebrae of the tail.
   c. The **xiphoid process,** the **last sternebra,** is longer than sternebrae 2–7 and flattened dorsoventrally.

2. **Cartilages of the sternum**
   a. The **intersternebral cartilages** are small cartilaginous discs positioned between each of the sternebrae (1–8). These cartilages frequently ossify in older animals.
   b. The **xiphoid cartilage** is a spade-shaped cartilage that extends caudally from the xiphoid process. This cartilage affords an attachment site for some abdominal musculature, but not for any bony elements.

C. Ribs form all of the lateral, as well as part of the dorsal and ventral, walls of the thoracic cage. **Thirteen pairs** of ribs are typically present in the dog. The **intercostal spaces** are the spaces between the pairs of ribs.

1. **Composition.** The ribs are composed of a **bony portion,** positioned dorsally and laterally, and a **cartilaginous portion** (i.e., the **costal cartilage),** positioned more ventrally. The relative proportion of each of these components varies considerably from cranial to caudal—the bony portion is proportionately larger in the cranial ribs.
2. **Size.** The ribs, both their bony and cartilaginous portions, undergo an increase and then a decrease in size progressing cranially to caudally along the thoracic cage.
3. **Shape**
   a. **Pairs 1–2.** The cranial two pairs of ribs are short; the bony portion is relatively straight, although the costal cartilages are quite curved.
   b. **Pairs 3–9.** The length and curvature of the ribs increase from pairs 3–9. Pair 9 is the longest, and has the longest costal cartilages.
   c. **Pairs 10–13.** The ribs caudal to pair 9 undergo a progressive decrease in size but retain a fairly pronounced curvature. The last ribs are about the same length as the first.

4. **Articulations**
   a. **Articulation with the sternum**
      (1) **Sternal ribs (pairs 1–9)** attach directly to the sternum. The **costal cartilages of the sternal ribs** articulate with the sternum as follows:
         (a) **Pair 1** articulates with the manubrium.
         (b) **Pairs 2–7** articulate with successive intersternebral cartilages.
         (c) **Pairs 8 and 9** share an articulation site on the last intersternebral cartilage.
      (2) **Asternal ribs (pairs 10–12)** attach, via their costal cartilages, to each preceding rib, forming a curving bridge of cartilage (i.e., the **costal arch)** that passes cranially and ventrally to attach to the sternum.
      (3) **Floating ribs (pair 13)** do not attach to the sternum; the distal ends of these ribs terminate freely in the abdominal musculature.

b. Articulation with the vertebral column

(1) **Pairs 1–10** articulate with **two vertebral bodies** and the **intervening intervertebral disc.** For example, pair 2 articulates with the caudal part of vertebra T1 and the cranial part of vertebra T2.

(2) **Pairs 11–13** articulate only with the vertebra of the same number.

5. Parts (Figure 33–1)

a. The **vertebral portion (vertebral extremity)** of the rib is specialized for articulation with the vertebrae. The vertebral portion presents the following features.

(1) The **head** is a rounded proximal portion that projects medially from the rib and articulates with the vertebral body of the thoracic vertebra. The heads of the ribs are largest and best developed on the cranial ribs.

(2) The **neck** is a constricted area adjacent to the head. The necks of the ribs decrease in prominence on the more caudal ribs.

(3) The **tubercle** is a projection from the proximal part of the rib, not far distal to the head, that protrudes dorsally and slightly cranially from the junction of the head and neck. The tubercles are specialized for articulation with the **transverse processes** of the vertebra of the same number. Like the heads and necks of the ribs, the tubercles become less prominent on the more caudal ribs.

b. The **body** of the rib is the elongate portion of the rib that extends between the vertebral portion and the costochondral junction. The body is roughly cylindrical in most ribs (although it is slightly flattened medial to lateral), and is slightly enlarged at the area of the costochondral junction.

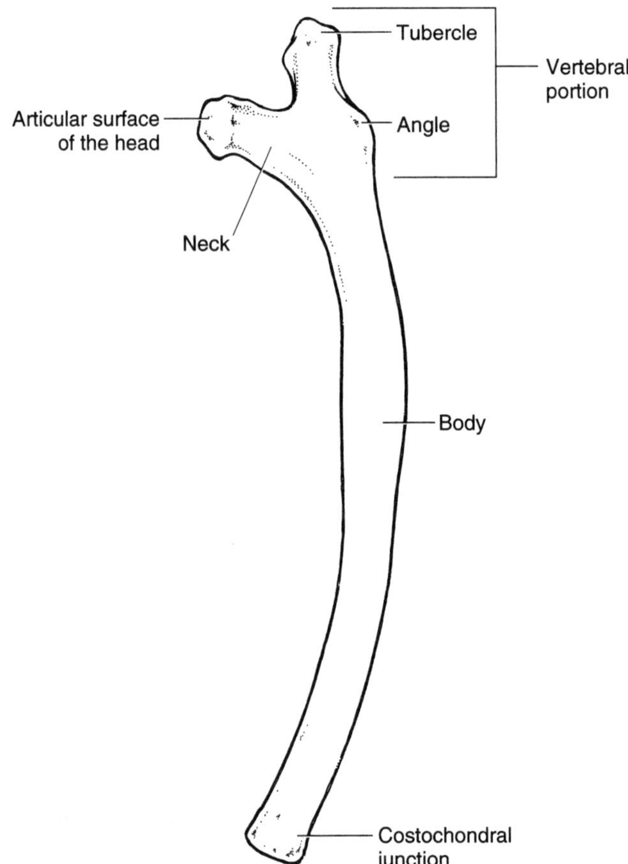

FIGURE 33–1. Bony parts of a rib. (Rib 3 is shown.)

(1) The **costochondral junction** is the junction of the bony and cartilaginous portions of the rib.

(2) The **costal groove** is a faint depression that passes along the caudal and medial surface of each rib, along which the intercostal vessels and nerves pass.

c. The **costal cartilage** continues distally from the ribs and articulates either directly or indirectly with the sternum. The costal cartilages are generally cylindrical in form, although many become compressed near their articulations with the sternum. They angle cranially, away from the costochondral junction. This angle is most pronounced in the cranial cartilages.

II. JOINTS AND LIGAMENTS

A. **Synchondroses** are present at the **costochondral junction.**

B. Synovial joints

1. The **costovertebral joints** are the articulations between the **ribs** and the **vertebral column.**
   a. **Portions.** The costovertebral joints have two portions, the:
      (1) Articulation of the **costal heads** with the **vertebral bodies**
      (2) Articulation of the **costal tubercles** with the **transverse processes** of the vertebrae
   b. **Ligaments.** Each costovertebral joint has four small ligaments.
      (1) The **ligament of the costal head** extends between the head of the rib and the intervertebral disc or the vertebral body just caudal to the head of the rib involved.
      (2) The **intercapital ligament** extends between the heads of most pairs of ribs, under the dorsal longitudinal ligament and over the dorsal surface of the intervertebral disc of the same level. The intercapital ligament holds the heads of the ribs tightly against the vertebral column.
         (a) A synovial sleeve extends along the length of the intercapital ligament, joining the joint capsules of the pair of involved costovertebral joints.
         (b) The intercapital ligaments are **absent between the first and the last two pairs of ribs.**

Canine Clinical Correlation

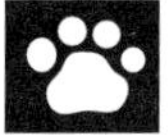

The presence of the intercapital ligaments in the thoracic region adds significantly to the ability of the annulus fibrosus of a given disc to retain its nucleus pulposus; as a result, disc ruptures and associated spinal cord trauma are relatively rare in the thoracic region.

      (3) The **ligament of the tubercle (costotransverse ligament)** extends between the tubercle and the dorsal surface of the transverse process of the same-numbered vertebra. The ligament of the tubercle is the strongest individual ligament uniting the ribs with the vertebral column.
      (4) The **ligament of the neck** extends between the neck of the rib and the ventral surface of the transverse process and adjacent vertebral body of the same-numbered vertebra.

2. The **sternocostal joints** are the articulations between the **ribs** and the **sternum.**
   a. **Location**
      (1) The first sternocostal joint is located between the **first sternebra** and the **first costal cartilage.**
      (2) The second through seventh joints are located between the **intersternebral cartilage** and the **associated costal cartilage.**
      (3) The last joint is located between the **last intersternebral cartilage** and the **eighth** and **ninth costal cartilages.**
   b. **Ligaments.** The associated ligaments are small and mostly of academic interest.

Chapter 34

Muscles and Fasciae of the Thoracic Region

I. MUSCLES. Some muscles with functions related primarily or even solely to the thorax have attachments outside of the bony thoracic wall. Because such muscles meet neither the definition of "intrinsic" or "extrinsic," muscles in the thoracic region (Figure 34–1) are most readily conceptualized according to function. Muscles in the thoracic region can be functionally associated with any one of the following five areas:

A. Neck and back. Muscles in this group are more fully described in Chapter 20.

1. The **thoracic part of the longus colli** [see Chapter 20 II B 3 b (2)] consists of small, overlapping bundles on the ventral surface of the cranial thoracic vertebral bodies.
2. The **scalenus** [see Chapter 20 II B 3 a (4)] consists of three bellies (two superficial and one deep) that are partially separated on the lateral surface of the cranial thorax. The bellies of the scalenus generally extend from ribs 1, 3, and/or 4, as well as from ribs 6–9, to the transverse processes of several cervical vertebrae.
3. **Epaxial musculature** [see Chapter 20 II A 2 b (1)]. Portions of the transversospinalis, longissimus, and iliocostalis muscle systems pass over the dorsal thoracic region.

B. Thoracic limb. Muscles in this group are more completely described in Chapter 28.

1. The **latissimus dorsi** (see Chapter 28 I G) covers a large portion of the craniodorsal thoracic wall as it sweeps from the thoracolumbar fascia along the lumbar and last 7 or 8 thoracic vertebrae to insert on the teres major tuberosity of the humerus.
2. The **trapezius** (see Chapter 28 I E) lies over a small portion of the craniodorsal thorax as it passes from its origin (the supraspinous ligament over vertebrae T3–T8 or T9) to its insertion (the spine of the scapula).
3. The **rhomboideus thoracis** (see Chapter 28 I F 3) passes over a small part of the craniodorsal thorax as it passes from its origin (the spinous processes of vertebrae T4–T6 or T7) to its insertion (the dorsal medial border of the scapula).
4. The **serratus ventralis thoracis** (see Chapter 28 I H) covers a considerable part of the cranioventral thoracic wall as it passes from its origin (the first seven or eight ribs) to its termination (the medial scapular surface).
5. The **deep pectoral** (see Chapter 28 I B) covers a large swathe of the cranioventral body wall as it extends from the sternum to insert on the lesser tubercle of the humerus.

C. Abdomen. These muscles are more completely described in Chapter 41.

1. The **costal part** of the **external abdominal oblique** (see Chapter 41 III B 2 a) passes over the ventrolateral portion of the thoracic cage.
2. The **costal part** of the **internal abdominal oblique** (see Chapter 41 III B 2 b) inserts on the last two ribs or costal cartilages.
3. The **costal part** of the **transversus abdominis** (see Chapter 41 III B 2 c) arises from the penultimate and last ribs as well as from the last few costal cartilages, and passes toward the ventral midline.
4. The **rectus abdominis** (see Chapter 41 IV A) arises from the first costal cartilage and rib and inserts on the pelvic brim.

D. Thoracic wall (Table 34–1)

1. The **cutaneous trunci,** the most superficial muscle associated with the thoracic wall, is an almost paper-thin muscle that closely adheres to the skin (it is, in fact, contained within the superficial truncal fascia and is usually removed with the fascia during dissection). The cutaneous trunci lies superficial to the latissimus dorsi and thoracic portion of

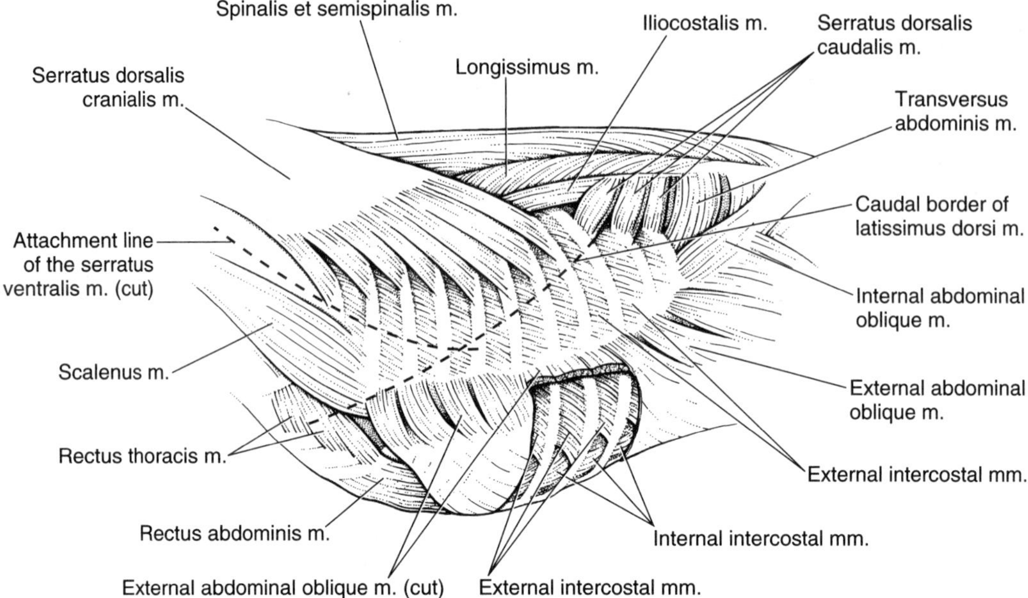

FIGURE 34–1. Muscles overlying the thoracic region and the intercostal muscles.

the trapezius, and covers most of the dorsal, lateral, and ventral surfaces of the thorax and abdomen.

2. The **serratus dorsalis cranialis** is a small muscle of the superficial craniodorsal thoracic wall. This muscle arises via a thin but strong and broad aponeurosis from the fibrous raphe of the neck, as well as the spinous processes of vertebrae T1–T6 or T8. The muscle inserts by distinct individual serrations onto the proximal, lateral surface of ribs 2–10.
3. The **serratus dorsalis caudalis** resembles its cranial namesake and occupies a similar (though more caudal) position in the superficial thoracic wall. This muscle also arises by a thin but strong and broad aponeurosis, but from the thoracolumbar fascia in the area of the external abdominal oblique muscle. The serratus dorsalis caudalis inserts by three distinct serrations on the lateral, proximal surface of ribs 11–13.
4. The **external intercostal muscles** fill most of the space between the ribs on the external surface. These muscles are robust; in large dogs, they can be as thick as 0.5 centimeter in their area of maximal development (i.e., over the central part of the thoracic cage). They originate on the caudal borders of ribs 1–12 and insert on the cranial borders of each adjacent rib.
   a. The external intercostal muscles are oriented caudoventrally, at a 90° angle to the internal intercostal muscles (see I D 6). It may help to think of the external intercostals as the "hand in the pocket" muscles—placing one's hands in one's pockets angles the forearm in a caudoventral direction, similar to the direction of these muscle fibers.
   b. The external intercostal muscles extend from the vertebral extremity of the rib ventrally to (or a short distance distal to) the costochondral junction.
   c. The portions of the external intercostal muscles that extend between the costal cartilages (as opposed to between the bony parts of the ribs) are technically called the **external interchondral muscles.**
5. The **rectus thoracis** is a flat muscle of the superficial thoracic wall, oriented somewhat obliquely on the ventral external thoracic wall.
6. The **internal intercostal muscles** fill most of the space between the ribs on the internal surface. These muscles are less substantial than their external counterparts.
   a. The internal intercostals are oriented at a 90° degree angle to their external fellows;

TABLE 34–1. Thoracic Wall Musculature Functionally Related to the Thoracic Wall

Muscle	Action	Innervation	Course
Cutaneous trunci	Twitches the skin over the thoracoabdominal region	Lateral thoracic nerve and the lateral branches of the adjacent intercostal nerves (thoracic region)	**Arises** from the dorsal region near the midline, parallel to the spinous processes of the thoracic and lumbar vertebrae **Courses** ventrally and cranially **Inserts** on the teres major tuberosity of the humerus and in the superficial fascia along the free edge of the pectoral muscle
Serratus dorsalis cranialis	Draws the ribs cranially on inspiration	Muscular branches of adjacent intercostal nerves	**Arises** from vertebrae T1–T6 or T8 **Courses** caudally and ventrally **Inserts** on ribs 2–10
Serratus dorsalis caudalis	Draws the ribs caudally on expiration	Muscular branches of adjacent intercostal nerves	**Arises** from the thoracolumbar fascia **Courses** cranially and ventrally **Inserts** on ribs 11–13
External intercostal muscles	Draw the ribs cranially on inspiration	Muscular branches of adjacent intercostal nerves	**Arise** from the caudal borders of ribs 1–12 **Course** obliquely caudoventrally **Insert** on the cranial border of the adjacent rib
Rectus thoracis	Draws the ribs cranially on inspiration	Muscular branches of adjacent intercostal nerves	**Arises** from the ventral part of the first rib (opposite the scalenus) **Courses** obliquely caudoventrally **Inserts** via an aponeurosis over the ventral regions of ribs 2–4
Internal intercostal muscles	Draw the ribs caudally on expiration	Muscular branches of adjacent intercostal nerves	**Arise** from the cranial borders of ribs 2–13 **Course** obliquely cranioventrally **Insert** on the caudal border of the adjacent rib
Transversus thoracis	Draws the ribs caudally on expiration	Muscular branches of adjacent intercostal nerves	**Arises** from the internal sternal surface (sternebra 2 through xiphoid process) **Courses** obliquely cranially **Inserts** on the internal surfaces of costal cartilages 2–7

therefore, the internal and external intercostal muscle form a grid. Think of the internal intercostals as the "hands-crossed-on-the-chest" muscles—placing one's hand on the opposite shoulder angles the forearm in the direction of these muscle fibers.

b. The internal intercostals extend from the vertebral extremity of each rib to the sternum. Thus, the most distal part of most internal intercostal muscles is visible through the small "window" left by the external intercostals where they do not extend fully to the sternum.

c. The portion of the internal intercostal muscles extending between the costal cartilages is technically called the **internal interchondral muscle.**

7. The **subcostal muscles,** largely of academic interest, are small, scattered bands of fibers positioned deep to the internal intercostal muscles near the dorsal ends of the ribs. The subcostals usually span several ribs.

8. The **transversus thoracis** is a muscle of the internal surface of the thorax. This flat though fleshy muscle consists of several distinct bundles that extend obliquely between the sternum and the more cranial costal cartilages.

E. Diaphragm (Figure 34–2)

1. **Structure.** The diaphragm has a **tendinous center** and a **muscular periphery.**
   a. The **central tendon** of the diaphragm is roughly "V"-shaped. The apex of the "V" is rather rounded and points ventrally and cranially. The arms of the "V" are directed dorsally and caudally.
   b. The **muscular portion** of the diaphragm entirely surrounds the central tendon and has recognizable regions.

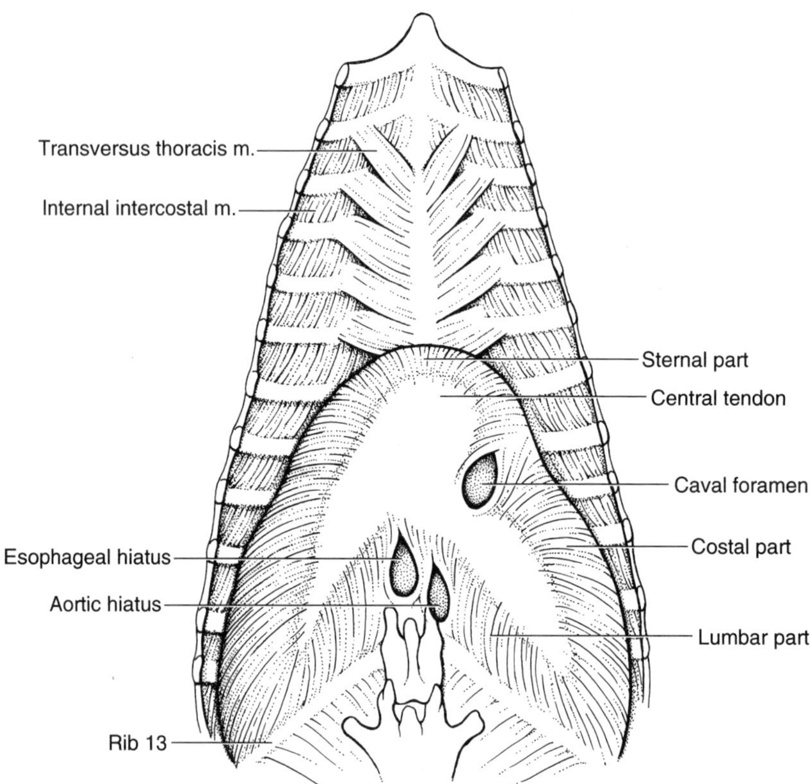

FIGURE 34–2. Dorsal view of the thoracic cavity, showing the diaphragm. (Modified with permission from Evans HE: *Miller's Anatomy of the Dog,* 3e. Philadelphia, WB Saunders, 1993, p 306.)

(1) The **sternal part** is the smallest portion, lying directly cranial to the apex of the "V" of the central tendon.
(2) The **costal parts,** one right and one left, are composed of muscle fibers that pass between ribs 8–13 and the central tendon. The line of attachment to the ribs is a gentle curve.
(3) The **lumbar part** consists of the right and left **diaphragmatic crura.** Each crus arises by a long and robust tendon from the ventral surfaces of vertebrae L3 and L4. Muscle fibers originate from the length of each crus, and radiate out to the central tendon.

2. **Innervation** is provided by the **phrenic nerve.**
3. **Action.** The diaphragm is a muscle of **ventilation.**
   a. When the diaphragm contracts, the dome of the diaphragm is drawn caudally, allowing the lungs to expand and inspiration to occur.
   b. As the diaphragm relaxes, the weight of the abdominal viscera tends to sag cranially, pushing the diaphragm passively back into the thorax. The size of the thoracic cavity decreases, and expiration occurs.

II. FASCIAE.

Two layers of fascia are present in the thoracic region. Both continue caudally into the abdomen.

A. The **external fascia** covers the external surface of the trunk, investing the muscles. In the thoracic region, this layer is referred to as the **external thoracic fascia.** The external fascia is divided into a **superficial** and a **deep layer** and is discussed in detail in Chapter 20 III B 1–2.

B. The **internal fascia** lines the deep surface of the muscles of the thoracic and abdominal walls, and adheres to the superficial surface of the serous membranes of the thoracic and abdominal cavities. In the thorax, this fascial layer takes the highly descriptive name of the **endothoracic fascia.**

Chapter 35

Vasculature of the Thoracic Region

I. ARTERIES OF THE THORACIC REGION

A. The **aortic arch** leaves the heart and courses first cranially, then dorsally, then caudally. The dorsally directed part of the arch gives rise to branches supplying the head, neck, thoracic limb, thoracic wall, and deep structures of the thorax (Figure 35–1).

1. The **brachiocephalic trunk** is typically the first of two large arteries arising from the aortic arch. This arterial trunk passes cranially and gives rise to a single branch before terminating by dividing into two other arteries.
   a. The **left common carotid artery** passes cranially along the neck to supply structures of the head and cranial cavity.
   b. The brachiocephalic trunk **terminates** by dividing into the **right common carotid artery** and the **right subclavian artery.**
2. The **left subclavian artery** also arises from the aortic arch. Its branching pattern is described in I C.

B. The **thoracic aorta** continues caudally from the descending portion of the aortic arch, taking a notably straight course just to the left of the vertebral column as far as the diaphragm. On reaching the diaphragm (approximately at the level of vertebra L2), the aorta passes between the crura of the diaphragm to continue caudal to it as the abdominal aorta.

1. **Parietal branches of the thoracic aorta**
   a. **Dorsal intercostal arteries 4 or 5–12** leave the thoracic aorta roughly at the level of the associated intervertebral foramen, course distally along the caudal border of the associated rib (giving off several branches *en route*), and anastomose with the corresponding ventral intercostal arteries. The course and branching of the dorsal intercostal arteries are described in detail in Chapter 21 II A 1 and in Figure 21–1.
   b. The **dorsal costoabdominal artery** (see Chapter 21 II A 2) arises from the thoracic aorta and follows rib 13 in a position similar to that of the intercostal arteries.
2. **Visceral branches of the thoracic aorta**
   a. The **bronchoesophageal artery** arises indirectly from the thoracic aorta, from the **right fifth intercostal artery.** The bronchoesophageal artery branches into the:
      (1) Bronchial arteries, right and left, the main nutritional arterial supply to the lungs
      (2) Esophageal arteries, which, via ascending and descending branches, supply most of the intrathoracic portion of the esophagus
   b. A few **mediastinal branches** usually leave the thoracic aorta and pass ventrally to supply structures located within the mediastinum, including the thymus.
   c. The **pericardial branches** are highly variable in their origin, but may originate from the thoracic aorta.

C. **Subclavian artery** (Figure 35–2). The branching patterns of the subclavian arteries, right and left, are typically identical. In a circular pattern, from cranial to caudal, the branches usually arise as follows:

1. The **vertebral artery** (see Chapter 21 I A 2) leaves the subclavian artery and courses cranially to supply the neck musculature. In addition, the vertebral artery makes a major contribution to the arterial supply of the cranial cavity, including the brain.
2. The **costocervical trunk** courses dorsolaterally from its origin near the vertebral artery. **Three main branches** arise from the costocervical trunk.
   a. The **first intercostal artery** leaves the costocervical trunk near its origin from the subclavian artery. The first intercostal artery passes caudally at approximately the mid-

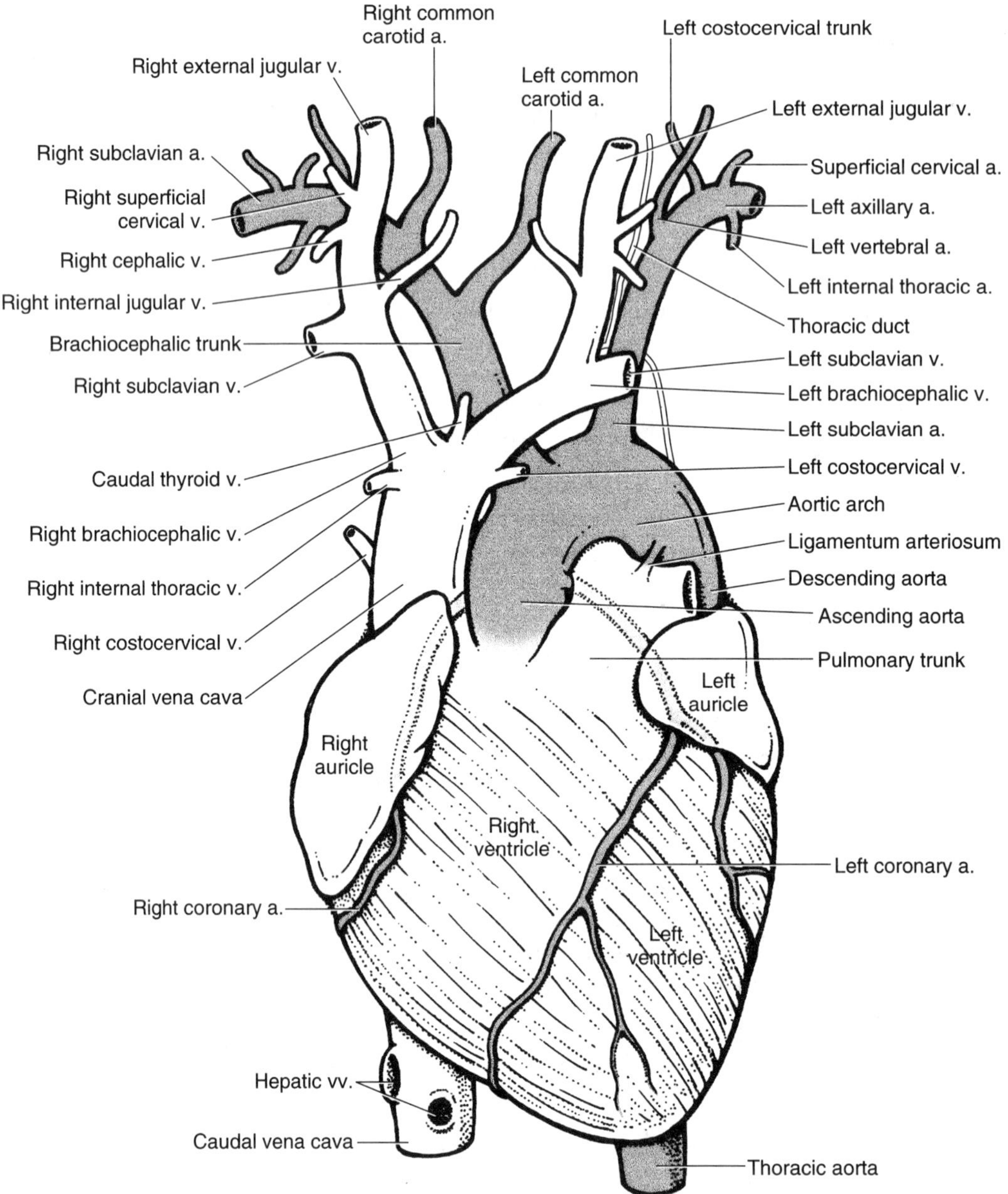

FIGURE 35–1. Great vessels of the heart, ventral view.

level of the first rib and provides the **major intercostal branches to ribs 1–3 or 4** by dividing into a dorsal and ventral branch for each rib.

(1) The dorsal branches of the first intercostal artery anastomose with the intercostal branches of the thoracic vertebral artery [see I C 2 c (2) (b)].

(2) The ventral branches of the first intercostal artery anastomose with the corresponding intercostal branches of the internal thoracic artery (see I C 5).

b. The **dorsal scapular artery** diverts slightly laterally from the trunk, continues dorsally, and exits the thoracic cavity cranial to the first rib. Along its course, it supplies the

serratus ventralis and **regional musculature,** and provides the **eighth cervical spinal branch** to the vertebral canal.

c. The **deep cervical artery,** the main continuation of the costocervical trunk, exits the thorax at the first intercostal space.

(1) **Structures supplied.** The deep cervical artery supplies the deep structures of the neck, and is particularly important in supplying the **cervical epaxial musculature.**

(2) **Branches**

(a) The deep cervical artery provides the **first thoracic spinal branch** to the vertebral canal.

(b) The **thoracic vertebral artery** branches from the deep cervical artery far dorsally, at the levels of the tubercles of the ribs. This artery provides small dorsal intercostal branches to the first three or four intercostal spaces; these branches pass ventrally to anastomose with the larger, dorsally directed intercostal branches from the first intercostal artery.

3. The **superficial cervical artery** courses cranially from the subclavian artery and plays an important role in supplying the **musculature of the shoulder,** as well as other structures. The superficial cervical artery is described in Chapter 29 I B 1.

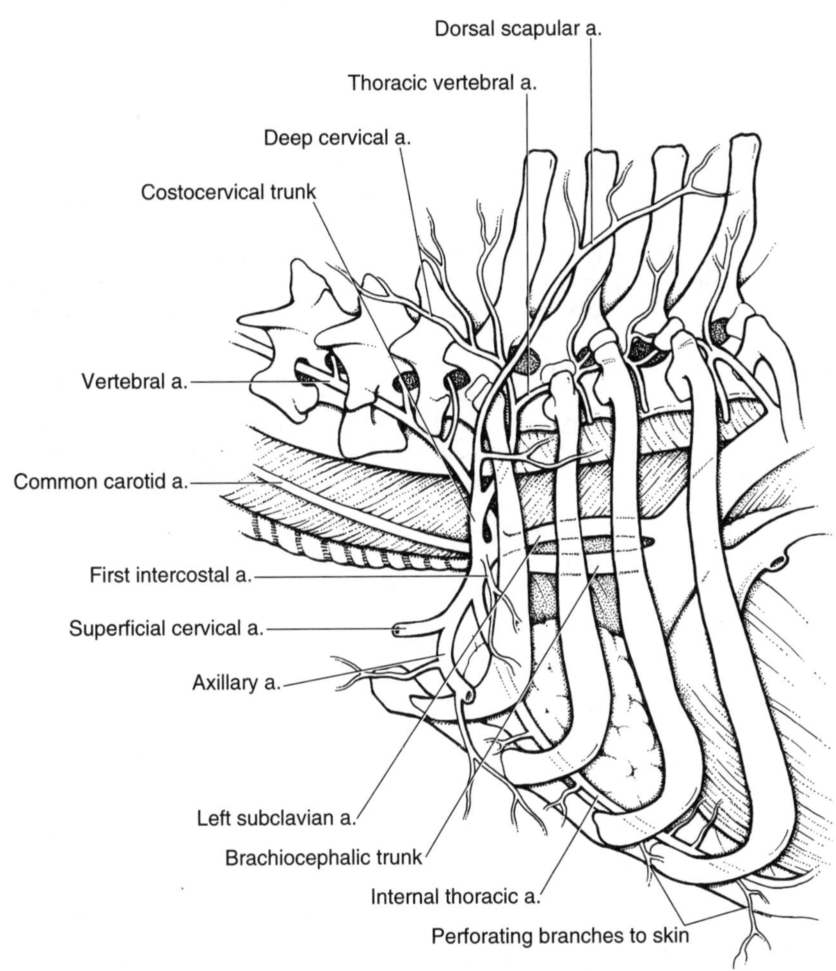

FIGURE 35–2. Branching of the left subclavian artery.

4. The **axillary artery** is the direct continuation of the subclavian artery outward into the thoracic limb (see Chapter 29 I B 2).
5. The **internal thoracic artery** passes caudally from the subclavian artery, coursing along the lateral side of the internal sternal surface and passing superficial to the transversus thoracis muscle.
   a. The internal thoracic artery gives rise to the **ventral intercostal arteries,** which supply the intercostal muscles, ribs, and pleura. The ventral intercostal arteries are usually present on **both sides of a given rib,** cranial as well as caudal. Those on the caudal costal border are larger, and are the ones that anastomose with the descending dorsal intercostal arteries. The cranial and caudal intercostal arteries anastomose with each other across the deep surfaces of the ribs.
      (1) **Ventral intercostal arteries 1–7** arise directly from the internal thoracic artery at each interchondral (i.e., -costal) space and ascend along the caudal border of the costal cartilage to anastomose with the dorsal intercostal artery descending in a similar position.
      (2) **Ventral intercostal arteries 8–12** arise from the **musculophrenic artery,** which is one of the terminal branches of the internal thoracic artery. These arteries follow a course similar to that of the more cranial ventral intercostal arteries.
   b. **Other branches** of the internal thoracic artery include the:
      (1) **Pericardiacophrenic artery,** which supplies the pericardium and the phrenic nerve
      (2) **Thymic branches,** major branches to the thymus
      (3) **Mediastinal branches,** which supply the mediastinal structures
      (4) **Perforating branches,** which pass through the body wall to supply adjacent muscles (including the intercostals and pectorals) and to provide mammary branches and ventral cutaneous branches
   c. The internal thoracic artery **terminates** by dividing into the musculophrenic and cranial epigastric arteries.
      (1) The **musculophrenic artery** continues inside the thorax, coursing caudodorsally in the gutter formed by the junction of the diaphragm and the thoracic wall. It perforates the diaphragm about one fourth of the way along the costal arch, and then ascends the caudal diaphragmatic surface. The musculophrenic artery supplies the **diaphragm** and **phrenic nerve** and **provides** the **ventral intercostal arteries** for intercostal spaces 8–10.
      (2) The **cranial (deep) epigastric artery,** an artery of considerable size, perforates the diaphragm at about the eighth interchondral (i.e., -costal) space, and passes caudally along the deep surface of the rectus abdominis. The **cranial superficial epigastric artery** arises from the cranial (deep) epigastric artery just caudal to the xiphoid cartilage, gains a position on the ventral (i.e., superficial) surface of the rectus abdominis, and passes caudally in that position.
         (a) The cranial superficial epigastric artery is important in the **blood supply to the mammary gland.**
         (b) Significant **cutaneous branches** also arise from the cranial superficial epigastric artery.

II. VEINS OF THE THORACIC REGION

A. The **cranial vena cava** is the unpaired, major vessel that delivers venous blood to the heart from the **head, neck,** and **thoracic limbs.**

1. The **subclavian** and **internal jugular veins** of each side flow together to form the right and left **brachiocephalic veins,** which become confluent to form the cranial vena cava just cranial to the thoracic inlet.
2. The cranial vena cava terminates by entering the right atrium of the heart.

B. The **caudal vena cava** ascends to the right atrium of the heart through the caudal part of the thorax. This vein drains the **pelvic region, pelvic limb,** and **abdominal viscera,** including the kidneys.

C. The **azygos vein system** originates in the abdomen, but the terminal part of its course is a prominent feature of the thorax. These veins **drain the body wall.**

1. The **right azygos vein,** often referred to as "the" azygos vein, is the dominant vein of this system in the dog.
   a. **Course.** After ascending from its origin in the abdomen (ventral to vertebra L3), the right azygos vein passes through the aortic hiatus of the diaphragm to enter the thorax. On entering the thorax, the vein inclines slightly to the right of the midline, and runs cranially between the vertebral bodies and the aorta. At the cardiac base, the vein curves sharply around the root of the lung to enter the **cranial vena cava.**
   b. **Tributaries** include the:
      (1) **Lumbar veins cranial to vertebra L3**
      (2) **Costoabdominal vein**
      (3) **Intercostal veins 12–3 or 4**
      (4) **Bronchoesophageal** and **esophageal veins**
2. The **hemiazygos vein** is highly variable in its presence as well as its formation.
   a. **Course.** When present, the hemiazygos vein is positioned on the left of the aorta and passes cranially through the aortic hiatus, terminating by entering the **ninth or tenth dorsal intercostal vein.**
   b. **Tributaries** include the **left costoabdominal veins** and the **last few dorsal intercostal veins.**

D. **Satellite veins.** Essentially all of the named arteries of the thorax have satellite veins.

III. LYMPHATIC VESSELS OF THE THORACIC REGION

A. The **parietal component** of the thoracic lymphatic system **drains the thoracic wall.**

1. The **ventral thoracic lymphocenter** is small and **highly variable** in both the number of nodes and the path of the efferent vessels. Occasionally, the nodes are absent, but the vessels are always present.
   a. The **cranial sternal lymph nodes** are usually present as one node on each side, or occasionally as a single median node.
      (1) The nodes lie immediately cranial to the transversus thoracis muscle, at the level of the second costal cartilage.
      (2) The cranial sternal lymph nodes drain the **ribs, sternum, pleura,** and **adjacent muscles.**
   b. The **efferent vessels** from the right node pass to the **right lymphatic duct,** and from the left node, to the **thoracic duct.** When the cranial sternal nodes are absent, the lymphatic vessels of this region pass into the **mediastinal lymph nodes.**
2. The **dorsal thoracic lymphocenter** is often absent.
   a. The **intercostal lymph nodes** may be present as a single paired set that lies at the vertebral end of intercostal space five or six. They receive afferent lymphatics from the **musculature of the neck, back, thorax,** and **abdomen,** as well as from the **ribs** and **vertebrae.**
   b. The **efferent lymphatics** from this center pass to the **mediastinal lymph nodes.**

B. The **visceral component** of the thoracic lymphatic system drains the **thoracic viscera.**

1. The **mediastinal lymphocenter,** the **larger** of the two lymphocenters that form the visceral component, is **constant in presence,** although the **associated nodes are variable** in number (1–6 on one side) and size (1–3 mm).
   a. The **mediastinal lymph nodes** are associated with the great vessels cranial to the heart in the cranial mediastinum. Some of the nodes may be embedded within the substance of the thymus, when this organ is large in young dogs. The mediastinal lymph nodes drain a significant portion of the body wall, even though they are included in the visceral group of nodes. Structures drained by these nodes include:

(1) The **musculature** of the **neck, thorax,** and **abdomen**
(2) The **cervical** and **thoracic vertebral column**
(3) The **ribs**
(4) **Soft tissue structures of the thorax,** including (but not limited to) the trachea, esophagus, thymus, and heart
(5) **Other lymph nodes of the thorax,** including the intercostal and sternal lymph nodes (when present), the deep cervical lymph nodes, and the pulmonary and tracheobronchial lymph nodes

b. The **efferent lymphatics** from the mediastinal lymph nodes pass to the **thoracic duct,** the **tracheal trunk,** or both.

2. The **bronchial lymphocenter** is associated with two groups of nodes.

a. The **pulmonary lymph nodes** are **often absent,** and, even when present, are normally not present on both sides.

(1) **Drainage.** When present, these nodes are positioned on the dorsal surface of the primary bronchi and drain the **lungs.**
(2) **Efferent vessels** pass to the **tracheobronchial lymph nodes.**

b. The **tracheobronchial lymph nodes** are **constant in presence** and **number (3).** Although their size is variable, they are nonetheless among the largest of the thoracic lymph nodes, and may be as long as 30 mm in an average-sized dog.

(1) **Position**

(a) The **right** and **left tracheobronchial lymph nodes** are positioned on the lateral surfaces of their respective primary bronchi at the level of the tracheal bifurcation.
(b) The **middle tracheobronchial lymph node** is consistently the largest. This node lies over the bifurcation of the trachea, and as a result, is usually "V" shaped.

(2) **Drainage.** The middle tracheobronchial lymph node receives afferents from **many soft tissue structures of the thorax,** including the pulmonary lymph nodes (when these nodes are present), bronchi, aorta, heart, thoracic esophagus and trachea, mediastinum, and diaphragm.
(3) **Efferent lymphatic vessels** from the tracheobronchial lymph nodes pass to **other nodes within the same group,** and to the **mediastinal lymph nodes.**

Chapter 36

Innervation of the Thoracic Region

I. NERVES OF THE PROXIMAL THORACIC LIMB. The shoulder region and some of the proximal brachial region overlie the lateral thoracic wall; therefore, the nerves of the proximal thoracic limb must be included when considering the innervation of the thoracic region. These nerves are discussed in Chapter 30.

II. THORACIC SPINAL NERVES (see also Chapter 22 III). Owing to the relatively simple structure of the thoracic wall, the thoracic nerves retain the simplest segmental pattern of distribution of all the spinal nerves. Each of the 13 pairs of thoracic spinal nerves exits the vertebral canal caudal to the vertebra of the same number. The **cutaneous innervation of the thoracic wall** is supplied by diverse sources (Table 36–1).

A. Dorsal primary branch. The dorsal primary branch of each thoracic spinal nerve passes dorsally into the region of the epaxial musculature and gives off a:

1. **Medial branch,** which is **motor** to the epaxial musculature
2. **Lateral branch,** which is **motor** to the iliocostalis thoracis and **sensory** to the skin of the dorsal third of the thoracic wall
3. **Dorsal cutaneous branch,** sensory to the skin near the dorsal midline

B. Ventral primary branch

1. **Intercostal nerves (ventral branches of spinal nerves T1–T12)***
   a. **Course.** The intercostal nerves continue distally from the division of the thoracic spinal nerve into dorsal and ventral branches, and take a position along the caudal border of the associated rib, much like the intercostal arteries and veins.
   b. **Branching pattern.** Most intercostal nerves follow a characteristic branching pattern.
      (1) The **proximal muscular branch** is **motor only,** and supplies the:
         (a) **Internal** and **external intercostal muscles**
         (b) **Serratus dorsalis cranialis** and **caudalis,** where the nerves are near these muscles
      (2) The **lateral branch** is **motor** and **sensory.** This branch perforates the thoracic wall about halfway down from the dorsal midline, and then passes distally with the same-named artery down the thoracic wall within the superficial fascia. The lateral branch is:
         (a) **Motor** to the **lateral parts of the abdominal musculature** near the thoracic wall
         (b) **Sensory** to the **skin over the lateral half of the thoracic wall** (via the **lateral cutaneous branch)** and the **mammary glands** (via the **lateral mammary branch)**
      (3) The **distal muscular branch** is **motor only,** and supplies the:
         (a) **Transversus abdominis**
         (b) **Rectus abdominis**
      (4) The **ventral cutaneous branch** is the **terminal continuation of the intercostal nerve.** This branch is present for all intercostal nerves except the first one and last two, and travels with its companion artery. It is **sensory** to the **skin on each side of the ventral midline** via the **medial mammary branch.**

---

*The ventral branch of T1 is usually referred to as an "intercostal nerve," even though it does not pass between two ribs—it continues distally from its origin cranial to the first rib. However, it is distributed largely like the "true" intercostal nerves.

TABLE 36–1. Cutaneous Innervation of the Thoracic Wall and Related Regions

Nerve	Source	Area Supplied
Proximal lateral cutaneous branches of the thoracic spinal nerves	Dorsal branches of the spinal nerves	Skin over the epaxial muscles near the dorsal midline
Lateral cutaneous branches of the intercostal nerves	Ventral branches of the spinal nerves	Skin over the ventral half of the thoracic wall, ventral to the edge of the latissimus dorsi
Ventral cutaneous branches of the intercostal nerves	Ventral branches of the spinal nerves	Skin along the ventral midline
Intercostobrachial nerve	Spinal nerve T2	Dorsal-to-ventral strip of skin over the triceps brachii and the long head of the triceps
Cranial lateral cutaneous branch	Axillary nerve of the brachial plexus	Skin over the deltoideus and the lateral head of the triceps brachii

2. **Costoabdominal nerve.** The ventral branch of spinal nerve T13 follows rib 13 in a position similar to that of the intercostal nerves.

III. NERVOUS STRUCTURES WITHIN THE THORAX (Figure 36–1)

A. Phrenic nerve. The phrenic nerve is the motor nerve to the diaphragm.

1. The roots of spinal nerves **C5, C6,** and **C7** emerge from their intervertebral foramina, pass caudoventrally over the superficial surface of the scalenus muscle, and merge to form the phrenic nerve.
2. The phrenic nerve enters the thoracic inlet and passes caudally through the thorax, across the lateral surface of the great vessels of the heart and the cardiac base (ventral to the hilus of the lung) to attain the diaphragm at its cranial surface (see Figure 36–1).

B. Vagus nerve. The vagus nerve provides the complete parasympathetic supply to the thorax, either directly or via its branch, the recurrent laryngeal nerve. The course of the vagus nerve through the thorax is described in detail in Chapter 10 II J and illustrated in Figure 36–1.

C. Sympathetic trunk. The sympathetic trunk passes along the ventrolateral surface of the vertebral bodies (see Figure 36–1).

1. Unspecialized **paravertebral ganglia** [see Chapter 4 III C 1 b (1) (a)] are present at each intervertebral space.
2. The **cervicothoracic ganglion** [see Chapter 4 IV B 3 a], the largest autonomic ganglion in the dog's body, is formed by the fusion of the last cervical and first thoracic ganglia. This ganglion is located at the cranial end of the sympathetic trunk (see Figure 36–1).
3. The **ansa subclavia** is a loop of sympathetic fibers that surrounds the subclavian artery on each side. The loop is formed by the passage of the sympathetic chain around the artery in its cranially directed course through the thorax.
4. The **middle cervical ganglion** [see Chapter 4 IV B 3 b] is another large sympathetic ganglion in the cranial thorax. This ganglion is formed from the fusion of several cervical ganglia (see Figure 36–1).

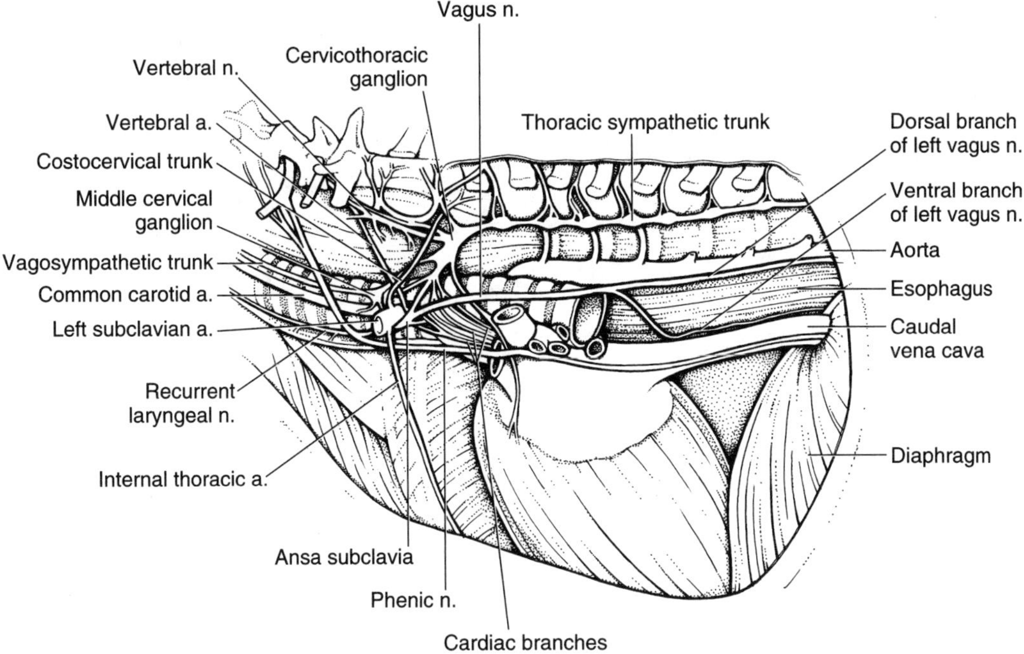

FIGURE 36–1. Nervous structures within the thorax. (Modified with permission from Anderson WD: *Atlas of Canine Anatomy.* Baltimore, Williams & Wilkins, 1994, p 489.)

D. **Cardiac nerves.** The heart receives both sympathetic and parasympathetic innervation. Individual cardiac nerves are named by position or origin, and differ from right to left. The details are mainly of academic interest.

1. The **sympathetic cardiac nerves** arise from the **cervicothoracic ganglion,** the **middle cervical ganglion,** the **ansa subclavia,** or all three.
2. The **parasympathetic cardiac nerves** arise from the **vagus nerve,** the **recurrent laryngeal nerve,** or both.

E. **Plexuses**

1. The **periarterial plexuses** are networks of autonomic fibers that surround the major arteries as they travel into the thoracic limb. These plexuses are named for the artery on which they travel, such as the axillary plexus or subscapular plexus.
2. The **pretracheal plexus** lies ventral to the tracheal bifurcation and supplies the atrial walls of the heart. It then continues as the coronary plexuses, which follow the right and left coronary arteries.
3. The **dorsal ventricular plexus** lies near the junction of the left atrium and ventricle, and supplies both sympathetic and parasympathetic fibers to the heart.
4. The **pulmonary plexus** carries autonomic fibers to the parenchyma and vasculature of the lungs. The two pulmonary plexuses (one left and one right) are located in the mediastinum.

Chapter 37

Pleura, Lungs, and Mediastinum

I. PLEURA

A. Pleural membranes line the thoracic cavity and cover the lungs and other structures within the thoracic cavity. Two separate pleural membranes are present in the thoracic cavity, one on the right side and one on the left.

1. **Structure.** The pleural membrane consists of a thin layer of mesothelial cells on top of a layer of smooth muscle and elastic fibers, anchored to a thin connective tissue layer (the endothoracic fascia in the thoracic area). The connective tissue layer supports the mesothelial layer and anchors it to the surrounding structures.
2. **Function.** The mesothelial cells produce a small amount of a thin, clear fluid that acts as a lubricant, permitting the structures within the thoracic cavity to move without friction.
3. **Regions.** Each pleural membrane is a continuous sheet that extends throughout its respective side of the thoracic cavity. Although all parts of the membrane are continuous with one another, several regions of the pleura can be identified (Figure 37–1):
   a. The **visceral (pulmonary) pleura** is intimately bound to the surface of the lung, and cannot be removed from it during dissection. The parenchyma of the lung is visible through the pleura.
   b. The **parietal pleura** lines the boundaries of the thoracic and pleural cavities. The parietal pleura has two named regions:
      (1) The **costal parietal pleura** lines the internal surface of the ribs and intercostal muscles (i.e., the lateral and much of the dorsal and ventral walls of the thoracic cavity).
      (2) The **diaphragmatic parietal pleura** covers the cranial surface of the diaphragm (i.e., the caudal wall of the thoracic cavity).
   c. The **mediastinal pleura** covers the mediastinum, the space between the lungs (see VI).
   d. The **pericardial pleura** covers the pericardial sac, which surrounds the heart.
4. **Specializations**
   a. The **pleural cupulae** (one right, one left) are small, cup-shaped "bubbles" of pleura at the cranial extent of each lung that protrude a short distance cranially through the thoracic inlet. The pleural cupulae form because the pleurae extend farther cranially than the lung tissue itself.
   b. The **pulmonary ligament** is a triangular, transparent, doubled fold of pleura, with a free border that extends between the caudal lobe of the lung and the caudal end of the lung's hilus. The pulmonary ligament forms where the mediastinal pleura reflects onto (i.e., becomes continuous with) the pulmonary pleura. The pulmonary ligament is best appreciated by gently reflecting the caudal lobe away from the hilus and peering under the lobe before it is displaced to a great extent.
   c. The **plica venae cavae** is a doubled fold of pleura that surrounds the caudal vena cava. (Despite the spelling of "venae cavae," only one plica is present.)

B. Pleural cavity. The continuous nature of the pleural membrane results in the formation of the pleural cavity, simply the space inside the walls of the pleura (see Figure 37–1).

1. The **two pleural cavities** (one right and one left) **do not communicate.**
2. **Both pleural cavities normally contain a small amount of serous fluid, but nothing else.** The mesothelial cells face the pleural cavity so that the serous fluid is elaborated into the potential space of the cavity. The lungs are not contained within the pleural cavity.

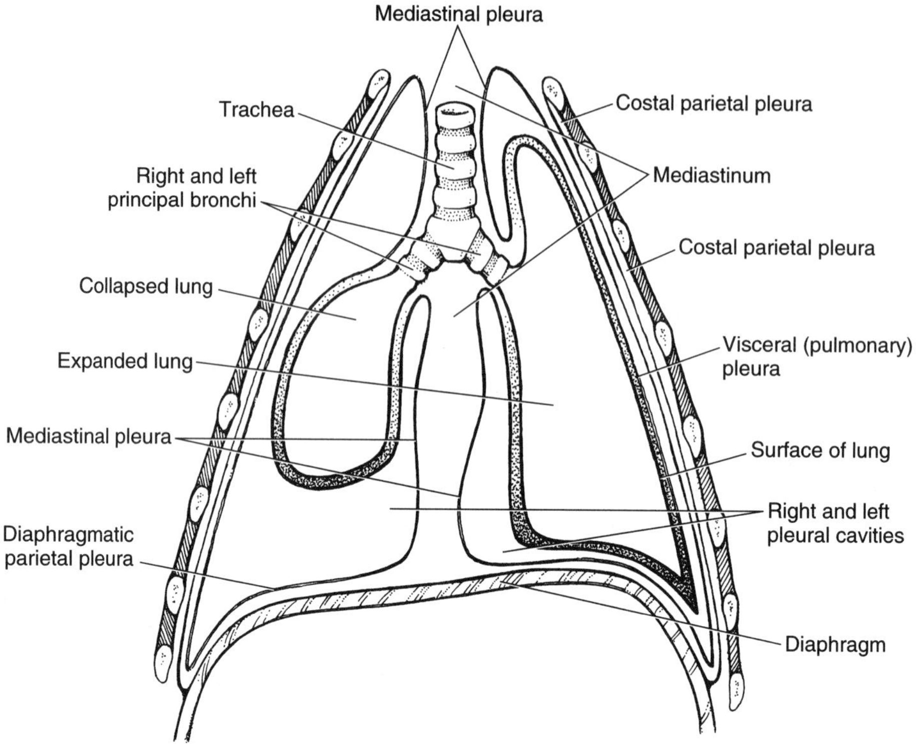

FIGURE 37–1. Schematized representation of the lungs, pleural membranes, pleural cavities, and thoracic cavity. The spaces between the pleural layers are expanded for demonstrative purposes. With the lung deflated (*left*), the continuous nature of the pleural regions is plain. With the lung inflated (*right*), the visceral (pulmonary) pleura and the parietal pleura are in close apposition, largely reducing the pleural cavity to a potential space. Note that this space does not contain the lungs—normally, it contains only a small amount of serous fluid.

II. LUNGS

A. Orientation.
Orientation. Each lung is oriented horizontally within the thorax, with its apex cranially and its base caudally.

1. The **apex** of each lung is the convex cranial end, directed toward the thoracic inlet.
2. The **base (diaphragmatic surface)** of each lung is the concave caudal portion that conforms to the dome of the diaphragm as it projects into the thoracic cavity.

B. Surfaces

1. The **costal surface** comprises all regions directly adjacent to the ribs and intercostal muscles; this convex area is largely the lateral surface of the lung. **Regularly spaced depressions formed by the ribs** mark the costal surface of each lung.
2. The **medial surface** is the flattened area that faces medially, toward the mediastinum and opposite lung. The **cardiac impression** is present on the medial surface of each lung, where the lungs nestle around the heart.
3. The **diaphragmatic (basal) surface** faces caudally and abuts the diaphragm.
4. The **interlobar surfaces** are the surfaces between neighboring lobes of the lungs, where the surface of one lobe is in direct contact with that of the adjacent lobe.

C. Margins (Figure 37–2)

1. The **ventral margin** of the lung is formed where the medial surface and the costal surface meet at an acute angle.

2. The **dorsal margin** is formed along the vertebral part of the lung.
3. The **basal margin** is formed along the acute angle where the costal surface becomes continuous with the diaphragmatic (basal) surface.

D. Structure

1. **Hilus.** The hilus of the lung is the general area where vascular, nervous, and airway structures enter or leave the lung.
2. **Root.** The root of the lung comprises the collected structures that pass into and out of the lung (via the hilus).
3. **Lobes.** Designation of the lung lobes is based on the division of the bronchi within the

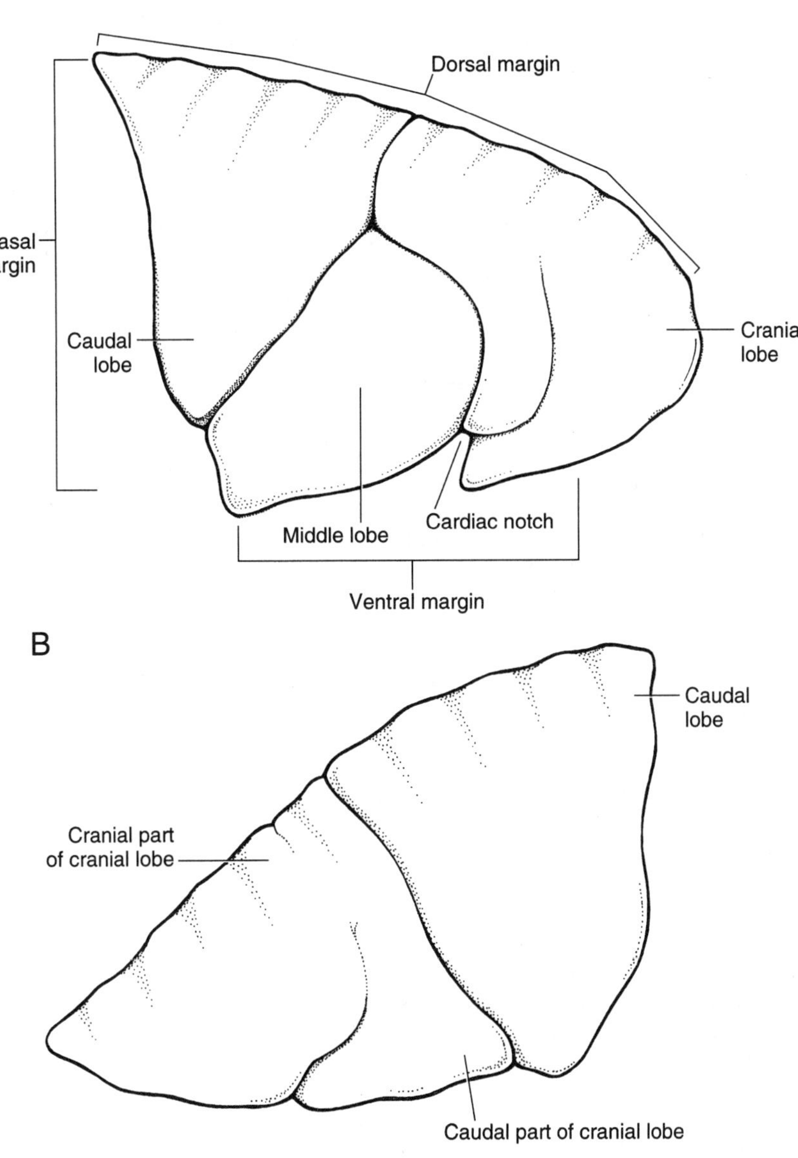

FIGURE 37–2. (*A*) Right lung, lateral view. The accessory lobe is not visible from the lateral surface. (*B*) Left lung, lateral view.

lung parenchyma, rather than any surface feature. Nonetheless, deep fissures on the surface of each lung generally correspond closely with the internal lobation of the lungs. The lobation of the lungs varies from right to left.

a. The **right lung** is somewhat larger than the left in volume, and has more lobes than the left (see Figure 37–2).
   (1) The **(right) cranial lobe** comprises approximately one third of the bulk of the right lung. The borders of the cranial lobe are rather irregular.
   (2) The **middle lobe** is a small, triangular lobe situated in the midventral region of the right lung. Viewed from the lateral surface, the middle lobe does not extend fully to the dorsal midline. A rather prominent projection dangles from its ventral border.
   (3) The **(right) caudal lobe** comprises almost half of the bulk of the right lung.
   (4) The **accessory lobe,** the smallest of the pulmonary lobes, is an irregularly shaped lobe that lies along the medial surface of the caudal lobe. The accessory lobe **surrounds the caudal vena cava** and the **right phrenic nerve** as these structures pass near the right atrium.

Canine Clinical Correlation

The pericardium and heart are accessible to needle puncture through the **cardiac notch,** a triangular space between the cranial and middle lobes of the right lung (see Figure 37–2A). Here, the borders of the associated lobes diverge from each other and leave a significant portion of the pericardial wall uncovered by lung tissue. Accessing the heart through this space avoids difficulties associated with puncturing the lung. The apex of the cardiac notch is positioned at the distal quarter of the fourth rib.

b. The **left lung** has only two lobes (see Figure 37–2).
   (1) The **(left) cranial lobe** has a **cranial** and a **caudal part.** In outline, the cranial lobe of the left lung is quite smooth and without projections, save for the surface fissure dividing its cranial and caudal parts.
   (2) The **(left) caudal lobe** is quite smooth along all of its borders.

III. RELATION OF THE PLEURAL CAVITY, LUNG, AND THORACIC CAVITY.

The relation of these structures is clinically relevant.

A. Line of pleural reflection.

The diaphragmatic parietal pleura reflects cranially as it becomes continuous with the costal parietal pleura along the line of pleural reflection. This region can be conceptualized as a gently curved line extending **from the last rib at the level of the epaxial muscles** to the **eighth costal cartilage** (Figure 37–3). This border does not follow the costal arch because the thoracic cavity does not extend as far caudally as the bony thorax.

B. Basal (caudal) border of the lungs.

Because the lungs do not fill the entire bony thorax, knowledge of their caudal borders is important in determining the area of the thorax over which lung sounds are audible, as well as for determining what areas of the thorax are safe for puncture.

1. **Auscultation.** The **auscultation triangle** (see Figure 37–3) is the area over the bony thorax where the lung is just deep to the thoracic wall, and thereby accessible to auscultation and percussion. The borders of the auscultation triangle are relatively easy to remember:

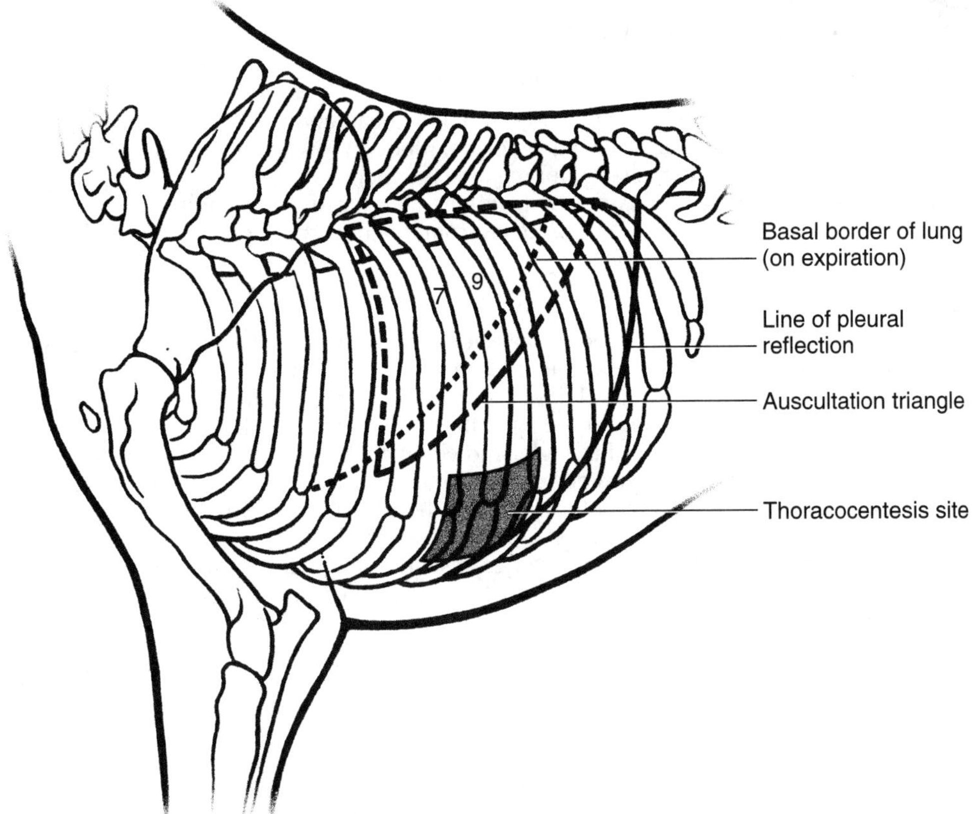

FIGURE 37–3. Basal border of the lung, line of pleural reflection, and the auscultation triangle. Thoracocentesis should access the space cranial to the line of pleural reflection and caudal to the basal border of the lung.

a. **Cranially,** a near-vertical line between the caudal angle of the scapula and the olecranon tuber
b. **Caudally,** an oblique, straight line from the olecranon tuber to the neck region of the penultimate rib (i.e., approximately the basal border of the lung)
c. **Dorsally,** a horizontal line from the neck region of the penultimate rib to the caudal angle of the scapula

2. **Thoracocentesis** is the clinical procedure used to access the pleural cavity to withdraw fluid (e.g., transudates, blood, pus, chyle) or air, either for diagnostic or therapeutic reasons.
   a. The basal border of the lung does not extend as far caudally as the line of pleural reflection (see Figure 37–3). This leaves an area where the lung and investing visceral pleura do not project between the costal and diaphragmatic pleura. Thus, the area between these two regions of parietal pleura (i.e., part of the pleural cavity) can be accessed by needle without risk of puncturing the lung.
   b. The **optimal site** for thoracocentesis in the standing dog is at the **costochondral junction, at the 7th or 8th intercostal space** (see Figure 37–3). Because fluids are heavy, they pool in the lower regions of the pleural cavity. Placement of the needle relatively low in the "safe" space increases the chance of acquiring samples of even a small amount of accumulated fluid. If air is suspected, the needle needs to be placed more dorsally.

IV. VASCULATURE OF THE LUNGS

A. Overview. Two sets of vascular beds are present in the lungs.

1. The **pulmonary vessels** carry blood between the heart and the lungs for the purposes of carbon dioxide removal and oxygen uptake. Blood in this system of vessels has little to do with providing gas exchange for the lung parenchyma itself.
2. The **bronchial vessels** are concerned with the delivery of oxygen and nutrients to, and the removal of metabolic waste products from, the more proximal regions of the lung parenchyma.

B. Pulmonary vessels

1. **Arteries.** The **pulmonary trunk and arteries** are **the only arteries in the adult body to carry deoxygenated blood.** [Recall that a vessel is designated as an artery or a vein based on the direction of blood flow within it (artery = away from the heart, vein = toward the heart), rather than according to the character of the blood within the vessel.]
   a. The **pulmonary trunk** is the single, undivided great artery that leaves the right ventricle of the heart and carries deoxygenated blood from the body toward the lungs for oxygenation and removal of carbon dioxide. The pulmonary trunk lies in close apposition to the aorta through most of the trunk's length.
   b. The **right** and **left pulmonary arteries** arise from the pulmonary trunk as it bifurcates (shortly after leaving the right ventricle), and course to their respective lungs. After entering each respective lung at the hilus, the arteries arborize to access all of the lobes of each lung.
      (1) The terminal branching of the pulmonary arteries continues distally to the alveoli so that gas exchange can take place for the blood destined for delivery to the remainder of the body.
      (2) In addition to delivering blood to the alveoli for gas exchange, the pulmonary arteries supply the more distal airways (i.e., the respiratory bronchioles, alveolar ducts, and alveoli) with metabolic nutrients and remove metabolic wastes. In these distal regions, oxygen is received directly from the airspaces surrounding the alveoli. (In the more proximal regions, metabolic exchange takes place via the bronchial arteries; see IV C 1).
   c. The **ligamentum arteriosum** is the fibrosed adult remnant of the fetal ductus arteriosus, the structure that permits most of the oxygenated blood arriving from the umbilical vein to bypass the lungs in the fetus. This structure is present near the termination of the pulmonary trunk into the pulmonary arteries, and extends between the trunk and the aorta.
2. **Veins.** The pulmonary veins are large, valveless veins that **return oxygenated blood from the lungs to the heart for distribution to the body.** Unlike the pulmonary arteries, which form a single vessel entering each lung, the pulmonary veins remain largely individualized until shortly before entering the right atrium. The usual pattern for each lung is as follows:
   a. **Right lung**
      (1) The pulmonary veins from the **cranial** and **middle lobes** become confluent and enter the right atrium as a single vessel.
      (2) The pulmonary veins from the **caudal** and **accessory lobes** become confluent and enter the right atrium together.
   b. **Left lung**
      (1) The pulmonary vein from the **cranial lobe** enters the right atrium as a single vessel.
      (2) The pulmonary vein from the **caudal lobe** enters the right atrium as a single vessel.

Canine Clinical Correlation

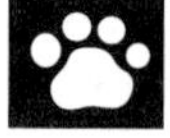

The pulmonary veins are variable in number and position, but this variation is of little clinical interest and likely to remain so, unless pulmonary surgery in dogs becomes more common in the future.

C. Bronchial vessels

1. **Arteries.** The **bronchial artery** [see Chapter 35 I B 2 a (1)] is variable in origin, but most commonly is the continuation of the bronchoesophageal artery (a branch of the thoracic aorta) after the bronchoesophageal artery provides a branch to the esophagus.
   a. The bronchial artery enters the lung at the pulmonary root, and follows the course of the branching bronchi. The bronchial branches deliver oxygenated, nutrient-rich blood to the more proximal airways and pulmonary parenchyma as far distally as the respiratory bronchioles.
   b. At the respiratory bronchiole, the bronchial arteries terminate by breaking up into a capillary bed that overlaps and communicates with the terminal capillary bed of the pulmonary arteries.
2. **Veins.** The bronchial veins are extremely variable, not only in branching pattern but also in occurrence.
   a. A set of bronchial veins corresponding to the bronchial arteries is often absent. When bronchial veins are absent, the communication between the terminal capillary beds of the bronchial and pulmonary arteries allows the pulmonary veins to return venous blood from the bronchial arteries to the heart. Dilution of the oxygen-rich blood in the pulmonary veins by the oxygen-depleted blood of the pulmonary parenchyma is physiologically negligible, owing to the overwhelmingly greater volume of pulmonary venous blood.
   b. A few bronchial veins are fairly reliably identifiable at the hilus of the lung, where they drain into the azygos or intercostal veins.

D. Lymphatic vessels.

The **bronchial lymphocenter** is discussed in Chapter 35 III B 2.

V. INNERVATION OF THE LUNGS

INNERVATION OF THE LUNGS consists of an autonomic (motor) component and a sensory component.

A. Efferent (motor) fibers

Efferent (motor) fibers pass to the smooth muscle of the arterioles and bronchioles, and to the bronchial glands. Mixed branches from the **pulmonary plexus** are distributed to the pulmonary parenchyma along the surfaces of the arteries traveling inward from the hilus.

1. The **sympathetic contribution** to the pulmonary plexus arrives largely from the **cervicothoracic ganglion.**
2. The **parasympathetic contribution** to the pulmonary plexus arrives from the **vagus nerve,** as the nerve travels dorsal to the root of the lung.

B. Afferent (sensory) fibers.

Sensory receptors have been demonstrated throughout the lung, as far distally as the alveoli. Pulmonary structures possessing sensory receptors include the:
   a. **Tracheal** and **bronchial epithelia** (responsible for the **cough reflex)**
   b. **Alveolar ducts** and **walls**
   c. **Arterial** and **venous vessels** within the parenchyma
   d. **Stretch receptors** within the parenchyma

VI. MEDIASTINUM.

The mediastinum is **the space between the lungs.** Therefore, it is roughly a median structure, extending along the midline from the thoracic inlet to the diaphragm. The mediastinum is bordered on essentially all sides by the mediastinal pleura.

A. Regions.

The heart divides the mediastinum into three portions.

1. The **cranial mediastinum** lies **cranial to the heart** and contains several structures:
   a. **Dorsal portion**
      (1) **Esophagus**
      (2) **Trachea**

(3) **Great vessels of the heart**
(a) **Brachiocephalic trunk** and the **left subclavian artery,** along with their branches
(b) **Cranial vena cava**

b. **Middle** and **ventral portions**
(1) **Thymus.** In young dogs, the thymus completely fills the middle and ventral portions of the cranial mediastinum and is indented by the great vessels of the heart. In mature dogs, little is present in this region of the mediastinum other than the fatty remnants of the regressed thymus. Once the thymus regresses, the cranial regions of the cranial lung lobes expand to fill the space.
(2) **Internal thoracic arteries** and **veins**
(3) **Cranial mediastinal lymph nodes**

2. The **middle mediastinum contains the heart,** as well as several other structures.
a. **Dorsal portion**
(1) **Esophagus,** as it continues toward the abdominal cavity
(2) **Termination of the trachea,** as it reaches the pulmonary hilus to divide into the primary bronchi
(3) **Root of the lung**
(4) **Tracheobronchial lymph nodes**
(5) **Aortic arch**

b. **Middle** and **ventral portions**
(1) **Heart** and **pericardium**
(2) **Folds of pleural tissue**

3. The **caudal mediastinum** lies **caudal to the heart** and is the smallest of the three regions.
a. The **dorsal portion** of the caudal mediastinum transmits the **aorta, right azygous vein,** and **esophagus.**
b. The **middle portion** of the caudal mediastinum transmits the **caudal vena cava.**
c. The **ventral portion** of the caudal mediastinum is reduced to the **potential space between the layers of pleura between the lungs.**

B. Vasculature. Because the mediastinum is actually a space, it is not accurate to refer to the mediastinum as being vascularized. However, the numerous structures within the mediastinum require arterial supply and venous drainage.

1. **Arteries**
a. The **mediastinal branches** of the **internal thoracic artery** [see Chapter 35 I C 5 b (3)] supply most mediastinal structures.
b. **Opportunistic branches** often arise from nearby arteries, as well.

2. **Veins.** The veins in the mediastinum are largely satellites of the regional arteries.
3. **Lymphatics.** The **mediastinal lymphocenter** consists of the **cranial mediastinal lymph nodes** and their associated lymphatic channels (see Chapter 35 III B 1).

Chapter 38

Pericardium and Heart

I. PERICARDIUM. The pericardium is the double-layered, fibroserous sheath that completely surrounds the heart and allows it to move freely within the thoracic cavity.

A. Attachments

1. **Dorsally,** the pericardium blends with the adventitia of the great vessels of the heart; thus, the pericardium extends slightly farther dorsally than the cardiac tissue.
2. **Ventrally,** the pericardium continues beyond the border of the heart as the **sternopericardiac ligament,** a bundle of elastic tissue that extends between the apex of the pericardium and the diaphragm.

B. Structure

1. The **fibrous pericardium,** the rugged **outer layer** of the pericardial sac, consists of irregularly arranged collagenous and elastic fibers. The fibrous layer of the pericardium takes part in the attachments of the pericardium, by blending with the adventitia of the great vessels dorsal and cranial to the heart, and by contributing to the sternopericardiac ligament.
   a. The **superficial surface** of the fibrous pericardium is covered by the pericardial mediastinal pleura.
   b. The **deep surface** of the fibrous pericardium is fused with the outer layer of the serous pericardium.
2. The **serous pericardium,** a thin, double-layered, continuous sheet composed mainly of a layer of serous cells supported by a thin connective tissue layer, is similar in form and function to other serous membranes throughout the body.
   a. **Regions.** The doubled layer is applied to the surface of the heart deeply, and the fibrous pericardium superficially. Two regions of the serous pericardium are thus identified:
      (1) The **parietal serous pericardium,** the **outer layer** of the serous pericardium, is intimately adherent to the inner surface of the fibrous pericardium.
      (2) The **visceral serous pericardium,** the **inner layer** of the serous pericardium, is intimately adherent to the external surface of the myocardium. Histologically, this layer is termed the **epicardium.**
   b. **Pericardial cavity.** The serous pericardial membrane is continuous with itself, thus forming a cavity that **normally contains only a small amount of serous fluid, and no structures.**

Canine Clinical Correlation

The fibrous layer of the pericardium is so tough that it holds against the pressure of great amounts of fluid in the cavity. If sufficient fluid accumulates, the fluid can interfere with the heart's ability to expand and fill with blood during diastole **(cardiac tamponade).** Fluids that can accumulate within the pericardial cavity include blood **(hemopericardium)** and pus **(pyopericardium). Pneumopericardium** results from the accumulation of gas produced by gas-forming bacteria.

II. HEART (Figure 38–1; see also Chapter 5 II)

A. Position. The heart occupies the **middle mediastinum** and is in intimate contact with the lobes of the lungs on essentially all sides. The heart is **oriented obliquely** in the thorax, so that its upper, attached portion (i.e., its **base)** is positioned dorsocranially, and its lower, free portion (i.e., its **apex)** is positioned caudoventrally. The heart lies **slightly to the left of the midline.**

Canine Clinical Correlation

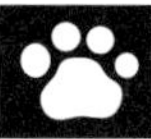

In the dog, the heart extends from approximately the third rib to the caudal border of the sixth rib. Given that in the standing dog, the olecranon tuber largely overlies the fifth intercostal space (i.e., between ribs 5 and 6), most of the heart lies medial to the thoracic limb and the mass of the triceps brachii muscle. The heart is thus doubly protected, by the bony cage of the thorax and by the thick substance of the proximal thoracic limb. In order to auscultate the heart, one must draw the limb cranially or place the stethoscope well medial to the thoracic limb.

B. Chambers (see Chapter 5, Figure 5–3)

1. **Atria.** The right and left atria are positioned dorsally on the heart, at its base. Each atrium needs to generate pressure sufficient to deliver blood to its respective ventricle, which is immediately adjacent to it. Thus, the required level of pressure is quite low, and the walls of the atria are rather thin and flaccid.
   a. The **right atrium** is positioned dorsocranially to the right ventricle.
   b. The **left atrium** is positioned dorsocaudally to the left ventricle.
   c. The **auricles** are blind-ended, roughly triangular pouches that extend from each atrium. The apices of the auricles point toward each other.
   d. The **interatrial septum** separates the right atrium from the left.
2. **Ventricles.** The right and left ventricles are positioned ventral to the atria, extending toward the apex of the heart. The ventricles must develop considerably higher pressure than the atria, and therefore, they have thicker walls.
   a. The **right ventricle** delivers blood to the **pulmonary capillary beds** and occupies the cranial portion of the ventricular region. The wall of the right ventricle, while many times thicker than the atrial walls, is nonetheless considerably thinner than that of the left ventricle, because the right ventricle must propel blood a shorter distance than the left ventricle. As a result of its thinner walls and lunate shape, the internal chamber of the right ventricle is more spacious than that of the left.
   b. The **left ventricle** delivers blood to the **systemic capillary beds.** Because of the force required to propel the blood throughout the body, the left ventricle has very thick walls. Despite the overall larger size of the left ventricle, its chamber is actually smaller than that of the right ventricle.

Canine Clinical Correlation

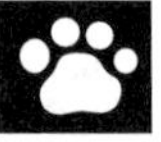

After death, the left ventricular wall typically maintains its normal form, while the walls of the other chambers collapse.

   c. The **interventricular septum** separates the right ventricle from the left. Two regions of the septum can be identified:
      (1) The **membranous part,** though not actually membranous, is noticeably thinner than the bulk of the septum. This small part is located closest to the atria.
      (2) The **muscular part,** which forms the bulk of the septum, is formed from the apposed and fused myocardial walls of the two ventricles.

C. **Surface features.** The **surface grooves of the heart** give an estimation of the position of most of the cardiac chambers.

1. The **coronary groove** encircles the dorsal part of the heart like a crown (*corona* = crown). The coronary groove:
   a. **Separates the atria from the ventricles**
   b. **Houses** the **coronary arteries** and the **great cardiac vein,** as well as the generous amount of **fat** that normally surrounds the vessels
2. The **paraconal interventricular groove** originates near the conus arteriosus. This relatively shallow groove:
   a. **Separates** the right and left ventricles
   b. **Houses** a **branch of the coronary arteries** and its **satellite vein**
3. The **subsinuosal interventricular groove** originates near the sinuatrial node of the cardiac conduction system. This relatively shallow groove:
   a. **Closely approximates** the internal position of the **interventricular septum**
   b. **Houses** a **branch of the coronary arteries** and its **satellite vein**

D. **Internal features**

1. **Right atrium.** The interior surface of the atrial wall is smooth, and is marked by several openings and other features.

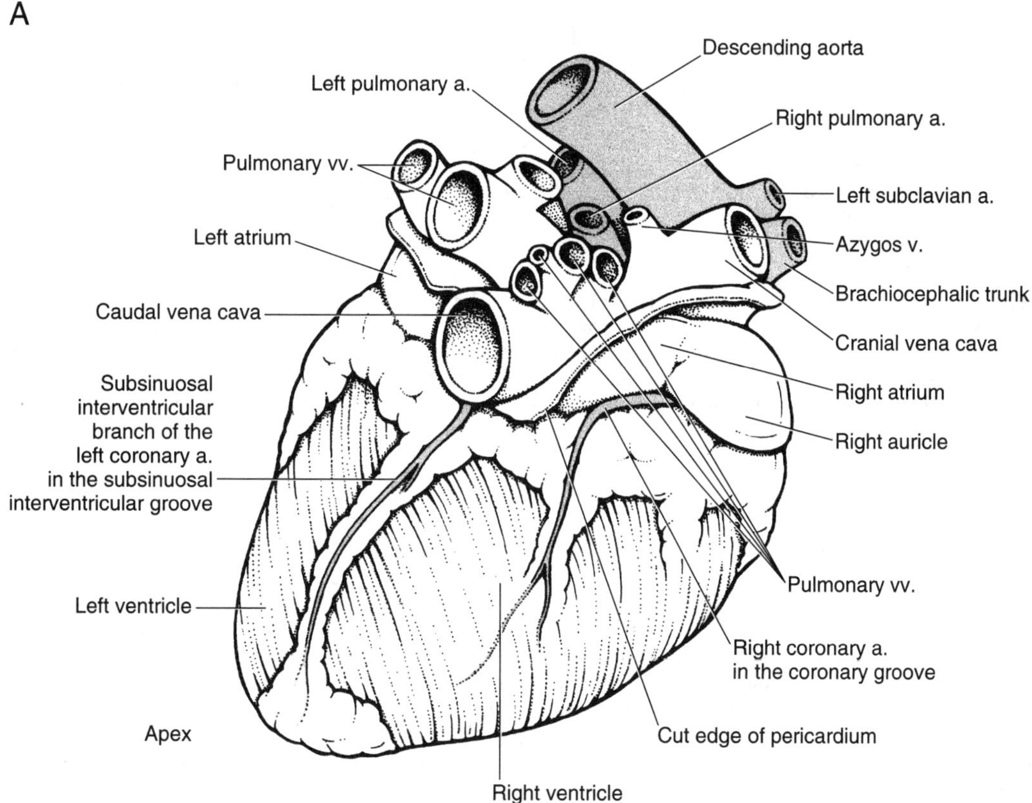

FIGURE 38–1. (*A*) The right lateral view of the heart presents mainly the right atrium, auricle, and ventricle. A significant portion of the left ventricle is also visible in this view, forming the apex of the heart. (*continued*)

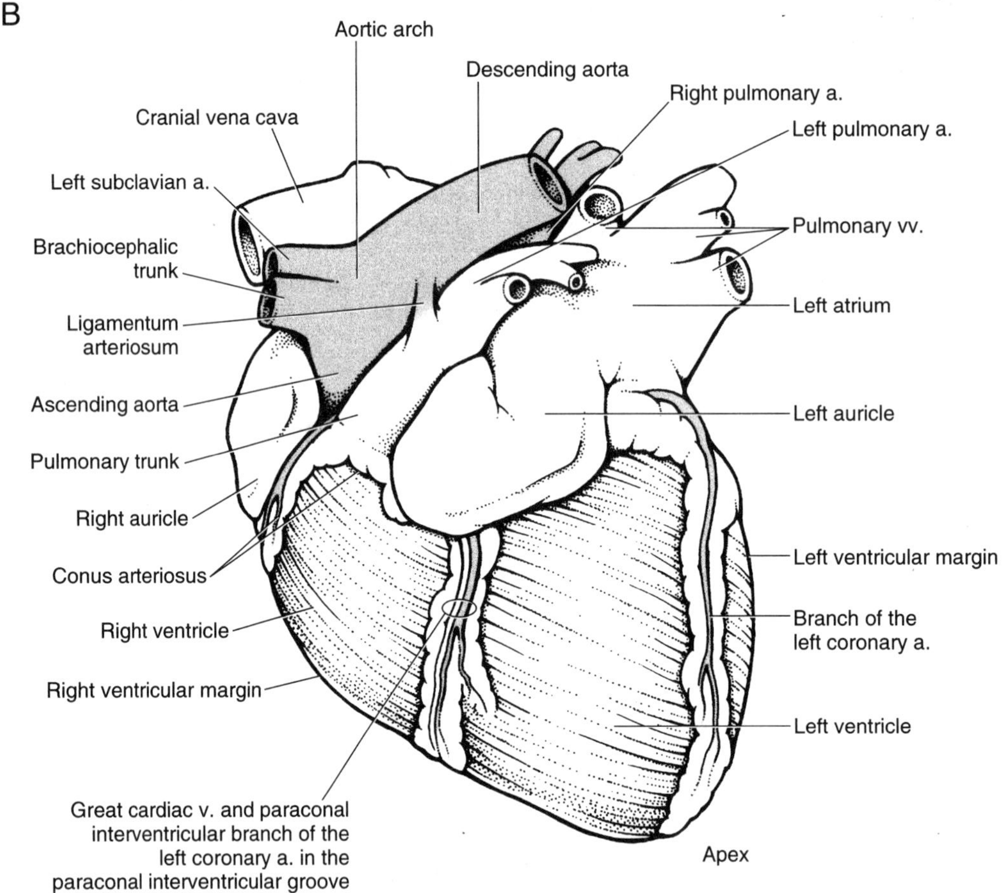

FIGURE 38–1—*continued* (*B*) The left lateral view of the heart presents a clear view of the left atrium, auricle, and ventricle. From this perspective, the left ventricle can be seen to form the entire cardiac apex. A significant portion of the right ventricle and the distal end of the right auricle are also visible. Note that the apex of the left auricle points fairly directly toward the paraconal interventricular groove. (Modified with permission from Anderson WD: *Atlas of Canine Anatomy.* Baltimore, Williams & Wilkins, 1994, pp 529, 530.)

a. Openings

(1) The **cranial vena cava** opens into the dorsocranial aspect of the right atrium, delivering blood to the heart from the head, neck, and thoracic limb, as well as the thoracic wall and lumbar region (via the azygos vein).

(2) The **caudal vena cava** opens into the dorsocaudal region of the right atrium, bringing blood to the heart from the abdominal viscera, pelvic limb, and part of the abdominal wall.

(3) The **coronary sinus** opens into the right atrium ventral to the caudal vena cava and drains blood from the heart itself.

(4) The **atrioventricular orifice (ostium),** the communication between the right atrium and the right ventricle, is located at the caudoventral margin of the right atrium.

b. The **intervenous tubercle** is an elevation on the internal right atrial wall positioned at the confluence of the cranial and caudal venae cavae. This "bump" serves to deflect the flow of blood from each vena cava smoothly into the atrioventricular orifice, thereby decreasing turbulence.

c. The **fossa ovalis,** the **remnant of the foramen ovale** of the fetal heart, is a depression just caudal to the intervenous tubercle on the interatrial septum.

d. The **pectinate muscles,** a prominent and extensive set of arborizing and interconnecting muscle fibers, mark the internal surface of the auricle of the right atrium. The appearance of the internal surface of the auricle contrasts sharply with the smooth appearance of the inner wall of the rest of the atrium.
e. The **crista terminalis,** a semilunar crest bordering the openings of the cranial vena cava and atrioventricular orifice, marks the boundary of the pectinate muscles and determines the margin between the atrium and the auricle.

2. **Left atrium.** The internal surface of the left atrium is similar to that of the right atrium, except for the following features:
   a. Approximately five **pulmonary veins** open into the left atrium, delivering oxygenated blood from the lungs.
   b. Instead of the fossa ovalis, the **valve of the foramen ovale** (the flap that covers and occludes the foramen ovale following pressure changes in the heart after birth) is present in the interatrial wall.
   c. **The left atrium does not have a crista terminalis or an intervenous tubercle.**

3. **Right ventricle**
   a. **Openings**
      (1) The **right atrioventricular orifice (ostium),** the communication between the right atrium and ventricle, is positioned at the dorsocranial margin of the right ventricle.
      (2) The **pulmonary orifice (ostium)** is the opening through which blood passes from the right ventricle to the pulmonary trunk.
   b. The **conus arteriosus** is the narrowing of the internal chamber of the right ventricle as it funnels toward the pulmonary trunk.
   c. The **papillary muscles** are prominent, blunt, cylindrical elevations of muscle that project freely from the ventricular wall into the chamber.
      (1) The number and form of the papillary muscles in the right ventricle vary. **Three is the usual number,** but only one or two may be present. When only one papillary muscle is present, it is compound, with multiple heads.
      (2) The free ends of the papillary muscles are usually smooth, although in some cases one or more may be bifid. **Chordae tendineae** are tough, fine strands of fibromuscular tissue that extend from the free end of the papillary muscles to the free edges of the atrioventricular valve leaflets. Occasionally, a small chorda tendinea arises directly from the ventricular wall.
   d. **Trabeculae carneae** are irregular elevations of muscle on most of the internal surface of the ventricle. Although the trabeculae are smooth-surfaced, rather low, and do not project freely for a great distance into the ventricular lumen, they are sufficiently prominent to render the interior of the ventricle quite uneven where they are present.
   e. The **trabecula septomarginalis** is a band of muscle that extends from the interventricular septum to the free marginal wall of the right ventricle.
      (1) The trabecula septomarginalis is **usually single,** but may also be branched or doubled.
      (2) The trabecula septomarginalis **transmits fibers of the conducting system of the heart to the free ventricular wall.**

4. **Left ventricle**
   a. **Openings**
      (1) The **left atrioventricular orifice (ostium),** the communication between the left atrium and ventricle, is positioned at the dorsocranial margin of the left ventricle.
      (2) The **aortic orifice (ostium)** is the opening through which blood passes from the right ventricle into the aorta.
   b. **Papillary muscles,** similar to those of the right ventricle, are present in the left ventricle.
      (1) Typically, the left ventricle has **two** large papillary muscles. Less variation is seen in the number than in the right ventricle.
      (2) **Chordae tendineae** are present on the papillary muscles of the left ventricle.
   c. **Trabeculae carneae** are prominent on the interior wall of the left ventricle.
   d. **The left ventricle does not have a trabecula septomarginalis.**

E. Internal structure

1. The **fibrous base (skeleton) of the heart,** a collection of fibrous tissue and bits of hyaline or fibrocartilage situated between the atria and the ventricles, provides a semirigid framework to support the contraction cycles of the heart. The fibrous cardiac base essentially consists of **four rings,** each surrounding one of the heart valves and connected to the others by fibrocartilaginous tissue that is more extensive in some areas than others. The rings are named for the valves which they support: the **aortic, pulmonary,** and **atrioventricular fibrous rings.**
2. **Valves.** The four major intracardiac openings through which blood passes when routing between the body and the lungs have valves, which regulate blood flow.
   a. The two **atrioventricular valves** are the **inflow valves of the ventricles.**
      (1) **Position.** The atrioventricular valves are positioned **between the atria** and **the ventricles,** over the atrioventricular orifice.
      (2) **Function.** The atrioventricular valves open to admit blood to the ventricles on diastole (i.e., when the ventricles relax) and close to prevent backflow of blood from the ventricles to the atria on systole (i.e., when the ventricles contract).

Canine Clinical Correlation

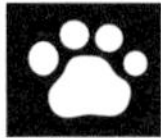

Closure of the atrioventricular valves produces the first ("lub") sound in the classic "lub-dup" sound of the heartbeat.

      (3) **Structure**
         (a) **General.** Each atrioventricular valve consists of **two** irregularly shaped **cusps (leaflets),** thin sheets composed largely of fibrous tissue.
            (i) The **attached ends** of the cusps are anchored to the **fibrous skeleton of the heart.**
            (ii) The **free ends** of the cusps attach to the **chordae tendineae.**
         (b) **Right atrioventricular valve.** Because the right atrioventricular valve has two leaflets, the term used to describe this valve in human anatomy ("tricuspid") cannot be used in veterinary medicine.
         (c) **Left atrioventricular valve.** The terms used to describe this valve in human anatomy **("bicuspid," "mitral")** are technically applicable in veterinary anatomy; however, because both atrioventricular valves have two leaflets, "bicuspid" is not a distinguishing term. Because the pressure generated by the left ventricle is about four times that of the right, the left atrioventricular valve and its associated structures (i.e., the chordae tendineae and papillary muscles) are more robust than those of the right atrioventricular valve.
   b. The **pulmonic** and **aortic valves** are the **outflow valves of the ventricles.**
      (1) **Position**
         (a) The **pulmonic valve** lies between the **right ventricle** and **pulmonary trunk,** over the pulmonary orifice.
         (b) The **aortic valve** lies between the **left ventricle** and the **aorta,** over the aortic orifice.

Canine Clinical Correlation

Closure of the outflow valves produces the second (or "dup") sound in the classic "lub-dup" sound of the heartbeat.

(2) **Function.** The outflow valves open to admit blood to the great arteries on diastole and close to prevent backflow of blood from the great arteries to the ventricles on systole.

(3) **Structure**

(a) **General.** Each outflow valve **(semilunar valve)** consists of three **half-moon–shaped cusps.** Because these outflow valves must withstand only the backflow pressure of the great arteries (as opposed to the pressure produced by ventricular contraction), they are simpler in form and lack chordae tendineae and other supporting structures.

(i) The **attached ends** of the cusps are anchored to the **fibrous skeleton of the heart.**

(ii) The **free ends** of the cusps of the outflow valves **have no supporting structures** similar to chordae tendineae.

(iii) The free edge of each cusp has a **nodule,** a small but prominent elevation in the center of the free edge. When the valve closes, the three nodules of each leaflet come into contact with each other at the center of the closed valve.

(b) The **pulmonic valve** is not as robust in structure as the aortic valve, because the right ventricle produces less pressure than the left.

(c) The **aortic valve** is associated with **aortic sinuses,** dilatations in the aortic wall just distal to the base of the aortic valve cusps (i.e., on the side away from the heart). The right and left **coronary arteries** arise from two of the aortic sinuses; their openings can be readily seen by reflecting the cusps of the aortic valve.

Canine Clinical Correlation

The sounds of each pair of valves closing tend to radiate through the chest to a fairly constant region on the lateral thoracic wall (Table 38–1). The **puncta maxima** are the points on the chest wall where the heart sounds can be best distinguished. With considerable practice, one can become skilled in distinguishing the sounds produced by each valve.

TABLE 38–1. Puncta Maxima for the Four Heart Valves

Valve	Point of Maximal Impulse
Right atrioventricular valve	**Right side, low** (i.e., at the costochondral junction) in the **fourth intercostal space**
Pulmonic valve	**Left side, low** in the **third intercostal space**
Aortic valve	**Left side, high** (i.e., one third of the way up the thoracic wall) in the **fourth intercostal space**
Left atrioventricular valve	**Low** in the **fifth intercostal space** on the **left side**

Canine Clinical Correlation

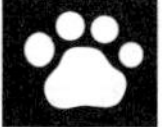

Interference with closure of any heart valve results in leakage or backflow of blood through the valve. This fluid movement produces sounds referred to as **heart murmurs.** The valve responsible for the murmur can be identified by the murmur's character and timing in the cardiac cycle and by clinical signs exhibited by the patient.

III. VASCULATURE OF THE HEART

A. Arteries. The **right** and **left coronary arteries** supply the heart with blood. The heart is the first organ to receive its arterial blood supply.

1. The **right coronary artery,** which is smaller than the left, supplies a proportionately smaller area of the myocardium.
   a. **Course.** The right coronary artery departs from an **aortic sinus,** and enters the **coronary groove** between the atria and ventricles. It then courses to the right and cranioventrally, giving off several named branches that need not be described here.
   b. **Structures supplied** include the:
      (1) **Right free ventricular wall** (approximately two thirds of it)
      (2) **Right atrium**
      (3) **Sinuatrial node**
      (4) **Proximal pulmonary trunk and aorta**

2. The **left coronary artery** supplies a greater proportion of the myocardium.
   a. **Branches**
      (1) The **left coronary artery proper** is a short trunk that departs from an aortic sinus and **almost immediately bifurcates into two constant branches.**
         (a) The **circumflex branch** of the left coronary artery, the larger of the two branches, enters the **coronary groove,** courses to the left and dorsocaudally, and eventually turns back to the right as it rounds the caudal border of the heart. On reaching the **subsinuosal interventricular groove,** the circumflex coronary artery enters the groove and becomes the **subsinuosal interventricular branch,** which passes essentially to the apex of the heart.
         (b) The **paraconal interventricular branch** of the left coronary artery enters the **paraconal interventricular groove** soon after arising from the left coronary artery. This vessel courses distally through the groove, typically extending beyond it to the cardiac apex and giving off several named branches along the way.
      (2) A **septal branch** frequently arises from the left coronary artery, as well. When present, this branch courses to and supplies the interventricular septum.
   b. Structures supplied by the left coronary artery include the:
      (1) **Free left ventricular wall**
      (2) **Interventricular septum**
      (3) **Left atrium**

B. Veins. The naming of the cardiac veins departs from the normal scheme of vein nomenclature in that, although many veins of the heart are essentially satellites of named arteries, the veins do not necessarily take the name of the arteries they accompany. In addition, **most of the cardiac veins are paired.**

1. The **great cardiac vein,** the major vein of the heart, is paired.
   a. **Course.** The great cardiac vein **originates near the cardiac apex** and ascends in the **paraconal interventricular groove** alongside the paraconal interventricular branch of the left coronary artery. Late in its course, the great cardiac vein lies in the **coronary groove** alongside the coronary arteries. The vein **terminates in the right atrium** at the **coronary sinus.**
   b. **Structures drained.** This vessel drains most of the myocardium. In its course proximally, the great cardiac vein receives as tributaries:
      (1) Many small tributaries from the **ventricular walls**
      (2) Small branches from the **left atrium**

2. The **middle cardiac vein** is also paired.
   a. **Course.** The middle cardiac vein **originates near the cardiac apex** and communicates with the great cardiac vein. It is positioned in the **subsinuosal interventricular groove,** alongside the subsinuosal interventricular artery.

b. **Structures drained.** The middle cardiac vein receives as tributaries many veins from **both ventricular walls.**

3. The **right cardiac veins** are a group of small veins that **drain the right ventricle** and typically empty directly into the right atrium.

4. The **small cardiac (Thebesian) veins** are microscopic venules in the myocardium that open directly into the associated heart chamber.

C. **Lymphatic vessels** drain into the **mediastinal lymphocenter;** therefore, they drain into the **cranial mediastinal lymph nodes** (see Chapter 35 III B 1).

IV. INNERVATION OF THE HEART

A. **Extrinsic innervation.** The extrinsic cardiac innervation is strictly **regulatory in nature,** because the heart is inherently rhythmic (i.e., the nervous impulses causing the heart to contract are generated within the cardiac tissue itself). The conducting tissues of the heart are normally regulated by input from the **autonomic nervous system (ANS).**

1. **Sympathetic innervation** arrives from the **cervicothoracic ganglion, middle cervical ganglion,** and **ansa subclavia.** Sympathetic tone **increases** heart rate and contractility.

2. **Parasympathetic innervation** arrives from the **recurrent laryngeal** and **vagus nerves.** Parasympathetic tone **decreases** heart rate and contractility.

B. **Intrinsic innervation.** The intrinsic cardiac innervation is the **cardiac conduction system,** which is composed of **specialized nervous (Purkinje) cells.** These cells are recognizable histologically but cannot be distinguished grossly; they form two intrinsically discharging nervous centers in the heart.

1. **Sinuatrial node**
   a. **Position.** The sinuatrial node is located in the internal right atrial wall, near the entrance of the cranial vena cava.
   b. **Function.** The sinuatrial node, which has the **faster discharge rhythm** of the two intrinsic nervous bundles of the heart, **controls the heart rate** (hence the clinical phrase, "normal sinus rhythm").

2. **Atrioventricular node**
   a. **Position.** The atrioventricular node is positioned in the interatrial septum just proximal to the ventricle. Fibers from the node pass through the fibrous skeleton of the heart, and divide into right and left septal branches. Each branch passes just deep to the endocardium (i.e., the inner single-cell layer of the heart) on the right and left sides of the ventricular septum. These **paired atrioventricular conduction fibers** are commonly referred to as the **bundle of His.**
      (1) The **right atrioventricular septal branch** is conducted across the right ventricular lumen as the **trabecula septomarginalis.**
      (2) The **left atrioventricular septal branch** is dispersed through the wall of the left ventricle more diffusely.
   b. **Function.** Normally, the sinuatrial node, which has a faster rate of discharge, controls the atrioventricular node. However, should disease or another disturbance interfere with the discharge of the sinuatrial node, the atrioventricular node takes control, causing the ventricles to contract at its own slower rate.

Canine Clinical Correlation

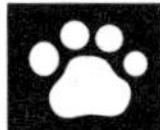

In certain clinical conditions, the coordination between the two conducting nodes is disturbed, so that the atrioventricular node overrides the sinuatrial node, causing **ventricular premature contractions (VPCs).** Treatment often successfully restores the normal rhythmicity of the heart.

Chapter 39

Prominent Palpable Features of the Thoracic Region

I. BONY STRUCTURES

A. The **scapula** is discussed in Chapter 31 I A 1.

B. The **spinous processes of the thoracic vertebrae** are palpable along the dorsal midline throughout the thoracic region, unless the animal is obese.

C. The **olecranon tuberosity** (see also Chapter 31 I C 3) is a readily palpable bony landmark of the lateral thoracic region, and in the normal standing animal may be used to approximate the level of the fifth intercostal space.

D. Most **ribs** (i.e., those caudal to rib 5) are palpated through the several flat muscles that overlie them (i.e., the latissimus dorsi, serratus dorsalis caudalis, serratus ventralis).

1. **Portions of ribs accessible to palpation**
   a. **Rib 1** is accessible along its cranial edge at the thoracic inlet, but the full body cannot be reached.
   b. **Ribs 2–5** are positioned medial to the proximal thoracic limb and the triceps brachii, and hence cannot be appreciated. However, gently abducting the thoracic limb increases the surface area of thoracic wall open to examination; the more ventral parts of ribs 2–5 can then be accessed by palpating in the axillary space.
   c. **Ribs 6–12** are normally palpable over most of their surface.
   d. **Rib 13** (i.e., the **floating rib)** is readily identifiable as terminating in the abdominal musculature without reaching the sternum.
2. The **bodies of the ribs** caudal to rib 5 are readily accessible from the ventral edge of the epaxial muscles to the sternum.
3. The **vertebral extremities of the ribs** (i.e., the head and tubercle) are normally not palpable, because they are deep to the epaxial muscles.
4. The **costal arch** formed by the costal cartilages of the ribs 10–12 is easily accessed passing cranioventrally toward the sternum.
5. The **intercostal spaces** are readily identified as the yielding areas between the bony ribs.

> **Canine Clinical Correlation**
>
> **Percussion of the thorax** is performed as follows:
>
> - Extend one finger over an intercostal space, ventral to the epaxial muscles.
> - Sharply tap the middle phalanx of the finger that you have placed against the thoracic wall with the middle fingertip of the other hand, evaluating the resulting sound.
>   1. Percussion of intercostal spaces 6–9 should produce a relatively hollow, resonant sound owing to the air-filled lung deep to that area of the thorax.
>   2. Percussion of the more caudal intercostal spaces should produce a duller sound, owing to the presence of fluid-filled digestive viscera deep to that area of the thorax.

E. **Sternum**

1. The **manubrium** is palpable along its cranial edge at the thoracic inlet, and over the ventral surface of its body along the ventral midline.

2. **Sternebrae 2–7** can be palpated along their ventral surfaces, along the ventral midline of the body caudal to the manubrium.
3. The **xiphoid process** and **xiphoid cartilage** can be palpated on the ventral midline at the caudal end of the sternum, in the angle between the converging costal cartilages.

II. SOFT TISSUE STRUCTURES.

Because the thoracic cage performs its function of protecting the structures within it so well, palpable soft tissue structures of the thoracic region are essentially limited to those of the lateral thoracic wall.

A. Muscles

1. The **epaxial musculature** is palpable as well-developed muscle masses along each side of the dorsal midline.
2. The **shoulder musculature** is palpable relative to the thoracic limb, over the craniolateral thoracic area.
3. The **pectoral muscles** are palpable in the ventral thoracic region, extending between the trunk and the thoracic limb.
4. The **intercostal muscles** are palpable as the yielding spaces between the bony hardness of the ribs.

B. The **axillary lymph nodes** are palpable only when enlarged.

Canine Clinical Correlation

The **precordial thrust** (i.e., the palpable "thud" of the heart valves closing during the cardiac cycle) is readily appreciated by placing the hands over the ventrolateral thoracic wall medial and caudal to the olecranon and triceps brachii muscle mass.

STUDY QUESTIONS

DIRECTIONS: Each of the numbered items or incomplete statements in this section is followed by answers or by completions of the statement. Select the ONE numbered answer or completion that is BEST in each case.

1. The defining characteristic that distinguishes the thoracic cavity from the thoracic cage is that the former has included in its boundaries the:

(1) ribs.
(2) sternum.
(3) diaphragm.
(4) thoracic vertebrae.

2. Which region of the rib is specialized for articulation with the transverse process of the corresponding vertebra?

(1) Tubercle
(2) Head
(3) Neck
(4) Transverse prominence

3. Which one of the following statements concerning the articulation of the ribs with the sternum is correct?

(1) The sternebrae articulate directly with the bony terminal part of each rib.
(2) The cranial ribs articulate with a single sternebra, whereas the caudal ribs share articulation sites on the last few sternebrae.
(3) No part of any rib articulates with the xiphoid cartilage.
(4) The first and last sternebrae are modified for muscular, but not bony, attachments.

4. Which statement regarding the sternocostal joints is true?

(1) They are synovial over the first six joints and synchondrotic for the remainder.
(2) They are positioned between the sternebrae and the corresponding costal cartilages.
(3) They are doubled on each sternebra to accommodate the greater number of ribs than sternebrae.
(4) They are absent on the last seven sternebrae.

5. Contraction of which one of the following muscles assists expiration?

(1) Diaphragm
(2) Serratus dorsalis cranialis
(3) Internal intercostals
(4) Rectus thoracis

6. Which ventilatory muscle consists of several distinct bundles, originates from the internal sternal surface and courses obliquely cranially to insert on the internal surfaces of the costal cartilages, and is innervated by intercostal nerves?

(1) Rectus thoracis
(2) Transversus thoracis
(3) Serratus ventralis cranialis
(4) Serratus ventralis caudalis

7. Which one of the following muscles of the thoracic wall has the potential to contribute to flexing of the shoulder?

(1) Cutaneous trunci
(2) Serratus dorsalis cranialis
(3) Serratus dorsalis caudalis
(4) Transversus thoracis

8. The external intercostal muscles are distinguished from the external interchondral muscles by:

(1) fiber direction.
(2) innervation.
(3) origin.
(4) action.

9. Which pair correctly matches the opening in the diaphragm with all of the structures that pass through it?

(1) Aortic hiatus—aorta and thoracic duct
(2) Aortic hiatus—aorta and azygos vein
(3) Esophageal hiatus—esophagus, dorsal and ventral vagus nerves
(4) Caval foramen—caudal vena cava

10. Which statement regarding the endothoracic fascia is correct?

(1) It is positioned deep to the musculature of the internal thoracic wall.
(2) It is positioned between the internal and external intercostal muscles.
(3) It is continuous with the central tendon of the diaphragm.
(4) It is also called the transversothoracic fascia.

11. The brachiocephalic trunk terminates by dividing inside the cranial thoracic cavity into the:

(1) right and left common carotid arteries.
(2) right and left brachiocephalic trunks.
(3) left and right subclavian arteries.
(4) right common carotid artery and right subclavian artery.

12. Which artery directly (or by its immediate branches) supplies the intercostal muscles, diaphragm, and mammary glands and is positioned deep to the transversus thoracis muscle?

(1) Internal thoracic artery
(2) Musculophrenic artery
(3) Cranial deep epigastric artery
(4) Ventral longitudinal intercostal artery

13. Which branch of the subclavian artery is most important in supplying the shoulder musculature?

(1) Axillary artery
(2) Vertebral artery
(3) Costocervical trunk
(4) Superficial cervical artery

14. Which statement regarding the cranial vena cava is true?

(1) It forms from the confluence of the right and left external jugular veins.
(2) It drains the head, neck, and thoracic limb.
(3) It is better developed on the right than on the left.
(4) It terminates in the right ventricle.

15. Which statement regarding the azygos vein is true?

(1) It terminates in the right atrium.
(2) It drains the digestive viscera and pelvic limbs.
(3) It is usually bilateral, but occasionally may be present only on the left.
(4) It includes the bronchoesophageal and esophageal veins among its tributaries.

16. Parasympathetic innervation to the thoracic viscera arrives through the:

(1) vagus nerves.
(2) vagus and recurrent laryngeal nerves.
(3) thoracic splanchnic nerves.
(4) cervicothoracic ganglion.

17. Which statement regarding the cardiac nerves is true?

(1) They arise from the vagus nerve.
(2) They arise from both the vagus and the recurrent laryngeal nerves.
(3) They are purely parasympathetic in nature.
(4) They form on the right, innervate the right side of the heart, and then pass to the left to innervate the left cardiac regions.

18. What are the normal contents of the cranial portion of the right and left pleural cavities?

(1) Nothing
(2) A small amount of serous fluid
(3) The thymus on the left and the cranial vena cava on the right
(4) The cranial and caudal parts of the cranial lobe of the left lung on the left and the cranial lobe of the right lung on the right

19. How might the pulmonary pleura be distinguished from the diaphragmatic parietal pleura?

(1) Position
(2) Thickness
(3) Fiber direction
(4) Histologic structure

20. What is the line of pleural reflection?

(1) The boundary between the visceral and parietal portions of the pleural membrane
(2) The boundary between the costal and diaphragmatic portions of the pleural membrane
(3) The site where the lungs enter the pleural cavity
(4) An imaginary line that forms as the lung volume decreases on expiration and is obliterated as the lungs expand on inspiration

21. The relation of the lungs and the line of pleural reflection results in:

(1) a recess caudal to the line of pleural reflection that can be accessed by needle diagnostically or therapeutically
(2) interdigitation between the basal border of the lung and the two layers of pleura on each side of the reflection
(3) two imaginary arcing lines that parallel each but do not overlap
(4) a triangular space on the ventrolateral thoracic wall that can be accessed to drain fluid

22. What is the best estimate for the line indicating the basal border of the lung?

(1) The costal arch
(2) A line between the olecranon tuber and the penultimate rib
(3) The curve of the ninth rib
(4) A line between the third intercostal space and the penultimate rib

23. Which statement regarding the anatomy of the lung is correct?

(1) The base of the lung corresponds to its diaphragmatic surface.
(2) The lobation of the lung is determined by the deep surface fissures that grossly divide the lungs into lobes.
(3) The cranial vena cava passes through a notch in the accessory lobe of the right lung.
(4) The root of the lung is the point where the lung is suspended from the internal dorsal thoracic wall by the pulmonary ligament.

24. Where should thoracocentesis to remove fluid from the pleural cavity be performed?

(1) At the third or fourth intercostal space at the costochondral junction
(2) At the fifth to eighth intercostal space at the level of the epaxial muscles
(3) At the seventh or eighth intercostal space at the costochondral junction
(4) At the seventh or eighth intercostal space halfway down the body of the rib

25. Which vessels associated with the lungs carry deoxygenated blood?

(1) Pulmonary veins
(2) Bronchial arteries
(3) Pulmonary arteries
(4) Pulmonary and bronchial arteries

26. The ligamentum arteriosum is associated with the:

(1) aorta and pulmonary trunk.
(2) aorta and left pulmonary vein.
(3) right and left bronchial arteries.
(4) pulmonary trunk and left atrium.

27. The pulmonary trunk divides into the right and left:

(1) pulmonary veins.
(2) pulmonary arteries.
(3) bronchial arteries.
(4) principal bronchi.

28. Most oxygen-depleted blood from the pulmonary parenchyma returns to the systemic circulation through the:

(1) bronchial veins.
(2) pulmonary veins.
(3) pulmonary venous sinuses.
(4) expanded lymphatic vessels peculiar to the lungs.

29. Why are the structures on the left side of the heart typically larger and stronger than the corresponding structures on the right side of the heart?

(1) The left lung, which is larger than the right, returns more blood to the heart than the right lung.
(2) The heart is displaced to the right side of the midline, and is therefore crowded by the thoracic cage.
(3) During development, more arteries anastomose to form the left side of the heart than contribute to formation of the right side.
(4) The left side of the heart has to pump blood further through the body than the right side of the heart.

30. Which artery supplies the greatest portion of the dog's heart?

(1) Left coronary artery
(2) Right coronary artery
(3) Great cardiac artery
(4) Subconal interventricular branch

31. The heart lies between which ribs?

(1) Ribs 2 and 6
(2) Ribs 3 and 6
(3) Ribs 4 and 7
(4) Ribs 5 and 7

32. Which heart valve can be best auscultated low in the fourth intercostal space on the right side?

(1) Aortic valve
(2) Pulmonic valve
(3) Left atrioventricular valve
(4) Right atrioventricular valve

33. What is the correct sequence for flow of conduction impulses through the heart?

(1) Sinuatrial node, atrioventricular node, trabecula septomarginalis, atrioventricular conduction fibers
(2) Sinuatrial node, atrioventricular node, atrioventricular conduction fibers, trabecula septomarginalis
(3) Atrioventricular node, trabecula septomarginalis, atrioventricular node, sinuatrial node
(4) Trabecula septomarginalis, atrioventricular conduction fibers, atrioventricular node, sinuatrial node

34. Which statement best describes the extrinsic innervation of the heart?

(1) It is provided solely by sympathetic nerves from the cervicothoracic ganglion.
(2) It is purely parasympathetic in nature.
(3) It serves to regulate the intrinsic cardiac innervation.
(4) It assumes the role of rhythmic contraction if the intrinsic system fails.

35. What is the coronary sinus?

(1) The dilatation at the base of the aorta where the coronary arteries arise
(2) The dilatation at the most proximal region of both coronary arteries that helps maintain pressure during cardiac diastole
(3) The opening of the cranial vena cava into the right atrium
(4) The opening of the great cardiac vein into the right atrium

36. Which structure is located in only two of the three regions of the mediastinum?

(1) Cranial vena cava
(2) Esophagus
(3) Aorta
(4) Lung

DIRECTIONS: Each of the numbered items or incomplete statements in this section is negatively phrased, as indicated by a capitalized word such as NOT, LEAST, or EXCEPT. Select the ONE numbered answer or completion that is BEST in each case.

37. Which statement regarding the intercostal nerves is FALSE?

(1) They are the dorsal branches of the thoracic spinal nerves.
(2) They are motor to the intercostal muscles.
(3) They are sensory to the mammary glands.
(4) They are motor to selected muscles of the ventral abdominal wall.

38. Which statement regarding the thoracic sympathetic ganglia is FALSE?

(1) They are relatively small and unspecialized along the length of the vertebral column.
(2) They are modified by fusions with certain cervical sympathetic ganglia in the cranial thoracic region.
(3) They directly supply sympathetic innervation to the heart.
(4) They are connected to the recurrent laryngeal nerve via the ansa subclavia.

39. Visceral branches of the thoracic aorta include arteries that supply all of the following organs EXCEPT the:

(1) heart.
(2) thymus.
(3) pericardium.
(4) mediastinal lymph nodes.

40. Assuming a typical branching pattern of the thoracic arteries, all of the following structures would be ultimately supplied by branches of the left subclavian artery EXCEPT the:

(1) brain.
(2) lungs.
(3) intercostal muscles.
(4) shoulder musculature.

41. Which of the following portions of the bony thoracic cage would NOT remain following decomposition of soft tissue after death?

(1) Costal body
(2) Costal arch
(3) Costal groove
(4) Costal tubercle

42. Which statement regarding the cardiac valves is INCORRECT?

(1) The inflow valves are specialized to withstand less pressure on systole.
(2) The outflow valves each have three leaflets.
(3) All four valves are anchored in the fibrous skeleton of the heart.
(4) On systole, the outflow valves open and the inflow valves close.

43. Which of the following is NOT a component of the pericardial sac?

(1) Mediastinal pleural layer
(2) Outer fibrous layer
(3) Outer serous layer
(4) Inner serous layer

44. Which statement regarding the coronary groove of the heart is INCORRECT?

(1) It separates the atria from the ventricles.
(2) It carries the right and left coronary arteries and veins.
(3) It encircles the base of the heart.
(4) Its contents are obscured by generous amounts of fat.

ANSWERS AND EXPLANATIONS

1. The answer is 3 [Chapter 32 I B 1]. The thoracic cage and the thoracic cavity differ only in their caudal boundaries, which in the case of the thoracic cavity is the diaphragm, and in the case of the thoracic cage is the thoracic outlet.

2. The answer is 1 [Chapter 33 I C 5 a (3)]. The tubercle of the rib articulates with the transverse process of the corresponding thoracic vertebra. The head of the rib articulates with the body of the corresponding vertebra, and the costal neck articulates with nothing. "Transverse prominence" is a fanciful term.

3. The answer is 3 [Chapter 33 I B 2 b, C 4 a]. The xiphoid cartilage projects freely from the caudal end of the xiphoid process, and has only muscular attachments. Option 2 is invalidated because only the first pair of ribs articulates with a sternebra (i.e., the manubrium); the remaining ribs articulate with the intersternebral cartilages. Because the first pair of ribs articulates with the manubrium, option 4 is invalidated.

4. The answer is 4 [Chapter 33 II B 2]. All sternocostal joints are synovial in nature. Only the first sternocostal joint is actually positioned on a sternebra—the remainder are singly placed on the intersternebral cartilages.

5. The answer is 3 [Chapter 34 I E 3; Table 34–1]. The internal intercostal muscles draw the ribs caudally on expiration. The serratus dorsalis cranialis and rectus thoracis act to draw the ribs cranially on inspiration. The diaphragm contracts to draw the dome of the diaphragm caudally, allowing the lungs to expand and inspiration to occur. Relaxation of the diaphragm pushes the digestive viscera cranially and decreases the size of the thoracic cavity, resulting in expiration; however, this is a passive occurrence.

6. The answer is 2 [Table 34–2]. The transversus thoracis, which is innervated by intercostal nerves, originates from the internal sternal surface and courses obliquely cranially to insert on the internal surfaces of the costal cartilages. The rectus thoracis is a muscle of the external thoracic wall, as opposed to the internal thoracic wall (like the transversus thoracis). The names "serratus ventralis cranialis" and "serratus ventralis caudalis" are fictional; the serratus dorsalis cranialis and serratus dorsalis caudalis lie high on the lateral thoracic wall and are unrelated to the sternum.

7. The answer is 1 [Table 34–1]. The cutaneous trunci, which functions mainly in twitching the skin over the thoracic wall, inserts on the teres major tuberosity in conjunction with the latissimus dorsi. Because the cutaneous trunci originates over the dorsolateral thoracic wall from the scapula and continues caudally, it can contribute (at least theoretically) to shoulder flexion.

8. The answer is 3 [Chapter 34 I D 4 c]. The external intercostal muscles and external interchondral muscles differ on the basis of origin. The external interchondral muscles are simply the continuation of the external intercostal muscles ventral to the costochondral junction. Thus, they share fiber direction, innervation, and action with the external intercostal muscles, but originate on the costal cartilages rather than the bony part of the rib.

9. The answer is 4 [Chapter 32 I B 1 a (3)]. The caudal vena cava passes through the caval foramen of the diaphragm. The thoracic duct, the aorta, and the azygos vein pass through the aortic hiatus. The dorsal and ventral vagal nerve trunks, not the nerves themselves, pass through the esophageal hiatus with the esophagus—the vagus nerves terminate cranial to the diaphragm, where they divide into dorsal and ventral branches which then recombine to form the dorsal and ventral vagal trunks.

10. The answer is 1 [Chapter 34 II B]. The endothoracic fascia is the name given to the portion of the internal fascia that lines the deep surface of the thorax. (The internal fascia also lines the deep surface of the abdomen.) The endothoracic fascia is positioned deep to the internal muscle layer and serves in part to adhere the parietal pleura to the internal thoracic wall.

11. The answer is 4 [Chapter 35 I A 1 b]. The brachiocephalic trunk, one of two large arteries arising from the aortic arch, terminates by dividing into the right common carotid artery and the right subclavian artery.

12. The answer is 1 [Chapter 35 I C 5]. The internal thoracic artery directly gives rise to the ventral intercostal arteries, and terminates by dividing into the musculophrenic artery, which supplies the diaphragm, and the cranial epigastric artery. Direct perforating branches from the internal thoracic artery, as well as branches from the cranial epigastric artery, supply the mammary gland. The placement of the artery deep to the transversus thoracis muscle clinches the identification.

13. The answer is 4 [Chapter 35 I C 3]. The superficial cervical artery plays an important role in supplying the musculature of the shoulder, including the trapezius, rhomboideus, supraspinatus, infraspinatus, and teres minor muscles. The axillary artery is not a branch of the subclavian; it is the continuation of the subclavian artery lateral to the first rib. The costocervical trunk supplies the serratus ventralis thoracis and many epaxial muscles. In addition, the costocervical trunk contributes to the supply of the first few intercostal spaces.

14. The answer is 2 [Chapter 35 II A]. The cranial vena cava, which is unpaired, forms from the confluence of the right and left brachiocephalic veins, and terminates in the right atrium. It drains (in part) the head, neck, and thoracic limb.

15. The answer is 4 [Chapter 35 II C 1]. The single, right azygous vein terminates in the cranial vena cava. It drains mainly the body wall, but also serves the bronchi and esophagus.

16. The answer is 2 [Chapter 36 III B]. Both the vagus and the cranial laryngeal nerves participate in delivery of parasympathetic innervation to the thoracic viscera (the recurrent laryngeal nerves are branches of the vagus nerves). Splanchnic nerves are not present in the thorax; furthermore, they are sympathetic rather than parasympathetic. The cervicothoracic ganglion is a sympathetic structure.

17. The answer is 2 [Chapter 36 III D]. The parasympathetic components of the cardiac nerves arise from the vagus and the recurrent laryngeal nerves. The cardiac nerves also have sympathetic components that arise from the cervicothoracic and middle cervical ganglia, as well as the ansa subclavia. The cardiac nerves form on both the right and left sides of the thorax.

18. The answer is 2 [Chapter 37 I B 2]. The pleural cavity contains a small amount of serous fluid, and nothing else. No structures are present in the pleural cavity, or any of the other serous cavities of the body. Serous cavities—freely sliding, lubricating structures that surround, but do not contain, the organs with which they are associated—contain only a small amount of serous fluid. Lack of this serous fluid is a pathologic condition.

19. The answer is 1 [Chapter 37 I A 3]. All parts of the pleura are essentially identical to each other, the differences among them being simply the structures they cover. Therefore, the visceral (pulmonary) pleura is distinguished form the diaphragmatic parietal pleura by position.

20. The answer is 2 [Chapter 37 III A]. The line of pleural reflection, which can be conceptualized as a gently curving line that extends from the last rib at the level of the epaxial muscles to the eighth costochondral junction, represents the boundary between the costal and diaphragmatic portions of the pleural membrane. The line of pleural reflection does not change appreciably with ventilatory movements, and the lungs are not contained within the pleural cavity.

21. The answer is 3 [Chapter 37 III; Figure 37–2]. The basal border of the lung and the line of pleural reflection parallel each other, separated by a considerable distance. The space between them is arciform and extends from the epaxial muscles to the diaphragm. The recess that is accessible to needle puncture lies cranial to the line of pleural reflection.

22. The answer is 2 [Chapter 37 III B 1 b; Figure 37–2]. The basal border of the lung is conceptualized as an oblique, straight line extending from the olecranon tuber to the neck region of the penultimate rib. The basal border of the lung forms the caudal border of the auscultation triangle, the area over the bony thorax where the lung is just deep to the thoracic wall, and thereby accessible to auscultation and percussion.

23. The answer is 1 [Chapter 37 II A 2]. The base (diaphragmatic surface) of the lung is the concave caudal portion that conforms to the dome of the diaphragm as it projects into the thoracic cavity. The lobation of the lung is determined by the internal branching of the bronchi, not by external features. The caudal vena cava, not the cranial vena cava, passes through the notch in the accessory lobe. The root of the lung consists of the vascular, nervous, and airway structures that pass into and out of the lung.

24. The answer is 3 [Chapter 37 III B 2 b]. In order to access fluid accumulated in the pleural cavity, the puncture site needs to be relatively ventral. Therefore, the ideal site for thoracocentesis would be at the costochondral junction, at the seventh or eighth intercostal space. The third or fourth intercostal spaces are largely inaccessible owing to the position of the thoracic limb. Intercostal spaces 5–8 at the level of the epaxial muscles are too high and too far cranial to render good results.

25. The answer is 3 [Chapter 37 IV B 1]. The pulmonary arteries deliver deoxygenated blood from the right ventricle to the lungs, and the pulmonary veins carry the freshly oxygenated blood back to the heart. The bronchial arteries deliver nutritional blood to the bronchi, pulmonary parenchyma, and airways as far distally as the respiratory bronchioles.

26. The answer is 1 [Chapter 37 IV B 1 c]. The ligamentum arteriosum is the fibrosed adult remnant of the ductus arteriosus. In the fetus, the ductus arteriosus shunts blood out of the pulmonary trunk (i.e., away from the lungs) and into the aorta. In the adult, the ligamentum arteriosum is located near the termination of the pulmonary trunk into the pulmonary arteries, and extends between the trunk and the aorta.

27. The answer is 2 [Chapter 37 IV B 1 a]. The pulmonary trunk, the great artery leaving the right ventricle of the heart, divides into the right and left pulmonary arteries. The pulmonary arteries deliver systemic blood to the lungs for the purpose of gas exchange.

28. The answer is 2 [Chapter 37 IV C 2 a]. Most of the oxygen-depleted blood from the pulmonary parenchyma returns to the heart via the pulmonary veins. Recall that the primary function of the pulmonary veins is to return oxygenated blood from the lungs to the heart for distribution to the body; however, because the bronchial veins of the lungs are few, they play only a negligible role in venous return from the pulmonary parenchyma. Instead, the distal capillary bed of the bronchial arteries overlaps and communicates with that of the pulmonary arteries, so that the majority of the oxygen-depleted blood from the bronchial branches gains entry to the capillary bed of the pulmonary arteries and returns to the heart together with the well-oxygenated blood in the pulmonary veins. Because the amount of well-oxygenated blood in the pulmonary veins far exceeds the amount of deoxygenated blood, the dilution effect is minimal.

29. The answer is 4 [Chapter 38 II B 2 b]. The left ventricle must propel blood through the systemic circulation, while the right ventricle only sends blood to the pulmonary circulation. Because the left ventricle must develop considerably more pressure than the right, its muscular walls are thicker and stronger.

30. The answer is 1 [Chapter 38 III A 2]. The left coronary artery supplies the left atrium, left ventricle (which is considerably larger than the right), and interventricular septum. The right coronary artery typically supplies mainly the right atrium and the relatively small right ventricle. The "great cardiac" vessel is a vein, not an artery. "Subconal artery" is a fanciful term.

31. The answer is 2 [Chapter 38 II A]. In a normal dog, the heart extends from approximately the third rib to the caudal border of the sixth rib.

32. The answer is 4 [Table 38–1]. The right atrioventricular valve is the only valve that can be auscultated on the right side of the thorax. It can be heard low in the fourth intercostal space. The aortic, pulmonic, and left atrioventricular valves are all auscultated on the left side of the thorax.

33. The answer is 2 [Chapter 38 IV B]. Normally, conduction impulses pass from the sinuatrial node, to the atrioventricular node, to the atrioventricular conduction fibers (i.e., the bundle of His), to the trabecula septomarginalis. The sinuatrial node has the fastest depolarization rate and therefore normally drives the heart's contraction.

34. The answer is 3 [Chapter 38 IV A]. The extrinsic cardiac innervation normally functions to regulate, rather than initiate, cardiac contractions. The extrinsic cardiac innervation controls the intrinsic conduction system. Both sympathetic and parasympathetic components contribute to extrinsic cardiac innervation.

35. The answer is 4 [Chapter 38 II D 1 a (3)]. The coronary sinus is the aperture where the largest vein of the heart (i.e., the great cardiac vein) enters the right atrium. The aortic sinuses are dilatations at the base of the aorta where the coronary arteries arise.

36. The answer is 3 [Chapter 37 VI]. The aorta is located in two of the three regions of the mediastinum—the aortic arch lies in the middle mediastinum, and the thoracic aorta, in the caudal mediastinum. The lungs are completely outside all mediastinal regions. The cranial vena cava is restricted to the cranial mediastinum, and the esophagus passes through all three regions.

37. The answer is 1 [Chapter 36 II B 1]. The intercostal nerves are the ventral branches of the thoracic spinal nerves. In addition to supplying motor innervation to the intercostal muscles, these nerves supply sensory innervation to the mammary glands (via their lateral mammary branches) and motor innervation to the rectus abdominis and transversus abdominis (via their distal muscular branches).

38. The answer is 4 [Chapter 36 III C]. The thoracic sympathetic ganglia (i.e., the paravertebral ganglia) are unspecialized structures present at each intervertebral space. In the cranial thoracic region, fusion of the last cervical and first thoracic ganglia results in the cervicothoracic ganglion, a large "star-shaped" structure located at the cranial end of the sympathetic trunk. The sympathetic cardiac nerves, which arise from the cervicothoracic ganglion, the middle cervical ganglion (another large collection of ganglia formed from members of the sympathetic chain), or the ansa subclavia, supply sympathetic innervation to the heart. The ansa subclavia passes between the middle cervical and the cervicothoracic ganglia. The ansa subclavia passes between the middle cervical and cervicothoracic ganglia and does not connect the thoracic sympathetic ganglia to the recurrent laryngeal nerve.

39. The answer is 1 [Chapter 35 I B 2]. The pericardium and structures within the mediastinum (e.g., the thymus gland, mediastinal lymph nodes) are usually supplied by small branches of the thoracic aorta. The heart itself is supplied by branches arising directly from the base of the aorta (i.e., the very first part of the aortic arch, as opposed to the thoracic aorta).

40. The answer is 2 [Chapter 35 I B 2 a (1), C] The lungs are supplied by the bronchoesophageal artery, which arises indirectly from the thoracic aorta, not the subclavian artery. Branches of the left subclavian artery are the vertebral artery (which supplies the brain), the internal thoracic artery (which supplies the intercostal muscles), and the superficial cervical artery (which supplies the shoulder musculature). The branching pattern of the left and right subclavian arteries are essentially the same.

41. The answer is 2 [Chapter 33 I C 4 a (2), 5 b (2)]. The costal arch is cartilaginous, whereas the costal body, the costal groove, and the costal tubercle are bony.

42. The answer is 1 [Chapter 38 II E 2]. The atrioventricular valves, which are the inflow valves, must withstand more pressure on systole (i.e., from ventricular contraction) than the pulmonic and aortic (i.e., outflow) valves, and are therefore more robust. On systole (i.e., on contraction of the ventricles), the outflow valves open and the inflow valves close. Each of the outflow valves has three leaflets, while each of the inflow valves has two. All four cardiac valves are anchored in the fibrous skeleton of the heart.

43. The answer is 1 [Chapter 38 I B]. The mediastinal pleural lies in direct contact with most of the superficial surface of the fibrous pericardium, but is not a part of the pericardial structure. The pericardium consists of an outer fibrous layer and a doubled serous layer.

44. The answer is 2 [Chapter 38 II C 1]. The coronary groove encircles the dorsal part (i.e., the base) of the heart like a crown, roughly separating the atria from the ventricles. The coronary groove houses the right and left coronary arteries and the great cardiac vein. (There are no right and left coronary veins.) These vessels are obscured by generous amounts of fat.

PART VI

ABDOMINAL REGION

Chapter 40

Introduction to the Abdominal Region

I. FUNCTION. The abdomen:

A. **Houses** and **protects** several major organs, either in their entirety or partially

B. **Provides a semirigid framework** and **compressive force** for movements requiring an abdominal press (e.g., urination, defecation, vigorous exhalation, loud vocalization, parturition).

II. MORPHOLOGY

A. **Internal morphology.** The abdominal region is roughly **cone-shaped.** The base of the cone is convex and directed cranially, and the apex of the cone is directed caudally. Note that both the thorax and the abdomen are cone-shaped, with their bases in contact with each other and their apices directed away from each other.

B. **External morphology.** In dogs of appropriate body weight, the abdomen tapers strongly dorsally from the xiphoid region. This contour is absent in overweight dogs, bitches in the advanced stages of pregnancy, and in lactating bitches.

III. BOUNDARIES, CONTENTS, AND OPENINGS

A. **Boundaries.** The abdominal region **extends from the diaphragm to the pelvic inlet** and is largely **bounded by muscle.**

1. The **cranial boundary** is the **diaphragm.** Recall that the diaphragm is convex cranially, and thus extends into the caudal portion of the thoracic cage (see Chapter 32 I B 1 b). As a result, part of the digestive viscera are actually found within the boundaries of the bony thorax, and are afforded the protection of the ribs.
2. The **caudal boundary** is the **pelvic inlet** (i.e., the bony ring surrounding the opening into the pelvic cavity). Because the pelvic inlet is **open,** the **abdominal** and **pelvic cavities are freely continuous.**
3. The **dorsal boundaries** include the:
   a. **Lumbar vertebrae** (bodies and transverse processes)
   b. **Sublumbar musculature**
   c. **Diaphragmatic crura** (i.e., the elongate attachment of the diaphragm to the dorsal body wall)
4. The **lateral boundaries** include the:
   a. **Diaphragm,** as well as the **last four pairs of ribs,** the **costal arch,** and the associated **intercostal muscles**
   b. **External** and **internal abdominal oblique muscles** and the **transversus abdominis muscle**
   c. **Iliac shaft** (a small portion)
5. The **ventral** boundary is the **rectus abdominis muscle.**

B. **Contents**

1. **Structures contained entirely within the abdomen** include the:
   a. Stomach
   b. Small intestine

c. Liver and gallbladder
d. Pancreas
e. Spleen
f. Kidneys and adrenal glands
g. Ovaries

2. **Structures contained partially within the abdomen** include the:
   a. Peritoneum and peritoneal cavity
   b. Large intestine
   c. Ureters
   d. Spermatic cord
   e. Uterus
   f. Urinary bladder (when very full)

Canine Clinical Correlation

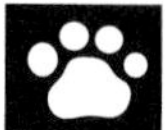

The excursion of the full urinary bladder onto the ventral abdominal wall is taken advantage of during the procedure known as **cystocentesis,** used to obtain a sterile urine specimen. The dog (with a full bladder) is placed in dorsal recumbency, and a needle is passed directly through the ventral midline a short distance cranial to the pubic brim. If the bladder is full, the needle will enter its lumen. Once the needle is withdrawn, no hemostasis or closure of the site is necessary.

C. Openings. The abdominal walls are characterized by a number of normal openings.

1. The **diaphragmatic openings** (i.e., the **aortic hiatus, esophageal hiatus,** and **caval foramen)** are discussed in Chapter 32 I B 1 a (3).
2. The **inguinal canals** are paired, slit-like openings in the ventrolateral abdominal walls. Various nervous and vascular structures, the vaginal process (in both sexes), and the testis and spermatic cord (in male dogs) pass through these openings. The inguinal canals extend between the deep and superficial inguinal rings.
   a. The **deep inguinal ring** opens to the interior of the abdominal cavity. The borders of the deep inguinal ring are the inguinal ligament (i.e., the caudal free tendon of the rectus abdominis muscle), the free caudal border of the internal abdominal oblique muscle, and the rectus abdominis muscle.
   b. The **superficial inguinal ring,** a slit in the aponeurosis of the external abdominal oblique muscle, opens to the subcutaneous tissues of the inguinal region.

Canine Clinical Correlation

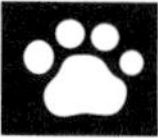

An **inguinal hernia** develops when a structure (e.g., a loop of jejunum) abnormally passes through the inguinal canal. Development of an inguinal hernia usually occurs only when some sort of trauma has artificially increased the size of the inguinal rings.

3. The **vascular lacunae** are paired openings at the junction of the thigh and abdomen that transmit nervous and vascular structures to and from the pelvic limb.
4. The **pelvic inlet** forms the caudal boundary of the abdominal cavity.
5. The **umbilical ring** is a **fetal structure** that transmits the umbilical cord. This opening may be pathologically retained in the adult (i.e., as an umbilical hernia).

IV. REGIONS.

To provide consistent reference points, the abdomen is arbitrarily divided into **nine** regions (Figure 40–1). Three main abdominal regions are each divided into three mi-

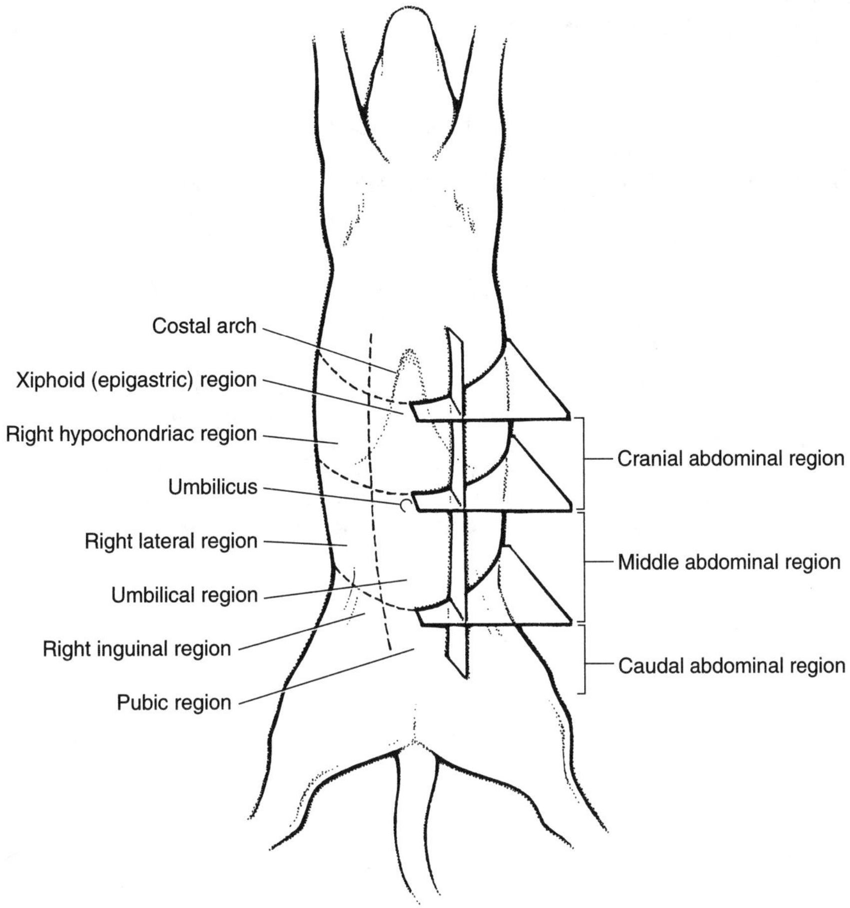

FIGURE 40–1. Nine regions of the abdomen.

nor regions (one unpaired central region with a unique name, and two paired lateral regions that share the same name).

A. The **cranial abdominal region** is divided into the:

1. **Xiphoid (epigastric) region,** unpaired
2. **Hypochondriac regions,** paired [note that in this case, "hypochondriac," refers to "under the (costal) cartilage," rather than to a dog overly concerned with its health!]

B. The **middle abdominal region** is divided into the:

1. **Umbilical region,** unpaired
2. **Lateral regions,** paired. Each lateral region includes a:
   a. **Paralumbar fossa,** a triangular area caudal to the costal arch, ventral to the lumbar vertebrae, and cranial to the ilium
   b. **Flank,** an area extending ventrally from the paralumbar fossa to the ventral midline

C. The **caudal abdominal region** is divided into the:

1. **Pubic region,** unpaired
2. **Inguinal regions,** paired

V. SUPERFICIAL STRUCTURES

A. **Mammae** (see Chapter 2 II)

1. The **abdominal mammae,** prominent features of the ventral abdominal wall, are the third and fourth (of five) pairs of mammae.
2. The **inguinal mammae** are the final pair of mammae. These mammae are located in the inguinal region, not far cranial to the pubis. The inguinal mammae are typically the largest of the five pairs of mammary glands seen in most bitches.

B.

The **umbilicus,** the closed scar of the umbilical ring, is located on the ventral midline at the level of a transverse plane across the last pair of ribs. The umbilicus is used as a landmark during many surgical procedures.

1. The umbilicus is usually **oval** and **varies in size** (from a few millimeters in small dogs, to 1 centimeter in large ones). It may be quite **flat or moderately raised.** This variability in size and contour must be recognized as normal during physical examination.
2. The umbilicus may be more visible in breeds with shorter or thinner hair. Regardless of the character of the dog's haircoat, the hair surrounding the umbilicus grows in a whorl directed toward the scar, forming a pattern referred to as a **vortex.**

Chapter 41

Abdominal Wall

I. INTRODUCTION

A. Skeletal component. Some vertebrae and ribs, as well as a part of the shaft of the ilium (see Chapter 50 I B 1), play a small role in the formation of the abdominal walls.

B. Soft tissue component. The abdominal wall is largely muscular in nature. Muscle contributes significantly to the dorsal wall, and together with its covering skin, forms the entirety of the lateral and ventral walls.

II. DORSAL ABDOMINAL WALL

A. Skeletal component. The bodies and transverse processes of all of the **lumbar vertebrae** contribute to the formation of the dorsal abdominal wall. Most of the muscles forming the lateral abdominal wall attach to these vertebrae.

B. Soft tissue component. The muscles of the dorsal abdominal wall are the **sublumbar muscles** (i.e., the hypaxial muscles of the lumbar and pelvic regions). These muscles (the **psoas minor, iliopsoas,** and **quadratus lumborum)** are described in Chapter 20 II C 2 b.

III. LATEROVENTRAL ABDOMINAL WALL

A. Skeletal component

1. The **bodies and costal cartilages of rib pairs 9–13** contribute to the lateral abdominal wall and provide attachment sites for much of the lateral abdominal wall musculature.
2. The **shaft of the ilium** (distal to the iliac wing and proximal to the acetabulum) forms a small part of the dorsal lateral abdominal wall.

B. Soft tissue component (Figure 41–1)

1. The **linea alba** is an elongate, tendinous structure extending along the ventral midline for the full length of the abdomen (i.e., from the xiphoid cartilage to the pubis).
   a. The **umbilicus** is contained within the substance of the linea alba. The linea alba is quite wide cranial to the umbilicus, where it can reach approximately 1 cm in width in large dogs. Caudal to the umbilicus, the linea alba becomes progressively attenuated, so that it is scarcely recognizable cranial to the pubis.

Canine Clinical Correlation

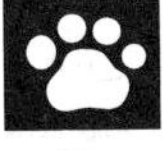

The tendinous composition of the linea alba and its position are important during abdominal surgery:

- Because it is collagenous, the linea alba lacks both an abundant blood supply and nerves; therefore, it is an advantageous site for entry into the abdominal cavity because the need for hemostasis and postoperative analgesia is minimized.
- The tendinous fibers of the linea alba offer tensile strength and are an opportune site for suture placement. Muscle holds suture poorly; the weight of the abdominal viscera on the ventral belly wall renders the muscle in this region even less suitable for suturing.

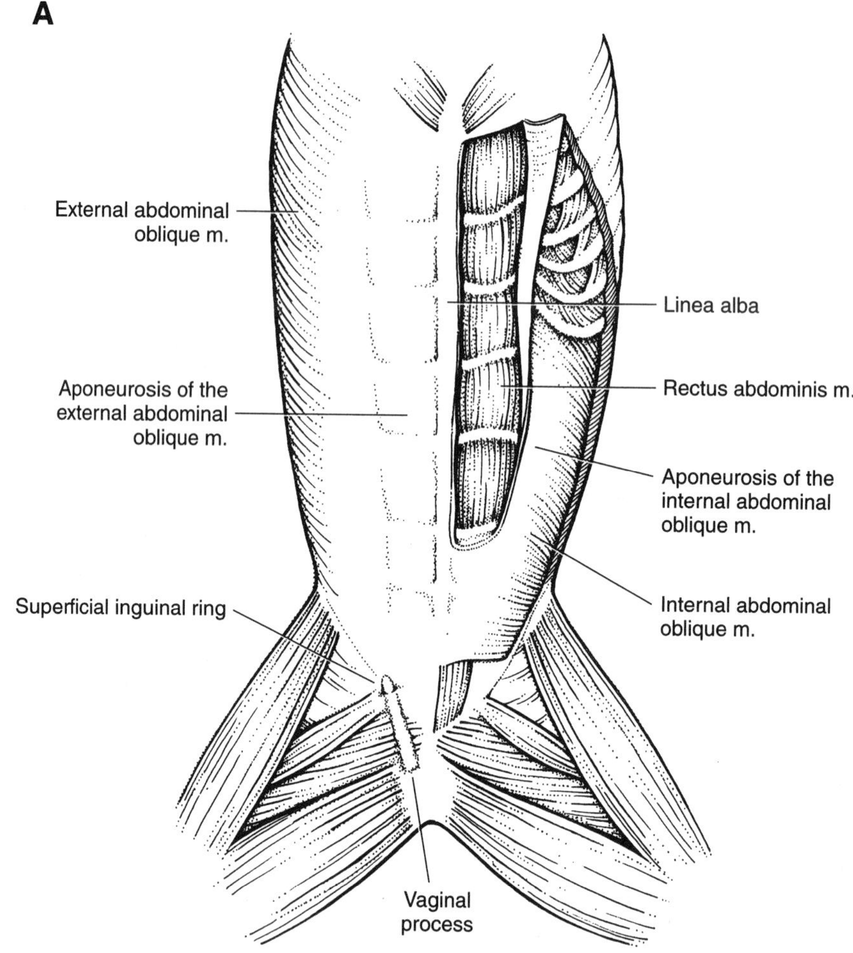

FIGURE 41–1. (*A*) Superficial muscles of the abdominal wall, ventral view. (*continued*)

b. The linea alba serves as an **attachment site for several muscles and ligaments:**
   (1) All of the **lateroventral abdominal wall muscles** attach to the linea alba.
   (2) The **falciform ligament** (a remnant of the ventral mesentery) attaches cranial to the umbilicus.
   (3) The **median ligament of the bladder** attaches caudal to the umbilicus.

2. The three **lateroventral abdominal muscles** (Table 41–1) are arranged so that their fibers form a grid that greatly increases the strength of the abdominal wall. These sheet-like muscles are fleshy dorsally and laterally; ventrally they become aponeurotic, and contribute to the formation of the **rectus sheath,** an aponeurotic sheath that surrounds the main muscle of the abdominal floor (i.e., the rectus abdominis).
   a. The **external abdominal oblique,** the most superficial of the lateral abdominal muscles, covers the ventral half of the bony thorax as well as most of the lateral surface of the abdominal wall. Its fibers travel at approximately right angles to those of the internal abdominal oblique. The external abdominal oblique has two parts:
      (1) The **costal part** arises along a gently curving line between ribs 4 or 5 and rib 12.
      (2) The **lumbar part** picks up where the costal part ends, arising from rib 13 and the thoracolumbar fascia (caudally from the ribs).
   b. The **internal abdominal oblique** is intermediate in position among the lateral abdomi-

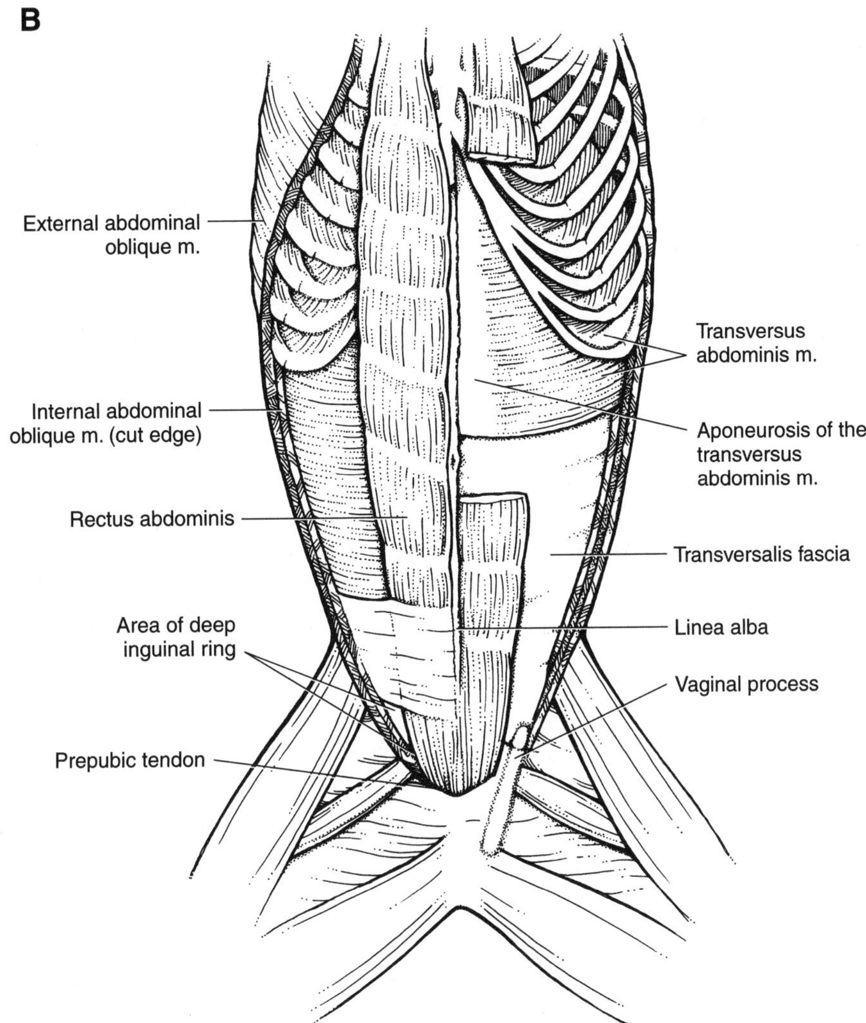

FIGURE 41–1—*continued* (*B*) Deep muscles of the abdominal wall, ventral view. Note how far the abdominal muscles extend over the ribs. (Modified with permission from Pasquini C, Spurgeon T: *Anatomy of Domestic Animals,* 7th ed. SUDZ Publishing, Pilot Point, TX, 1995, pp 200, 201.)

nal muscles. The internal abdominal oblique is essentially covered by its external fellow, and its fibers run approximately at right angles to those of the external oblique. It has three parts.

(1) The **costal part** inserts on the last two ribs or costal cartilages.

(2) The **abdominal part** inserts on the linea alba by means of an aponeurosis.

(3) The **inguinal part** also inserts on the linea alba. In males, the **cremaster muscle,** associated with the spermatic cord, is derived from the caudal-most portion of the inguinal part of the internal abdominal oblique.

c. The **transversus abdominis,** the deepest of the lateral abdominal muscles, fills the space between the costal arch and the pelvis and is often quite thick (up to 4 mm in large dogs). This is the only lateral abdominal muscle to take a **straight** (rather than an oblique) **course.** The transversus abdominis is marked by several distinct **tendinous intersections** that course in the same direction as the muscle fibers.

TABLE 41–1. Abdominal Wall Musculature*

Muscle	Action	Innervation	Course
Lateroventral abdominal muscles			
External abdominal oblique	Supports and compresses the abdominal viscera Flexes the vertebral column laterally and twists trunk side-to-side (unilateral contraction) Flexes the vertebral column ventrally (bilateral contraction)	Lateral branches of the last several intercostal nerves Lateral branches of the last thoracic and first three lumbar nerves	**Arises** from ribs 4 or 5 through rib 12 (costal part); from rib 13 and thoracolumbar fascia (lumbar part) **Courses** caudoventrally toward the inguinal region **Inserts** on the linea alba after forming a broad aponeurosis
Internal abdominal oblique	Supports and compresses the abdominal viscera Flexes the vertebral column laterally and twists trunk side-to-side (unilateral contraction) Flexes the vertebral column ventrally (bilateral contraction)	Lateral branches of the last several intercostal nerves Lateral branches of the last thoracic and first three lumbar nerves	**Arises** from the tuber coxae and the thoracolumbar fascia (caudal to the last rib) **Courses** cranioventrally toward the ventral midline **Inserts** on the last two ribs or costal cartilages (costal part), and the linea alba (abdominal and inguinal parts)
Transversus abdominis muscle	Supports and compresses the abdominal viscera	Lateral branches of the last several intercostal nerves Lateral branches of the last thoracic and first three lumbar nerves	**Arises** from the medial surfaces of costal cartilages 8–11 and ribs 12–13, the transverse processes of the lumbar vertebrae, and the tuber coxae **Courses** ventrally toward the ventral midline **Inserts** on the linea alba
Ventral abdominal muscles			
Rectus abdominis	Supports and compresses the abdominal viscera Flexes the vertebral column laterally (unilateral contraction) Flexes the vertebral column ventrally (bilateral contraction) Draws the pelvis cranially	Medial branches of the intercostal nerves Medial branches of the last thoracic and first three lumbar nerves	**Arises** from the first costal cartilage and rib (tendinous portion) and from the ninth costal cartilage (fleshy portion) **Courses** caudally toward the pelvis **Inserts** by means of the prepubic tendon on the pecten of the pubis (at the pelvic brim)

*The hypaxial back muscles of the lumbar and pelvic regions (i.e., the psoas minor, iliopsoas, and quadratus lumborum) also contribute to the dorsal abdominal wall. These muscles are summarized in Table 20–5.

d. The **cutaneous trunci,** located superficially over much of the lateral and ventral abdominal walls, contributes mainly to the structure of the skin (rather than to the abdominal wall). The cutaneous trunci is listed here for the sake of completeness; a detailed description is given in Chapter 34 I D 1.

3. The **inguinal ligament** is a stout ligamentous band that arises from the tuber coxae (i.e., the cranial end of the ilium) and passes medially to blend with the prepubic tendon, a ligamentous structure formed on each side from the tendons of the rectus abdominis muscle and the pectineus muscle (a muscle of the pelvic limb). The inguinal ligament forms the caudal border of the origin of the transversalis fascia, the caudal border of the deep inguinal ring, and part of the caudal attachment point of the external abdominal oblique muscle.

IV. VENTRAL ABDOMINAL WALL.

The **abdominal floor** is essentially formed by the paired **rectus abdominis muscles** and the **rectus sheath.** The sheath, which surrounds the rectus abdominis, is formed from the aponeurotic terminations of the lateroventral abdominal musculature.

A. Rectus abdominis

Rectus abdominis (see Table 41–1, Figure 41–1). These paired muscles extend from the cranial part of the bony thorax to the pubis. They form a wide band that extends laterally from each side of the linea alba.

1. The rectus abdominis originates by two parts, one tendinous and one fleshy.

2. Several transversely oriented **tendinous intersections,** reminiscent of the somites of the early embryo, mark the rectus abdominis.

- **a.** The intersections of the rectus abdominis run at right angles to the muscle fibers.
- **b.** By breaking the long course of the muscle into shorter segments and providing strong tendinous attachment points, these tendinous intersections increase the strength of the rectus abdominis.

B. Rectus sheath

Rectus sheath. The rectus abdominis muscle is surrounded by aponeurotic sheets over much of its length, both dorsally (i.e., deeply or internally) and ventrally (i.e., superficially or externally). The aponeuroses of each side blend with the linea alba; thus, each rectus muscle is ensheathed throughout most of its length. However, the muscle is attached to its sheath only in the regions of the tendinous intersections in the muscle.

1. Formation. The aponeuroses of the lateroventral muscles of the abdominal wall contribute to the sheath. Three regions are identifiable passing cranially to caudally.

- **a.** The **aponeurosis** of the **external abdominal oblique muscle** forms the most superficial layer of the rectus sheath, extending from the costal arch to the pubis.
- **b.** The contribution of the **aponeurosis** of the **internal abdominal oblique muscle** to the rectus sheath varies regionally.
  - **(1) Cranially,** from the xiphoid cartilage to approximately the end of the costal arch, the aponeurosis of the internal abdominal oblique splits. One of its leaves passes ventral to the rectus abdominis, and the other passes dorsal to it.
  - **(2) In the midregions and caudally,** the full substance of the aponeurosis of the internal abdominal oblique muscle passes along the ventral surface of the rectus abdominis.
- **c.** The contribution of the **aponeurosis** of the **transversus abdominis muscle** to the rectus sheath also varies regionally.
  - **(1) Cranially** and **through the mid-abdominal region** (to approximately the junction of the middle and caudal thirds of the abdomen), the aponeurosis of the transversus abdominis passes along the ventral surface of the rectus abdominis.
  - **(2) Caudally** (approximately at the level of the inguinal pair of mammae), the aponeurosis of the transversus abdominis passes ventral to the rectus abdominis, leaving the caudal-most part of the inner surface of the rectus abdominis covered only by the transversalis fascia.

2. **Layers.** The rectus sheath has two layers.
   a. The **superficial layer** of the rectus sheath is formed:
      (1) **Cranially and in its midregions,** by the aponeuroses of the external and internal abdominal oblique muscles
      (2) **Caudally,** by the aponeuroses of all three lateroventral abdominal muscles
   b. The **deep layer** of the rectus sheath is formed:
      (1) **Cranially,** by the aponeuroses of the internal abdominal oblique and the transversus abdominis muscles
      (2) **In its midregions,** by the aponeurosis of the transversus abdominis
      (3) **Caudally,** by nothing (the prepelvic region of the rectus abdominis is covered only by the transversalis fascia and peritoneum)

Canine Clinical Correlation

The rectus sheath, which has strong layers both dorsal and ventral to the rectus abdominis in the cranial and middle abdominal regions, is useful during abdominal surgery when the body wall incision strays from the linea alba. The surgeon can place sutures in the two layers of the rectus sheath (rather than in the rectus abdominis muscle). Because the rectus sheath is incomplete caudally, incisions in the ventral abdominal wall just cranial to the pubis (e.g., for urinary bladder surgery), must be carefully made, since the option of suturing into the rectus sheath is no longer available.

V. VASCULATURE OF THE ABDOMINAL WALL

A. Arteries

1. **Dorsal abdominal wall.** The dorsal-most portions of the lateral abdominal wall are supplied by the **costoabdominal** and **lumbar arteries.**
   a. The paired **costoabdominal arteries** are essentially the final intercostal arteries (see Chapter 20 II A 1 and Chapter 35 I B 1). They pass along the caudal border of the last rib, supplying the adjacent areas of the caudal-most thoracic and cranial-most abdominal areas.
   b. The paired **lumbar arteries** arise from the dorsal surface of the aorta adjacent to their respective lumbar vertebrae. Their course and distribution is detailed in Chapter 21 II A 3.
2. **Lateral abdominal wall.** Because the lumbar arteries end so far proximally, the vascularization of the lateral abdominal wall is accomplished by other vessels (Figure 41–2).
   a. The **phrenicoabdominal artery** is paired.
      (1) **Origin.** The phrenicoabdominal artery arises from the **lateral surface of the abdominal aorta,** ventral to the diaphragmatic crura (i.e., within the abdomen), approximately at the level of vertebra L2.
      (2) **Branches.** As its name suggests, the phrenicoabdominal artery supplies parts of both the diaphragm and the abdomen.
         (a) The **caudal phrenic artery** courses to the caudal surface of the diaphragm.
         (b) The **cranial abdominal artery** continues into the abdomen, toward the costal arch. This branch **supplies most of the lateral abdominal wall.**
   b. The **deep circumflex iliac artery,** which arises directly from the **abdominal aorta,** is also paired. The **deep branch** of this artery supplies **most of the dorsocaudal parts of the lateral abdominal wall.**
   c. The **caudal abdominal artery,** also paired, is a small vessel arising from the **external iliac artery,** usually just distal to the departure of the deep femoral artery. The caudal abdominal artery supplies a relatively small portion of the **caudolateral abdominal wall,** just cranial to the thigh.
3. **Ventral abdominal wall.** The ventral abdominal wall receives arterial supply from four sets of paired arteries, all designated "epigastric." The four epigastric arteries form a pat-

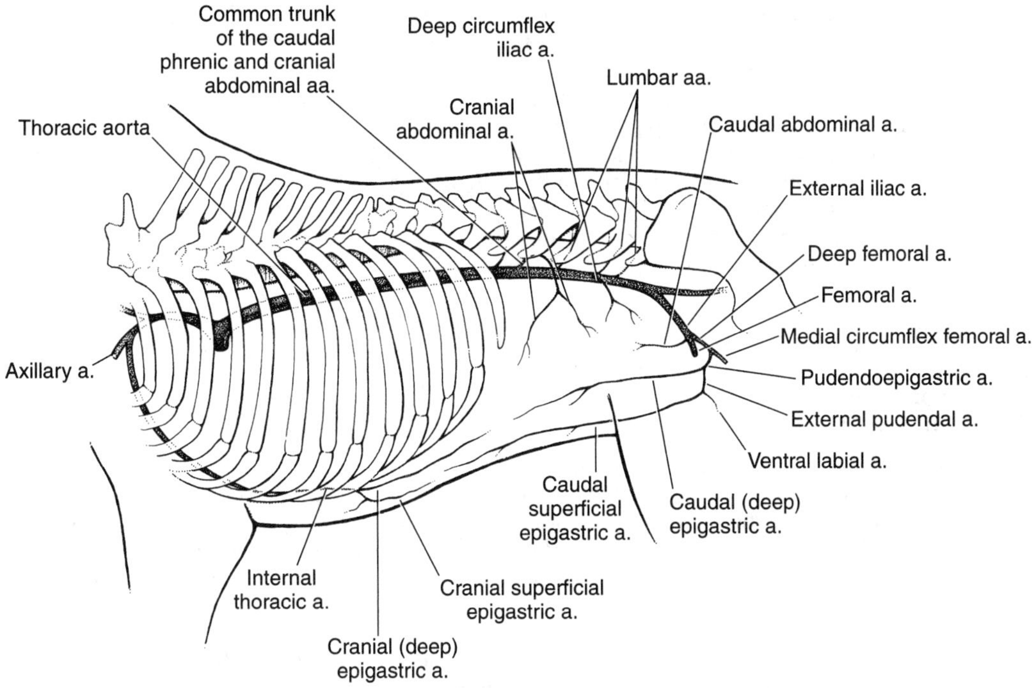

FIGURE 41–2. Arteries of the lateral and ventral abdominal walls. Note how little the lumbar arteries contribute to the supply of the lateral abdominal wall. The rectus abdominis muscle is "sandwiched" between the two sets of epigastric arteries.

tern, with one set (the deep epigastric arteries) coursing along the deep (internal) surface of the rectus abdominis muscle, and a second set (the superficial epigastric arteries) running on the superficial (external) surface of the rectus abdominis muscle just deep to the skin.

a. The **deep set** of vessels is always robust.

(1) Cranial (deep) epigastric artery

(a) Source. The cranial (deep) epigastric artery is one of the two **terminal branches** of the **internal thoracic artery** (see Chapter 35 I C 5 c).

(b) Course. The cranial (deep) epigastric artery **passes along the deep surface of the rectus abdominis muscle,** positioned between the muscle and the deep layer of the rectus sheath, and generously **supplies the muscle.** The terminal part of its field of distribution overlaps that of its caudal fellow (i.e., the caudal (deep) epigastric artery), and numerous anastomoses between these vessels take place.

(2) Caudal (deep) epigastric artery

(a) Source. The caudal (deep) epigastric artery is a direct branch of the **pudendoepigastric trunk.**

(b) Course. The caudal (deep) epigastric artery passes cranially in a position mirroring that of its cranial fellow (i.e., along the deep surface of the rectus abdominis between the muscle and the deep layer of the rectus sheath; see Figure 41–2).

b. The **superficial set** of vessels is always present but variably developed; this set of arteries reaches maximal development in lactating bitches.

(1) Cranial superficial epigastric artery

(a) Source. The cranial superficial epigastric artery is a branch of the **cranial (deep) epigastric artery.**

(b) **Course.** The cranial superficial epigastric artery **pierces the rectus abdominis to course caudally along its superficial surface.** Like the cranial (deep) epigastric artery, the cranial superficial epigastric artery anastomoses with its caudal fellow (i.e., the caudal superficial epigastric artery).

(2) **Caudal superficial epigastric artery**

(a) **Source.** The caudal superficial epigastric artery is a branch of the **external pudendal artery,** a branch of the pudendoepigastric trunk.

(b) **Course.** The position and course of the caudal superficial epigastric artery mirrors that of the cranial superficial epigastric artery, passing cranially along the superficial surface of the rectus abdominis muscle just deep to the skin (see Figure 41–2).

B. **Veins.** The veins of the abdominal region are essentially satellites of the named arteries.

C. **Lymphatic vessels.** Multiple lymphocenters, some constant and others not, drain the abdominal wall.

1. The **lumbar lymphocenter** is inconstant.

a. The **lumbar aortic lymph nodes** are small nodes of varying number, potentially distributed along the length of the aorta from the diaphragm to the deep circumflex iliac arteries. Although one set of paired nodes, the **cranial lumbar lymph nodes,** is fairly constant near the diaphragm, the remainder are unpredictable in their development, and are easily overlooked owing to their small size and similarity in color to the fat in which they are embedded.

(1) **Drainage area.** The lumbar aortic lymph nodes drain the lumbar vertebrae and the last ribs; the musculature of the intercostal, lumbar, and abdominal regions; the urogenital organs located in the abdominal region; the abdominal aorta; the peritoneum; the adrenal glands; and some structures cranial to the diaphragm (i.e., the mediastinum and pleura).

(2) **Efferent vessels** from the constant node near the diaphragm pass to the cisterna chyli; those of the less constant nodes enter the lumbar lymphatic trunks.

b. The **renal lymph nodes** are quite small, and not constant.

(1) **Drainage area.** When present, the renal lymph nodes drain the kidneys.

(2) **Efferent vessels** pass to any regional lumbar aortic lymph nodes that may be present, or alternately, directly into the lumbar lymphatic trunks.

2. The **iliosacral lymphocenter** can include several sets of lymph nodes, some constant and others not.

a. The **medial iliac lymph nodes,** which are paired, large, and **constant,** are positioned adjacent to the aorta between the deep circumflex iliac and external iliac arteries.

(1) **Drainage area.** These nodes receive drainage from many structures, including the abdominal wall, the abdominal cavity, the pelvic walls and viscera, the tail, and the pelvic limb.

(2) **Efferent vessels** pass to the adjacent lumbar aortic nodes (when these nodes are present); otherwise, the efferent vessels of the medial iliac lymph nodes pass cranially and associate with each other to form the lumbar lymphatic trunks.

b. The **hypogastric lymph nodes** are small, paired nodes positioned between the internal iliac and median sacral arteries.

(1) **Drainage areas** of these nodes include the sublumbar muscles, as well as muscles of the abdominal wall, pelvic limb, and tail; the viscera of the abdomen, pelvis, and reproductive systems; and the deep inguinal lymph nodes.

(2) **Efferent vessels** pass to the more cranially situated medial iliac lymph nodes.

c. The **sacral lymph nodes** are small and inconstant; when present, they lie ventral to the sacral body, close to the hypogastric nerves.

3. The **superficial inguinal (inguinofemoral) lymphocenter,** which is **constant** in occurrence, drains the inguinal and femoral regions.

a. **Nodes.** The **superficial inguinal lymph nodes,** usually two on each side, lie in the fat that fills the groove where the abdominal wall meets the medial surface of the thigh. The right and left superficial inguinal lymph nodes communicate with each other via direct connections.

b. **Drainage.** Areas drained by the superficial inguinal lymphocenter include the ventral half of the abdominal wall (including the regional mammary glands) and pelvis; the medial thigh, stifle, and crus; and the popliteal lymph node.

c. **Efferent vessels** from the superficial inguinal lymph nodes form one or two major lymphatic trunks that pass into the abdomen through the inguinal canal to enter the medial iliac lymph nodes.

4. The **deep inguinal (iliofemoral) lymphocenter** is highly variable among dogs. One or two paired lymph nodes, both of which are highly inconstant, compose this center. If present, they may only be present on one side.
   a. The **iliofemoral lymph node** (when present) lies in the area of the internal and external iliac veins.
   b. The **femoral lymph node,** rarely present, is small and buried in the fat of the femoral triangle.

VI. INNERVATION OF THE ABDOMINAL WALL

A. Costoabdominal nerve. The costoabdominal nerve is the ventral branch of the last thoracic spinal nerve (nerve T13). This nerve passes ventrally, supplying the area immediately caudal to the last rib as well as a strip of muscle and skin of the cranial-most region of the abdominal wall.

B. Lumbar spinal nerves. The innervation of the abdominal wall is largely accomplished by the **seven paired lumbar spinal nerves,** which have a branching pattern similar to that of the segmental thoracic spinal nerves (see Chapter 36 II). Three main branches arise from each lumbar nerve.

1. The **meningeal branch,** like that of the thoracic nerves, is small and variable, and enters the spinal canal to innervate the meninges there.
2. The **dorsal branches** are important when considering the innervation of structures intrinsic to the back. These branches are discussed in Chapter 22 IV A.
   a. The dorsal branches of **nerves L1–L3 or L4,** like the dorsal branches of the thoracic spinal nerves, divide into a:
      (1) **Medial branch** that is **motor** to the epaxial muscles
      (2) **Lateral branch** that is both **motor** and **sensory** and supplies the adjacent epaxial muscles before terminating in the **dorsal cutaneous branches**
   b. The dorsal branches of **nerves L4 or L5–L7** simply arborize in the epaxial musculature.
3. The **ventral branches** of the lumbar nerves participate in the innervation of the abdominal wall.
   a. The ventral branches of **nerves L1** and **L2** usually continue in a segmental manner into the lateral abdominal wall.
      (1) The ventral branches of nerves L1 and L2 have specific names.
         (a) The **cranial iliohypogastric nerve** is the ventral branch of nerve L1.
         (b) The **caudal iliohypogastric nerve** is the ventral branch of nerve L2.
      (2) Each of the iliohypogastric nerves travels ventrally through the abdominal musculature.
         (a) Each nerve has a **motor branch** that is **motor** to certain sublumbar muscles.
         (b) Each nerve has a **lateral branch** that is **motor** to the two abdominal oblique muscles. The lateral branch terminates as the **lateral cutaneous branch** of the abdominal wall, which is **sensory** to the skin. The field of nerve L1 reaches the ventral midline; that of nerve L2 does not pass quite so far ventrally.

(c) Each nerve has a **medial branch** that runs along the deep surface of the transversus abdominis muscle, sending **motor** fibers to the muscle and **sensory** fibers to the peritoneum.

b. The ventral branches of **nerves L3–L7** contribute to the **lumbosacral plexus** (similar to the brachial plexus) and also innervate the lateral abdominal wall. The **ilioinguinal nerve** is the name given to the portion of the ventral branch of nerve L3 that innervates the abdominal wall. This nerve provides:

(1) Motor branches to certain sublumbar muscles

(2) Lateral and **medial branches** that are similar in distribution and function to those of the ventral branches of nerves L1 and L2

Chapter 42

Peritoneum of the Abdominal Region

I. PERITONEUM. The peritoneum is a serous membrane similar in structure and function to the pleura and pericardium.

A. Structure. Like the other serous membranes, the peritoneum is a single layer of mesothelial cells supported by a thin layer of elastic and collagenous fibers. The peritoneum adheres to the muscle and bone of the abdominal wall via the **transversalis fascia.**

B. Function. The mesothelial cells produce a serous fluid that permits the organs within the abdominal cavity to move without friction.

C. Location

1. **Abdominal cavity.** Most of the peritoneum is contained within the abdominal cavity.
2. **Pelvic cavity.** The peritoneum extends caudal to the termination of the abdomen to enter the pelvis. Peritoneal pouches are formed as the perineum reflects cranially around the pelvic viscera (see Chapter 51).

D. Specializations

1. The **vaginal process** is a blind-ended evagination of peritoneum through the inguinal canal. The vaginal process forms during normal development in **both sexes.**
   a. In male dogs, the process specializes to provide a serous cavity associated with the testes and the spermatic cords.
   b. In female dogs, the process ceases development soon after it begins. However, in most females, the vaginal process remains recognizable as a fat-filled "finger" of peritoneum of varying length just under the skin of the inguinal region.
2. The **vaginal ring** marks the boundary where the parietal peritoneum lining the abdominal wall becomes continuous with the vaginal process (i.e., the part of the peritoneum that passes through the inguinal canal).

II. PERITONEAL CAVITY. Like the pleura and the pericardium, the peritoneum is a continuous sheet that forms a closed cavity, the peritoneal cavity.

A. The peritoneal cavity is the **potential space** between the layer of peritoneum that covers the body wall and the layer of peritoneum that covers the abdominal organs.

B. No organs are located within the peritoneal cavity. Only the minimal secretions of the serous cells accumulate within the cavity.

Canine Clinical Correlation

When serous fluid is not present in the cavity, movement of the abdominal organs is impaired and the two regions of the membrane bind together, forming **adhesions.** Adhesions can also form when the peritoneum becomes inflamed. Adhesions are painful and impair organ function, and they can be life-threatening.

III. REGIONS. As with the pleura and pericardium, regions of the peritoneum can be identified.

A. The **parietal peritoneum** is the portion of the peritoneum that lines the abdominal wall. The parietal peritoneum adheres tightly to the inner abdominal musculature and the diaphragm, by virtue of the transversalis fascia. A considerable amount of fat can be stored between the parietal peritoneum and the body wall.

B. The **visceral peritoneum** consists of extensive folds of peritoneum that cover the abdominal viscera. The visceral peritoneum is intimately applied to the surface of the abdominal organs, and cannot be removed from them.

1. **Classification of abdominal organs related to the peritoneum**
   a. **Retroperitoneal organs** (e.g., kidneys) have one surface tightly applied to the body wall (Figure 42–1); therefore, only one surface is covered with peritoneum.
   b. "Intraperitoneal" organs (e.g., liver, gonads, uterus) are covered on almost all sides by peritoneum. These organs have long mesenteries and are suspended deep within the abdominal cavity (see Figure 42–1). Although these organs are referred to as "intraperitoneal," they do not lie within the peritoneal cavity, as the term would suggest.
2. **Development of the visceral peritoneum** depends on the organ.
   a. In **most abdominal organs,** the visceral peritoneum forms as the developing organ extends down from the dorsal body wall, pushing the parietal peritoneum in front of it. In this way, the parietal peritoneum is transformed into the visceral peritoneum of the organ in question.
   b. The visceral peritoneum of the **intestine** develops in a different manner. In the very early embryo, a right and left peritoneal sheet are present. When these two layers meet longitudinally along the midline, they form a midsagittal divider between the right and left halves of the abdominal cavity. The simple, straight gut tube of the very early embryo develops between these two layers of peritoneum, and thus is surrounded on nearly all sides by this portion of the visceral peritoneum. When most of the ventral portion of the midline partition eventually degenerates, the gut tube is surrounded by peritoneum on all sides, except for a small area along its dorsal border when the two layers of visceral peritoneum reflect off the organ to travel to the dorsal body wall.

C. The **connecting peritoneum** extends between organs or between an organ and the abdominal wall. There are specific types of connecting peritoneum.

1. A **mesentery** extends **between an abdominal organ** and the **body wall.** Mesenteries are **wide,** and **conduct vessels** and **nerves** to and from the organs they suspend.
   a. Specific mesenteries are named by prefixing the name of the organ with "meso-" (e.g., **mesocolon, mesoduodenum, mesorectum, mesoileum, mesogastrium).**
   b. The **dorsal common ("great") mesentery (mesojejunoileum)** is an elongate mesentery that suspends the jejunum and ileum from the dorsal body wall. It is continuous with the mesogastrium and mesoduodenum cranial to it, and the mesocolon caudal to it. The **root of the mesentery** is the attachment point of the great mesentery to the dorsal body wall (see Figure 42–1).
      (1) The root of the mesentery is **positioned** at the **level of vertebrae L2–L3.** Here, the mesentery reflects back onto the structures of the dorsal body wall (i.e., the crura of the diaphragm and the aorta).
      (2) The root of the mesentery **surrounds** the large **cranial mesenteric artery** and **vein,** the **intestinal lymphatic vessels,** and the **mesenteric nerve plexus.**
2. A **peritoneal ligament** extends **between two abdominal organs.** Peritoneal ligaments, like pulmonary ligaments, are simply doubled folds of peritoneum; they bear no resemblance to the stout, dense collagenous collections associated with the skeleton.
   a. Peritoneal ligaments are **narrow,** and **conduct few or no vascular or nervous structures.**

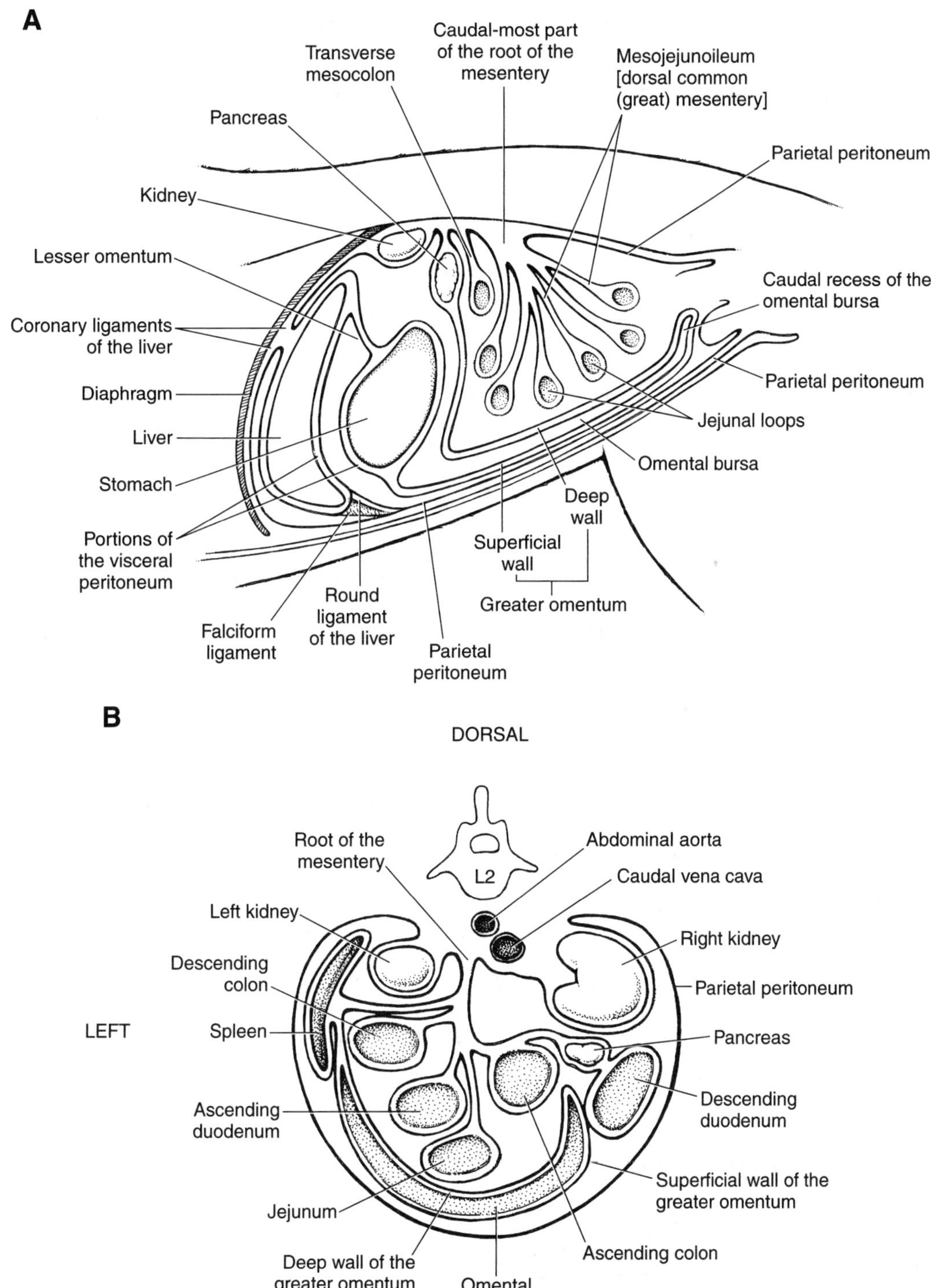

FIGURE 42–1. (*A*) The parietal and visceral peritoneum and associated peritoneal structures, left parasagittal view. Note how the two layers of visceral peritoneum reflect off the stomach to form the superficial wall of the greater omentum. (*B*) Cross-section through the abdomen at the level of vertebra L2.

b. Peritoneal ligaments are named for the two organs between which they extend (e.g., the **gastrosplenic ligament** extends between the stomach and the spleen; the **hepatoduodenal ligament** extends between the liver and the duodenum).

D. The **greater omentum** is a continuous, doubled fold of peritoneum that is elaborated from the greater curvature of the stomach.

1. The greater omentum contains a **lacy network** of fine vessels surrounded by fat. The lacy appearance is most prominent in dogs of proper body weight; in emaciated animals, insufficient fat is present to make the pattern outstanding, and in obese dogs, the fat obscures the branchings of the vessels and fills the intervascular areas.

Canine Clinical Correlation

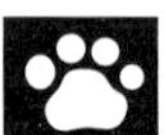

The greater omentum is highly vascular and very mobile, features often advantageous during abdominal surgery—surgeons often tack bits of the greater omentum over sites where the viscera have been opened; this way, any adhesions that form are more likely to form between the organ and the very mobile omentum, rather than between an organ and the immobile body wall.

2. The greater omentum extends from the greater curvature of the stomach along the ventral belly wall, reflects back on itself near the pelvic inlet, and travels back along its own outer layer, passing caudal to the stomach. After passing the stomach, it surrounds part of the pancreas, and then gains the dorsal body wall. At this point, the peritoneum (of which the greater omentum is formed) continues on as parietal peritoneum until it reflects onto the next organ as a portion of visceral peritoneum (see Figure 42–1).
   a. The **superficial wall** of the greater omentum is its superficial layer, which itself is a doubled fold of peritoneum (see Figure 42–1).
   b. The **deep wall** of the greater omentum is its deeper layer, which reflects forward in the region of the pelvic inlet.
   c. The **omental bursa** is the space between the superficial and deep walls of the greater omentum.
      (1) The omental bursa is a **subdivision of the peritoneal cavity.**
      (2) The **epiploic foramen** is the communication between the omental bursa and the larger part of the peritoneal cavity. The epiploic foramen is bounded dorsally by the caudal vena cava and ventrally by the hepatic portal vein.

E. The **lesser omentum** is a smaller stretch of peritoneum that extends between the lesser curvature of the stomach and the liver (see Figure 42–1).

1. Like the greater omentum, the lesser omentum is laced with vessels and fat.
2. The lesser omentum envelops the papillary process of the caudate lobe of the liver.

IV. EMBRYOLOGIC DEVELOPMENT

A. Dorsal and ventral mesenteries

1. **Foregut.** The **primitive stomach** is supported both dorsally and ventrally by mesenteries (i.e., the **dorsal** and **ventral mesogastria).**
   a. The **dorsal mesogastrium** undergoes more specialization than the remainder of the dorsal mesentery. The **spleen** develops in the midregion of the dorsal mesogastrium, dividing it into two parts.
      (1) The portion of mesogastrium between the spleen and the stomach is the **gastrosplenic ligament.**

(2) The portion of mesogastrium between the spleen and the dorsal body wall is the region of the peritoneum that **gives rise to the greater omentum.**

b. The **ventral mesogastrium** is the only portion of the ventral mesentery that is retained into the definitive form. The **liver** develops in the midregion of the ventral mesentery, dividing it into two parts.

(1) The **lesser omentum** is the portion of the ventral mesogastrium that extends between the liver and the lesser curvature of the stomach.

(2) The **falciform ligament** is the portion of the ventral mesogastrium that extends between the liver and the ventral body wall.

(a) The falciform ligament attaches to the **linea alba.**

(b) The falciform ligament carries the **umbilical vein** in the fetus. In the adult, the umbilical vein degenerates to form the **round ligament of the liver,** which is sometimes visible as a thickening in the caudal free edge of the falciform ligament.

(c) The falciform ligament **stores significant amounts of fat,** even in lean animals. In overweight animals, the falciform ligament can resemble a shapeless lump of fat on the ventral body wall.

Canine Clinical Correlation

The fat-filled ligament can complicate closure of abdominal incisions in the cranial part of the abdomen.

2. **Hindgut.** The **primitive gut tube** is a straight tube extending from the head to the tail region of the embryo. Early in development, the gut tube is no longer than the body cavity (i.e., it is not coiled) and it is supported along its full length by a complete dorsal and ventral mesentery.

a. The **dorsal mesentery** is located between the dorsal body wall and the dorsal edge of the developing gut tube. The full length of the dorsal mesentery is retained into the definitive form as the **dorsal common mesentery** (i.e., the mesogastrium, -duodenum, -jejunum, -ileum, -colon, and -rectum).

b. The **ventral mesentery** associated with the intestine degenerates.

B. Length of the mesenteries

1. **Herniation and retraction of the gut tube.** During normal development, the pace of growth of the gut tube exceeds that of the body wall, causing most of the length of the gut tube to herniate through the incomplete body wall. While the gut loops are external to the body cavity, the entire mass undergoes two rotations (reflected in the final form as the passage of the gut from right to left, and then from left to right). As the body cavity acquires sufficient size, the gut loops are eventually retracted back inside. The sequence of retraction begins at the cranial- and caudal-most ends of the tube; the region of the stomach, duodenum, and colon are retracted early, while the jejunum is retracted late.

2. **Crowding of the viscera.** The portions of gut that are retracted early are crowded by the portions coming in later.

a. **Fixed viscera.** The parts retracted early are packed tightly against the body wall by the portions of the gut that enter later, causing their mesenteries to partially fuse with the body wall. Therefore, these mesenteries are quite short in the definitive form. The viscera with short mesenteries, called fixed viscera, include the:

(1) Stomach and duodenum (cranially)

(2) Ileum, cecum, and all three parts of the colon (caudally)

b. Mobile viscera. The regions of gut that are retracted late, mainly the jejunum, are not crowded and retain their longer mesenteries.

Canine Clinical Correlation

The length of the mesentery affects the ease with which various regions of the intestine can be mobilized and removed from the abdominal cavity during surgery. Access to the jejunum is easily achieved through a relatively small incision, while access to the stomach or colon requires a longer incision.

Canine Clinical Correlation

"Landmark" mesenteries. Many of the fixed viscera are reliably located, an advantage during surgery.

- On the right and left sides, the **broad ligaments of the uterus** are the lateral-most mesenteries in the abdomen of the bitch. The consistent placement of these mesenteries allows the surgeon to readily locate the uterine horn during **ovariohysterectomy.**
- The short mesenteries of the **descending colon** (on the left side) and the **descending duodenum** (on the right side) give these organs a constant position.

Canine Clinical Correlation

The descending mesocolon and the descending mesoduodenum are short enough to retain the gut portion in place, but are long enough to serve as **physiologic retractors** for the jejunum. Retraction of any gut loops during surgery must be carefully performed in order to avoid irritation of the gut surface, leakage of serum, and the possibility of adhesions after surgery. Should the surgery in question require the jejunal mass to be retracted from the right side, the descending duodenum can be raised and drawn toward the midline—the descending mesoduodenum will gently retract the jejunum, so that it is not necessary to handle the loops of the jejunum directly. Similarly, should it be necessary to access the left dorsal abdominal wall, the descending colon can be raised and drawn toward the midline, and most of the jejunal mass will be retracted medially by the descending mesocolon.

Chapter 43

Gastrointestinal Organs and Spleen

I. TUBULAR GASTROINTESTINAL ORGANS

A. Esophagus. The terminal esophagus joins the stomach immediately after passing the diaphragm, high on the dorsal left side of the abdomen, at about the level of the eighth rib.

B. Stomach. The stomach's main function is the storage, acidification, and manipulation of ingesta for periodic passage to the intestines.

1. **Relations** (Figure 43–1). The relations of the stomach are the liver (cranially) and the pancreas, spleen, and transverse colon (caudally).
   a. The **parietal surface** of the stomach faces cranially, toward the liver.
   b. The **visceral surface** of the stomach faces caudally, toward the remainder of the abdominal viscera.
2. **Shape.** The stomach, a highly distensible organ, **varies** in shape according to its degree of fullness. When completely full, the stomach is quite round; when completely empty, it is reduced to a small, flattened tube.
3. **Position.** The stomach is oriented transversely across the body. The position of the stomach **varies** according to its degree of fullness.
   a. The **completely empty** stomach retracts into a deep depression of the caudal surface of the liver, and has no contact with any part of the abdominal wall.
   a. The **moderately full** stomach is positioned under the last four ribs (see Figure 43–1) and lies mostly to the left of the median plane, although its terminal portions extend across the midline to the right in order to meet the duodenum.
   c. When the stomach is **greatly distended,** the cranial border projects caudal to the costal arch and the caudal border may reach nearly to the pelvic brim! The fully distended stomach passes from the right to the left body walls.

Canine Clinical Correlation

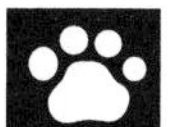

Gastric dilatation-volvulus (GDV) is a potentially fatal condition that most commonly occurs in large-breed dogs. GDV occurs when the accumulation of gas within the stomach causes it to rotate. This twisting occludes the normal outflow path for ingesta, causing the ingesta to undergo rapid fermentation in the stomach and leading to the production of more gas and more distention. The combination of the twisting and pathologic stretching of the stomach compromises gastric blood supply and leads to death of large parts of the gastric wall, which can lead to the death of the dog in a surprisingly short period of time.

---

4. **Regions** (Figure 43–2). Dimensions and positions given refer to those of a moderately full stomach.
   a. The **cardia** of the stomach is a small area surrounding the esophageal entrance.
   b. The **fundus** of the stomach is a blind region that extends to the left and dorsally of the cardia. Of all the gastric regions, the fundus is positioned farthest left of the midline.
      (1) The fundus is the **first portion of the stomach to fill with ingesta.** The fundus is relatively small in the empty stomach, but is capable of remarkable distention.
      (2) The **cardiac incisure** is a relatively sharp angle formed at the junction of the cardia and the fundus. This incisure varies in prominence with the degree of gastric dilatation.

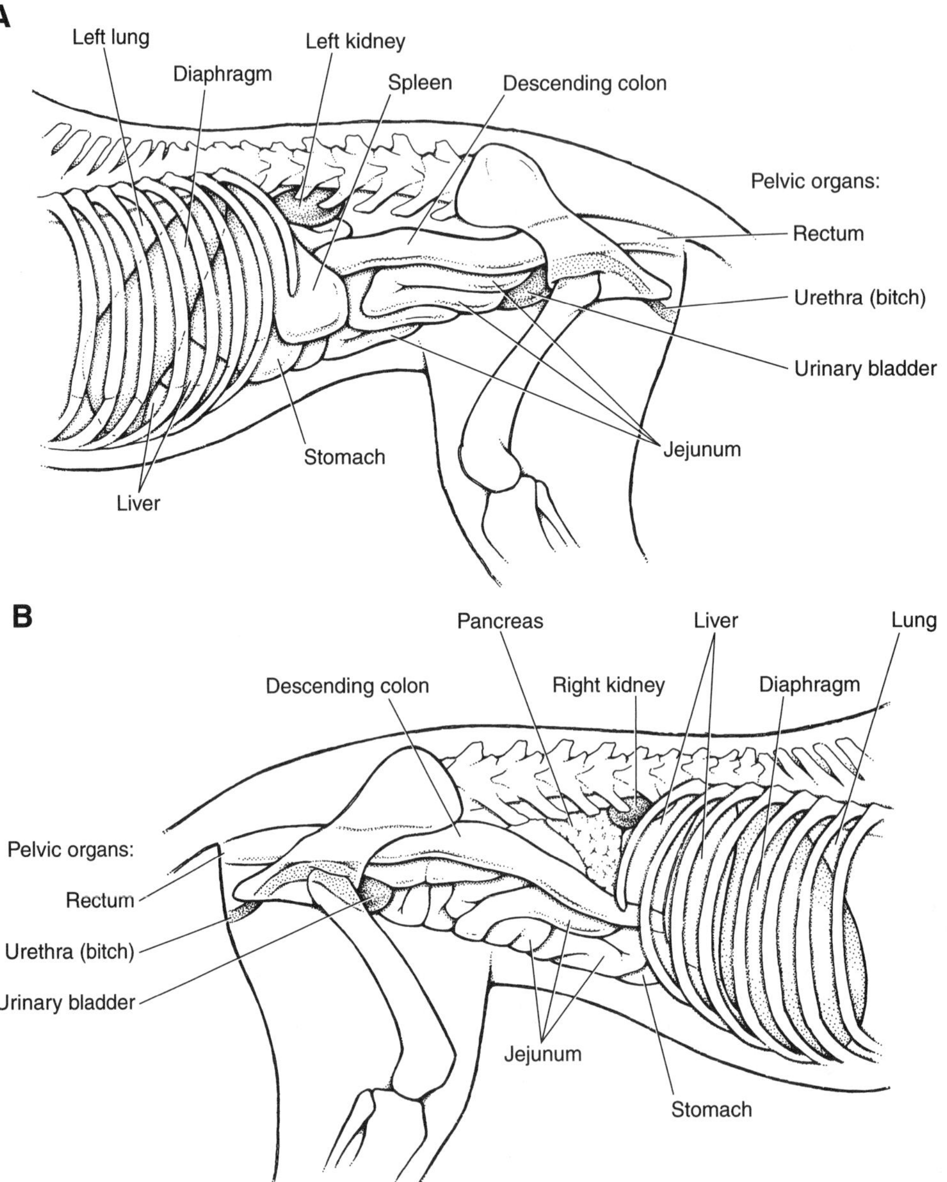

FIGURE 43–1. Abdominal organs *in situ.* (*A*) Left lateral view. (*B*) Right lateral view. (*continued*)

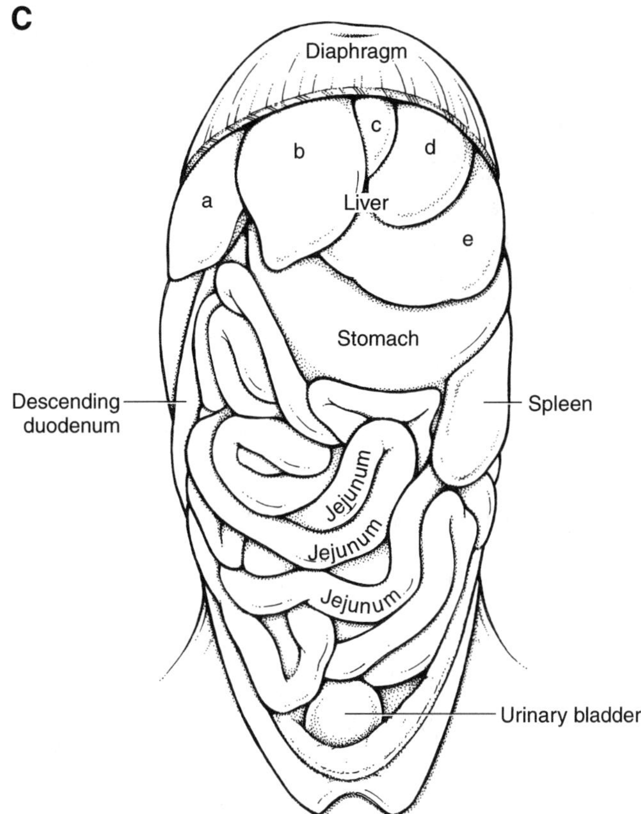

FIGURE 43–1—*continued* (*C*) Ventral view. The lobes of the liver are identified with lowercase letters: *a* = right lateral lobe; *b* = right medial lobe; *c* = quadrate lobe; *d* = left medial lobe; *e* = left lateral lobe. (Modified with permission from Dyce KM, Sack WO, Wensing CJG: *Textbook of Veterinary Anatomy,* 2nd ed. Philadelphia, WB Saunders, 1996, pp 132, 421.)

c. The **body** of the stomach is its largest region. The body communicates directly with both the cardia and the fundus.

(1) Most of the gastric body lies to the left of the midline, with its terminal portions extending across the midline to blend with the next area of the stomach, the pyloric region.

(2) The body of the stomach fills with ingesta after the fundus is full.

d. The **pyloric region** of the stomach, the terminal portion of the stomach, extends between the body and the duodenum. The pyloric region normally undergoes relatively little distention compared with the fundus and body, and is the last region to fill during a meal. The pyloric region has two divisions:

(1) The **pyloric antrum** (i.e., the continuation from the gastric body) forms the first two-thirds of the pyloric region. This portion of the pyloric region is the widest, although it narrows as it funnels into the next segment.

(2) The **pyloric canal** tapers to approximate the diameter of the duodenum. The **pylorus** is the muscular sphincter that surrounds the pyloric canal where it joins the duodenum. **The terms "pylorus" and "pyloric region" are not synonymous**—"pylorus" refers to the sphincter that is a part of the pyloric canal, while "pyloric region" refers to the gastric region that includes the pyloric antrum, pyloric canal, and the pylorus.

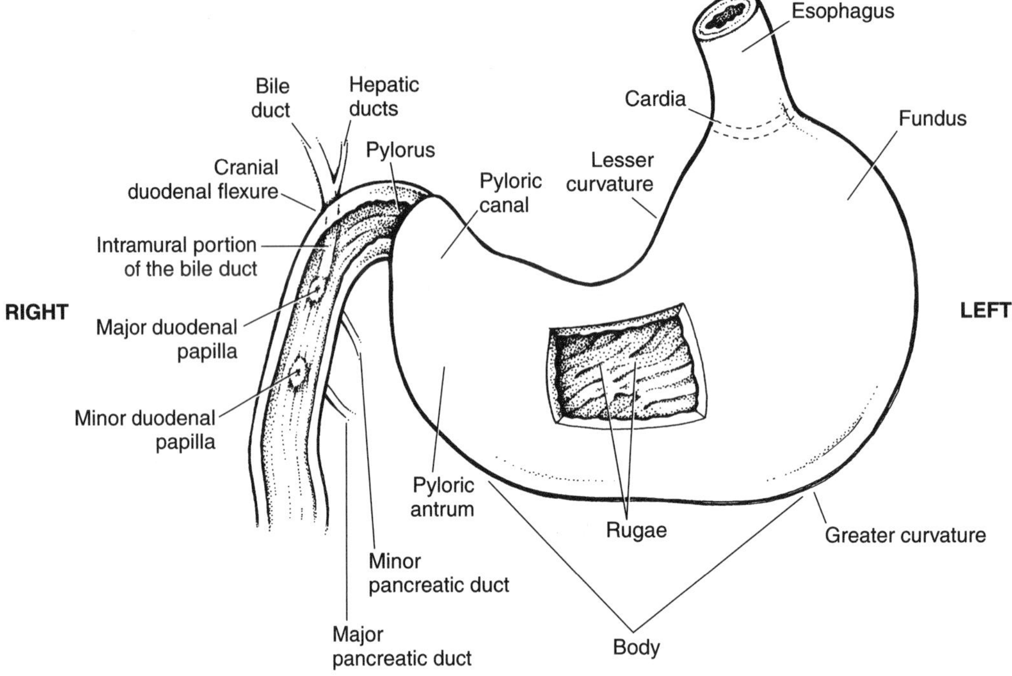

FIGURE 43–2. Parietal surface of the stomach.

5. **Borders**
   a. The **greater curvature** of the stomach is its **caudal border.** The greater curvature extends from the cardia to the pylorus, passing along the fundus, body, and pyloric region (see Figure 43–2). The greater curvature of the stomach provides an attachment line for most of the superficial wall of the **greater omentum.**
   b. The **lesser curvature** of the stomach is its **cranial border.** The lesser curvature extends from the cardia along the body and pyloric region, to end at the pylorus. (Note that it does not include the fundus; see Figure 43–2).
      (1) The **angular incisure** is the pronounced notch at the junction of the body and pyloric region on the lesser curvature. The **papillary process of the caudate lobe of the liver** [see II B 4 c (6) (a)] is nestled within the angular incisure.
      (2) The lesser curvature of the stomach provides the attachment site for the caudal edge of the **lesser omentum.**
6. **Structure**
   a. **Muscular coat.** The muscular wall of the stomach is composed of three major layers, based on fiber direction. These layers are visible on careful gross dissection.
      (1) The **outer longitudinal layer** of gastric muscle fibers is continuous with the outer longitudinal layer of both the esophagus and duodenum.
      (2) The **inner circular layer** of gastric muscle fibers is denser and more organized than the outer layer, and has two notable condensations in its substance.
         (a) The **cardiac sphincter** is a weak condensation of inner circular muscle fibers in the cardiac region of the stomach.
         (b) The **pylorus** is a dense, strong condensation of inner circular muscle fibers at the junction of the pyloric canal and the duodenum.
      (3) The **innermost oblique layer** of gastric muscle is an incomplete muscle layer internal to the circular layer and adjacent to the submucosa. The fibers of this layer fan out from the area of the cardia across the body toward the greater curvature and pyloric region.

b. Internal surface. In the moderately full stomach, the internal gastric surface is marked by parallel, tortuous ridges of mucosa called **rugae** (see Figure 43–2). The rugae are quite pronounced, and in the nearly empty stomach may be as high as 1 centimeter. The numerous rugae are generally arranged along the long axis of the body.

C. **Small intestine.** The small intestine comprises, from cranial to caudal, the **duodenum, jejunum,** and **ileum.**

1. The **duodenum,** a small-bore muscular tube with a smooth external surface, begins just caudal to the pylorus and ends at the duodenojejunal flexure (Figure 43–3).
   a. **Position.** The duodenum lies to the right of the midline, and is held close to the dorsal abdominal wall by its short mesentery.
   b. **Course.** The duodenum leaves the stomach close to the dorsal body wall at about the level of the ninth rib. After an initial brief cranial turn, it courses caudally to the level of the tuber coxae. At the tuber coxae, the duodenum makes a hairpin loop, and travels cranially again to become continuous with the jejunum at the level of the root of the mesentery.
   c. **Regions**
      (1) The **cranial portion** of the duodenum continues directly from the pylorus and is short. Almost immediately after leaving the pylorus, the duodenum passes through the tight **cranial duodenal flexure** and is redirected into a caudal course.
      (2) The **descending duodenum** (see Figure 43–3) courses directly caudally adjacent to the right body wall. This long region of the duodenum extends nearly to the pelvic inlet.

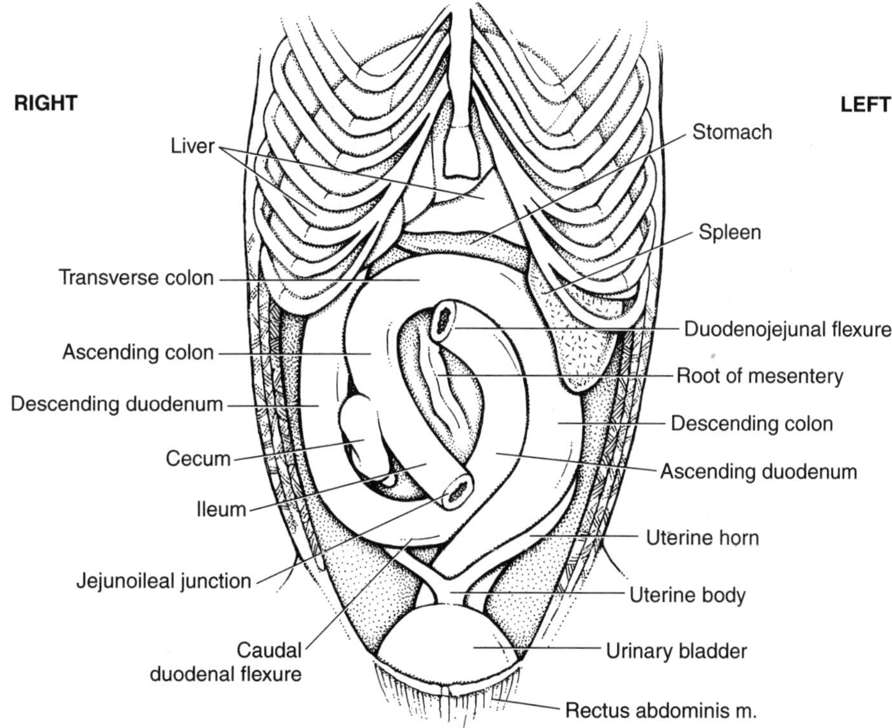

FIGURE 43–3. Removal of the jejunum reveals the duodenum, ileum, cecum, and colon. (*In situ,* ventral view.) (Modified with permission from Pasquini C, Spurgeon T: *Anatomy of Domestic Animals,* 7th ed. SUDZ Publishing, Pilot Point, TX, 1995, p 274.)

(a) The **right lobe of the pancreas** lies in direct contact with the medial side of the descending duodenum.

(b) The **duodenal papillae** (see Figure 43–2), small elevations in the duodenal wall, are present in the initial part of the descending duodenum. Ducts of the liver and pancreas open on these papillae, which are often not visible unless the mucosa is scraped away.

(i) The **major duodenal papilla** is the more cranial of the two, and provides the openings for both the **bile duct** and the **pancreatic duct.**

(ii) The **minor duodenal papilla** lies slightly caudal to its major fellow. The **accessory pancreatic duct** opens here.

(c) At the **caudal duodenal flexure,** approximately at the level of the tuber coxae, the duodenum assumes a cranial course.

(3) The **ascending duodenum** takes a somewhat oblique course cranially, angled slightly toward the midline, to almost reach the greater curvature of the stomach.

(4) The **duodenojejunal flexure** is the point at which the duodenum joins the jejunum. This junction is marked by a change in mesentery length from short to longer, and by a change in the pattern of blood supply (i.e., from short, straight vessels to arcades).

2. The **jejunum** is the longest and most mobile portion of the small intestine. The jejunum begins at the duodenojejunal flexure, and ends at the jejunoileal junction.

a. **Appearance.** The jejunum, like the duodenum, is a smooth-surfaced, small-bore tube. The jejunum is distinguished from the duodenum by its long mesentery and arterial arcades.

b. **Position.** The jejunum occupies most of the free space within the abdominal cavity (see Figure 43–1). It lies ventral to nearly all of the other abdominal organs and structures, with the exception of the greater omentum, which is positioned between the jejunal coils and the ventral belly wall. The length of the great mesentery allows the jejunum to be disposed as a series of loops throughout the abdominal cavity. These loops freely mingle with the other abdominal viscera.

c. **Course.** From the duodenojejunal flexure, the jejunum passes toward the left. Most of the jejunum is disposed openly in the abdominal cavity; however, as the jejunum nears its junction with the succeeding portion of the intestinal tract (the ileum, at approximately the level of the midregion of the abdomen), the mesentery shortens.

3. The **ileum** is the short, terminal portion of the small intestine. The ileum, which begins at the jejunoileal junction and ends at the ileocolic sphincter (see Figure 43–3), measures 10–15 cm.

a. **Appearance.** The gut wall of the ileum is largely indistinguishable from that of the jejunum or duodenum. However, the mesentery and the pattern of blood supply differ from the immediately preceding segment: the mesentery is notably shorter, and the arcades of vessels characteristic of the jejunum are replaced by short, straight vessels that enter the ileal wall. In addition, an artery is present along the antimesenteric border of the ileum that is not found in any other segment of the small intestine.

b. **Position.** The termination of the ileum is positioned near the dorsal body wall, just lateral to the ascending duodenum.

c. **Course.** The ileum angles dorsally from the jejunum, and approximates the dorsal abdominal wall just cranial to the caudal duodenal flexure. Here the ileum enters the large intestine at the **ileocolic orifice.** This junction is guarded by the **ileocolic sphincter,** a thickening of the inner circular muscle layer of the ileum.

D. Large intestine. The large intestine comprises the **cecum, colon, rectum,** and **anal canal;** it begins at the ileocolic sphincter and ends at the anus. The rectum and anal canal are located within the pelvic cavity and are discussed more completely in Chapter 51 III A–B.

1. The **cecum** is a blind-ended pouch at the junction of the small and large intestines (see Figure 43–3). In the dog, it is essentially a diverticulum of the most proximal part of the colon. Just distal to the ileocolic sphincter, the cecum diverts from the colon at the **cecocolic orifice,** which is guarded by the **cecocolic sphincter.**

a. **Appearance.** The cecum is variable in size and form. Generally, it takes the form of a truncate cone, and usually is rather corkscrewed in the adult.
   (1) The **body** of the cecum occupies the greatest part of its length; its blind end is referred to as its **apex.**
   (2) The cecum is normally **oriented with its long axis parallel to the vertebral column,** with its apex pointing caudally.

b. **Position**
   (1) The cecum is located to the right of the midline in the cranial abdomen, close to the dorsal body wall (in the region of the transverse processes of vertebrae L2–L4), and dorsal to the jejunal loops.
   (2) The cecum is closely attached to the ileum by fascia and peritoneum through nearly all its length. The free end of its peritoneal attachment is termed the **ileocecal fold.** This fold is sometimes used to identify the point where the small intestine changes from the jejunum to ileum.

2. The **colon** is the major part of the large intestine, extending from the region of the ileocecal junction to the anus (see Figure 43–3).
   a. **Appearance.** The colon is larger in diameter than the small intestine, but the difference is only moderate. The surface of the colon is also smooth, although somewhat more irregular than that of the small intestine.
   b. **Position.** The colon is positioned along the dorsal body wall.
   c. **Course.** The colon begins in the cranial region to the right of the midline, crosses from right to left, and then passes caudally near the left body wall to enter the pelvic cavity.
      (1) The **ascending colon,** the initial and shortest part of the colon, extends from the area of the ileocecal junction to the right colic flexure. The ascending colon passes cranially along the dorsal body wall just ventral to the right kidney, reaches the greater curvature of the stomach, and then turns to the left.
      (2) The **right colic flexure** is the angle at which the ascending colon becomes continuous with the transverse colon. Depending on the disposition of the colon as a whole, the flexure may be more or less pronounced.
      (3) The **transverse colon** extends from the right colic flexure to the left colic flexure. The transverse colon passes from the right to the left just cranial to the root of the mesentery, in a position just caudal to the greater curvature of the stomach. The transverse colon is intermediate in length among the three colic regions.
      (4) The **left colic flexure** is the angle at which the transverse colon becomes continuous with the descending colon. As with the right colic flexure, the degree of angularity of this flexure varies.
      (5) The **descending colon** is the longest portion of the colon. It continues caudally from the left colic flexure, in a straight course parallel to the left body wall, to the pelvic inlet. At the pelvic inlet, the intestine changes name from colon to rectum.

II. GLANDULAR GASTROINTESTINAL ORGANS

A. Pancreas

1. **Function**
   a. **Exocrine gland.** The exocrine portion of the pancreas, its largest part, produces enzymes essential for the digestion of carbohydrates, fats, and proteins.
   b. **Endocrine gland.** The endocrine portion produces insulin and glucagon, essential in regulating the sugar content of the blood.

2. **Appearance**
   a. The pancreas is a "V"-shaped, rather flat organ consisting of a **body** and two elongate lobes; the **right lobe** is longer, thinner, and narrower than the **left lobe.**
   b. The surface of the pancreas is **lobulated,** giving it a cobbled look.

3. **Position.** The pancreas is positioned largely caudal to the stomach.

a. The **body** is settled into the angle formed by the pyloric region of the stomach and the duodenum.
b. The **left lobe** lies against the deep wall of the greater omentum. This lobe passes across the caudal surface of the stomach, and ends against the left kidney.
c. The **right lobe** lies in the mesoduodenum, and courses caudally along the full length of the descending duodenum so that its rounded caudal end fits into the loop formed by the caudal duodenal flexure.

4. **Ducts.** Usually, in dogs, two ducts are present, one leading mainly from the right pancreatic lobe and one from the left. The ducts from both lobes intercommunicate within the substance of the pancreas.
   a. The **pancreatic duct,** the more cranial and usually the smaller of the two ducts, opens into the cranial part of the descending duodenum on the **major duodenal papilla** (along with the bile duct from the liver). The pancreatic duct is occasionally absent.
   b. The caudally positioned **accessory pancreatic duct,** despite its name, is the main conduit of the gland, and is constant. This larger duct opens on the **minor duodenal papilla.**

B. Liver. The liver is the largest gland of the body.

1. **Function.** The liver has both exocrine and endocrine functions. In addition, it plays a role in the metabolism of food and the detoxification of numerous substances.
2. **Position**
   a. The liver is positioned **immediately caudal to the diaphragm,** and covers all of the caudal diaphragmatic surface, with the exception of a small portion of the dorsal left corner.
      (1) The **diaphragmatic (parietal, cranial) surface** is **convex** (because it molds intimately to the diaphragm) and quite smooth.
      (2) The **visceral (caudal) surface** of the liver is **concave** and irregular in contour because it is marked by the impressions of the several abdominal organs that crowd against it. Chief among these is the stomach.
   b. The liver **lies almost entirely within the part of the abdomen covered by the bony thorax.**

3. **Appearance.** The liver is composed of six lobes that are deeply separated from each other. Its extremely vascular nature renders the fresh liver firm to the touch, but highly friable. Removed from the body and placed on a firm surface, the liver tends to assume a rectangular shape. *In situ,* the liver somewhat resembles a valentine heart with one short shoulder (Figure 43–4).
   a. Almost the entire surface of the liver is **covered by peritoneum,** owing to its development within the ventral mesogastrium. Only the portal region and the area where the gall bladder is fused to the liver lack a peritoneal covering.
   b. The **borders of the liver** (i.e., the peripheral edges of the lobes) are normally **quite sharp.** Rounding of the borders implies a pathologic condition.

4. **Features** (see Figure 43–4)
   a. **Porta.** The porta of the liver (i.e., its **hilus)** transmits the hepatic vessels, nerves, and bile duct. The porta is positioned on the visceral surface.
   b. **Groove for the caudal vena cava.** The caudal vena cava deeply grooves the **dorsal surface** of the liver as it passes across the organ *en route* to the heart.
   c. **Lobes.** The six lobes of the canine liver are mostly named for position; only one is named for its shape.
      (1) The **right lateral lobe** is moderately large, and is positioned against the right lateral body wall. The right lateral lobe lies entirely to the right of the median plane, and a portion of it projects dorsally as far as the dorsal body wall. This bit of the right lateral lobe forms a small part of the deep, distinct **renal impression,** which houses the cranial pole of the right kidney.
      (2) The **right medial lobe** is roughly the same size as the right lateral lobe, and also

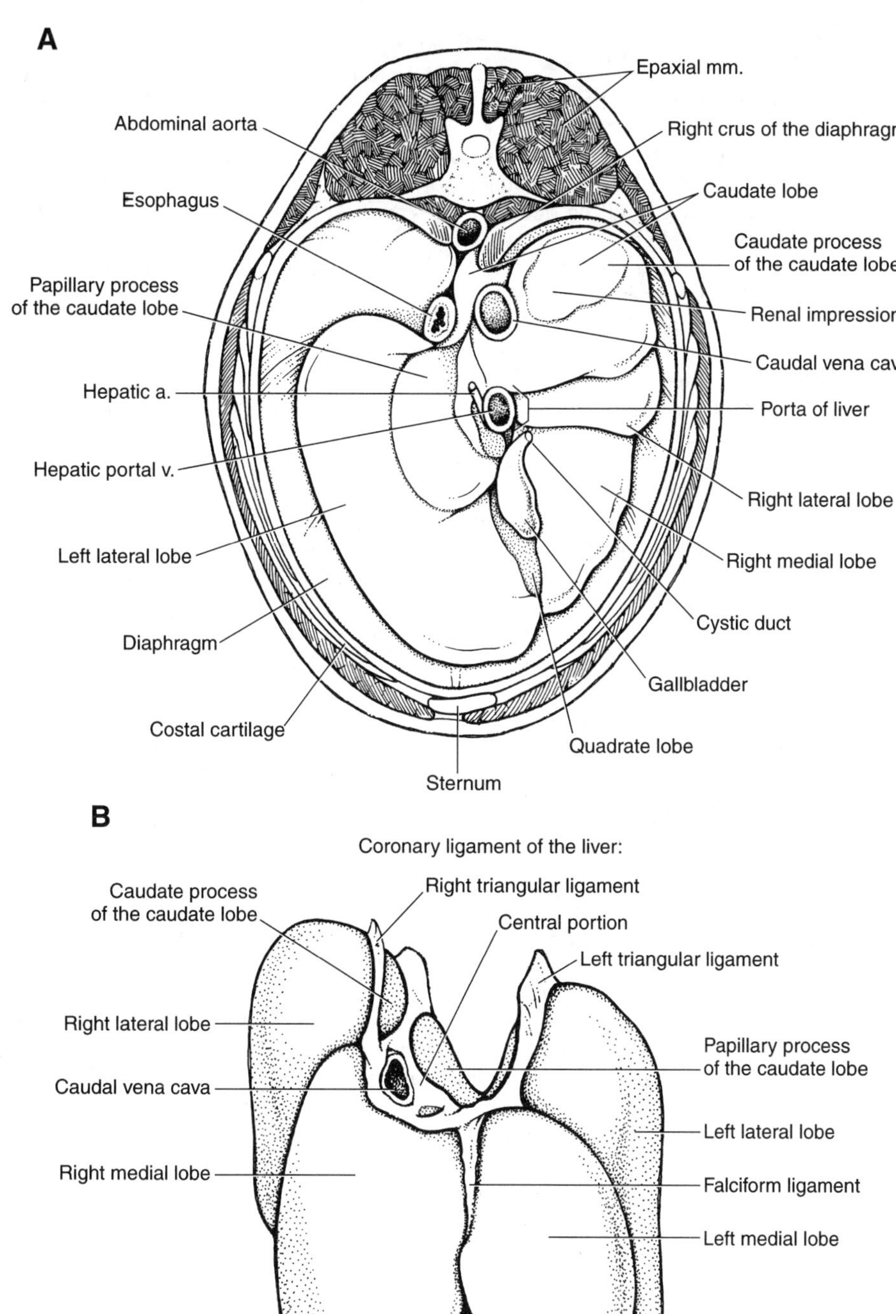

FIGURE 43–4. The liver *in situ.* (*A*) Caudal view (i.e., visceral surface). (*B*) Cranial view (i.e., diaphragmatic surface). [Part *A* modified with permission from Pasquini C, Spurgeon T: *Anatomy of Domestic Animals,* 7th ed. SUDZ Publishing, Pilot Point, TX, 1995, p 293; Part *B* modified with permission from Schummer A, Nickel R, Sack WO: *The Viscera of the Domestic Mammals,* 2e. New York, Springer-Verlag, 1979, p 135.]

lies entirely on the right side of the body. The right medial lobe extends from the right lateral lobe to nearly the midsagittal plane.

(3) The roughly rectangular **quadrate lobe** is the only lobe named for its shape. This relatively small liver lobe lies along the midline, directly between the right and left medial lobes. The quadrate lobe forms a landmark for two other structures related to the liver:

(a) The **gallbladder** lies between the quadrate and the right medial lobes.

(b) The **falciform ligament** (and thus the round ligament when this structure is recognizable in the free edge of the falciform ligament) lies between the quadrate and left medial lobes.

(4) The **left medial lobe,** another relatively large lobe, is interposed between the quadrate and left lateral lobes. Most of the lobe lies to the left of the midline.

(5) The **left lateral lobe,** also rather large, is located between the left medial lobe and the left lateral body wall. The left lateral lobe lies entirely to the left of the midline.

(6) The **caudate lobe** is a small, irregularly shaped lobe with two processes.

(a) The **papillary process of the caudate lobe** extends from the small central part of the caudate lobe to the angular incisure on the lesser curvature of the stomach. The papillary process is enveloped by the lesser omentum.

(b) The **caudate process of the caudate lobe,** the largest part of the lobe, projects caudally, along the dorsal body wall from the central part of the caudate lobe. The caudate process of the caudate lobe forms the majority of the **renal impression.**

d. Ligaments. The development of the liver within the ventral mesogastrium results in a peritoneal covering over most of its surface, as well as the thin but strong fibrous layer that attaches the peritoneum to the surface of the liver.

(1) **Coronary ligament of the liver.** On the diaphragmatic surface of the liver, the fibroserous layer reflects onto the surface of the diaphragm, providing the only attachment of the liver to any wall of the abdomen. This "U"-shaped attachment is called the coronary ligament of the liver.

(2) **Triangular ligaments.** Like the pulmonary ligaments, the triangular ligaments are nothing more than thin, transparent folds of peritoneum at the right and left termination of the coronary ligament of the liver.

(3) **Falciform ligament.** The falciform ligament (i.e., the ventral portion of the remnant of the ventral mesogastrium) extends between the liver and the ventral body wall [see Chapter 42 IV A 1 b (2)].

(4) **Lesser omentum.** The lesser omentum, the dorsal portion of the persistent part of the ventral mesogastrium, extends between the liver and the lesser curvature of the stomach [see Chapter 42 IV A 1 b (1)].

(5) **Hepatorenal ligament.** The hepatorenal ligament is a delicate, doubled layer of peritoneum that extends between the renal fossa of the liver and the right kidney.

5. Gallbladder and bile passages. The gallbladder stores the bile produced by the hepatic cells. The biliary passages transmit bile either from the liver to the gallbladder, or from the gallbladder to the duodenum.

a. Gallbladder

(1) **Position.** The gallbladder resides in the **fossa for the gallbladder,** which deeply indents the facing surfaces of the quadrate and right lateral lobes of the liver, approximately at the level of the eighth intercostal space.

(2) **Appearance.** The gall bladder is capable of tremendous changes in size. Generally, it can be described as a **pear-shaped** organ, with a rounded **fundus** at its cranial end, a gradually narrowing **body,** and a narrow **neck** directed toward the duodenum.

b. Biliary passages

(1) The **cystic duct** arises from the neck of the gallbladder and carries bile toward the duodenum. In addition, it receives the hepatic ducts from the hepatic parenchyma. The term "cystic" in its name denotes its direct attachment to the gallbladder.

(2) The **hepatic ducts** receive the smaller ducts within the liver that originate from the microscopic bile canaliculi. Usually, three to five hepatic ducts are present, receiving bile from multiple lobes and carrying it to the cystic duct.

(3) The **(common) bile duct** is the continuation of the cystic duct following the entrance of the last hepatic duct. The common bile duct passes caudal to the duodenum in the region of the most cranial part of the descending duodenum to enter the duodenal lumen on the **major duodenal papilla,** along with the pancreatic duct.

III. SPLEEN.

The spleen is associated with the immune system, but is considered with the digestive organs because of its physical proximity to the stomach, with which it shares vascular supply and drainage.

A. Appearance

1. **Size.** The size of the canine spleen varies widely, because dogs have the "storage" type of spleen—the spleen is capable of either pooling large volumes of blood, or actively contracting to quickly deliver that blood into the systemic circulation.
2. **Shape.** The highly vascular spleen takes the shape of an **elongate oblong.** A slight constriction is sometimes present about halfway along its length. Transversely sectioned, the spleen is triangular. The spleen is gently curved as it follows the greater curvature of the stomach.
3. **Surface.** The surface is generally smooth, but close inspection reveals a finely reticulated appearance caused by considerable amounts of connective tissue within the substance of the organ.

B. Position.

The spleen generally **follows the contour of the greater curvature of the stomach.** Thus, the spleen is located **largely on the left of the midline** (see Figure 43–1C).

1. The **visceral surface** of the spleen faces the greater gastric curvature.
2. The **parietal surface** faces the diaphragm and the left lateral body wall.

C. Features

1. **Hilus.** The visceral surface presents the splenic hilus, which is rather unusual in that it is elongate rather than focal. The splenic hilus extends along nearly the entire length of the visceral splenic surface.
2. **Dorsal extremity.** The rounded dorsal extremity is typically positioned rather far dorsally, between the gastric fundus and the left kidney. This portion varies the least with gastric distention, because it is tacked in place by its association with the relatively immobile left kidney.
3. **Ventral extremity.** The rounded ventral extremity varies widely in position, being entirely intrathoracic in the maximally contracted spleen, and well outside the bony thorax and even moved across the midline when the spleen is maximally engorged.

Chapter 44

Vasculature of the Gastrointestinal Organs and Spleen

I. ARTERIES OF THE GASTROINTESTINAL ORGANS AND SPLEEN. The arterial supply to the gastrointestinal organs and spleen arrives through **three unpaired ventral branches of the aorta:** the **celiac artery,** the **cranial mesenteric artery,** and the **caudal mesenteric artery.** In the abdomen, as in all other regions of the body, the **arteries are named according to the structures they supply** (Table 44–1).

A. Celiac artery. The celiac artery is a large artery, about 4 mm in diameter in a 20-kg dog.

1. **Structures supplied.** The celiac artery supplies a large portion of the cranial digestive tract, including the **esophagus, liver, stomach, lesser** and **greater omenta, spleen, duodenum,** and much of the **pancreas.**
2. **Origin.** The celiac artery typically **arises immediately caudal to the diaphragm** as the **first visceral branch of the abdominal aorta** (Figure 44–1).
3. **Branches.** The celiac artery has **three branches:** the **left gastric, splenic,** and **hepatic arteries.**
   - **a.** The **left gastric artery** is the smallest and typically the first branch of the celiac artery. Occasionally it is doubled or it arises from a common trunk with the splenic artery. The left gastric artery courses cranially along the dorsal gastric surface toward the cardia of the stomach (see Figure 44–1). At this point, the left gastric artery gains the ventral gastric surface.
     - **(1)** After gaining the ventral gastric surface, the left gastric artery sends **branches** to the **esophagus,** the **lesser omentum,** and to the **parietal** and **visceral surfaces of the fundic region of the stomach.**
     - **(2)** It then **continues along the lesser curvature of the stomach,** retaining its name as the left gastric artery.
     - **(3)** The left gastric artery **anastomoses** on the lesser curvature **with the terminal branches of the right gastric artery,** which takes a similar course, but from the right instead of the left [see I A 3 c (2)].
   - **b.** The **splenic artery** departs from the celiac artery and turns to the left to travel toward the spleen (see Figure 44–1).
     - **(1)** Initially, the splenic artery travels close to the surface of the left lobe of the pancreas, giving rise to **pancreatic branches.** These branches provide the major arterial supply to the left pancreatic lobe.
     - **(2)** The splenic artery continues toward the spleen, which it supplies via the **splenic branches.**
       - **(a)** The splenic artery forms several branches as it approaches the elongate hilus of the spleen. These branches repeatedly branch to enter the elongate splenic hilus along its full length.
       - **(b)** The splenic branches traveling to the proximal end of the spleen (typically the last two splenic branches) make an almost 180-degree turn and provide the **short gastric arteries** to the caudal part of fundus of the stomach.
     - **(3)** After giving off the splenic branches, the main trunk of the splenic artery makes a "U"-turn, changing its name to the **left gastroepiploic artery.**
       - **(a)** The left gastroepiploic artery **courses back toward the right** in the substance of the **gastrosplenic ligament,** a centimeter or so from the greater curvature of the stomach.
       - **(b)** The left gastroepiploic artery gives **branches to the greater omentum** and the **greater curvature of the stomach,** and then continues along its course to anastomose with the right gastroepiploic artery [see I A 3 c (a)].
   - **c.** The **hepatic artery,** the largest of the celiac artery's branches, supplies the **liver** and **parts of the stomach, duodenum,** and **pancreas.** The hepatic artery is essentially the

Canine Clinical Correlation

Splenectomy (removal of the spleen) is a fairly common surgery in dogs, necessitated by trauma or a pathologic condition (e.g., lymphosarcoma, hemangiosarcoma, ehrlichiosis). Splenectomy would be simplified if one could ligate the splenic artery proximal to the origin of the splenic branches, but this would result in loss of arterial supply to a major part of the stomach (because the short gastric and left gastroepiploic arteries arise after the splenic branches). Thus, the splenic artery must be followed along its course until the origins of the short gastric and left gastroepiploic artery are identified, and the individual branches of the splenic artery ligated distal to those points.

TABLE 44–1. Arterial Supply of the Gastrointestinal Organs and Spleen

Organ	Main Arterial Supply	Parent Artery
Stomach	Left gastric	Celiac
	Right gastric	Hepatic (celiac)
	Left gastroepiploic	Splenic (celiac)
	Right gastroepiploic	Hepatic (celiac)
	Short gastric	Splenic (celiac)
Spleen	Splenic	Celiac
Duodenum	Cranial pancreaticoduodenal	Gastroduodenal (hepatic, celiac)
	Caudal pancreaticoduodenal	Ileocolic (cranial mesenteric)
Jejunum	Jejunal arteries	Cranial mesenteric
Ileum	Ileal	Cranial mesenteric
	Mesenteric ileal	Cranial mesenteric
	Antimesenteric ileal	Ileocecal (cranial mesenteric)
Cecum	Ileocecal	Ileocolic (cranial mesenteric)
Ascending colon	Right colic	Ileocolic (cranial mesenteric)
Transverse colon	Middle colic	Ileocolic (cranial mesenteric)
Descending colon	Left colic	Caudal mesenteric
	Overlap from middle colic	Cranial mesenteric
Pancreas	Splenic	Celiac
	Cranial pancreaticoduodenal	Hepatic (celiac)
	Caudal pancreaticoduodenal	Cranial mesenteric
	Hepatic (occasionally)	Celiac
Liver	Proper hepatic arteries	Hepatic (celiac)

continuation of the celiac artery after the left gastric and splenic arteries have arisen (see Figure 44–1).

(1) The hepatic artery courses toward the right, through a groove in the surface of the pancreas. As it reaches the hepatic porta, it provides three to five **proper hepatic branches** into the liver.

- **(a)** The proper hepatic branches have specific names and their typical courses have been described, but these details are mainly of academic interest.
- **(b)** The proper hepatic branches branch into the hepatic parenchyma, delivering oxygenated blood to the hepatic cells. Oxygen delivery is their primary function, because nutrient-laden blood arrives directly from the hepatic portal veins.

(2) After detaching the proper hepatic branches, the hepatic artery continues toward the right. The **right gastric artery** arises as **one of two terminal branches of the hepatic artery.**

- **(a)** This vessel turns cranially and courses toward the pylorus, attaining a course along the right side of the lesser curvature of the stomach. It follows this course until it anastomoses with the left gastric artery.

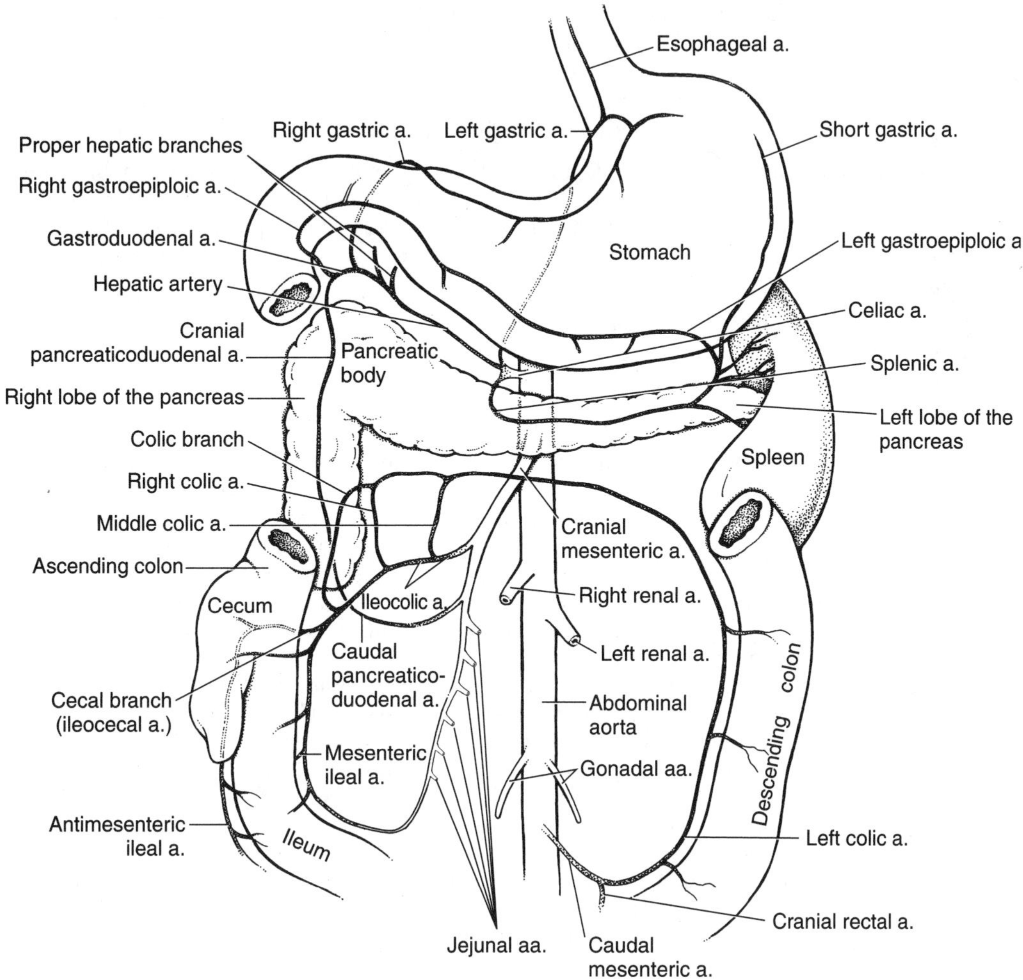

FIGURE 44–1. Schematized ventral view of the arteries of the gastrointestinal organs and spleen. (Redrawn with permission from Evans HE, 1993, *Miller's Anatomy of the Dog,* 3e. Philadelphia, WB Saunders, p 651.)

(b) In its course, the right gastric artery **supplies** the **parietal** and **visceral surfaces of the pyloric region of the stomach,** as well as the **lesser omentum.**

(3) The **gastroduodenal artery** is the **other terminal branch of the hepatic artery.** Before **terminating as the right gastroepiploic artery** and the **cranial pancreaticoduodenal artery,** the gastroduodenal artery provides a large branch to the left lobe of the pancreas, as well as small branches to the pyloric antrum, the pyloric canal, and the pylorus.

(a) The **right gastroepiploic artery** makes a "U"-turn as it arises from the gastroduodenal artery, to course back toward the right in the greater omentum about a centimeter from the greater curvature of the stomach to anastomose with the left gastroepiploic artery. Like its fellow from the left, the right gastroepiploic artery gives branches to the greater omentum and the greater gastric curvature.

(b) The **cranial pancreaticoduodenal artery** courses caudally in the substance of the pancreas near its duodenal border.

(i) Along its course, the cranial pancreaticoduodenal artery supplies multiple

pancreatic branches to the right lobe of the pancreas, as well as multiple **duodenal branches** to the duodenum.

(ii) The cranial pancreaticoduodenal artery **terminates by anastomosing** within the pancreatic parenchyma **with one or more branches of the caudal pancreaticoduodenal artery** (see I B 3 b).

B. The **cranial mesenteric artery** (see Figure 44–1) is the largest of all of the visceral branches of the aorta (about 5 mm in diameter in a 20-kg dog). The cranial mesenteric artery is sometimes referred to as the **axis of the mesentery,** because it provides the focal point around which the mass of the small and large intestine rotates during development.

1. **Structures supplied** include the gut tube from the **ileum through the greatest part of the descending colon,** as well as part of the **pancreas.**
2. **Origin.** The cranial mesenteric artery arises from the ventral surface of the abdominal aorta at approximately the level of vertebra L1 or L2, a few millimeters caudal to the celiac artery.
3. **Branches**

a. The **ileocolic artery** (see Figure 44–1), typically the first branch of the cranial mesenteric artery, takes an oblique course toward the right and somewhat cranially.

(1) Branches. The ileocolic artery, formerly known as the ileocecocolic artery, provides several major branches to the **colon, cecum,** and **ileum.** Although the branching of these arteries from the ileocolic artery is variable, the arteries consistently course through the associated mesocolon parallel to their respective colonic regions (supplying branches along the way) and terminate by anastomosing through terminal arcades with the arteries preceding and following them.

(a) The **middle colic artery** usually arises shortly after the ileocolic artery departs from the cranial mesenteric artery, and passes almost directly cranially toward the transverse colon. Typically, it has two large divisions.

(i) Left branch. The branch directed toward the left follows the curve around the left colic flexure and terminates at an indefinite point along the descending colon by anastomosing with the ascending branch of the left colic artery. This branch usually arises directly from the ileocolic artery.

(ii) Right branch. The branch directed toward the right supplies the right portion of the transverse colon, and terminates by anastomosing with a branch of the right colic artery.

(b) An **accessory middle colic artery** is often present, leaving the ileocolic shortly after the middle colic artery.

(c) The **right colic artery** arises near the cecocolic junction, and courses cranially through the mesocolon supplying the ascending colon and the early part of the transverse colon. The right colic artery terminates by anastomosing with the middle colic artery.

(2) After giving off the right colic artery, the ileocolic artery continues to the left while inclining caudally, providing several arteries to the ileum and cecum.

(a) The **colic branch** courses cranially, supplying the proximal part of the ascending colon.

(b) The **cecal branch** (formerly called the **ileocecal artery)** arises around the dorsal surface of the cecum, providing the major arterial supply to this organ. The **antimesenteric ileal branch** is the continuation of the ileocecal artery past the end of the cecum, where it courses along the antimesenteric surface of the ileum until it terminates by ramifying in the intestinal tissue near the jejunoileal junction. The termination point of the antimesenteric ileal artery is one characteristic that can be used to estimate the junction of the ileum and jejunum.

(3) After giving off the cecal branch, the much-reduced ileocolic artery continues as the **mesenteric ileal artery** along the mesenteric surface of the ileum. The mesenteric ileal artery turns cranially along the mesenteric surface of the ileum and terminates by anastomosing with the remainder of the cranial mesenteric artery, after the cranial mesenteric gives off the last jejunal artery.

b. The **caudal pancreaticoduodenal artery** (see Figure 44–1) arises from the cranial mesenteric artery shortly after the origin of the ileocolic artery.

(1) The caudal pancreaticoduodenal artery courses caudally and toward the right, passing through the great mesentery toward the caudal duodenal flexure.

(2) This vessel provides branches to both the **right lobe of the pancreas** and the **descending duodenum.** These branches terminate by anastomosing with similar branches that originate from the cranial pancreaticoduodenal artery.

c. Twelve to fifteen **jejunal arteries** arise from the caudal surface of the cranial mesenteric artery (see Figure 44–1).

(1) These vessels are not necessarily equal in size, nor do they progressively decrease in size in a regular manner.

(2) These vessels pass into the dorsal common (great) mesentery, where they branch and then join with the branches of neighboring jejunal arteries to form primary and secondary **arterial arcades** (Figure 44–2). The secondary (terminal) arcades are generally formed close to the intestinal wall. Short, straight vessels **(vasa recti)** leave the terminal arcades to travel directly to the jejunal wall.

d. One or two **ileal arteries** typically arise just after the last jejunal artery, and pass to the wall of the ileum. These vessels pass directly to the intestinal wall without branching within the mesentery.

4. Termination. The **mesenteric ileal artery** is the continuation and termination of the greatly reduced cranial mesenteric artery after it has given off the last jejunal branch. This portion of the parent artery continues along the mesenteric border of the ileum, providing short, direct arteries to this region of the intestine.

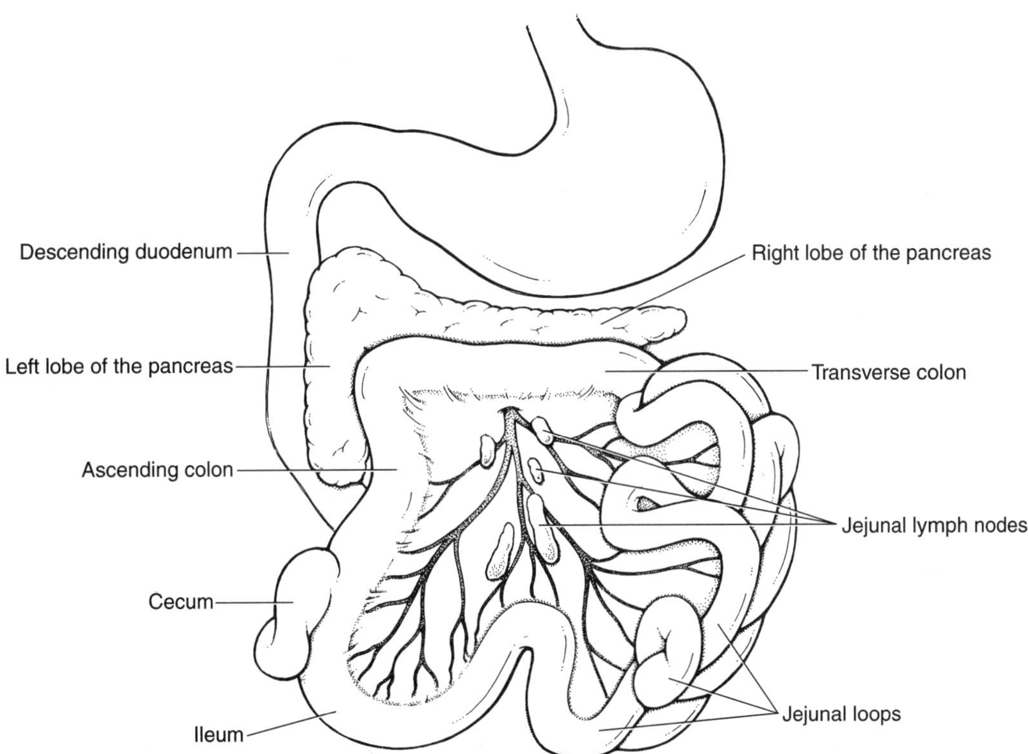

FIGURE 44–2. Arcade pattern associated with the vascularization of the jejunum, and the jejunal lymph nodes. The unique arcade pattern of arterial supply and venous drainage of the jejunum is one characteristic used to identify the jejunoileal junction.

C. The **caudal mesenteric artery** is relatively small.

1. **Origin.** The caudal mesenteric artery arises unpaired from the **ventral aortic surface at approximately the level of vertebra L5;** therefore, a considerable distance separates the cranial and caudal mesenteric arteries (see Figure 44–1). Two sets of paired visceral branches (renal and gonadal) and several sets of parietal branches (lumbar and deep circumflex iliac) arise from the abdominal aorta between the origins of the cranial and caudal mesenteric arteries.
2. **Course.** The caudal mesenteric artery passes caudoventrally through the mesentery, slightly toward the left, to gain the mesenteric border of the descending colon.
3. **Branches.** On approximating the intestinal wall, the caudal mesenteric artery **bifurcates** into the left colic artery and the cranial rectal artery.
   a. The **left colic artery** passes cranially along the mesenteric border of the descending colon and terminates by anastomosing with the descending branch of the middle colic artery.
   b. The **cranial rectal artery** passes caudally along the mesenteric border of the caudal descending colon and on to the rectum.

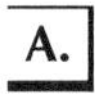

II. VEINS OF THE GASTROINTESTINAL ORGANS AND SPLEEN

A. **Overview.** With the exception of the hepatic veins, the veins of the gastrointestinal organs and spleen are **largely tributaries of the hepatic portal vein,** rather than of the caudal vena cava.

1. The blood drained from the gastrointestinal tract is laden with nutrients derived from the digestion of food; these nutrients need to be processed by the liver before the blood enters the systemic circulation. After entering the liver (via the hepatic portal vein), blood from the gastrointestinal tract courses into the hepatic parenchyma, is processed through a second capillary bed and is then collected from the parenchyma into the hepatic veins, which carry the blood back to the general systemic circulation.
2. Portal veins, by definition, deliver blood from one capillary bed to another prior to the blood entering a vein that delivers it to the systemic circulation. In the case of the hepatic portal vein, the first capillary bed is that of the gut tube, and the second is that of the liver.

Canine Clinical Correlation

The nitrogen content of the blood returning from the capillary bed of the intestinal tract is very high (owing to the digested amino acids it contains). The direct introduction of this nitrogen-rich blood into the systemic circulation, such as occurs with **portacaval shunt,** causes life-threatening seizures. Portacaval shunt is a developmental anomaly in which the umbilical vein fails to close after birth, causing most blood drained from the intestinal tract to pass directly into the caudal vena cava and immediately into the systemic circulation. This anomaly, left untreated, leads to the death of the animal at a young age. Surgical (definitive) treatment of a large shunt is difficult due to the necessity of searching the friable and blood-rich hepatic parenchyma to identify and ligate both ends of the shunt.

B. **Satellite veins** accompany most of the named arteries that are branches of the celiac artery, the cranial mesenteric artery, and the caudal mesenteric artery. There are some notable exceptions.

1. The **caudal mesenteric vein** does not parallel the caudal mesenteric artery in its course to the hepatic portal vein (see II C 2 b).
2. The **hepatic veins,** which drain the blood from the liver parenchyma after it has entered the hepatic portal system and passed through the capillary beds of the liver, are **independent of the hepatic arteries.** These veins are **direct tributaries of the caudal vena cava.**

a. **Three major** hepatic veins are usually present:
   (1) One very large vein drains the entire left side of the liver and a small part of the right side of the liver.
   (2) A second vein drains the right side of the liver.
   (3) A third vein drains mainly the caudate lobe of the liver.

b. **Approximately 20 small veins** (1 mm in diameter) serve focal areas of the liver parenchyma.

C. Hepatic portal system

1. **Definition.** The hepatic portal system is a series of named veins that drains most of the tubular digestive tract (i.e., the stomach, small intestine, and large intestine, with the exception of the anal canal), as well as the pancreas and spleen. The veins of the hepatic portal system drain into the **hepatic portal vein.** This vein takes its final form near the body of the pancreas, at the confluence of the cranial mesenteric, caudal mesenteric, and splenic veins.
2. **Tributaries.** Although the smaller branches of the two mesenteric arteries and the celiac artery have fairly faithful satellite veins, the confluence of the larger veins into the named tributaries of the hepatic portal system is subject to marked variation. Only the larger veins that are usually formed and contribute to the hepatic portal system are discussed here.
   a. The **cranial mesenteric vein** is consistently the largest of the hepatic portal system tributaries. This vein largely parallels its companion artery, and typically receives the **jejunal, caudal pancreaticoduodenal, caudal mesenteric,** and **ileocolic veins** before entering the hepatic portal vein.
   b. The **caudal mesenteric vein** drains veins corresponding to the branches of the same-named artery (i.e., the **cranial rectal** and **left colic veins)** as would be expected, but it courses far more cranially into the abdomen. It receives a portion of the drainage of the **middle colic vein** and enters the cranial mesenteric vein in a cranial position, opposite the ileocolic vein.
   c. The **ileocolic vein** parallels the same-named artery, and receives the **mesenteric ileal, right colic,** and **middle colic veins** and the **cecal** and **colic branches** before entering the cranial mesenteric vein.
   d. The **splenic vein** enters the hepatic portal vein not far from the liver, dorsal to the pyloric region of the stomach. The splenic vein drains the spleen, part of the pancreas, and the stomach, by **receiving** the **left gastroepiploic** and **left gastric veins** and the unnamed **pancreatic branches.**
   e. The **gastroduodenal vein** is typically the last tributary of the hepatic portal vein, entering a short distance cranial to the splenic vein. The gastroduodenal vein receives the **cranial pancreaticoduodenal, right gastroepiploic,** and **right gastric veins.** Some variability exists in their pattern of confluence.

III. LYMPHATIC VESSELS OF THE GASTROINTESTINAL ORGANS AND SPLEEN.

Usually, three lymphocenters are associated with the gastrointestinal tract: the **celiac, cranial mesenteric,** and **caudal mesenteric lymphocenters.**

A. The **celiac lymphocenter** drains the organs supplied by the celiac artery (i.e., the liver, stomach, spleen, pancreas, and duodenum). This center potentially comprises the hepatic, splenic, gastric, and pancreaticoduodenal lymph nodes.

1. The **hepatic lymph nodes** are always present, although they may vary considerably in number and size. They are usually paired, with one large node lying on each side of the entrance of the hepatic portal vein at the porta of the liver.
   a. **Drainage area.** The hepatic nodes drain the **liver, stomach, duodenum,** and **pancreas.** The nodes are also extensively interconnected with each other.
   b. **Efferent lymphatics** from the hepatic nodes pass to the **intestinal lymphatic trunk.**

2. The **splenic lymph nodes** are reliably positioned along the course of the splenic artery and its satellite vein.
   a. **Drainage area.** The relatively small splenic lymph nodes drain the **esophagus, stomach, liver, pancreas, greater omentum,** and **diaphragm.**
   b. **Efferent lymphatic vessels** from the splenic nodes pass to the **intestinal lymphatic trunk.**

3. The **gastric lymph nodes** are an inconstant set of small nodes located in the lesser omentum near the pylorus.
   a. **Drainage area.** Structures drained include the **esophagus, stomach, lesser omentum,** and **peritoneum.**
   b. **Efferent lymphatic vessels** drain into either **hepatic** or **splenic nodes,** or both.

4. The **pancreaticoduodenal lymph nodes** are a small group that includes a slightly larger constant node and potentially some smaller inconstant nodes. These nodes are located in the mesentery between the pyloric region of the stomach and the right lobe of the pancreas.
   a. **Drainage area.** The pancreaticoduodenal lymph nodes receive drainage from the **duodenum, pancreas,** and **omentum.**
   b. **Efferent vessels** pass to the **hepatic nodes** or the **right colic node** (of the cranial mesenteric lymphocenter; see III B 2).

B. The **cranial mesenteric lymphocenter** contains the **jejunal** and **colic lymph nodes.**

1. The **jejunal lymph nodes** (see Figure 44–2) are the largest lymph nodes of the abdomen. These nodes are positioned along the branching of the jejunal vessels near their origin from the cranial mesenteric artery.

Canine Clinical Correlation

The jejunal lymph nodes tend to be larger in dogs that forage or hunt—in a 20-kg dog with an "open" diet, the nodes may reach dimensions of 6 cm by 2 cm by 0.5 cm! Very large nodes may be mistaken for a pathologic mass.

   a. **Structures drained** include the **jejunum, ileum,** and **pancreas.**
   b. **Efferent vessels** play a major role in the formation of the **intestinal lymphatic trunk.**

2. The **colic lymph nodes** are consistently present.
   a. **Nodes**
      (1) The **right colic node** is usually single, but as many as five small nodes may be present. The node lies close to the ileocolic junction.
      (2) The **middle colic node** is usually single, but may be doubled. The node lies near the transverse colon, approximately halfway along its right-to-left extent.
   b. **Drainage area.** The right and middle colic nodes drain the **ileum, cecum,** and associated **parts of the colon;** the middle colic node also receives efferent vessels from the left colic lymph node.
   c. **Efferent vessels** pass to the **intestinal lymphatic trunk.**

C. The **caudal mesenteric lymphocenter** comprises the **left colic lymph nodes.** These small but constant nodes number from two to five, and are positioned near the terminal branching of the cranial mesenteric artery (i.e, where the cranial mesenteric artery branches into the left colic and cranial rectal arteries).

1. **Drainage area.** The left colic lymph nodes drain the **descending colon.**
2. **Efferent vessels** pass independently from each node to the **intestinal lymphatic trunk,** the **middle colic lymph node,** the **medial iliac lymph node,** or the **lumbar lymph nodes.**

Chapter 45

Innervation of the Gastrointestinal Organs and Spleen

I. INTRODUCTION.

Innervation of the gastrointestinal tract is accomplished entirely by the **autonomic nervous system (ANS).**

A. **Prevertebral ganglia** and **plexuses** supply motor and limited sensory input to the gastrointestinal organs and spleen.

1. The **prevertebral ganglia,** so named because they are positioned ventral to (and thus, in humans, "in front of") the vertebral column, are **associated with the large, unpaired visceral branches of the aorta.**
   - **a. Celiac and cranial mesenteric ganglia.** Often, partially owing to the close physical proximity of the celiac and cranial mesenteric arteries, the celiac and cranial mesenteric ganglia fuse to form the **celiacomesenteric ganglion.**
     - (1) The **celiac ganglion** is positioned near the celiac artery.
     - (2) The **cranial mesenteric ganglion** is positioned near the cranial mesenteric artery.
   - **b.** The **caudal mesenteric ganglion** is positioned near the caudal mesenteric artery.
2. The **prevertebral plexuses** are dense networks of sympathetic and parasympathetic fibers surrounding the associated prevertebral ganglia.
   - **a.** The networks represent the branching and reassociation of the postganglionic sympathetic fibers (which have synapsed within the prevertebral ganglion) with the preganglionic parasympathetic fibers (which are arriving to the prevertebral ganglion).
   - **b.** The plexuses are located on the surfaces of the associated visceral aortic branches; fibers are distributed to the viscera by coursing directly along the surfaces of the arteries traveling to those viscera. Considering the arterial supply to an organ suggests which major plexus sends autonomic fibers to the organ.
     - **(1) Celiacomesenteric plexus**
       - **(a)** The **celiac part** supplies the stomach, the liver, the spleen, most of the pancreas, and the duodenum.
       - **(b)** The **cranial mesenteric part** supplies a small part of the pancreas, the jejunum, the ileum, the cecum, the ascending and transverse colon, and a small part of the descending colon.
     - **(2) Caudal mesenteric plexus.** The caudal mesenteric plexus supplies the descending colon and the rectum.

B. **Sympathetic innervation** of the gastrointestinal organs and spleen is provided by the **sympathetic trunk.** The **thoracic** and **lumbar splanchnic nerves,** specialized nerves leading from the late thoracic and most of the lumbar regions of the sympathetic trunk (see Chapter 4, Figure 4–5), carry mostly **preganglionic sympathetic input to the prevertebral ganglia.** The splanchnic nerves also carry the **limited afferent fibers from the gastrointestinal organs.**

1. The paired **major thoracic splanchnic nerves** arise from spinal cord segment T13, pass into the abdomen lateral to the crus of the diaphragm, and course to the **celiacomesenteric ganglion** and **plexus.**
   - **a.** The nerve is often larger than the continuation of the sympathetic trunk!
   - **b.** There is only one pair of greater thoracic splanchnic nerves.
2. The paired **minor thoracic splanchnic nerves** leave the sympathetic trunk just caudal to the major thoracic splanchnic nerve and pass to the **celiacomesenteric ganglion** and **plexus.** There may be one or two pairs of lesser splanchnic nerves.
3. The paired **lumbar splanchnic nerves** are variable in number, but usually there is one pair associated with each lumbar segment. These nerves simply leave the associated segment and pass to their allied ganglia.

a. **Lumbar splanchnic nerves 1–4** typically course to the **cranial mesenteric** or **gonadal ganglia** and **plexuses,** as well as to the **intermesenteric** and **aorticorenal plexuses.**
b. **Lumbar splanchnic nerves 5–7** typically pass to the **caudal mesenteric ganglion** and **plexus.**

C. Parasympathetic innervation

1. The **vagus nerve** supplies parasympathetic innervation to the gastrointestinal tract from the esophagus as far caudally as the left colic flexure.
   a. The **ventral vagal trunk** is **distributed fairly directly,** without passing through a plexus. Fibers from this trunk supply mainly the liver, stomach, and pancreas.
      (1) **Liver.** Direct branches from the ventral vagal trunk pass through the lesser omentum to innervate the liver.
      (2) **Stomach.** The ventral vagal trunk sends branches to the ventral surface of the stomach (i.e., the lesser curvature and the pyloric region).
      (3) **Pancreas.** A few branches from the ventral vagal trunk are also distributed to the right lobe of the pancreas, along the course of the cranial pancreaticoduodenal artery.
   b. The **dorsal vagal trunk** is associated with the **celiacomesenteric plexus.** From the plexus, the fibers of the dorsal vagal trunk are distributed (along with the sympathetic fibers) along the branches of the celiac and cranial mesenteric arteries. The dorsal vagal trunk plays the largest role in innervation of the gut because it supplies the dorsal surface of the **stomach,** as well as the **intestines** as far caudally as the left colic flexure.
2. The **pelvic nerve,** from the **pelvic plexus** (see Chapter 54 I B), provides parasympathetic fibers to the **caudal mesenteric plexus.** Fibers originate in the sacral region, gain the lateral surface of the rectum, and ascend to supply the **descending colon;** some fibers also contribute to the innervation of the more cranial colic regions. The pelvic nerve is the only source of parasympathetic fibers to most of the descending colon.

II. INNERVATION OF THE ORGANS.

In general, an organ receives its autonomic fibers from the ganglion or plexus most closely associated with its blood supply. For example, the jejunum receives its autonomic fibers mainly from the cranial mesenteric part of the celiacomesenteric plexus, rather than from the celiac part of that plexus, or the caudal mesenteric plexus.

A. Stomach

1. **Sympathetic fibers** to the stomach arrive via branches of the **celiac part** of the **celiacomesenteric plexus.**
2. **Parasympathetic fibers** arrive from the dorsal and ventral vagal trunks.
   a. The **ventral vagal trunk** supplies the lesser curvature of the stomach and the pyloric region **directly.**
   b. The **dorsal vagal trunk** supplies a few branches to the lesser curvature and dorsal wall of the stomach before continuing to the **celiac part** of the **celiacomesenteric plexus.** Fibers from the plexus supply the portions of the stomach that do not receive parasympathetic innervation directly from the ventral vagal trunk or the dorsal vagal trunk.

B. Small intestine.

The **duodenum, jejunum,** and **ileum** receive innervation from the same sources.

1. **Sympathetic fibers** to the small intestine arrive via branches from both the **celiac** and **cranial mesenteric parts** of the **celiacomesenteric plexus.**
2. **Parasympathetic fibers** arrive from the **dorsal vagal trunk** via the **celiacomesenteric plexus.**

C. Colon. The colon receives its sympathetic and parasympathetic innervation from two sources, with the left colic flexure being a watershed area for determining source. However, just as the arterial supply to the descending colon is supplied by both the cranial and caudal mesenteric arteries, the innervation of the descending colon is supplied by both the cranial and caudal mesenteric ganglia and plexuses.

1. **Sympathetic fibers**
   a. **Ascending** and **transverse colon.** Sympathetic innervation arrives mainly through the **cranial mesenteric part** of the **celiacomesenteric plexus.**
   b. **Descending colon.** Sympathetic innervation arrives mainly through the **caudal mesenteric plexus.** The nerve fibers that leave the cranial portion of the caudal mesenteric plexus to travel to the colon are often large enough to be recognized and have been named the **lumbar colonic nerve.**
2. **Parasympathetic fibers**
   a. **Ascending** and **transverse colon.** Parasympathetic innervation arrives mainly through the **dorsal vagal trunk** via the **cranial mesenteric part** of the **celiacomesenteric plexus.**
   b. **Descending colon.** Parasympathetic innervation arrives mainly through the **pelvic nerve** and **pelvic plexus** via the caudal mesenteric plexus.

D. Pancreas

1. **Sympathetic fibers** arrive from the **celiacomesenteric plexus,** mainly from the celiac part, but also from the cranial mesenteric part.
2. **Parasympathetic fibers** arrive from the **dorsal vagal trunk,** also via the **celiacomesenteric plexus.**

E. Liver and biliary tree

1. **Sympathetic fibers** arrive from the **celiac part** of the **celiacomesenteric plexus.**
2. **Parasympathetic fibers** arrive directly from **two large branches** of the **ventral vagal trunk** and **one branch** of the **dorsal vagal trunk.**

Chapter 46

Female Reproductive Organs

I. INTRODUCTION

A. Organs. The **ovaries,** the **uterine tubes,** the **uterine horns,** and **part of the uterine body** reside within the abdominal cavity. The caudal-most part of the female reproductive tract (i.e., a portion of the uterine body, the uterine cervix, and the vagina) is found within the pelvic cavity and is discussed in Chapter 51 IV A.

B. Peritoneum. The **broad ligament,** a specialized, doubled fold of peritoneum, links and supports the ovaries and uterus and transmits vessels and nerves. The broad ligament is a paired structure.

1. **Composition.** Each broad ligament contains **smooth muscle** and is capable of storing considerable amounts of **fat.** In a specimen from a thin dog, the ligament is paper-thin and translucent, while in an obese dog, it is thick and opaque.
2. **Position.** The broad ligament extends from the dorsolateral body wall (near the junction of the transversus abdominis and psoas major muscles) to the ovaries, uterine horns, and uterine body.
3. **Regions**
   a. The **mesovarium** is the portion of the broad ligament that supports the ovary.
   b. The **mesosalpinx** is the portion of the broad ligament that supports the uterine tube (salpinx).
   c. The **mesometrium** is the area of the broad ligament that supports the uterine horns and body; it is the largest region.
      (1) The **free fold of the broad ligament** is a sheet of peritoneum that extends at approximately a right angle from the lateral surface of the mesometrium.
      (2) The **round ligament of the uterus** courses down the free (lateral-most) edge of the broad ligament's free fold, and passes through the inguinal canal to end in the vaginal process.

II. OVARIES. The ovaries are the paired female gonads.

A. Position (Figure 46–1)

1. The ovaries lie **near the dorsal body wall,** just caudal to the caudal pole of the associated kidney (the ovary develops from the same mesodermal ridge as the kidney).
2. The ovaries lie **several centimeters caudal to the last rib.** In a pregnant bitch, the ventral displacement of the uterus draws the ovary somewhat caudal and ventral to this position.

B. Shape. The ovary is a **flat, ovoid structure** with **cranial** and **caudal poles.** The ovary is smaller and smoother in the non-cycling bitch, and slightly larger and markedly more irregular in the cycling bitch.

C. Attachments (Figure 46–2)

1. The **suspensory ligament** is a well-defined, dense, rather long collection of collagenous fibers and smooth muscle that extends between the cranial pole of each ovary and the dorsal body wall in the region just caudal to the last rib (see Figures 46–1 and 46–2).

2. The **proper ligament of the ovary** is another dense band of ligamentous tissue that extends between the ovary and the tip of the uterine horn. The proper ovarian ligament is

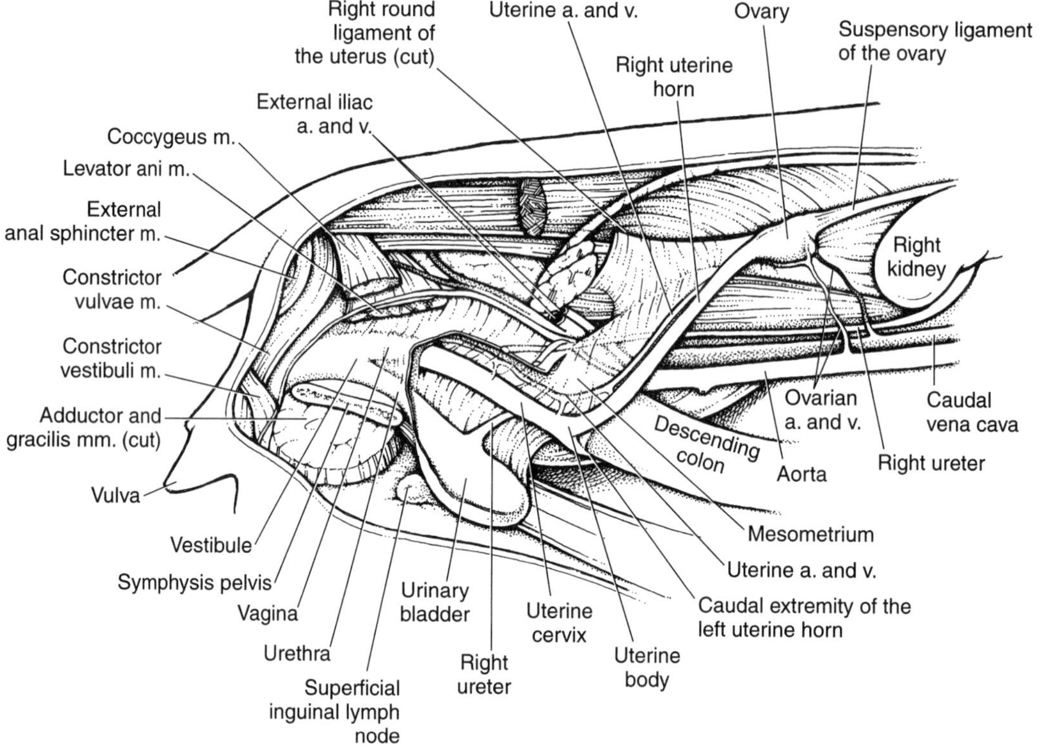

FIGURE 46–1. The ovary, uterus, and associated structures (right lateral view). [Redrawn with permission from Evans HE, 1993, *Miller's Anatomy of the Dog,* 3e. Philadelphia, WB Saunders, p 534.]

Canine Clinical Correlation

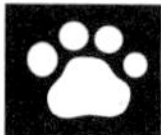

During **ovariohysterectomy,** rupture of the suspensory ligament, which contains a small artery, is necessary. In small dogs, ligation of the ligament is not necessary before rupturing it; however, in very large breeds, ligation of the ligament is prudent.

continuous cranially with the suspensory ligament of the ovary and caudally with the round ligament of the uterus (see Figure 46–2).

3. The **ovarian bursa** is an envelope of broad ligament that nearly surrounds the ovary. The **opening of the ovarian bursa** is a tiny slit on the medial side of the bursa that communicates with the peritoneal cavity. The **mesovarium** and **mesosalpinx** contribute to the formation of the ovarian bursa (see Figure 46–2).
   a. The **mesovarium** extends between the ovary and the remainder of the broad ligament along the medial side of the ovary.
   b. The **mesosalpinx** covers the lateral side of the ovary with a peritoneal fold. The uterine tube courses caudally over the lateral ovarian surface (see Figure 46–2), bringing the mesosalpinx over the lateral side of the ovary.

D. Vasculature

1. **Arteries.** The paired **ovarian arteries** are direct branches of the **abdominal aorta.**
   a. **Course.** The ovarian artery takes a fairly direct course to the ovary. Distally, the ovarian artery anastomoses with the uterine artery as that vessel ascends the broad ligament along the uterine horn.

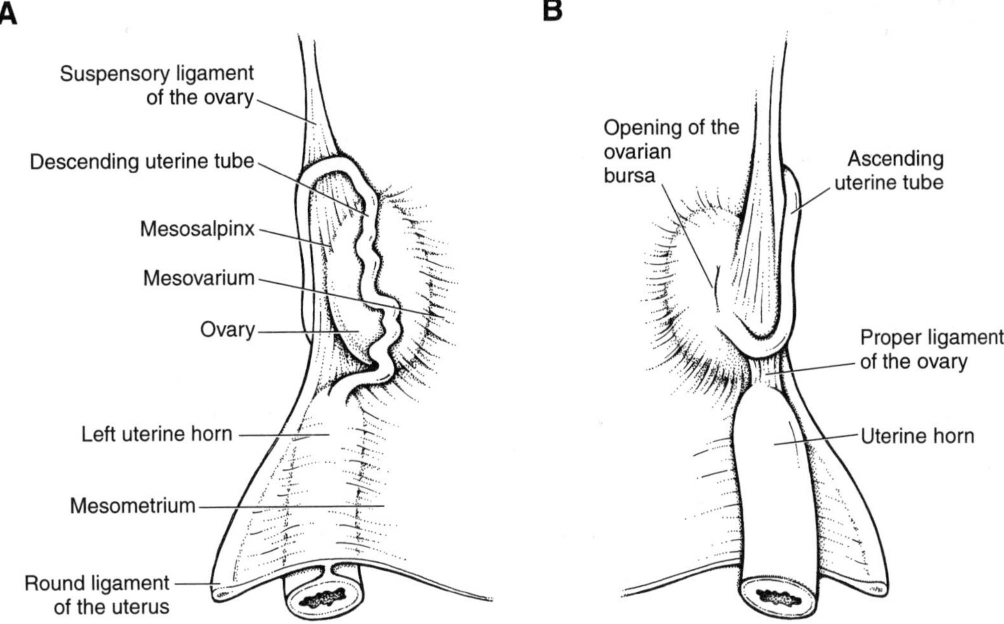

FIGURE 46–2. The ovary, uterine tube, mesovarium, mesosalpinx, and ovarian bursa. (*A*) Lateral view. (*B*) Medial view.

Canine Clinical Correlation

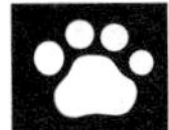

In parous bitches (i.e., those that have borne a litter), the course of the artery is sinuous as it approaches the ovary. This "stretch room" prevents rupture of the artery as the ovary and uterus are displaced with advancing pregnancy.

b. **Structures supplied.** In addition to supplying the **ovary,** the ovarian artery sends branches to the **renal capsule, uterine tube,** and **cranial part of the uterine horn.**

2. **Veins.** The **right** and **left ovarian veins** are largely satellites of the ovarian arteries, although they terminate differently.
   a. The **right ovarian vein** enters the **caudal vena cava.**
   b. The **left ovarian vein** enters the **left renal vein.**
3. **Efferent lymphatics** from the ovaries drain to the **lumbar lymph nodes.**

E. **Innervation. Sympathetic nerves** from the **aorticorenal plexuses** are carried to the ovary along the surface of the ovarian artery.

III. UTERINE TUBE (SALPINX).

Fertilized eggs pass from the ovary to the uterus through the uterine tube, an extremely fine-bore tubular structure extending from the ovary to the uterine horn.

A. **Position.** Each uterine tube originates on the medial surface of the ovary, passes cranially, and then turns around the cranial ovarian pole to course caudally along the lateral ovarian surface to gain the tip of the uterine horn (see Figure 46–2). The uterine tube is surrounded by the mesosalpinx.

B. Regions

1. The **infundibulum** is the funnel-shaped portion of the uterine tube that embraces the ovary.
   a. **Fimbriae** (villous projections from the infundibulum) massage the surface of the ovary at ovulation to facilitate the retrieval of oocytes.
   b. **Fertilization** normally takes place near the junction of the infundibulum and segment that follows, the ampulla. While passing through the tortuous, long course of the uterine tube, the zygote undergoes sufficient development to ensure successful implantation in the uterine horn.
2. The **uterine ostium** is the site where the uterine tube opens into the uterine horn.

C. Vasculature

1. **Arteries and veins.** The **ovarian** and **uterine arteries** and **veins** serve the uterine tube.
2. **Efferent lymphatics,** like those of the ovary, pass to the **lumbar lymph nodes.**

D. Innervation

1. **Sympathetic innervation** arrives from the **aorticorenal plexuses.**
2. **Parasympathetic innervation** arrives from the **pelvic plexus.**

IV. UTERUS. The uterus is a muscular organ in female mammals that houses the fetuses during development and contracts to expel them during parturition.

A. Position. The uterus extends through the abdomen in a longitudinal, cranial-to-caudal orientation. The uterus extends from near the ovary to the pelvic inlet (see Figure 46–1).

1. In a nonparous bitch, the uterus mingles with the jejunal loops, relatively near the dorsal body wall.
2. In a pregnant bitch, the uterus gradually sinks ventrally as the pregnancy advances. Much of the fully gravid uterus lies directly on the ventral belly wall, and displaces the digestive viscera dorsal to it.
3. Following parturition, the uterus involutes and once again attains a position not far ventral to the dorsal body wall, intermingled with the intestines.

B. Shape. The uterus resembles a capital "Y." The arms of the "Y" are the uterine horns, which are directed cranially in the abdomen; the tip of each arm is adjacent to an ovary. The upright of the "Y" represents the uterine body and cervix and is directed caudally toward the perineum (see Figure 46–1).

C. Regions. From cranial to caudal, the regions of the uterus are the **uterine horns, uterine body,** and **uterine cervix.** The uterine tube (salpinx) is not considered part of the uterus.

1. The **uterine horns** are the most elongate portion of the uterus, reflecting the minimal fusion of the paired embryonic primordia characteristic of litter-bearing animals. Gestation occurs in the uterine horns.
   a. The uterine horns extend from a point just caudal to the last rib to a point just cranial to the pelvic brim (see Figure 46–2). The uterine horns are continuous cranially with the uterine tube, and caudally with the uterine body.
   b. The uterine horns are attached to the ovary by the proper ovarian ligament.
2. The **uterine body** is short in litter-bearing species, because its main function is to direct fetuses to the cervix for delivery, rather than to provide space for gestation.
   a. Typically, the uterine body is positioned mainly in the caudal abdominal region, although a small part of it may extend into the cranial pelvic region.
   b. The uterine body is displaced cranially in advanced pregnancy. In bitches that have borne many litters, it may lie entirely within the abdomen, even between pregnancies.
3. The **uterine cervix** is an obliquely positioned, thickened partition at the junction of the

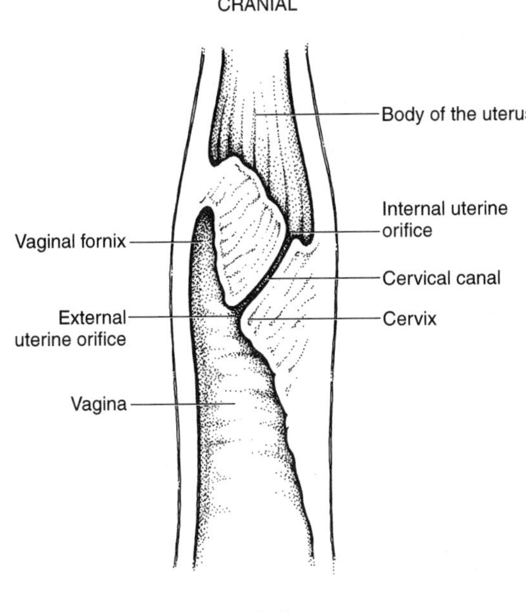

FIGURE 46–3. Sagittal section through the uterine cervix. Note the oblique position of the cervix and cervical canal, and the blind-ended vaginal fornix. The oblique positioning of the cervical canal and the vaginal fornix must be considered when trying to access the uterus (e.g., for artificial insemination, sample retrieval, or therapeutic administration of materials).

uterus and vagina (Figure 46–3) that acts as a **muscular sphincter.** The cervix holds the uterus closed at all times (other than during estrus and parturition) to preserve the sterile condition of the uterus. The cervix is typically located within the cranial pelvic region (see Figure 46–1), but is discussed here for the sake of continuity.

a. The **cervical canal** (see Figure 46–3) is positioned obliquely within the muscular mass of the cervix.

  (1) The **external uterine orifice** is the opening between the cervical canal and the vagina.

  (2) The **internal uterine orifice** is the opening between the cervical canal and the uterine body.

b. The **vaginal fornix** is a blind pocket at the cranial end of the vagina formed by the oblique positioning of the cervix at the uterovaginal junction (see Figure 46–3).

D. Vasculature

1. Arteries

a. The **uterine artery** (a branch of the vaginal artery; see Chapter 56) supplies the **uterine cervix, body,** and **horns.** The uterine artery courses cranially in the mesometrium, close to the uterine wall, from its origin in the pelvic region.

b. The **ovarian artery** (see II D 1) courses caudally from the ovarian region to anastomose with the uterine artery within the broad ligament. The ovarian artery contributes to the arterial supply of the **cranial regions of the uterine horn.**

2. Veins. Satellite veins follow the uterine and ovarian arteries. The termination of the ovarian veins is described in II D 2.

3. Efferent lymphatics from the uterus enter the **hypogastric** and **lumbar lymph nodes.**

E. Innervation.

Autonomic fibers are distributed to the uterus along the branches of the vaginal artery.

1. Sympathetic innervation arrives via the right and left **hypogastric nerves.** The hypogastric nerves extend from the caudal mesenteric plexus to the pelvic plexus.

2. Parasympathetic innervation arrives more directly from the **pelvic nerve** of the **pelvic plexus.**

Chapter 47

Kidneys, Ureters, and Adrenal Glands

I. KIDNEYS

A. Function. In addition to the role they play in excreting nitrogenous waste, the kidneys:

1. Function in vitamin D metabolism
2. Recover proteins, sugars, and water from the filtrate, and play an essential role in electrolyte balance and mineral conservation
3. Produce vasoactive substances (agents that play a role in blood pressure regulation) and erythropoietin (a hormone that stimulates red blood cell production)

B. Appearance. The canine kidneys are elongate, smooth-surfaced, dark reddish-brown, and bean-shaped.

Canine Clinical Correlation

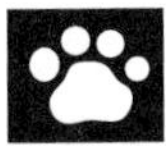

Each kidney is approximately 2–2.5 times as large as vertebra L2. This feature may be used during radiographic evaluation of the kidneys to estimate appropriateness of renal size.

C. Position. The kidneys lie along the dorsal abdominal wall to the right and left of the vertebral column, just ventral to the sublumbar muscles.

1. The kidneys are typically **staggered in position,** with the right lying more cranial than the left by about half the length of the organ (Figure 47–1). The right kidney extends from vertebrae T12 or T13 to vertebrae L2 or L3; the left kidney extends from vertebrae L1 to L3.
2. The right kidney is more firmly fixed than the left, but both are **somewhat mobile.** Renal position may vary slightly with deep ventilatory movements or postural changes. In addition, the kidney may be slightly displaced by a full stomach or gravid uterus.
3. **Relations**
   a. The **right kidney** lies with its cranial pole embedded in the renal impression in the caudate process of the caudate lobe of the liver. Its relations are:
      (1) **Cranially,** to the liver and right adrenal gland
      (2) **Medially,** to the caudal vena cava
      (3) **Ventrally,** to the descending duodenum, pancreas, and full stomach
      (4) **Laterally,** to the last rib (it may lie largely under cover of the rib) and the abdominal wall
      (5) **Dorsally,** to the sublumbar musculature
   b. The **left kidney** lies about one-half a kidney length caudal to the right kidney. Its relations are:
      (1) **Cranially,** to the spleen, pancreas, and full stomach
      (2) **Medially,** to the left adrenal gland and aorta

Canine Clinical Correlation

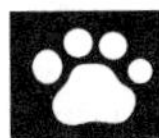

Failure of the kidneys to "ascend" from their original, more caudal position during normal embryologic development can cause one or both kidneys to lie more caudally than normal.

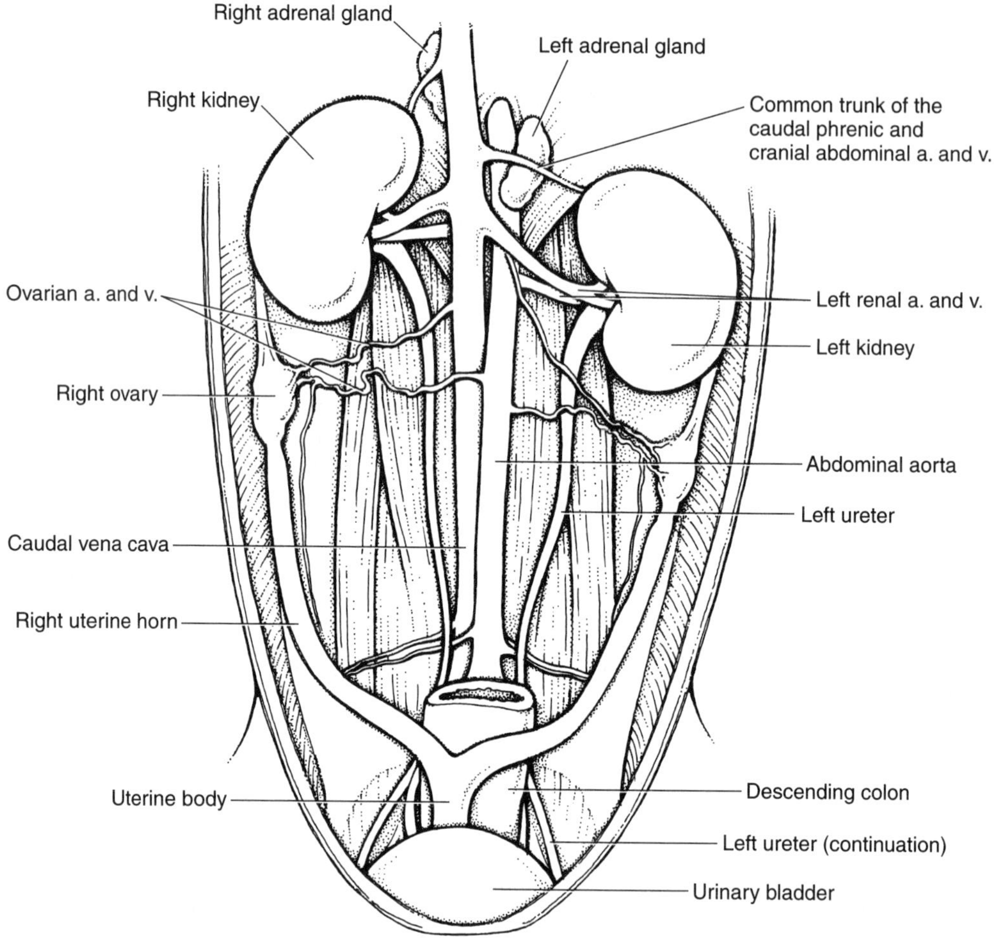

FIGURE 47–1. Kidneys *in situ* and associated structures (female dog). [Redrawn with permission from Evans HE, 1993, *Miller's Anatomy of the Dog,* 3e. Philadelphia, WB Saunders, p 495.]

(3) **Ventrally,** to the descending colon
(4) **Laterally,** to the spleen and abdominal wall
(5) **Dorsally,** to the spleen and full stomach

D. Surface features

1. **Renal hilus.** Structures enter and leave the kidney at the renal hilus, an indentation on the medial border of the kidney (in the same position as the "eye of the bean"). Structures passing through the renal hilus include the:
   a. Renal artery and vein
   b. Renal nerves
   c. Renal lymphatic vessels
   d. Ureter
2. **Fibrous capsule.** A thin, strong connective tissue sheet intimately surrounds all external surfaces of the kidney and extends inward through the hilus to line the walls of the renal sinus. The fibrous capsule invests the vessels and nerves passing through the hilus.
3. **Perirenal fat.** The kidneys, retroperitoneal organs, are embedded in perirenal fat. This adipose capsule extends through the renal hilus into the sinus.

Canine Clinical Correlation

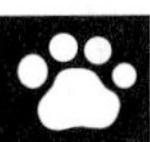

The fibrous renal capsule should strip easily from the surface of the kidney; adherence of the capsule to the renal surface (even at small points) indicates a pathologic process.

Canine Clinical Correlation

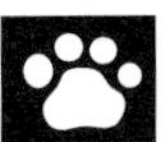

The adipose capsule can obscure visualization of the hilus and caudal pole. Perirenal fat is among the last fat reserves to be lost during disease or starvation.

E. Internal features (Figure 47–2)

1. **Renal sinus.** The renal sinus is a **cavity** within the kidney that opens to the exterior at the renal hilus.
   a. Structures. The renal sinus houses the following structures:
      (1) **Branches of the renal artery**
      (2) **Tributaries of the renal vein**
      (3) The **renal pelvis** (i.e., the dilated proximal portion of the ureter), before it narrows distally to form the ureter
      (4) **Renal nerves** and **lymphatic vessels**
   b. **Fat** fills the space that is not occupied by structures.

2. **Renal parenchyma**
   a. **Histology.** The **nephron** is the **subgross structural unit of the kidney.** Understanding the structure of the nephron simplifies understanding of the regions visible on the internal cut surface of the kidney. Each nephron has several parts.
      (1) The **renal corpuscle** is comprised of a **glomerulus** (a capillary tuft) surrounded by a double-layered **glomerular (Bowman's) capsule.**
      (2) The **proximal convoluted tubule** continues from the glomerular capsule. This tubule, as the name suggests, is highly convoluted and tortuous in its course.
      (3) The **nephric loop (loop of Henle)** leaves the proximal convoluted tubule, takes a straight course into the deeper region of the kidney, makes a hairpin turn, and returns in a course immediately adjacent to its descending limb, to reach a point near the parent renal corpuscle.
      (4) The **distal convoluted tubule** continues from the end of the nephric loop, and, like the proximal convoluted tubule, has a tortuous course. The nephron terminates as the distal convoluted tubule joins the collecting duct.
   b. **Divisions.** Grossly, the sectioned kidney presents a **cortex** and a **medulla.** The boundary where the cortex meets the medulla is the **corticomedullary junction.**
      (1) The **cortex,** the **outer region** of the kidney, is usually paler than the deeper sections. The cortex consists mainly of proximal convoluted tubules, distal convoluted tubules, peritubular capillary networks, and renal corpuscles. The renal corpuscles and convoluted tubules give the cortex a characteristic finely granular appearance.
      (2) The **medulla,** the **inner region** of the kidney, is comprised mainly of nephric loops, collecting ducts, and long, looped capillaries. The medulla has two regions.
         (a) The **outer medulla** is dark reddish-purple. Extensions from the outer medulla, **medullary rays,** extend superficially into the cortex.
         (b) The **inner medulla,** a paler grayish-red, displays radial striations of variable distinctness.
   c. **Subdivisions.** A **renal lobe** consists of a renal pyramid and its overlying cortical cap. The lobe is relatively difficult to appreciate owing to the large degree of fusion among adjacent lobes.

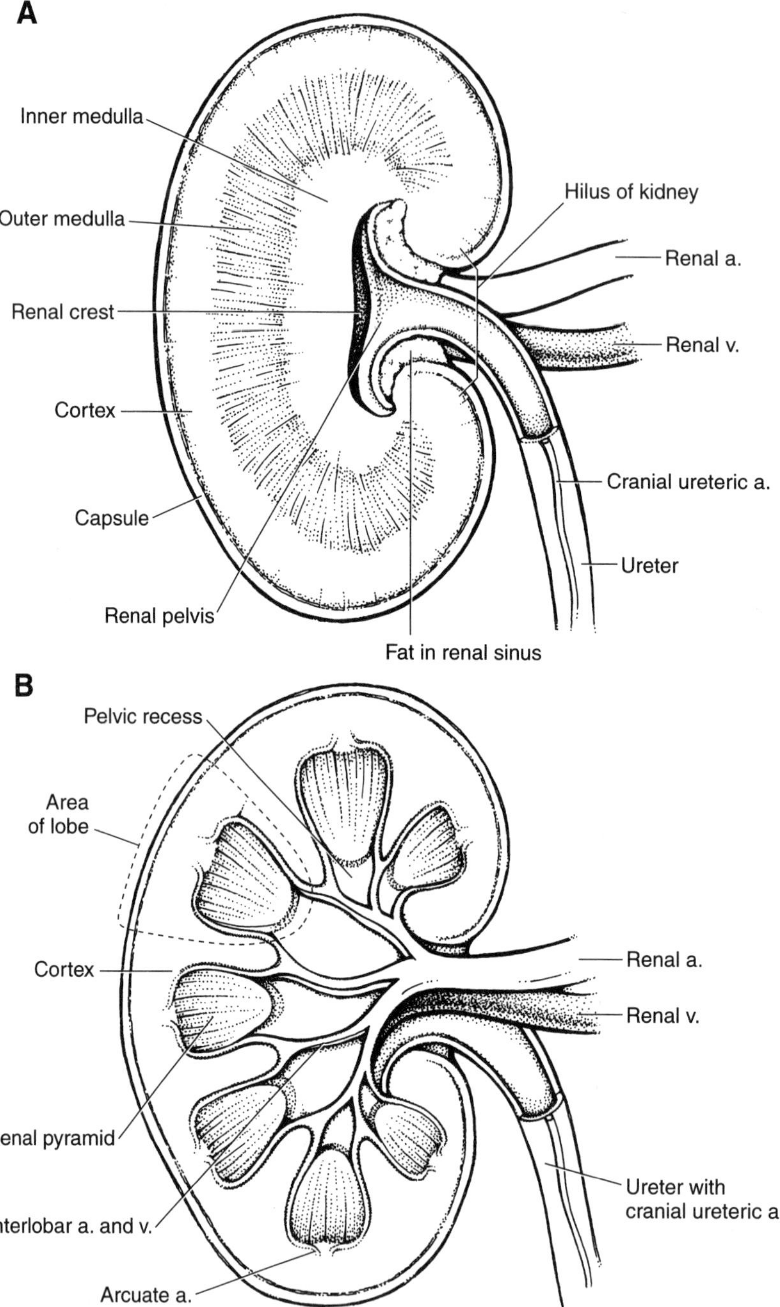

FIGURE 47–2. (*A*) Kidney, midline section. (*B*) Kidney, parasagittal section.

(1) The **renal pyramids** are triangular portions of the medulla that are best appreciated on parasagittal sections. The apices of each triangle point toward the renal hilus, where they fuse with each other along the midline to form the **renal crest.**
   (a) **Renal papilla** is a term sometimes applied to the area of the apex of each adjacent pyramid.
   (b) **Renal columns** are dark **cortical extensions** that project into the medulla, between the paler renal pyramids.
   (c) The **cortical cap** of the pyramid is the cortical region that covers the pyramid.

(2) The **renal crest** is formed by the fusion of the apices of adjacent renal pyramids. Because the papillae fuse to form the renal crest, the dog kidney is described as **unipyramidal.** This structure is best appreciated on the midline section.

d. Collecting system. The collecting system is best considered from proximal to distal, beginning in the kidney and ending at the urinary bladder.

(1) The **collecting ducts** pass from the distal convoluted tubule through the medulla, becoming progressively larger as adjacent tubules join.

(2) As the collecting ducts become larger and approach the renal papillae, they are referred to as **papillary ducts.** The papillary ducts open on the renal crest.

(3) The **area cribrosa** is the region on the renal crest where the papillary ducts open. The area cribrosa gives the renal crest a finely perforated appearance.

(4) The **renal pelvis,** the dilated proximal portion of the ureter, occupies much of the space within the renal sinus. Renal **pelvic recesses** project from the periphery of the renal pelvis into the medulla and toward the cortex, between the renal pyramids.

(5) The **ureter,** the tubular continuation of the renal pelvis, exits the kidney at the hilus, and passes directly caudally toward the urinary bladder in the pelvis (see Chapter 51 V B).

F. Vasculature

1. Arteries. The kidneys are copiously supplied with arterial blood; together, the two kidneys receive 25% of the cardiac output under normal conditions.

a. Origin and course. Each **renal artery** is a **direct branch of the aorta.** The renal arteries take a direct course to their respective kidneys.

(1) The **right renal artery** arises approximately at the level of vertebrae L1 and L2 and passes dorsal to the caudal vena cava *en route* to the right kidney.

(2) The **left renal artery** arises somewhat caudal to the right renal artery.

Canine Clinical Correlation

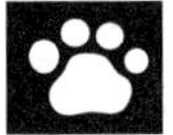

Typically, one artery is present on each side. However, the embryologic development of the kidney involves renal "ascent" from a more caudal position, during which time the kidney is progressively supplied by newly developing arteries. Therefore, multiple renal arteries may supply the same kidney. During surgery, care must be taken when searching the hilar fat for arteries to be certain that all have been located.

b. Branches

(1) **Extrarenal branches.** Typically, each renal artery gives rise to branches supplying the:
   (a) **Adrenal gland** (caudal adrenal branch)
   (b) **Ureter** (cranial ureteric branch)
   (c) **Adipose capsule**
   (d) **Hilar region** (branches pass into the sinus and then to the poles and midregion of the kidney)

(2) **Interlobar arteries** arise from the branches within the sinus, and are grossly visible. These arteries pass into the renal parenchyma in the spaces between the re-

nal pyramids. The interlobar arteries radiate toward the cortex and terminate at the corticomedullary junction.

(3) **Arcuate arteries** arise from the corticomedullary termination of the interlobar arteries and take an arching course over the curved surface where the medullary pyramids meet the cortex. These grossly visible arteries simplify identification of the corticomedullary junction.

(4) **Other arteries** within the renal parenchyma include (in sequence) the **interlobular arteries,** the **afferent arterioles,** the **glomerulus,** the **efferent arterioles,** and the **peritubular capillary network.**

2. **Veins.** The veins of the kidney largely parallel the arteries, with the exception of the glomerulus and the afferent and efferent arterioles. Thus, **straight venules** and **interlobular, arcuate, interlobar,** and **renal veins** are present. The renal veins are tributaries of the **caudal vena cava.**

G. Innervation. Autonomic nerves form dense plexuses surrounding the renal vasculature.

1. **Efferent (motor) pathways.** Sympathetic innervation arrives through the splanchnic nerves and supplies mainly the vasculature. Sympathetic tone decreases blood supply during the "fight or flight" response.
2. **Afferent (sensory) pathways** pass to the spinal cord via the splanchnic nerves.

II. URETERS.

The ureters are tubes of smooth muscle that carry urine from the kidney to the urinary bladder.

A. Position. Like the kidneys, the ureters are retroperitoneal in position. Because the right kidney lies more cranial that the left, the right ureter is slightly longer than the left. Ureters are also longer in males than in females, because in males the ureter passes through the penis.

Canine Clinical Correlation

Should the integrity of the ureter be breached (e.g., by **ureteral trauma),** urine pools in a retroperitoneal position, rather than diffusing throughout the abdominal cavity. This pooling causes a localized fluid density that is readily recognizable radiographically.

B. Course. The ureters course caudally and slightly medially *en route* to the urinary bladder.

1. The **abdominal part** of the ureter courses on the ventral surface of the psoas muscles. This portion of the ureter lies ventral to the caudal vena cava and iliac arteries, but dorsal to the arteries supplying the gonads.
2. The **pelvic part** of the ureter differs according to gender.
   a. In **females,** the ureter continues its slightly oblique course directly to the urinary bladder.
   b. In **males,** the ureters pass dorsal to the ductus deferens, and each ductus deferens loops around its respective ureter *en route* to the urethra.
3. The ureters **enter the urinary bladder** at its dorsolateral surface, just caudal to the neck

Canine Clinical Correlation

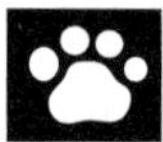

The fairly common condition of **ectopic ureters** results from faulty embryonic development in which the ureters open at abnormal sites such as the vagina or urethra.

Canine Clinical Correlation

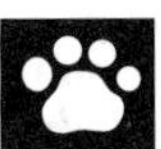

Because of the proximity of the ureter to the uterine vessels, it is necessary to meticulously evaluate the tubular structures to be ligated and cut during ovariohysterectomy.

of the bladder. The oblique course of the ureters through the urinary bladder's musculature assists in preventing urinary reflux into the ureter as the bladder fills.

C. Vasculature

1. **Arteries.** Typically, a **cranial ureteral artery** (arising from the renal artery) and a **caudal ureteral artery** (arising from the vaginal or prostatic artery) supply the ureter, anastomosing partway along the length of the ureter. Variations in the origin of the ureteric arterial supply are common, and twigs to the ureter may arise from essentially any nearby larger artery.
2. **Veins.** Each ureteral artery has a companion vein of the same name.

Canine Clinical Correlation

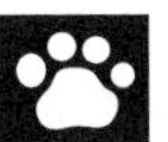

The ureteral vasculature is delicate in nature, and excessive mobilization or traction on the ureter should be avoided during abdominal surgery. Compromise of the delicate blood supply can result in **ischemic ureteral necrosis.**

D. Innervation.

The ureters are inherently peristaltic, and receive **sympathetic** and **parasympathetic** innervation from the **celiac** and **pelvic plexuses,** respectively. Both **motor pathways** and **visceral afferent (sensory) pathways** are present.

Canine Clinical Correlation

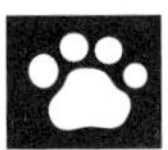

The **inherent peristaltic activity** of the ureters is visible during **intravenous pyelography.**

III. ADRENAL GLANDS.

The adrenal glands are paired primary endocrine organs that lie along the craniomedial border of each kidney. A thick layer of retroperitoneal fat surrounds each adrenal gland.

A. Function, appearance, and position.

The function, appearance, and position of the adrenal glands are discussed in detail in Chapter 6 II E.

B. Vasculature

1. **Arteries.** The arterial supply arrives through **numerous, small branches** of the **caudal phrenic, cranial abdominal, lumbar,** and **renal arteries,** as well as the **aorta.** Numerous arterioles from each of these branches approach the adrenal gland from many directions, course through the fibrous capsule that surrounds the gland, and branch within the parenchyma.
2. **Veins.** The adrenal glands possess a complex pattern of **venous sinuses.** From the si-

nuses, the **adrenal vein** forms and leaves the gland at the hilus. (Note that the adrenal hilus differs from the hilus of many other organs, in that although the adrenal vein exits here, the organ's arteries do not enter via the same route!)

3. **Lymphatic vessels.** Extensive **lymphatic plexuses** are present through much of the substance of the adrenal glands. These plexuses drain into the **lumbar aortic lymph nodes.**

C. Innervation

1. The innervation of the **adrenal cortex** is not well-characterized.
2. The **adrenal medulla,** which produces epinephrine and norepinephrine (hormones that affect the sympathetic nervous system), is considered a **sympathetic ganglion.** Preganglionic fibers arrive to the medulla via the **celiac** and **adrenal ganglia.**

Chapter 48

Prominent Palpable Features of the Abdominal Region

I. ABDOMINAL WALL

A. Bony structures. Few bony structures are associated with the abdominal wall.

1. **Caudal lumbar vertebrae.** The **transverse processes** of the caudal lumbar vertebrae are palpable in emaciated dogs, and may be palpable in some healthy but thin dogs.
2. **Ribs 10–13.** The ribs contributing to the craniolateral boundaries of the abdomen are palpable, from the point where they emerge from under the cover of the epaxial musculature distally to the sternum via the costal arch.
3. **Costal arch.** The costal arch is palpable.
4. **Xiphoid process** and **xiphoid cartilage.** These structures contribute to a small part of the ventral abdominal wall and are palpable.
5. **Pubic brim.** The pubic brim is palpable between the thighs (along the midline and to each side of it).

B. Soft tissue structures. The musculature forming most of the lateral and ventral abdominal walls can be appreciated just deep to the skin. However, the specific muscles are not distinguishable as individual entities.

1. The **external intercostal muscles,** located in intercostal spaces 10–12, bridge the spaces between the ribs that form a part of the abdominal wall.
2. The **external abdominal oblique muscle** forms most of the lateral abdominal wall. This muscle lies under the skin and extends from the level of the lumbar transverse processes to the area where the lateral wall blends with the ventral wall. In addition, by means of its aponeurosis, the external abdominal oblique extends fully to the ventral midline.
3. The **rectus abdominis muscle** forms most of the ventral abdominal wall.

II. ABDOMINAL CAVITY.

Palpating the contents of the abdominal cavity is an art and a science. The soft tissue structures within the abdominal cavity are mostly covered with peritoneum and are highly mobile; therefore, distinguishing one organ from another can be difficult. Furthermore, many of these structures are inaccessible to palpation, either because they are protected by the caudal part of the bony thorax, or they are too deep to access. However, regular palpation of normal abdomens imparts an understanding of the degree of "normal ambiguity" of the region, so that when an abnormality is encountered in the form of a more distinctly palpable structure or an identifiable mass, the aberrance is recognizable as such.

A. Gastrointestinal organs

1. **Stomach.** Much of the empty or moderately full stomach is protected by the ribs. However, when moderately full, the caudal edge of the stomach becomes palpable on the left side, just caudal to the ribs.
2. **Spleen.** The spleen normally can be recognized as an elongate, firm structure on the left side. Because of its close association with the greater curvature of the stomach, the position of the spleen can vary according to the fullness of the stomach.
   - **a.** With an undistended stomach, the spleen should be palpable just caudal to the costal arch on the left side.
   - **b.** When the stomach is full, the spleen will be displaced caudal to the costal arch on the left side.
3. **Liver.** Normally, none (or only a small part) of the liver is palpable because the liver is

largely protected by the ribs. The small part of the liver that may be palpable is detected just caudal to the costal arch near the midline. The ability to palpate more of the liver is considered a clinically significant abnormality.

4. **Jejunum.** The jejunum can be appreciated mainly as loose, fluctuant, ill-defined soft masses within the abdominal cavity. The loops slip smoothly through the fingers on palpation. If filled with gas, the jejunum may feel hard and distinctly tubular.
5. **Descending colon.** The descending colon is often readily palpable, although its prominence varies according to whether the colon is relatively empty or filled with fecal matter.
   a. The empty descending colon cannot be distinguished from the other intestinal loops.
   b. A full descending colon can be readily distinguished as a moderately firm tubular structure, discernable on the left side or toward the midline of the abdomen. A very firm descending colon implies constipation.

B. **Female reproductive organs.** In the nonpregnant state, the uterus is not palpable. In the **early stages of pregnancy,** the multiple swellings along the length of the **uterine horns** distinguish these structures from the jejunal loops. Once the swellings of the conceptuses become confluent, the uterine horns blend imperceptibly with the jejunal loops. **Near parturition,** the uterine horns can be appreciated as large, firm masses.

C. **Urinary organs**

1. **Kidneys**
   a. The **left kidney** is usually palpable over most of its length from the cranial to the caudal poles. This kidney is detected as a mass with an even, smooth surface and uniform firmness in the dorsocranial abdomen, just caudal to the ribs.
   b. The **right kidney,** which is positioned much further cranially and nestled into the caudate process of the caudate lobe of the liver, is generally not palpable, although its caudal pole may be palpable.
2. **Urinary bladder.** When moderately full, the urinary bladder can be palpated as a roundish mass that "floats" midway along the dorsal-to-ventral dimension of the caudal abdomen. When very full, the heavy bladder sinks to the ventral abdominal wall, where it is readily palpable.

STUDY QUESTIONS

DIRECTIONS: Each of the numbered items or incomplete statements in this section is followed by answers or by completions of the statement. Select the ONE numbered answer or completion that is BEST in each case.

1. Which statement best describes the inguinal region of the abdomen?

(1) Its superficial features include the caudal two pairs of mammae.
(2) It extends over the caudal third of the abdomen, from the ventral midline to the dorsal-most boundary of both the right and left sides of the abdomen.
(3) It is partially obscured by the caudal thigh musculature.
(4) It is covered by the external abdominal oblique muscle.

2. Which statement correctly describes the inguinal canal in female dogs?

(1) It develops in all females and transmits structures both into and out of the abdomen.
(2) It develops in obese females when the increased weight of the abdomen stretches the inguinal rings.
(3) It develops in hermaphroditic females and transmits rudimentary testis.
(4) It does not normally develop in females.

3. Which muscle of the abdominal wall has fibers that course caudoventrally and contributes to the superficial layer of the rectus sheath?

(1) The external abdominal oblique muscle
(2) The internal abdominal oblique muscle
(3) The transversus abdominis muscle
(4) The rectus abdominis muscle

4. Which one of the following muscles is the most internal of the muscles on the lateroventral body wall?

(1) Rectus abdominis muscle
(2) Transversus abdominis muscle
(3) Internal abdominal oblique muscle
(4) External abdominal oblique muscle

5. The strength of the abdominal wall, which is mostly composed of soft tissue, is attributable to the:

(1) particularly dense collagen fibers in the skin overlying the area.
(2) thin fibrocartilaginous plates strategically located in the muscles.
(3) angled orientation of the muscle fibers relative to each other.
(4) transverse tendinous intersections placed at intervals along the full length of the muscles

6. Which one of the following statements regarding the relation of the abdominal structures and peritoneum to the abdominal cavity is correct?

(1) The peritoneal cavity contains the abdominal organs, and the abdominal cavity contains the peritoneal cavity.
(2) The abdominal cavity contains the abdominal organs and the peritoneal cavity.
(3) The omental bursa contains the abdominal organs, the peritoneal cavity contains the omental bursa, and the abdominal cavity contains both the omental bursa and the peritoneal cavity.
(4) The peritoneal cavity contain serous fluid, the omental bursa contains the abdominal organs, and the abdominal cavity contains both the peritoneal cavity and omental bursa.

7. The length of mesentery of a given region of intestine depends on:

(1) the developmental origin of the intestinal segment.
(2) whether the intestinal segment herniated through the belly wall during development.
(3) the order in which the region of intestine was retracted back into the body cavity.
(4) the degree of rotation the intestine underwent during development.

8. Which of the following abdominal organs has a long mesentery and is fairly mobile?

(1) Descending duodenum
(2) Descending colon
(3) Jejunum
(4) Ileum

9. Which one of the following is a remnant of the ventral mesentery that persists in the definitive form?

(1) The lesser omentum
(2) The round ligament of the liver
(3) The falciform ligament
(4) The gastrosplenic ligament

10. What is the pylorus?

(1) An opening at the caudal duodenal flexure
(2) The terminal region of the stomach that precedes the duodenum
(3) The muscular sphincter that controls the passage of ingesta from the ileum to the colon
(4) A specialization of the muscle fibers of the stomach

11. Which one of the following characteristics can help distinguish the duodenum from the jejunum?

(1) Diameter of the gut tube
(2) Surface appearance of the gut tube
(3) Pattern of blood supply
(4) Pattern of innervation

12. The major duodenal papilla provides an opening site for the:

(1) pancreatic and accessory pancreatic ducts.
(2) accessory pancreatic duct and the bile duct.
(3) pancreatic duct and the bile duct.
(4) bile duct.

13. The two liver lobes positioned on each side of the gallbladder are the:

(1) right and left medial lobes.
(2) right medial and quadrate lobes.
(3) right medial and right lateral lobes.
(4) quadrate and caudate lobes.

14. The major arteries supplying the gastrointestinal tract are unusual among the branches of the aorta in that they:

(1) are retroperitoneal.
(2) course within an associated, specific subdivision of the mesentery.
(3) are unpaired and leave the ventral surface of the aorta.
(4) turn at 90 degrees and take a directly ventral course after leaving the lateral surface of the aorta to gain the gut wall.

15. If the caudal pancreaticoduodenal artery becomes occluded, which artery could supply collateral flow to the duodenum?

(1) Hepatic artery
(2) Jejunal arteries
(3) Right gastric artery
(4) Cranial mesenteric artery

16. Which visceral branch of the abdominal aorta supplies the greatest number of gastrointestinal organs?

(1) Celiac artery
(2) Cranial mesenteric artery
(3) Middle mesenteric artery
(4) Caudal mesenteric artery

17. How does venous drainage of the gastrointestinal tract differ from that of most other regions of the body?

(1) Most of the veins are doubled or tripled.
(2) Satellite veins of named arteries are largely absent.
(3) Blood does not directly re-enter the systemic circulation.
(4) The veins have thick muscular walls to assist in moving blood at low pressure.

18. The hepatic portal vein is designated as "portal" because it:

(1) enters the hepatic porta.
(2) is positioned ventral to the caudal vena cava.
(3) carries blood directly between two capillary beds.
(4) carries blood at such low pressure.

19. The largest lymph nodes associated with the gastrointestinal tract are typically the:

(1) hepatic nodes.
(2) splenic nodes.
(3) jejunal nodes.
(4) cranial mesenteric nodes.

20. Which statement regarding the prevertebral ganglia is true?

(1) They are parasympathetic in composition.
(2) They give rise to the thoracic and lumbar splanchnic nerves.
(3) They take the place of the sympathetic trunk within the abdomen.
(4) They are associated with the major arteries that supply the gastrointestinal organs and spleen.

21. What is the function of the splanchnic nerves?

(1) They supply sympathetic fibers to the abdominal wall.
(2) They carry sympathetic fibers from the prevertebral ganglia to the gastrointestinal organs and spleen.
(3) They deliver parasympathetic input to the pelvis from the caudal mesenteric ganglion.
(4) They deliver sympathetic fibers to the celiac, cranial mesenteric, and caudal mesenteric ganglia.

22. Which statement regarding the arterial supply of the ovary is true?

(1) It arrives through direct branches of the abdominal aorta.
(2) It provides branches to the adjacent regions of the ureter.
(3) It forms a plexus on the superficial surface of the ovary.
(4) It arrives through branches of the renal artery.

23. Which one of the following statements regarding the suspensory ligament of the ovary is true?

(1) It is a thin, doubled fold of peritoneum that extends between the ovary and the salpinx.
(2) It attaches the ovary to the dorsal body wall.
(3) It attaches the ovary to the tip of the uterine horn.
(4) It is a subdivision of the broad ligament.

24. Surgery of the kidney requires temporary occlusion of the renal artery and vein. What feature of the kidney and surrounding structures can make the occlusion of these vessels difficult?

(1) The thickness of the fibrous renal capsule
(2) The retroperitoneal position of the kidney
(3) The abundance of perirenal fat
(4) The medially directed orientation of the renal hilus

25. What is the renal sinus?

(1) The area of the kidney through which structures enter and leave the organ
(2) The space containing renal vessels and nerves and the renal pelvis
(3) The space in which urine is collected prior to passage through the ureter
(4) A blind-ended diverticulum of the renal pelvis located at each renal pole

26. A veterinarian palpates the full length of a firm, oblong structure in the dorsocranial region of the abdomen, just caudal to the ribs on the right side. This structure is most likely:

(1) the right kidney.
(2) an abnormal mass.
(3) the ascending colon.
(4) the caudal-most projection of the liver.

DIRECTIONS: Each of the numbered items or incomplete statements in this section is negatively phrased, as indicated by a capitalized word such as NOT, LEAST, or EXCEPT. Select the ONE numbered answer or completion that is BEST in each case.

27. Which statement regarding the internal subdivision of the kidney is FALSE?

(1) The cortex is the site where the glomeruli and convoluted tubules reside.
(2) The internal division of the kidney into lobes is not reflected on the surface of the kidney.
(3) The renal pyramids are portions of the cortex.
(4) The medulla has an inner and an outer region.

28. A clot lodged in the celiac artery would be LEAST likely to compromise arterial flow to which one of the following organs?

(1) Stomach
(2) Duodenum
(3) Gallbladder
(4) Transverse colon

29. Which one of the following statements does NOT correctly describe the mesentery?

(1) It is formed of a doubled fold of peritoneum.
(2) It has a visceral and a parietal surface.
(3) It suspends the small and large intestines from the dorsal body wall.
(4) It conducts vessels and nerves through its substance to the gut wall.

30. Which one of the following groups of lymph nodes does NOT receive drainage from the abdominal wall?

(1) Renal lymph nodes
(2) Hypogastric lymph nodes
(3) Medial iliac lymph nodes
(4) Cranial lumbar lymph nodes

31. The internal abdominal oblique muscle, the external abdominal oblique muscle, and the rectus abdominis muscle share all of the following actions EXCEPT:

(1) drawing of the bony pelvis cranially.
(2) supporting and compressing the abdominal viscera.
(3) flexing the vertebral column ventrally.
(4) flexing the vertebral column laterally.

32. All of the following bones contribute to some portion of the abdominal wall EXCEPT the:

(1) shaft of the ilium.
(2) bodies and costal cartilages of ribs 9–13.
(3) bodies and transverse processes of lumbar vertebrae 1–7.
(4) bodies and transverse processes of thoracic vertebrae 9–13.

33. Which one of the following types of structure does NOT normally pass through the inguinal canal?

(1) Peritoneal
(2) Reproductive
(3) Vascular
(4) Digestive

34. Which one of the following body systems is NOT represented within the abdomen?

(1) Immune system
(2) Respiratory system
(3) Endocrine system
(4) Reproductive system

35. A veterinarian makes an incision in the ventral abdomen. Her intent is to make the incision along the linea alba, but she misses. Fortunately, she can use the rectus sheath to assist in closing the incision, UNLESS the incision is at which one of the following levels?

(1) Just caudal to the xiphoid cartilage
(2) Just cranial to the umbilicus
(3) Between the xiphoid cartilage and the mid-abdominal region
(4) In the caudal abdominal region, cranial to the pelvic brim

36. The ventral branches of several of the lumbar nerves take individual names. All of the following are ventral branches of a lumbar nerve EXCEPT the:

(1) costoabdominal nerve.
(2) cranial iliohypogastric nerve.
(3) caudal iliohypogastric nerve.
(4) ilioinguinal nerve.

37. Which one of the following structures is NOT associated with the descending duodenum?

(1) The left lobe of the pancreas
(2) The major duodenal papilla
(3) The minor duodenal papilla
(4) The opening of the bile duct

38. Which one of the following structures does NOT receive autonomic innervation via the celiacomesenteric plexus?

(1) Cecum
(2) Spleen
(3) Pancreas
(4) Descending colon

39. The stomach receives autonomic fibers from all of the following EXCEPT the:

(1) celiac part of the celiacomesenteric plexus.
(2) lumbar splanchnic nerves.
(3) thoracic sympathetic trunk.
(4) ventral vagal trunk.

40. Which one of the following statements regarding the uterine tube is INCORRECT?

(1) It is supported by a portion of the uterine broad ligament.
(2) It courses between the ovary and the uterine horn.
(3) It is the normal site of fertilization.
(4) It is the initial part of the uterus.

ANSWERS AND EXPLANATIONS

1. The answer is 4 [Chapter 40 IV C 2; Figure 40–1; Chapter 41 III B 2 a; Table 41–1]. The external abdominal oblique muscle, which attaches to the inguinal ligament, extends over the inguinal region of the abdomen. The other statements regarding the inguinal region are false: the inguinal region does not extend to the midline (the pubic region intervenes between the two inguinal side regions), only the last pair of mammae are located in the inguinal region, and the inguinal region is partially obscured by the cranial, not the caudal, thigh musculature.

2. The answer is 1 [Chapter 40 III C 2]. The inguinal canal is a normal feature in both sexes, transmitting the vaginal process, the external pudendal artery, the external pudendal vein, and the genitofemoral nerve. Structures pass both into and out of the abdominal cavity via the inguinal canal. In males, the inguinal canal also provides passage for the testes and spermatic cord.

3. The answer is 1 [Chapter 41 IV B 1 a; Table 41–1]. The muscle described is the external abdominal oblique—its fibers course caudoventrally toward the inguinal region, and its aponeurosis contributes to the superficial layer of the rectus sheath. The fibers of the internal abdominal oblique muscle pass cranioventrally. Those of the transversus abdominis muscle pass directly dorsal to ventral, and those of the rectus abdominis muscle pass directly cranial to caudal.

4. The answer is 2 [Chapter 41 III B 2 c]. The transversus abdominis muscle is the deepest muscle of the lateroventral body wall. The external abdominal oblique muscle is the most external, and the internal oblique is intermediate in position between the external oblique and the transversus abdominis muscles. The rectus abdominis occupies only the ventral abdominal wall.

5. The answer is 3 [Chapter 41 III B 2]. The fibers of the two oblique abdominal muscles and the transverse abdominal muscle form a grid, which significantly increases the strength of the muscular abdominal wall. Transverse tendinous intersections increase the strength of the rectus abdominis muscle, which does not contribute to the lateral body wall. (The tendinous intersections of the transversus abdominis muscle run parallel to the muscle fibers, and do not act to increase the strength of that muscle.)

6. The answer is 2 [Chapter 42 I–II]. The abdominal cavity contains the abdominal organs and the peritoneal cavity. The peritoneal cavity, the potential space between the layer of peritoneum that covers the body wall and the layer of peritoneum that covers the abdominal organs, normally contains only a small amount of serous fluid. No organs are located within the peritoneal cavity or the omental bursa.

7. The answer is 3 [Chapter 42 IV B 2]. Essentially all regions of the intestinal tube, from the duodenum through the descending colon, normally herniate through the body wall during development and are later retracted. Those gut regions nearest the cranial and caudal regions of the tube are withdrawn into the cavity first, and because they are crowded near the body wall by the intestines entering later, their mesenteries are shortened by the crowding. Therefore, the length of mesentery of a given region of intestine depends on the order in which the region of intestine was retracted into the body cavity.

8. The answer is 3 [Chapter 42 IV B 2 b]. The jejunum possesses the longest mesentery of all regions of the gut tube, and as a result, is fairly mobile. The descending duodenum, ileum, and descending colon have shorter mesenteries and are considered "fixed" viscera.

9. The answer is 3 [Chapter 42 IV A 1 b (2)]. The falciform ligament is the remnant of the ventral mesentery of the foregut (i.e., the ventral mesogastrium), which extends between the liver and the ventral body wall. The ventral mesentery associated with the hindgut (i.e., the intestine) degenerates. The gastrosplenic ligament is a remnant of the dorsal mesogastrium, and the round ligament of the liver is a remnant of the umbilical vein.

10. The answer is 4 [Chapter 43 I B 6 a (2) (b)]. The pylorus is a muscular sphincter of the stomach, positioned at the junction of the stomach with the duodenum. It is formed from the inner circular muscle fibers of the stomach wall. The term "pylorus" describes only this sphincter, not the entire terminal region of the stomach, which is referred to as the pyloric region. The pyloric regions is composed of the pyloric antrum (adjacent to the gastric body), the pyloric canal, and the pylorus.

11. The answer is 3 [Chapter 43 II C 2 a]. The jejunum is supplied by long arcades of vessels passing through the supporting mesentery; although the duodenum's vessels also pass through the mesentery, the vessels pass directly to the duodenal wall as short, straight vessels.

12. The answer is 3 [Chapter 43 II A 4 a]. The pancreatic duct and the hepatic bile duct open on the major duodenal papilla. The accessory pancreatic duct opens on the minor duodenal papilla.

13. The answer is 2 [Chapter 43 II B 4 b (3); Figure 43–4A]. The gallbladder lies between the quadrate and right medial lobes.

14. The answer is 3 [Chapter 44 I]. The major arteries supplying the gastrointestinal tract (i.e., the celiac, cranial mesenteric, and caudal mesenteric arteries) are the only unpaired, ventrally directed arteries in the body.

15. The answer is 1 [Chapter 44 I A 3 c]. The cranial pancreaticoduodenal artery, which supplies multiple branches to the duodenum, is a branch of the gastroduodenal artery, which in turn is one of the terminal branches of the hepatic artery. The right gastric artery is the other terminal division of the hepatic artery, but this artery passes to the lesser curvature of the stomach without supplying the duodenum. The jejunal arteries do not supply the duodenum. The cranial mesenteric artery is the source of the caudal pancreaticoduodenal artery, which is the artery specified as compromised in the leader.

16. The answer is 2 [Chapter 44 I B]. The cranial mesenteric artery, the largest visceral branch of the abdominal aorta, supplies the duodenum, pancreas, jejunum, ileum, cecum, and the ascending, transverse, and descending colons. The caudal mesenteric artery supplies only the descending colon and rectum. The celiac artery supplies the stomach, liver, pancreas, duodenum, and spleen. The "middle mesenteric artery" does not exist.

17. The answer is 3 [Chapter 44 II A 1]. Venous drainage of the gastrointestinal tract differs from that of most other regions of the body in that the blood from the gastrointestinal organs passes to the liver via the hepatic portal vein, before being returned to the systemic circulation. Satellite veins of most named arteries are indeed present.

18. The answer is 3 [Chapter 44 II A 2]. A portal vein is defined as one that carries blood from one capillary bed to another before the blood is returned to the systemic circulation. Blood from the capillary bed of the gut wall passes through the hepatic portal vein to the capillary bed of the liver before gaining the caudal vena cava. Although the hepatic portal vein does enter the hepatic porta and is positioned ventral to the caudal vena cava, these are not the criteria for designating it as a "portal" vein.

19. The answer is 3 [Chapter 44 III B 1]. The jejunal lymph nodes, arranged along the origin of the jejunal arteries from the cranial mesenteric artery, are the largest lymph nodes associated with the gastrointestinal tract. Sometimes they are so large, they can be mistaken for an abnormal mass.

20. The answer is 4 [Chapter 45 I A 1]. The prevertebral ganglia (i.e., the celiacomesenteric and the caudal mesenteric ganglia) are associated with the large, unpaired visceral branches of the aorta that supply the gastrointestinal organs and spleen. These ganglia receive (as opposed to give rise to) the splanchnic nerves, and provide the site for synapse of the sympathetic (not the parasympathetic) component of the gastrointestinal nerves. (Although the parasympathetic nerves pass through the ganglia, they do not synapse within them.) The sympathetic trunk continues intact throughout the length of the abdomen, and is the source of the sympathetic fibers that travel to the prevertebral ganglia.

21. The answer is 4 [Chapter 45 I B]. The splanchnic nerves (i.e., the major splanchnic nerves, the minor splanchnic nerves, and the lumbar splanchnic nerves) deliver preganglionic sympathetic fibers to the celiac, cranial mesenteric, and caudal mesenteric ganglia. The major and minor splanchnic nerves deliver sympathetic fibers to the celiacomesenteric ganglion, and the lumbar splanchnic nerves deliver preganglionic sympathetic fibers to the cranial and caudal mesenteric ganglia, as well as some other ganglia related to the abdomen (e.g., the gonadal and aorticorenal ganglia). Fibers from the ganglia travel via the plexuses to the gastrointestinal organs and spleen, not to the abdominal wall.

22. The answer is 1 [Chapter 46 II D 1]. The ovarian arteries leave the lateral surface of the abdominal aorta and course directly to each ovary to enter it. The arteries do not form a plexus. The ovarian arteries supply the ovary, the uterine tube, the cranial part of the uterine horn and the renal capsule, but not the ureter. The origin of the ovarian arteries is independent of the renal arteries, despite the similar embryologic relations and physical proximity ovary and kidney.

23. The answer is 2 [Chapter 46 II C 1]. The suspensory ligament of the ovary is a dense collection of collagenous and smooth muscle fibers that extends from the cranial pole of each ovary to the dorsal body wall in the region of the last rib. The proper ligament of the ovary attaches the ovary to the tip of the uterine horn. The mesosalpinx is the peritoneal fold related to the ovary and salpinx. The subdivisions of the broad ligament are the mesosalpinx, mesovarium, and mesometrium.

24. The answer is 3 [Chapter 47 I E 3]. The perirenal fat is so abundant that it often completely obscures the renal hilus and the structures passing through it. The fibrous capsule and peritoneum offer no significant resistance to accessing the kidney and its vessels. The medially directed orientation of the hilus is not a hindrance to accessing the vessels.

25. The answer is 2 [Chapter 47 I F 1]. The renal sinus is a cavity within the kidney that opens to the exterior at the renal hilus. The renal sinus houses the renal vessels, the renal nerves, and the renal pelvis. The renal pelvis is the space where urine collects prior to passing through the ureter. There are no blind-ended diverticula at each renal pole in the dog.

26. The answer is 2 [Chapter 48 II C 1]. The structure palpated by the veterinarian is an abnormal mass. The full length of the left kidney, not the right, can be palpated as a firm, oblong structure in the dorsocranial region of the abdomen, just caudal to the ribs. Only a small portion, if any, of the right kidney is palpable. The ascending colon, although positioned on the right, is not palpable, and the tiny portion of the liver that normally can be appreciated on palpation is located in relation to the ventral midline.

27. The answer is 3 [Chapter 47 F 2 c (1)]. The renal pyramids are portions of the medulla, not the cortex. The cortex is the site where the glomeruli and convoluted tubules reside. The medulla does have an inner and outer region, and the internal division of the kidney into lobes is not reflected on the surface of the kidney.

28. The answer is 4 [Table 44–1]. The transverse colon receives its arterial blood from the ileocolic artery, a branch of the cranial mesenteric artery. Therefore, the transverse colon would be minimally (if at all) affected by a clot in the celiac artery. The left gastric and hepatic arteries of the celiac artery supply the stomach, duodenum, and gallbladder, so these organs could be affected by a clot in the celiac artery.

29. The answer is 2 [Chapter 42 III C]. Organs, not mesenteries, are described as having parietal and visceral surfaces. A mesentery is a portion of the connecting peritoneum, a subdivision of the peritoneum. A mesentery extends between an abdominal organ and a body wall and is formed of a doubled fold of peritoneum. Mesenteries are wide, and conduct vessels and nerves to and from the organs they suspend.

30. The answer is 1 [Chapter 41 V C 1 b]. The renal lymph nodes drain only the kidney. The hypogastric lymph nodes drain the muscles of the abdominal wall, as well as other structures. The medial iliac lymph nodes drain structures of the abdominal wall and the abdominal cavity, the pelvic walls and viscera, the tail, and the pelvic limb. The cranial lumbar lymph nodes drain the last few ribs and the musculature of the abdominal region.

31. The answer is 1 [Table 41–1]. Only the rectus abdominis muscle attaches to the pelvic brim and is therefore able to draw the pelvis cranially. The rectus abdominis and the abdominal oblique muscles all support and compress the abdominal viscera, flex the vertebral column ventrally (when contracted unilaterally), and flex the vertebral column laterally (when contracted bilaterally).

32. The answer is 4 [Chapter 41 II A; III A]. The diaphragm attaches to the bodies of vertebrae L1 and L2. Therefore, all of the thoracic vertebrae are positioned cranial to the diaphragm, and thus are not contained within the abdomen. The bodies and transverse processes of all of the lumbar vertebrae (L1–L7) contribute to the dorsal abdominal wall. The bodies and costal cartilages of ribs 9–13 contribute to the lateral abdominal wall. The shaft of the ilium makes a nominal contribution to the dorsal abdominal wall.

33. The answer is 4 [Chapter 40 III C 2]. Passage of a digestive structure through the inguinal canal is indicative of an inguinal hernia! The vaginal process is a peritoneal structure, the testis and spermatic cord are reproductive structures, and the external pudendal artery and vein are vascular structures that normally pass through the inguinal canal.

34. The answer is 2 [Chapter 40 III B]. The respiratory system is the only major body system not represented in the abdomen. The immune system is represented by the spleen, the endocrine system by the adrenal glands, and the reproductive system by the uterus and ovaries.

35. The answer is 4 [Chapter 41 IV B 1 c (2), 2 b (3)]. The rectus sheath is double-layered through the cranial and mid-regions of the abdomen. However, in the caudal regions just cranial to the pelvic brim, the rectus sheath lacks a deep layer, because the aponeurosis of the transversus abdominis muscles passes ventral to the rectus abdominis muscle, leaving the caudal-most part of the inner surface of the rectus abdominis muscle covered only by the transversalis fascia. Therefore, the veterinarian could use the rectus sheath to hold sutures if the incision was caudal to the xiphoid cartilage, cranial to the umbilicus, or between the xiphoid cartilage and the mid-abdominal region, but not if the incision was in the caudal abdominal region, cranial to the pelvic brim.

36. The answer is 1 [Chapter 41 VI]. The costoabdominal nerve is the last thoracic spinal nerve. The cranial iliohypogastric nerve is the ventral branch of spinal nerve L1; the caudal iliohypogastric nerve is the ventral branch of spinal nerve L2; and the ilioinguinal nerve is the ventral branch of spinal nerve L3.

37. The answer is 1 [Chapter 43 I C 1 c (2)]. The right lobe of the pancreas, not the left lobe, courses parallel to the descending duodenum, along essentially its full length. The major and minor duodenal papillae and the opening of the bile duct are present on the descending duodenum.

38. The answer is 4 [Chapter 45 II C 1 b, 2 b]. The dorsal vagal trunk is associated with the celiacomesenteric plexus. Innervation of the gut tube via the vagus nerve stops at the level of the left colic flexure (i.e., at the junction of the transverse and descending colons). The descending colon receives sympathetic innervation from the caudal mesenteric plexus, and parasympathetic innervation from the pelvic plexus.

39. The answer is 2 [Chapter 45 II A]. The lumbar splanchnic nerves deliver preganglionic sympathetic fibers to the cranial mesenteric and caudal mesenteric plexuses, which do not supply the stomach with autonomic innervation. The major splanchnic nerve, from sympathetic trunk segment T13, carries preganglionic sympathetic fibers to the celiac part of the celiacomesenteric plexus; these fibers are distributed to the stomach along the surfaces of the arteries that supply the stomach and arise from the celiac artery. The ventral vagal trunk supplies the stomach with parasympathetic innervation directly.

40. The answer is 4 [Chapter 46 III]. The uterine tube (salpinx) is not considered part of the uterus. This structure, the normal site of fertilization, extends from the ovary to the uterine horn and is supported by a portion of the broad ligament (mesosalpinx).

PART VII

PELVIC AND PERINEAL REGIONS

Chapter 49

Introduction to the Pelvic and Perineal Regions

I. PELVIC REGION. The pelvic region extends from the caudal border of the abdominal region to the caudal end of the body. The pelvic region comprises the **bony pelvis** and **its associated musculature,** as well as the **pelvic cavity** and **its contents.**

A. Bony pelvis

1. **Bones.** The bony pelvis is a bony ring formed around the pelvic cavity by the articulated **pelvic girdle, sacrum,** and **vertebrae Cd1–Cd2.** The bony pelvis is integral to both the caudal trunk and the pelvic limb.
   a. **Pelvic girdle (pelvis).** The pelvic girdle (i.e., the fused **ilium, ischium, pubis,** and **acetabular bones)** forms the lateral and ventral walls of the bony pelvis.
   b. **Sacrum** and **vertebrae Cd1–Cd2.** These bones, discussed in Chapter 18 III D–E, form the dorsal wall (roof) of the bony pelvis.
2. **Associated musculature.** Many of the proximal attachments of the gluteal muscles and the muscles of the cranial and caudal thigh are on the bony pelvis. Distally, these muscles attach to the bones of the pelvic limb.

B. Pelvic cavity

1. **Boundaries.** The pelvic cavity is **directly continuous with the abdominal cavity.**
   a. The **pelvic inlet** is the bony ring that surrounds the entrance to the pelvic cavity. The **borders of the pelvic inlet** are:
      (1) **Dorsally,** the promontory of the sacrum (see Chapter 18 III D 2 b)
      (2) **Laterally,** the arcuate line along the medial surface of the iliac shaft
      (3) **Ventrally,** the cranial border of the pubis (i.e., the pecten of the pubis)
   b. The **pelvic outlet** is the bony ring that designates the caudal border of the pelvic cavity. The **borders of the pelvic outlet** are:
      (1) **Dorsally,** vertebra Cd1
      (2) **Laterally,** the sacrotuberous ligament and middle gluteal muscle
      (3) **Ventrally,** the ischial arch
2. **Contents** of the pelvic cavity include the:
   a. Rectum and anal canal
   b. Neck of the urinary bladder and the urethra
   c. Caudal part of the uterine cervix and the vagina (in females)
   d. Ducti deferentia and the prostate gland (in males)

II. PERINEAL REGION (PERINEUM). The perineal region is the **caudal body surface** between the tail and the vulva or scrotum, and the immediately surrounding areas. The perineal region surrounds the pelvic outlet and presents features related mainly to the terminal gastrointestinal tract and the terminal (in females) or late (in males) parts of the reproductive tract.

A. The **anus** (i.e., the exit site from the body for the gastrointestinal tract) occupies the dorsal perineal region in both sexes.

B. The **vulva** (i.e., the exit site for the urinary and reproductive tracts) lies at the ventral perineal border in females.

C. The **root of the penis** lies just deep to the perineal skin in males.

Chapter 50

Bones, Joints, Ligaments, and Muscles of the Pelvic Region

I. BONES OF THE PELVIC REGION

A. Overview. The bones found within the pelvic region are all part of the skeleton of other body regions. The **bony pelvis** is a bony ring formed around the pelvic cavity by the articulated **pelvic girdle, sacrum,** and **vertebrae Cd1–Cd2** (Figure 50–1A).

1. The **pelvic girdle** comprises two symmetrical halves, the **ossa coxarum ("hip bones;"** singular, **os coxae).** The ossa coxarum fuse intimately with each other across the ventral midline to form a single strong bone. Each os coxae is composed of four bones (i.e., the **ilium,** the **ischium,** the **pubis,** and the **acetabular bone),** which are recognizable in puppies, but fused in adults.
2. The **sacrum** and **vertebrae Cd1–Cd2** are discussed in Chapter 18 III D–E.

B. Bones of the pelvic girdle

1. The **ilium** is the largest of the four bones that form the os coxae.
   - **a.** The **iliac wing,** the cranial-most part of the ilium, is broad both dorsoventrally and craniocaudally, and markedly compressed laterally (see Figure 50–1A).
     - **(1)** The **iliac crest,** the **cranial border of the iliac wing,** is notably thickened compared with the remainder of the iliac wing.

Canine Clinical Correlation

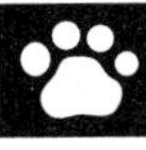

Rarely, the iliac crest does not fuse with the remainder of the iliac wing. Careful radiographic evaluation is necessary to avoid misinterpretation as a fracture.

     - **(2)** The **tuber sacrale,** the **dorsal border of the iliac wing,** is the area most closely associated with the sacrum.
     - **(3)** The **tuber coxae** is the **ventral border of the iliac wing.**
     - **(4)** The **iliac spines** are **small projections on the dorsal and ventral borders of the iliac wing** (Figure 50–1B). These spines are positioned at the cranial and caudal margins of the iliac wing, one dorsally and one ventrally.
     - **(5)** The **auricular surface** of the ilium is a "C"-shaped region on the medial surface of the iliac wing that articulates with the sacrum.
   - **b.** The **iliac body (shaft)** tapers caudoventrally from the iliac wing (see Figure 50–1).
     - **(1)** The **greater ischiatic (sciatic) notch** is a subtle, gently sloping concavity along the caudal part of the dorsal border of the iliac shaft (see Figure 50–1). In the intact state, the **sciatic nerve** and the **cranial** and **caudal gluteal artery, vein,** and **nerve** pass over this region.
     - **(2)** The **ischiatic spine** is a small elevation on the dorsal surface of the ilium, **where the ilium joins the ischium** (see Figure 50–1). The ischiatic spine marks the caudal limit of the greater ischiatic notch.
     - **(3)** The **tuberosity for the rectus femoris** is a thickened protuberance on the ventral surface of the iliac shaft near its caudal end, from which the rectus femoris muscle originates (see Figure 50–1B). The tuberosity lies just cranial to the acetabulum.

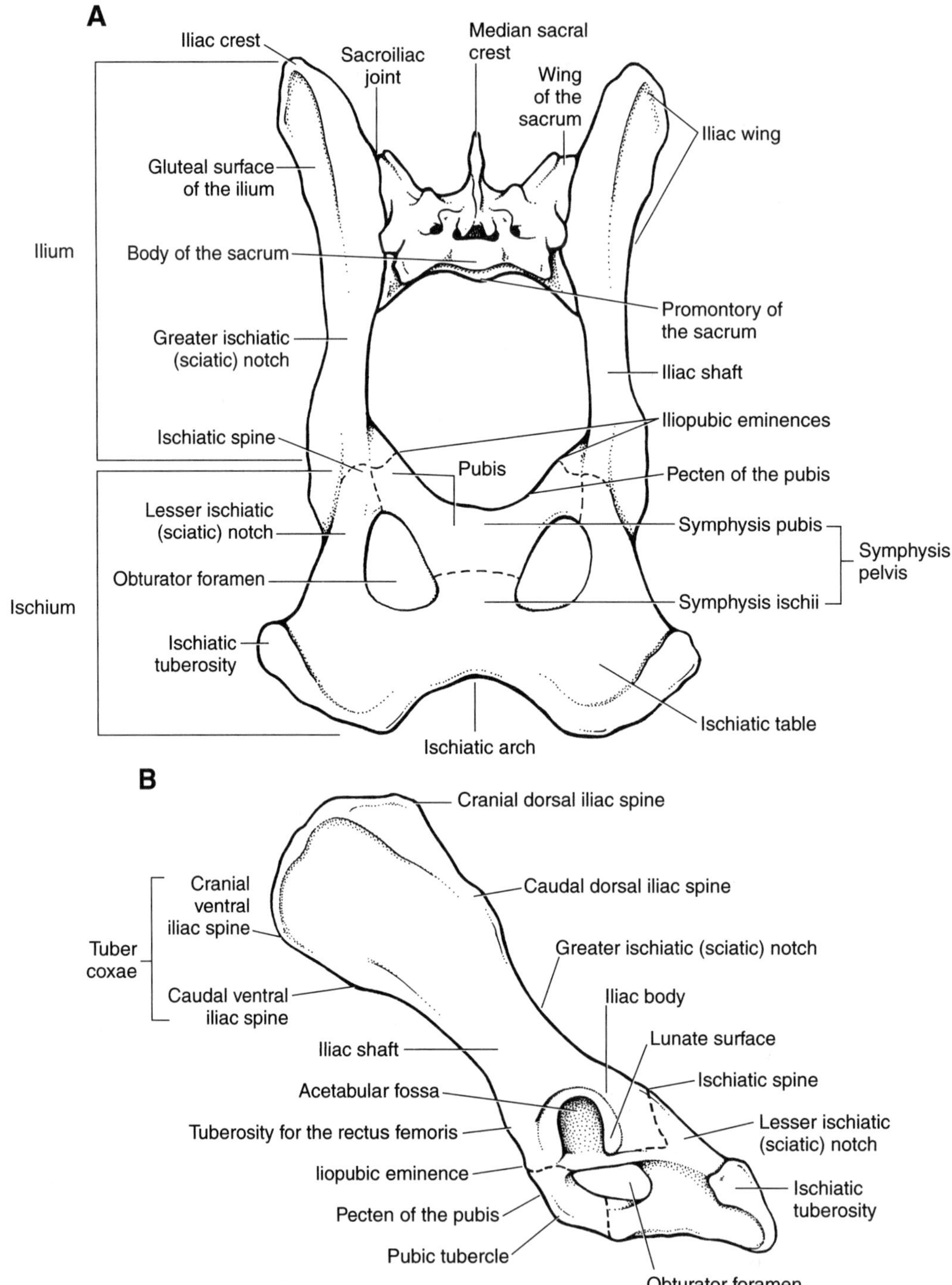

FIGURE 50–1. (*A*) The bony pelvis. The ossa coxarum (i.e., the two halves of the pelvic girdle) and the sacrum are shown; the first two caudal vertebrae also contribute to the bony pelvis. Each os coxae is formed by the ilium, the ischium, the pubis, and the acetabular bone; these four bones blend imperceptibly into one. The region of the acetabular bone is not visible in this view. (*B*) The left os coxae, lateral view.

(4) The **iliopubic eminence** is a subtle elevation positioned at the termination of the iliac shaft on its ventral surface, **where the ilium fuses with the pubis** (see Figure 50–1).

(5) The **arcuate line** is a low ridge of variable prominence passing along the ventral side of the medial surface of the iliac shaft; this line takes part in designating the end of the abdominal cavity and the beginning of the pelvic cavity.

c. The **gluteal surface of the ilium** is essentially its **lateral surface,** to which the middle and deep gluteal muscles attach (see Figure 50–1A).

2. The **ischium** forms most of the caudolateral as well as a portion of the caudomedial part of the pelvic girdle. This bone resembles a wide letter "U" (see Figure 50–1A) and is roughly horizontal *in situ.*

a. The **body of the ischium** extends cranially to fuse laterally with the caudal extremity of the iliac body.

(1) The **ischiatic spine** marks the **junction** of the **ischiatic body** and the **iliac body.**

(2) The **lesser ischiatic (sciatic) notch** is a faint depression along the dorsal edge of the ischiatic body caudal to the ischiatic spine.

(a) The proximity of the sacrotuberous ligament dorsal to this notch creates the impression of a complete border, referred to as the **lesser sciatic foramen.**

(b) In the intact state, the **tendon of the internal obturator muscle** passes across the lesser ischiatic notch *en route* to its insertion site.

b. The **ramus of the ischium** extends medially from the body, almost at a right angle. The ramus extends to the midline, where it fuses with its fellow from the opposite side at the symphysis pelvis.

c. The **ischiatic tuberosity** is a prominent convexity on the caudolateral-most area of the bone (see Figure 50–1). The sacrotuberous ligament (see II B 2) attaches to the ischiatic tuberosity.

3. The **pubis** forms the craniomedial part of the pelvic girdle and is roughly "L"-shaped (see Figure 50–1A).

a. The **body** of the pubis is positioned at the craniomedial edge of the ox coxae. The body of each pubis fuses with that of its fellow from the other side to contribute to the formation of the symphysis pelvis.

b. The **cranial ramus** extends craniolaterally from the body to fuse with the caudal part of the iliac shaft. The **iliopubic eminence** is positioned at the junction of the ilium and pubis.

c. The **caudal ramus** of the pubis extends caudally along the midline to fuse with the ischium and contribute to the formation of the symphysis pelvis.

4. The **acetabular bone,** the smallest of all the pelvic bones, forms most of the acetabulum (see I C 1) and does not extend beyond the borders of the acetabular cup. The acetabular bone fuses early with the remaining bones of the pelvic girdle and is the first to lose its identity.

C. Articulated pelvic girdle

1. The **acetabulum,** a deep hemispherical cup on the lateral surface of the pelvis, is formed by contributions from all four bones of the girdle (see Figure 50–1B). The **acetabular lip** is a rim of cartilage that encircles the open edge of the acetabulum, considerably deepening the cavity. The acetabulum provides the socket where the head of the femur articulates with the trunk. However, the entire acetabular surface does not actually contact the femoral head.

a. The **lunate surface** of the acetabulum is the large, crescent-shaped smooth surface within the cup of the acetabulum that provides the actual articular surface for the femoral head. The ligament to the head of the femur passes adjacent to the concave part of the crescent.

b. The **acetabular fossa** is the smaller, nonarticular surface in the depths of the acetabular cup.

2. The **pecten of the pubis (pecten ossis pubis)** is the cranial border of the fused pelvic girdle, formed by the fused cranial rami of the right and left pubes. The pecten extends from one iliopubic eminence to the other (see Figure 50–1A).

3. The **symphysis pelvis** (see Figure 50–1A) is the midline border where the two halves of the pelvic girdle articulate.
   a. The **pubis** and **ischium** fuse with their fellows from the opposite side and with each other to form the symphysis. Thus, the symphysis pelvis is formed by the combination of the **symphysis ischii** and the **symphysis pubis.**
   b. The **pubic tubercle** (an elevation on the ventral surface of the symphysis pelvis) and the **pecten of the pubis** (see Figure 50–1B) provide part of the attachment site for the **prepubic tendon,** a ligamentous structure that plays an important role in the attachment of all of the abdominal muscles, except for the transversus abdominis.
4. The **obturator foramen** is a large paired hole in the caudal part of the pelvic girdle. The obturator foramen is bordered by the pubis (craniomedially), the ischium (caudomedially), and the ilium (craniolaterally).
   a. In the intact state, the obturator foramen is closed by a membrane, and covered on both its dorsal and ventral surfaces by the **internal** and **external obturator muscles,** respectively.
   b. The **obturator nerve** and **obturator branch of the medial circumflex femoral artery** and **vein** pass over the craniomedial border of the obturator foramen.
5. The **ischiatic arch** (see Figure 50–1A) is a deep, broad, "U"-shaped concavity formed at the caudal-most extremity of the pelvis where the ramus of one ischium meets the other.

II. JOINTS AND LIGAMENTS OF THE PELVIC REGION

A. Joints

1. The **symphysis pelvis** is fibrocartilaginous in young animals, but normally ossifies as the animal matures.
   a. The age of onset and completion of ossification varies, even among individuals of the same breed.
   b. The joint is thought to soften near parturition to facilitate expulsion of the fetus through the pelvic outlet, but this feature is less important in species that bear litters of smaller fetuses (as opposed to species that bear a single, larger fetus).
2. The **sacroiliac joints** (one dorsal and one ventral) are partly synovial and partly fibrous. This combination permits secure attachment of the pelvic girdle (i.e., the proximal-most portion of the pelvic limb) to the axial skeleton at the sacrum, while enabling the joint to absorb the shock waves transmitted from the pelvic limb to the trunk.

B. Ligaments

1. The **sacroiliac ligaments** (one dorsal and one ventral on each side) extend between the wing of the ilium and the dorsal and ventral surfaces of the sacrum, respectively.
2. The **sacrotuberous ligament** is a stout bundle of collagenous fibers extending between the caudal part of the sacrum and the ischiatic tuberosity (Figure 50–2). This ligament provides attachment for the middle gluteal muscle, and the caudal gluteal vessels course along its ventral surface.

III. MUSCLES OF THE PELVIC REGION

A. Muscles of the pelvic limb. Many muscles of the pelvic limb (particularly the gluteal muscles) have extensive attachments to the pelvic girdle. Because the function of these muscles is related to the pelvic limb, these muscles are discussed in Chapter 59.

B. Muscles of the pelvic diaphragm. The pelvic diaphragm is a set of muscles that closes the caudal end of the pelvic cavity (i.e., the pelvic outlet). Because dogs are quadrupeds, most of the weight of the abdominal and pelvic viscera is borne by the muscles of the ventral

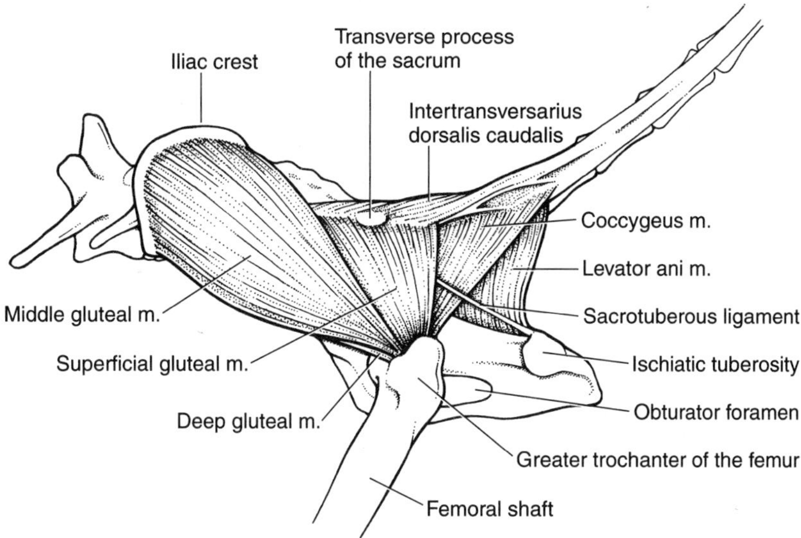

FIGURE 50–2. Muscles of the left pelvic diaphragm, lateral view. Note that the cranial part of the coccygeus muscle is covered by part of the superficial gluteal muscle, and that the coccygeus passes medial to the sacrotuberous ligament in its course.

belly wall; therefore, complete closure of the pelvic outlet by the pelvic diaphragm muscles is unnecessary. In species that walk erect, more complete closure is necessary, and the muscles more closely resemble a diaphragm in primates. The pelvic diaphragm is composed of two muscles, the coccygeus and the levator ani, both of which attach to the pelvic girdle and pass to the base of the tail.

1. The **coccygeus muscle** (see Figure 50–2) is a paired, "V"-shaped muscle that passes between the ischial spine and the tail base.
   a. **Course.** The coccygeus muscle originates from the **ischiatic spine** by a narrow tendon (the point of the "V") and courses dorsocaudally, fanning out cranially and caudally (like the arms of the "V") toward the lateral surface of the tail. The coccygeus muscle inserts on the **transverse processes of vertebrae Cd2–Cd5.**
   b. **Innervation.** The coccygeus muscle is innervated by the **ventral branch of the third sacral nerve (S3).**
   c. **Action.** The coccygeus muscle **depresses the tail.**
2. The **levator ani muscle,** also "V"-shaped, is thinner but broader than the coccygeus muscle, extending beyond the borders of the coccygeus cranially as well as caudally (see Figure 50–2). The levator ani lies medial to the coccygeus muscle.
   a. **Course**
      (1) **Origin.** The levator ani originates along the **medial border of the iliac body,** the **inner surface of the pubic ramus,** and the **full length of the symphysis pelvis.**
      (2) **Insertion.** From its broad origin, the levator ani passes toward the **hemal process of vertebra Cd7.** Along the way, its fibers converge to form a distinct, stout tendon.
   b. **Innervation.** The levator ani is innervated by the **ventral branches of spinal nerves S3** and **Cd1.**
   c. **Action.** Acting bilaterally, the levator ani muscle **depresses the tail** and **compresses the rectum** (assisting in defecation). Acting unilaterally, it **draws the tail laterally.**

Chapter 51

Peritoneum and Viscera of the Pelvic Region

I. INTRODUCTION

A. Viscera. The terminal parts of three organ systems are located within the pelvic cavity. Dorsal to ventral, these organ systems are the **gastrointestinal, reproductive,** and **urinary systems** (Figure 51–1A).

B. Peritoneum. The abdominal and pelvic cavities are continuous; therefore, the peritoneum enters the pelvic cavity and passes over the surfaces of the pelvic viscera. As within the abdomen, the layer of peritoneum within the pelvis has **parietal** and **visceral** portions.

1. The peritoneum **does not extend to the caudal pelvic wall;** instead, it reflects back on itself when it reaches its caudal limit, forming five blind-ended pouches. Two of these pouches are paired.
2. Because the organs pass through the full length of the pelvic cavity but the peritoneum does not, only the cranial portion of **some organs** (e.g., the rectum) **is covered by peritoneum** (see Figure 51–1A).

II. PERITONEUM

A. Pouches

1. The **pararectal fossae** are the paired extensions of peritoneum that pass laterally along each side of the rectum (see Figure 51–1).
2. The **rectogenital pouch** lies between the rectum and the uterus or prostate gland (see Figure 51–1).
3. The **vesicogenital pouch** lies between the urinary bladder (*vesico* = hollow organ) and the uterus (in females) or the ducti deferentia (in males).
   a. In **females,** the vesicogenital pouch is **well-developed** (see Figure 51–1).
   b. In **males,** the vesicogenital pouch is **poorly developed** or **absent** because the tubular part of the reproductive tract consists of the paired, narrow ducti deferentia rather than the large uterus. The **rectogenital** and **vesicogenital pouches may blend together to form the rectovesical pouch** between the rectum and the bladder.
4. The **pubovesical pouch** is positioned most ventrally, between the pubis and the neck of the urinary bladder (see Figure 51–1).
   a. In **males,** the pubovesical pouch is intimately related to the prostate gland, which surrounds the neck of the urinary bladder.
   b. In **females,** the pubovesical pouch is smaller (or even absent) because the peritoneum reflects directly from the bladder to the ventral abdominal wall.

B. Ligaments

1. The **mesometrial portion** of the **broad ligament of the uterus** continues from the abdominal cavity into the pelvic cavity, along with the uterus (see Chapter 46 I B 3 c and Figure 51–1B).
2. The **ligaments of the urinary bladder** are three peritoneal folds that attach the bladder to the surrounding pelvic walls. **Vessels, nerves, portions of the ureters** and **ducti deferentia,** some **embryonic remnants,** and generous amounts of **body fat** are sandwiched between the layers of the ligaments.
   a. The **lateral ligaments of the bladder,** which are paired and triangular, extend be-

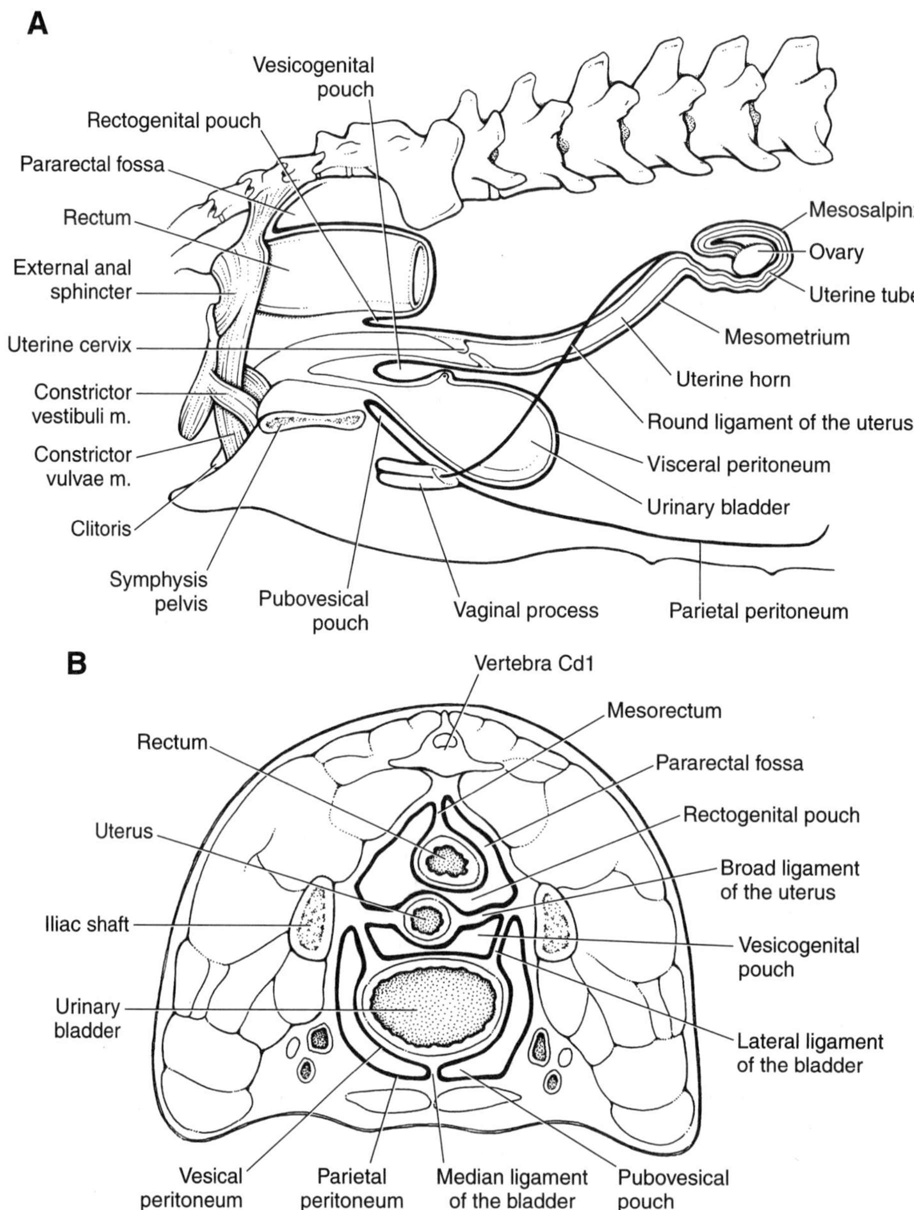

FIGURE 51–1. Peritoneum of the pelvic region in the female. (*A*) Right parasagittal view. Note the location of the gastrointestinal, reproductive, and urinary systems in the pelvic region. (*B*) Transverse section, showing the ligaments of the bladder and the five peritoneal pouches. (Part *A* modified with permission from Evans HE, 1993, *Miller's Anatomy of the Dog*, 3e. Philadelphia, WB Saunders, p 532. Part *B* modified with permission from Evans HE, deLahunta A: *Miller's Guide to the Dissection of the Dog*, 4e. Philadelphia, WB Saunders, 1996, p 218.)

tween each lateral surface of the bladder and the lateral pelvic wall (see Figure 51–1B).

(1) In **females,** each of the bladder's lateral ligaments **blends with the broad ligament of the uterus.**

(2) During development, the paired **umbilical arteries** of the fetus course through the lateral edges of the lateral ligaments of the bladder and exit the abdominal cavity at the umbilicus.

(a) After birth, the umbilical arteries fibrose and form thickened cords (i.e., the **round ligaments of the bladder).** The round ligaments of the bladder are contained in the lateral edge of the bladder's lateral ligaments, between the umbilicus and the cranial part of the body of the urinary bladder.

(b) The portions of the umbilical arteries between the aorta and the internal iliac arteries remain patent. After birth, the arteries arising from the internal iliac arteries retain the name of umbilical arteries; as the umbilical arteries gain the surface of the urinary bladder, their name changes to **cranial vesical arteries.**

b. The unpaired **median ligament of the bladder** extends between the bladder and the ventral body wall. The ligament extends along the full length of the ventral wall of the bladder.

III. GASTROINTESTINAL VISCERA

GASTROINTESTINAL VISCERA in the pelvic region include the **rectum** and the **anal canal.** The **anorectal line** is the visible demarcation between the rectum and the anal canal.

A. The **rectum** (see Figure 51–1A) is the direct continuation of the descending colon in the pelvic region.

1. **Position.** The rectum extends in a straight course from the **pelvic inlet to the anal canal,** which begins at the level of vertebrae Cd1–Cd2.
2. **Musculature.** The paired **rectococcygeus muscles** sweep from the lateral surfaces of the rectum and pass dorsally and medially onto the ventral surface of the tail. The rectococcygeus muscles pass as far caudally as vertebra Cd6, and assist in defecation by drawing the rectum and anal canal caudally.
3. **Vascularization.** The **cranial, middle,** and **caudal rectal arteries** supply the rectum. These arteries are branches of the **caudal mesenteric, vaginal** or **prostatic,** and **internal pudendal arteries,** respectively.
4. **Innervation** is autonomic, provided by the **pelvic plexus.** Fibers leave the pelvic plexus and follow the arteries to the target organs.
   a. The **hypogastric nerves** deliver **sympathetic fibers** to the pelvic plexus.
   b. The **pelvic nerve** delivers **parasympathetic fibers** to the same plexus.

B. The **anal canal** is the 1-inch-long terminal portion of the gastrointestinal tract. The anal canal has three zones.

1. The **columnar zone** is the most cranial region of the anal canal, measuring only about 1 centimeter in length.
   a. This band is characterized by **anal columns** (i.e., columnar ridges of mucosa oriented longitudinally or somewhat obliquely). The anal columns are irregular in size and length, but as a group begin at the anorectal line and extend caudally to the next region of the anal canal, the intermediate zone.
   b. **Anal sinuses** are small blind pouches formed between the elevations of adjacent anal columns.
2. The **intermediate zone (anocutaneous line)** is approximately 1 millimeter wide. This region separates the innermost region of the anal canal (i.e., the columnar zone) from the outermost region (i.e., the cutaneous zone).
3. The **cutaneous zone,** the most caudal portion of the anal canal, has an **internal** and **ex-**

ternal region. The **anus** (i.e., the terminal opening of the gastrointestinal tract) lies at the junction of the internal and external regions of the cutaneous zone.

a. The **internal region** of the cutaneous zone extends from the anocutaneous line caudally to the anus. This region has a **moist surface** and houses the openings of the **anal sacs.**

b. The **external region** of the cutaneous zone is the relatively hairless region of skin surrounding the anus. Although technically part of the perineum, this region is discussed here for the sake of continuity.

  (1) This region is covered in **dry skin** and houses the openings of the **circumanal glands,** which form small elevations on the skin's surface (see Chapter 2; Figure 2–2).

  (2) The external region of the cutaneous zone is **wider in intact, older male dogs** (owing to the testosterone-driven continuous growth of the circumanal glands beneath the skin).

Canine Clinical Correlation

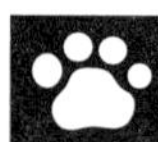

Because of the responsiveness of the circumanal glands to testosterone, benign tumors (adenomas) of these glands are common in older intact males. Castration is often the simplest treatment.

C. The **anal region** comprises the anal canal and the associated structures.

1. **Musculature**

  a. The **internal anal sphincter** is a condensation of the fibers of the inner circular layer of the caudal-most rectum and the anal canal. This sphincter is composed of **smooth muscle.**

  b. The **external anal sphincter** is a circular layer of **skeletal muscle** positioned external to the internal anal sphincter. Because the external anal sphincter is formed from skeletal muscle, it is under voluntary control and plays the greatest role in inhibiting or initiating defecation.

2. **Vascularization**

  a. **Arterial supply** is provided mostly by the **caudal rectal artery,** a branch of the **internal pudendal artery.**

  b. **Venous drainage** is via **satellite veins** of the caudal rectal and internal pudendal arteries.

  c. **Lymphatic drainage** passes mainly to the **internal iliac lymph nodes;** when the **sacral lymph nodes** are present, they, too, receive drainage from the anal region.

3. **Innervation**

  a. **Autonomic innervation** is provided by the **pelvic plexus.**

  b. **Somatic innervation** of the external anal sphincter is provided by the **pudendal nerve.**

4. **Anal sacs** are paired saccular structures positioned between the internal and external anal sphincter muscles (see Chapter 2, Figure 2–2).

  a. The **glands of the anal sac** are numerous microscopic glands located within the walls of the anal sacs.

    (1) These glands **produce a serous to gummy secretion** that functions in individual recognition and territorial marking.

    (2) The ducts of these glands **open directly into the anal sacs.**

  b. The **anal sacs open onto the internal region of the cutaneous zone of the anal canal** by means of a single duct for each sac. The anal sacs vary in size according to the amount of secretion contained within them.

    (1) The positioning of the anal sacs between the external and internal anal sphincters

normally assists with the expulsion of the contents of the anal sacs with each bowel movement.

(2) The secretions of the anal sac glands may become inspissated when the normal emptying mechanism does not operate properly and the sacs are not regularly evacuated.

Canine Clinical Correlation

Despite the positioning of the anal sacs between the two anal sphincters, many dogs have difficulty with emptying them. Various complications can result, including enlargement of the sacs, obstruction, abscessation and associated constipation, and rupture. Owners of dogs with abnormally emptying anal sacs may report that the dog "scoots" its rear along the ground. Manual expression of the sacs is usually sufficient treatment for dogs with enlarged (or sometimes even impacted) sacs; animals with abscessed or ruptured glands may require surgical removal of the anal sacs (anal sacculectomy).

5. **Glands.** Three groups of glands are associated with the anal region.
   a. The **glands of the anal sac** are discussed in III C 4 a.
   b. The **anal glands** are distinct from the glands of the anal sac. These microscopic glands discharge a fatty secretion by means of ducts opening at the anocutaneous line.
   c. The **circumanal glands** are positioned subcutaneously and circumferentially around the anus [see III B 3 b (1)].

IV. REPRODUCTIVE VISCERA in the pelvic region include mainly the **vagina** in females, and the **prostate gland** in males.

A. Female

1. The **vagina,** a muscular, distensible portion of the tubular female reproductive tract, extends from the caudal end of the cervix to the cranial end of the vestibule. The vagina thus extends beyond the pelvic cavity both cranially and caudally (Figure 51–2A).
   a. **Features.** The mucosal surface of the vagina presents **longitudinal folds** that contribute to the distensibility of the vaginal wall.
   b. **Vascularization**
      (1) **Arterial supply** to the vagina is provided through the paired **vaginal arteries,** which are branches of the internal pudendal arteries.
      (2) **Venous drainage** occurs via **satellite veins.**
      (3) **Lymphatic drainage** passes to the **internal iliac lymph nodes.**
   c. **Innervation**
      (1) **Autonomic innervation** (both sympathetic and parasympathetic) arrives from branches of the **pelvic plexus.**
      (2) **Somatic innervation** is provided by the **pudendal nerve.**
2. The **vestibule** is the final common passageway from both the uterus and the urinary bladder to the exterior of the body. Although the vestibule is not technically part of the reproductive system, it is discussed here because of its intimate association with the caudal part of the vagina.
   a. **Features**
      (1) The **urethral tubercle,** more of a ridge along the vestibular floor than a discrete elevation, marks the point where the vagina and urethra enter a final common passageway (i.e., **where the vestibule originates).**
      (2) The mucosa of the vestibule is **smooth,** rather than longitudinally ridged like that of the vagina.

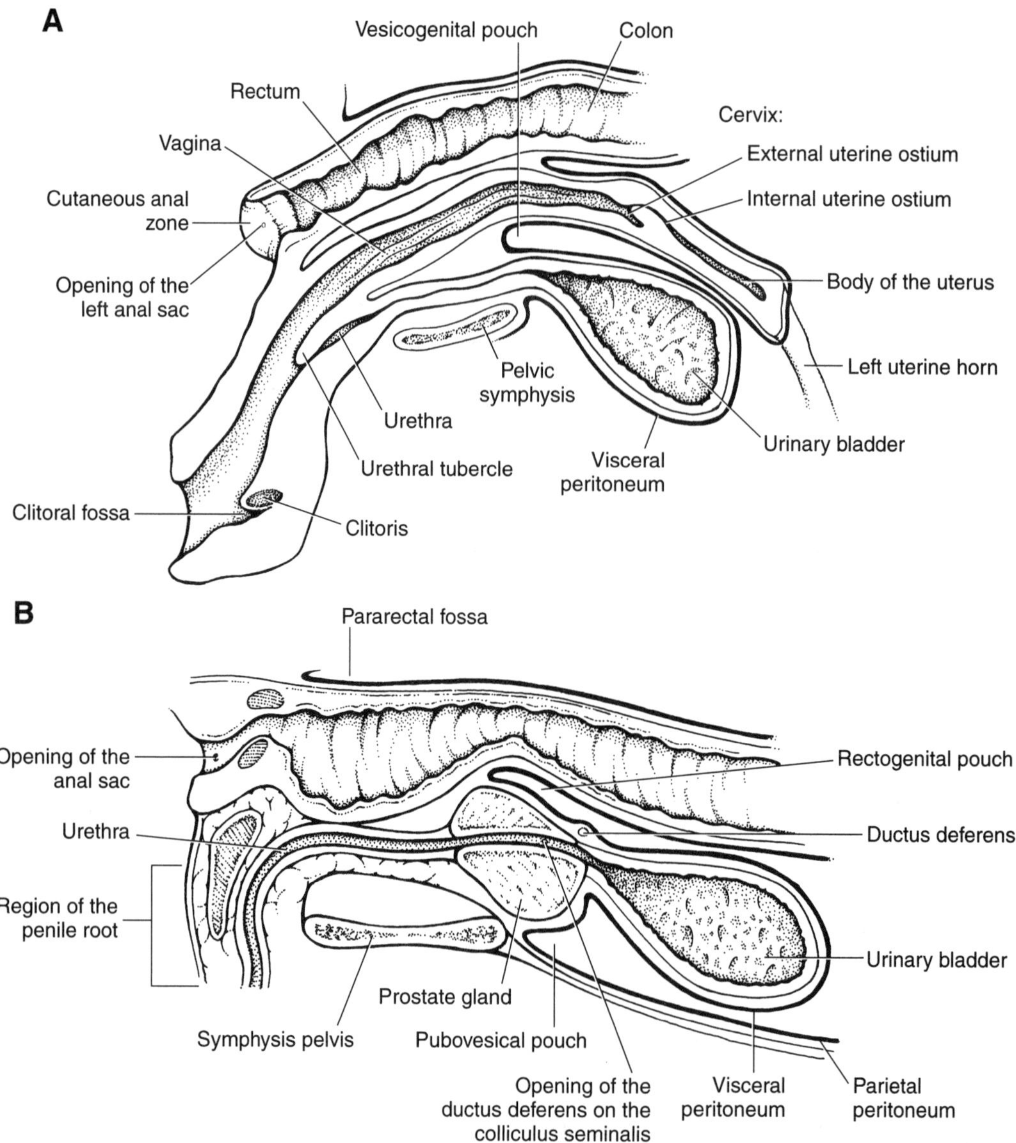

FIGURE 51–2. Pelvic viscera in (A) the female (left view, median section) and (B) the male (left parasagittal view). [Part *A* modified with permission from Evans HE, 1993, *Miller's Anatomy of the Dog,* 3e. Philadelphia, WB Saunders, p 542. Part *B* modified with permission from Evans HE, deLahunta A: *Miller's Guide to the Dissection of the Dog,* 4e. Philadelphia, WB Saunders, 1996, p 217.]

b. **Vascularization** and **innervation** are the same as the vascularization and innervation of the vagina.

B. Male

1. The **prostate gland,** a **bilobed organ** surrounding the neck of the urinary bladder and the urethra, is the **only accessory sex gland in the dog.** (Unlike other domestic mammals, the dog lacks bulbourethral and vesicular glands.)
   a. **Position**
      (1) The prostate gland rests against the pelvic symphysis ventrally, and the rectum dorsally (Figure 51–2B).

Canine Clinical Correlation

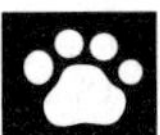

The proximity of the rectum and the prostate gland together with the thinness of the rectal wall facilitates digital palpation *per rectum* of the prostate gland. This procedure should be part of the physical examination of intact male dogs, regardless of age.

Canine Clinical Correlation

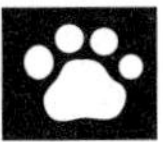

Primary prostatic disease (e.g., benign hyperplasia, abscessation, malignant neoplasia) is often manifested clinically with signs related to other nearby body systems, such as constipation and dysuria.

(2) The entire prostate gland resides within the pelvic cavity until the dog becomes sexually mature. Under the influence of testosterone, the gland enlarges, so that in an intact young adult dog, a large portion of the prostate gland lies in the abdominal cavity. In elderly intact dogs with prostatic hyperplasia, nearly all of the enlarged gland may reside within the abdominal cavity.

Canine Clinical Correlation

Castration of a dog of any age will cause a marked decrease in the size of the gland by removing the influence of testosterone. The incidence of prostatic disease is greatly reduced in dogs who are neutered at an early age.

Canine Clinical Correlation

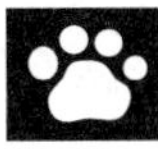

Castration is often employed as part of the treatment for various forms of prostatic disease, and is highly effective in reducing benign forms of enlargement.

b. Function. The secretions of the prostate gland contribute to the seminal fluid. Because the prostatic portion of the male urethra [see V C 1 b (1)] passes through the prostate gland, the **ducts of the prostate gland** open directly into the lumen of the prostatic urethra.

c. Vascularization

(1) Arterial supply arrives via the **prostatic artery,** a branch of the **internal pudendal artery.**

(2) Venous drainage departs via **satellite veins** of the prostatic arteries.

(3) Lymphatic drainage from the prostate gland passes to the **iliac lymph nodes.** This fact is important to know when evaluating and treating prostatic carcinoma.

d. Innervation. The prostate gland receives **sympathetic** and **parasympathetic** fibers from the **pelvic plexus.** The central part of the pelvic plexus, the region most directly associated with the prostate gland, is sometimes referred to as the **prostatic plexus.**

2. Ducti deferentia. The **ducti deferentia** pass through the pelvic cavity, but originate and terminate outside of the cavity. Their course through the pelvic cavity and their relation to other intrapelvic organs is discussed in Chapter 52 III D 1.

V. URINARY VISCERA

A. Ureters. The ureters enter the pelvic cavity as they continue caudally from the kidneys. Each ureter crosses ventral to the external iliac artery, passes between the two layers of the lateral ligament of the bladder, and enters the dorsal surface of the urinary bladder relatively far cranially, a few centimeters caudal to the bladder's neck. After entering the urinary bladder at an oblique angle, the ureters tunnel through the musculature for a short distance before entering the bladder's lumen. This oblique course through the bladder's walls assists in preventing urine reflux into the ureter.

1. In **females,** the ureters are related to the uterine broad ligament through the more caudal portion of their course.
2. In **males,** the ductus deferens loops around the ureter near the neck of the bladder.

B. Urinary bladder

1. **Position.** The most terminal part of the urinary bladder (i.e., the neck) is always located within the pelvic cavity. The position of the rest of the bladder varies according to its size.
   a. When distended, much of the urinary bladder lies within the abdominal cavity.
      (1) Dorsally, relations include the jejunum, the descending colon, and the caudal parts of the tubular reproductive organs (i.e., the uterine body and cervix in females and the ducti deferentia in males).
      (2) Ventrally, the distended bladder lies on the ventral abdominal wall, or on the dorsal surface of the deep wall of the greater omentum when that structure has moved caudally.
   b. When contracted, the bladder normally rests on the pelvic brim, and is entirely intrapelvic.

2. **Structure.** The urinary bladder is a muscular structure possessing an apex, a body, and a neck. The wall of the urinary bladder comprises three muscular layers—a circular middle layer interposed between two longitudinal layers. These layers are sometimes referred to collectively as the **detrusor muscle.**
   a. The **apex** of the urinary bladder is its blind, rounded **cranial end.** When maximally distended, the apex may reach cranially as far as the umbilicus. Distention to this degree is painful.
   b. The **body,** the **main part** of the bladder, is notable for its distensibility. Like the apex, the body is highly mobile according to degree of fullness.
   c. The **neck** is the **terminal portion** of the urinary bladder, where it narrows to join the urethra. The neck is relatively fixed in its intrapelvic position, even when the bladder is maximally distended.
      (1) The **internal urethral sphincter** (see also V C 2) is positioned at the caudal end of the bladder's neck.
      (2) The **prostate gland** surrounds the neck of the bladder in male dogs.

3. **Features**
   a. The **trigone** is a triangular region on the internal surface of the dorsal wall of the bladder.
      (1) An imaginary line drawn between the points where the ureters enter the bladder and from each ureter entrance point to the urethral orifice denotes the triangular area of the trigone.
      (2) The mucosa of the trigone presents ill-defined ridges directed toward the urethra, but lacks the mucosal folds characteristic of the rest of the bladder's internal surface.
   b. The **urachus** is a fetal structure (the allantoic stalk) that extends between the lumen of the urinary bladder and the umbilical cord. Occasionally, a slight thickening in the free edge of the bladder's median ligament remains as a reminder of the original position of the urachus.

Canine Clinical Correlation

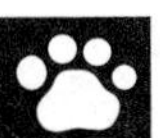

Occasionally the urachus remains patent, causing urine to drip continually from the umbilical cord in the neonate. Treatment of **patent urachus** is surgical and is associated with an excellent prognosis.

Canine Clinical Correlation

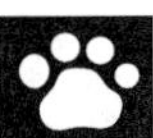

Persistence of a widened area at the original site of the urachal exit is referred to as a **vesicourachal diverticulum.** This area typically does not empty completely during urination, leading to a small, static pool of urine. This condition can predispose the dog to lower urinary tract infections, as well as complicate treatment of these infections. Surgical intervention is sometimes necessary to remove the diverticulum.

4. **Vascularization**
   a. **Arterial supply.** The paired **cranial vesical** and **caudal vesical arteries** deliver arterial blood to the urinary bladder.
      (1) The **cranial vesical artery,** a branch of the **umbilical artery,** supplies the cranial region of the bladder's body.
      (2) The **caudal vesical artery,** a branch of the **vaginal** or **prostatic artery,** supplies the neck region of the bladder.
   b. **Venous drainage.** The urinary bladder is drained by a **venous plexus** located on its surface. The plexus drains into the **internal pudendal veins.**
   c. **Lymphatic drainage.** The efferent lymphatic vessels of the urinary bladder drain into the **hypogastric** and **lumbar lymph nodes.**

5. **Innervation.** The urinary bladder receives **sympathetic** and **parasympathetic innervation** via the **pelvic plexus,** and **somatic innervation** via the **pudendal nerve.**
   a. Sympathetic innervation
      (1) Sympathetic fibers travel mainly to the region of the **trigone** and to the bladder's **apex;** a few fibers are present over the bladder's neck and body.
      (2) Sympathetic tone relaxes the bladder and constricts the internal urethral sphincter, favoring the **retention of urine.** In addition, sympathetic fibers carry the afferent nerves that convey the **pain** of an overfull bladder.
   b. **Parasympathetic innervation**
      (1) Parasympathetic fibers are widely distributed over the **detrusor muscle,** which forms much of the substance of the bladder's neck and body.
      (2) Parasympathetic tone contracts the detrusor muscle, leading to the **voiding of urine.**
   c. **Somatic innervation.** The pudendal nerve supplies fibers to the external sphincter of the bladder, as well as to the striated urethral musculature. These fibers carry impulses necessary for **voluntary withholding** and **voiding of urine.**

C. **Urethra.** The urethra is a tubular organ that extends from the neck of the urinary bladder to the external body surface.

1. **Form.** Because the urethra functions as part of the reproductive system as well as part of the urinary system in the male, considerable differences in the form of the urethra exist between the sexes.
   a. The **female urethra** is shorter and simpler in form, because it functions only in the elimination of urine. The urethra of the bitch arises from the neck of the urinary bladder (near the pelvic brim) and courses caudally with a slight ventral inclination, terminating at the junction of the vagina and the vestibule. (Throughout its course, the urethra lies just ventral to the vagina; see Figure 51–2A.)

b. The **male urethra** is divided into three regions (see Figure 51–2B):
   (1) The **prostatic urethra** is the most proximal region, where the organ is surrounded by the prostate gland. The prostatic urethra presents several features.
      (a) The **urethral crest** is a low longitudinal ridge of tissue along the urethra's dorsal midline. The numerous, minute **prostatic ducts** open into the prostatic urethra around the urethral crest.
      (b) The **colliculus seminalis** is a small, elliptical knob at approximately the midpoint of the urethral crest.
         (i) Each **ductus deferens** opens just lateral to the colliculus seminalis.
         (ii) When present, the **prostatic utricle (uterus masculinus)** opens onto the center of the colliculus seminalis. This tiny, blind tubular structure is a remnant of the paramesonephric ducts (the primordia of the uterus).
   (2) The **pelvic urethra** succeeds the prostatic part and extends as far caudally as the pelvic outlet.
   (3) The **penile urethra** is the part of the urethra that extends from the pelvic outlet through the full length of the penis, to open to the exterior of the body at the distal tip of the glans penis.

2. **Musculature.** Two **urethral sphincters** are recognized.
   a. The **internal urethral sphincter** (sometimes called the "internal sphincter of the bladder") is located at the junction of the neck of the bladder and the urethra and is similar in both sexes. The internal urethral sphincter is formed of **smooth muscle** and is under strictly **autonomic** control.
   b. The **external urethral sphincter** is formed of **skeletal muscle** (i.e., the **urethralis muscle)** and is under **voluntary** control.
      (1) In **females,** the external urethral sphincter is positioned near the junction of the urethra and the vestibule.
      (2) In **males,** the external urethral sphincter extends from near the neck of the bladder (just caudal to the prostate gland) to the root of the penis.

3. **Vascularization** of the urethra differs somewhat between males and females, although the pattern is similar in the proximal-most regions because this area is supplied by the gender-specific branch of the internal pudendal artery.
   a. **Arterial supply and venous drainage**
      (1) **Females.** The urethra is supplied by the (paired) **urethral branch of the vaginal artery,** and drained by its satellite vein.
      (2) **Males**
         (a) The **prostatic** and **pelvic urethra** is supplied by the (paired) **urethral branch of the prostatic artery,** and drained by its satellite vein.
         (b) The **penile urethra** is supplied by the (paired) **urethral branch of the artery of the penile bulb,** and drained by its satellite vein.
   b. **Lymphatic drainage** of the ureter passes to the **iliac, hypogastric, superficial inguinal,** and **sacral lymph nodes.**

4. **Innervation** of the urethra varies according to the type of muscle.
   a. **Smooth muscle** is innervated by **autonomic fibers** from the **pelvic plexus.** This innervation is **mainly sympathetic.**
   b. **Skeletal muscle** receives **sympathetic innervation** from the **pelvic plexus** and **somatic innervation** from the **pudendal nerve.**

Chapter 52

Genitalia in the External Pelvic and Perineal Regions

I. HOMOLOGOUS STRUCTURES. The clitoris and penis are homologous structures, as are the labia and the scrotum. The gender-specific differences observed in the external pelvic region relate mainly to two factors:

A. The degree of development of the erectile organ

B. The positioning of the male gonad external to the abdominal cavity and the extension and fusion along the ventral midline of paired skin folds (which originate from the same region as the bitch's vulva) to provide the pouch that houses the gonads (i.e., the scrotum)

II. FEMALE EXTERNAL GENITALIA. The external genitalia of the bitch comprises the **vulva** and the **clitoris.***

A. Vulva. The vulva is the only external female genital structure that is visible to the eye without manipulating the genitalia.

1. **Position.** The vulva is positioned on the external body surface, at the caudal termination of the vestibule. The vulva lies considerably ventral to the pelvic outlet (see Chapter 51, Figure 51–2A).
2. **Form.** The vulva is composed of paired **labia,** which meet at the **dorsal** and **ventral commissures.**
   a. The **labia,** which are thick and fleshy, are composed of connective tissue containing abundant elastic fibers, smooth muscle, and fat. The labia are relatively small and firm in anestrus, but large and soft during estrus.
   b. The **dorsal commissure** is relatively rounded, but hidden by a skin fold.
   c. The **ventral commissure** is quite pointed, and may bear a small tuft of hair.
3. **Musculature**
   a. **Smooth muscle.** The smooth muscles of the vulva are mainly continuations of the smooth muscle coats of the vagina and vestibule.
   b. **Skeletal muscle.** Three skeletal muscles are associated with the vulva. These muscles are homologous with the skeletal muscles of the penis in male dogs (see III F 3 a).
      (1) The **ischiourethralis muscle** is smaller in females than in males. In males, this muscle plays an essential role in copulation, but in females, contraction of this muscle is not necessary for normal copulation to occur.
      (2) The **ischiocavernosus muscle** arises from the ischial arch and inserts on the crura of the clitoris.
      (3) The **constrictor vestibuli** and **constrictor vulvae muscles** are homologous with the bulbospongiosus muscle of the male.
         (a) The **constrictor vestibuli,** a muscle of considerable substance, is positioned relatively cranially and surrounds the urethra, vestibule, and caudal part of the vagina.
            (i) The **vestibular bulb** [homologous to the bulb of the penis; see III F 2 a (1) (a)] is a mass of erectile tissue within the wall of the cranial vestibular region, deep to the constrictor vestibuli muscle.

*Although the female urethra is listed as part of the female external genitalia in the *Nomina Anatomica Veterinaria,* this structure most intuitively fits with the urinary tract and was discussed in Chapter 51 V C 1 a.

(ii) During copulation, contraction of the constrictor vestibuli muscle and engorgement of the vestibular bulb functions to compress the penis caudal to the bulbus glandis, allowing completion of erection.

(b) The **constrictor vulvae,** a thinner muscle positioned more caudally, encircles the vulva and vestibule just caudal to the urethral tubercle. This muscle functions during copulation to raise the vulva prior to intromission, facilitating entry of the penis.

4. **Vascularization**
   a. **Arterial supply.** The vulva is supplied by branches of the **vaginal artery.** In addition, the **internal pudendal artery** supplies the vestibular bulb, and the **external pudendal artery** supplies the labia.
   b. **Venous drainage** occurs through **satellite veins.**
   c. **Lymphatic drainage** passes to the **superficial inguinal lymph nodes.**

5. **Innervation**
   a. **Autonomic innervation.** Both **sympathetic** and **parasympathetic** fibers pass from the **pelvic plexus** to the musculature and blood vessels of the vulva.
   b. **Somatic innervation**
      (1) The **pudendal** and **genitofemoral nerves** provide somatic **sensory** innervation to the **labia.**
      (2) The **pudendal nerve** supplies **motor** innervation to the **ischiourethralis, constrictor vestibuli,** and **constrictor vulvae muscles.**

B. Clitoris. The clitoris is the female erectile organ. Despite being erectile, the clitoris plays no essential role in the mechanics of copulation.

1. **Position.** The **clitoral fossa** is a depression in the ventral wall of the labia, just proximal to the ventral commissure, into which the free part of the clitoris projects. The clitoral fossa is readily visualized by gently parting the labia.
2. **Form.** The clitoris, like the penis, is composed of paired **roots,** a **body,** and a **glans.** An **os clitoridis,** homologous to the os penis, may be present in the clitoral body. These structures are discussed in detail in III F.

Canine Clinical Correlation

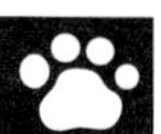

Common clinical procedures (e.g., passage of an instrument into the vagina, urinary catheterization) necessitate an understanding of the positions of the vulva, clitoral fossa, vestibule, external urethral orifice, and caudal part of the vagina relative to the position of the bony pelvic outlet and the cranial continuation of the vagina (see Chapter 51, Figure 51–2A).

- **Accessing the vagina.** Direct cranial passage of an instrument through the vulva will lodge the instrument in the clitoral fossa, an event that is both futile and painful. In order to successfully access the vagina, the instrument must be passed dorsally along the caudal vestibular wall until it is past the pelvic outlet; after reaching the dorsal wall of the vestibule, the instrument may be angled cranially and dorsally to access the vagina.
- **Accessing the urethra.** First, the catheter must be passed dorsally along the cranial wall of the vestibule, and then it can be angled cranially and ventrally to access the external urethral orifice.

3. **Vasculature.** The clitoris is supplied by the **artery of the clitoris;** venous drainage occurs via the **satellite vein.** Lymphatic drainage is via the **superficial inguinal lymph nodes.**
4. **Innervation.** The **dorsal nerve of the clitoris,** a branch of the **pudendal nerve,** provides **somatic sensory innervation** to the clitoris. This pattern of innervation is the same as that of the penis.

III. MALE EXTERNAL GENITALIA

A. Scrotum. The scrotum, a pouch of skin carried high between the thighs in the caudal inguinal region, houses the testes. Various features of the scrotum allow it to control testicular temperature by either facilitating or inhibiting heat loss.

1. **Form**
   a. **Layers.** All layers of the abdominal wall are represented in the scrotal wall, which is an outpouching of the abdominal wall.
      (1) **Skin** covers the external scrotal surface. This **variably pigmented** skin is relatively **thin** (facilitating heat loss), **slightly oily,** and **sparsely covered by fine hairs.** Little subcutaneous fat is present, which also facilitates heat loss.
      (2) **Muscle.** The **tunica dartos,** a thin layer of smooth muscle, elastic fibers, and collagenous fibers, lies just deep to the skin. The tunica dartos contracts the scrotal skin when the cremaster muscle draws the testes near the body, as occurs in cold temperatures or under sympathetic drive.
      (3) **Fascia.** The **internal spermatic fascia** lies deep to the dartos muscle and is the **continuation** of the **transversalis fascia** of the abdominal cavity. (The external spermatic fascia is described in III E 4 b).
      (4) **Peritoneum.** The **parietal layer of the vaginal tunic** forms the inner lining of the scrotum. This tunic is a modification of the peritoneum of the vaginal process, and is directly continuous with the parietal peritoneum of the abdominal cavity.
   b. **Septum**
      (1) A **median septum** divides the internal cavity of the scrotum in half; each half houses one testis, one epididymis, and one proximal ductus deferens.
      (2) The **scrotal raphe,** a line extending the full length of the scrotum along the midline, marks the internal position of the median septum. The scrotal raphe results from the fusion of the two skin folds that form the scrotum.

2. **Vascularization**
   a. **Arterial supply** to the scrotum is provided directly by the **scrotal arteries** and indirectly by the **perineal branches;** both the scrotal arteries and the perineal branches originate from the **external pudendal artery.**
   b. **Venous drainage** occurs via satellite veins of the arterial branches.
   c. **Lymphatic drainage.** Efferent lymphatic vessels from the scrotum pass to the **superficial inguinal lymph nodes.**

3. **Innervation.** The **superficial perineal nerve** (a branch of the pudendal nerve) supplies **sensory innervation** to the **skin,** as well as **sympathetic innervation** to the **tunica dartos.**

B. Testis. The paired testes produce spermatozoa, which are stored in the epididymis, a tubular structure located on the dorsolateral surface of each testis (Figure 52–1; see also III C).

1. **Position.** The **oval** testis lies horizontally within the scrotum (i.e., with its **long axis parallel to the vertebral column).** Owing to its shape and positioning within the scrotum, the testis is described as having:
   a. **Cranial** and **caudal poles**
   b. **Dorsal** and **ventral borders**
   c. **Medial** and **lateral surfaces**

2. **Layers**
   a. The **tunica albuginea** is a stout, white fibrous capsule that invests the surface of the testis. The tunica albuginea is continuous with the **mediastinum testis,** a collagenous connective tissue cord that passes through the midregion of the testis from its cranial to its caudal end. From the mediastinum testis, connective tissue divides and redivides to form the microscopic supportive structures for the testicular lobules that contain the seminiferous tubules.

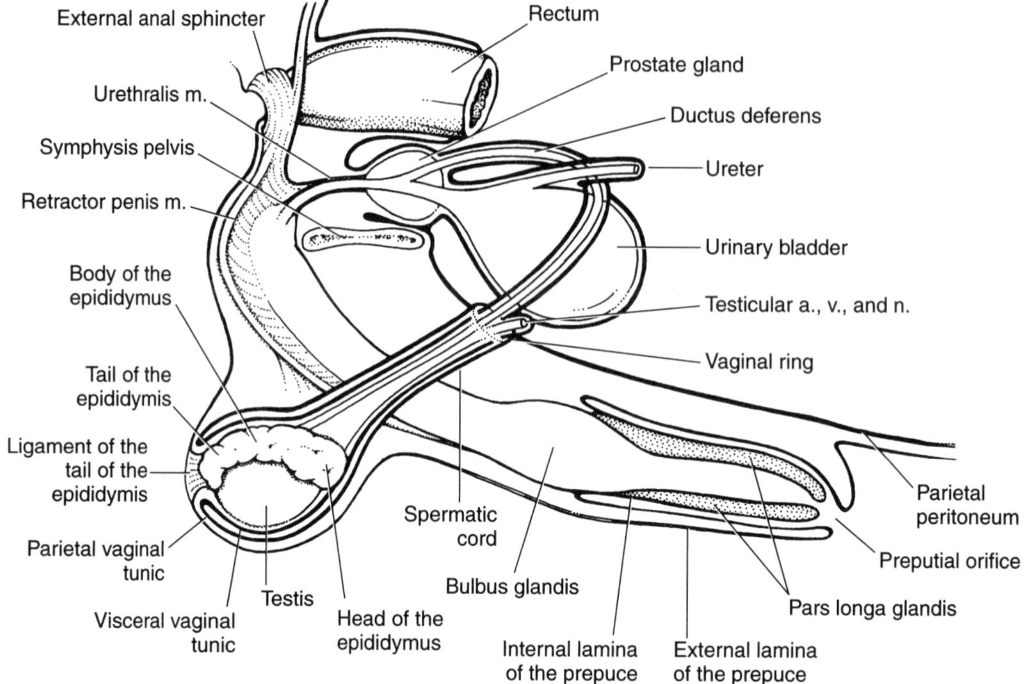

FIGURE 52–1. The male genital organs, right lateral view. The vaginal ring and vaginal tunics are also depicted. (Redrawn with permission from Evans HE, 1993, *Miller's Anatomy of the Dog,* 3e. Philadelphia, WB Saunders, p 512.)

b. The **parietal** and **visceral vaginal tunics** of the testis are the peritoneal layers that permit testicular mobility within the scrotum. The parietal and visceral vaginal tunics **develop from the vaginal process.**

(1) The **vaginal process** is an outpocketing of the abdominal peritoneum that exits the abdomen through the inguinal canal (see Chapter 44 I D 1). In male embryos, the vaginal process enters the scrotum.

(2) The **testes** develop within the abdominal cavity, just caudal to the kidneys. Although the testes remain retroperitoneal, they **descend** from their abdominal position to take up residence within the scrotum.

(a) As the testis continues distally into the scrotum, it passes alongside (but not into) the vaginal process. Thus, the vaginal process envelops it, forming two layers: one directly against the testis, and one directly against the internal wall of the scrotum. These layers are designated the visceral and parietal vaginal tunics, respectively (see Figure 52–1).

(b) The two layers of the tunic are separated by a space continuous (in domestic animals) with the peritoneal cavity. This space contains a small amount of serous fluid, which facilitates motion of the testis within the scrotum.

(c) The vaginal process remains continuous with the parietal peritoneum into the definitive form. Thus, the full length of the inguinal canal and the space between the superficial inguinal ring and the cranial pole of the testis are provided with parietal and visceral layers of peritoneum as well (see Figure 52–1).

3. Vascularization

a. Arterial supply arrives mainly through the **testicular artery,** a direct branch of the **abdominal aorta.** The **artery of the ductus deferens** (a branch of the internal pudendal artery) also contributes a small amount of arterial blood to the testis.

Canine Clinical Correlation

Cryptorchidism (*crypto* = hidden; *orchid* = testis) is the clinical condition in which one or both testes fail to fully descend into the scrotum. The retained testis may lie at any level, from the original sublumbar position to a subcutaneous position just cranial to the scrotum. The retained testis is able to successfully produce testosterone, but not viable sperm, leading to normal sexual behavior but reduced fertility in affected dogs. Retained testes are prone to neoplasia, so surgical correction of the condition is necessary. Although surgical replacement of the testes into the scrotum is feasible, cryptorchidism tends to be heritable; thus, castration is the ethical treatment.

b. **Venous drainage** is provided by the **testicular veins** and the **vein of the ductus deferens.** Differences between the arteries and their satellite veins include the following:
   (1) The right testicular vein is a tributary of the caudal vena cava, but the **left testicular vein** drains into the **left renal vein.**
   (2) **Pampiniform plexus** (see also III E 4 c). Although the testicular arteries take a relatively direct course, the testicular veins widen and form a tortuous and extensive network surrounding the testicular arteries. This arrangement forms a heat exchanger that cools the arterial blood entering the testes and warms the venous blood returning to the body core.

c. **Lymphatic drainage.** Efferent lymphatic vessels from the testis drain into the **lumbar lymph nodes.**

4. **Innervation** of the testis is provided by **sympathetic fibers** that leave the **lumbar sympathetic trunk** and travel along the surface of the testicular arteries. The fibers form a plexus on the surface of the testis referred to as the **testicular plexus;** fibers from this plexus innervate the smooth muscle of the testis (including that of the vasculature).

C. **Epididymis.** The epididymis is the convoluted tubular structure that stores maturing and mature sperm following their production by the testis and prior to their ejaculation. The convolutions increase the length of the epididymis. The length of the epididymis provides sufficient opportunity for the sperm to continue their maturation before ejaculation.

1. **Position.** The epididymis is tightly applied to the dorsolateral surface of the testis.
2. **Regions.** Three regions are identifiable along the length of the epididymis.
   a. The **head,** which lies at the cranial head of the testis, is slightly wider dorsally to ventrally than the more distal portions of the epididymis. The head of the epididymis is continuous with the internal duct system of the testis.
   b. The **body** continues caudally from the head, and passes along the dorsolateral region of the testis. The **epididymal sinus (testicular bursa)** is a potential space between the body of the epididymis and the surface of the testis over which it lies.
   c. The **tail** is the caudal extremity of the epididymis. The tail of the epididymis is continuous with the ductus deferens.
3. **Ligaments**
   a. The **ligament of the tail of the epididymis** attaches the epididymal tail to the vaginal tunic and the internal spermatic fascia (i.e., to the innermost layer of the scrotum).
   b. The **proper ligament of the testis** attaches the tail of the epididymis to the caudal pole of the testis.
4. **Vascularization** of the epididymis is essentially the same as that of the testis.
5. **Innervation** of the epididymis is mainly **parasympathetic,** arriving via the **pelvic plexus.**

D. **Ductus deferens.** The ductus deferens is the tubular organ that conducts sperm from the tail of the epididymis to the prostatic portion of the urethra.

1. **Course** (see Figure 52–1)
   a. **Testis.** A direct continuation of the epididymis, the ductus deferens passes from the

lateral to the medial surface of the caudal testicular pole. From here, the ductus deferens straightens and passes **cranially** along the dorsomedial border of the testis toward the cranial testicular pole.

b. **Spermatic cord.** At the cranial testicular pole, the ductus deferens passes obliquely craniodorsally as one of the components of the spermatic cord (see III E). As a member of the spermatic cord, the ductus deferens passes through the inguinal canal to gain the interior of the abdominal cavity.

c. **Abdominal cavity.** Once inside the abdominal cavity, the ductus deferens courses slightly more cranially, making a wide arc that carries it across the **lateral surface of the bladder** cranial to the ureter.

(1) After looping around the **ureter,** the ductus deferens approaches the **dorsal surface of the bladder.**

(2) The **ampulla of the ductus deferens** is a thickening in the wall of the ductus deferens that forms shortly after the ductus deferens gains the dorsal surface of the bladder.

d. **Prostate gland.** After gaining the dorsal surface of the bladder, the ductus deferens turns caudally and courses toward the prostate gland. The **genital fold** is a triangular fold of peritoneum extending between the two deferent ducts along the midline shortly before they enter the prostate gland.

e. **Prostatic urethra.** Each ductus deferens pierces the respective lobe of the prostate gland and passes through the substance of the gland for a short distance before opening into the lumen of the prostatic urethra, one on each side of the colliculus seminalis.

2. **Vascularization**

a. **Arterial supply** and **venous drainage** is provided by the **artery of the ductus deferens** (a branch of the **prostatic artery)** and its **satellite vein.**

b. **Lymphatic drainage.** Efferent lymphatics pass to the **hypogastric** and **medial iliac lymph nodes.**

3. **Innervation.** The **pelvic plexus** provides **sympathetic** and **parasympathetic** fibers.

E. Spermatic cord. The spermatic cord is a collection of structures passing to and from the testis. These structures are carried through the inguinal canal as the testis descends to the scrotum.

1. **Position.** The spermatic cord extends from the deep inguinal ring to the testis.
2. **Components** of the spermatic cord include vascular, nervous, and reproductive structures:

a. **Testicular artery** and **vein**

b. **Efferent testicular lymphatic vessels**

c. **Testicular nerve**

d. **Ductus deferens** and its **associated artery** and **vein**

3. **Mesenteries.** The components of the spermatic cord are invested by the visceral layer of the original vaginal process. This visceral layer is modified according to the structures invested.

a. The **mesoductus deferens** is the portion of the visceral layer that invests the deferent duct, artery, and vein.

b. The **mesorchium** invests the testicular artery, vein, nerves, and efferent lymphatics.

4. **Associated structures**

a. The **cremaster muscle** is a band of muscle originating from the caudal edge of the internal abdominal oblique muscle and passing onto the external surface of the spermatic cord. The cremaster muscle **elevates the testis** in response to cold or to sympathetic drive.

b. The **external spermatic fascia,** a combination of the superficial and deep abdominal fascia, arises from the superficial surface of the external abdominal oblique muscle. This fascial layer reflects onto and invests the external surface of the internal spermatic fascia and the cremaster muscle.

c. The **pampiniform plexus,** a specialization of the testicular veins [see III B 3 b (2)], surrounds the spermatic cord immediately adjacent to the cranial pole of the testis and extends along the cord for a considerable distance.

F. Penis. Dogs, like primates and horses, have a **musculocavernous penis,** characterized by a **predominance of cavernous tissue** (i.e., tissue containing a myriad of small spaces that fill with arterial blood to achieve erection of the penis).

1. **Regions**
   a. **The** root is the most **proximal portion** of the penis, located in the region of the ischial arch. Two paired regions (the crura) and one median region (the bulb) form the root of the penis; more distally (i.e., cranially), the three regions blend into a single unit.
   b. The **body** is the **intermediate portion** of the penis, extending from the root to the beginning of the glans. The penile body, which is rather compressed laterally, is the narrowest region of the penis.
   c. The **glans,** the most **distal portion** of the penis, comprises the greatest part of the free portion of the penis. The glans is slightly larger than the body in the nonerect state, and increases in dimension the most when the penis becomes erect. The glans has two portions:
      (1) The **bulbus glandis** is globular in shape and entirely surrounds the proximal end of the glans. On erection, the bulbus glandis (the most distensible part of the penis) increases dramatically in size, owing to its role in forming the "tie" or "lock" characteristic of canine copulation.
      (2) The **pars longa glandis** is the elongate distal portion of the glans.
2. **Cavernous tissue and associated structures** (Figure 52–2)
   a. The **corpus spongiosum** may be described as the cavernous tissue that **surrounds the urethra.**
      (1) The **corpus spongiosum penis** contributes to the formation of the root, body, and glans of the penis.
         (a) The **bulb of the penis (penile bulb)** is a large, partially bilobed, expanded region of the corpus spongiosum that surrounds the urethra in the region of the ischial arch. The penile bulb forms a portion of the **penile root.**

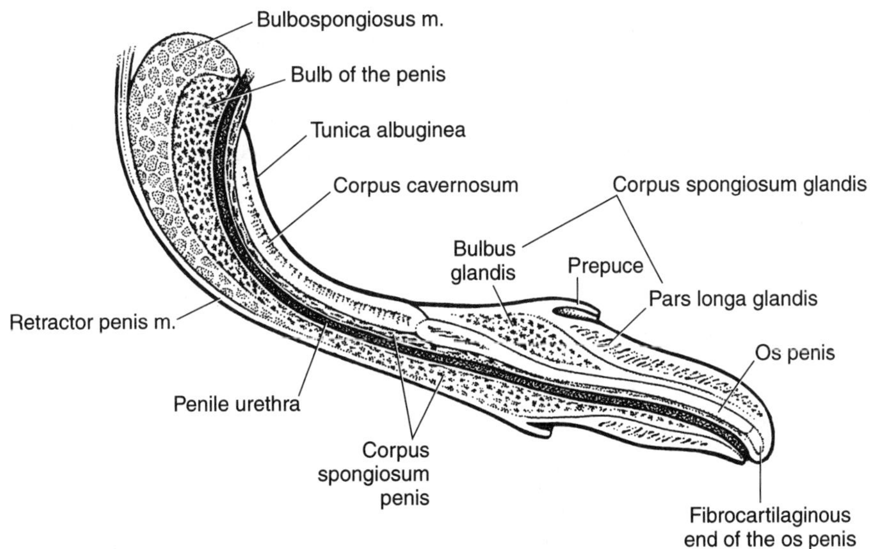

FIGURE 52–2. The internal structure of the penis, right median view. (Redrawn with permission from Evans HE, 1993, *Miller's Anatomy of the Dog,* 3e. Philadelphia, WB Saunders, p 517.)

(b) Distally, the bulb of the penis becomes a **narrow band** that surrounds the urethra throughout the remainder of its length, contributing to the formation of the **penile body** and **glans.**

(2) The **corpus spongiosum glandis** is the portion of the corpus spongiosum comprising the two parts of the penile glans (i.e., the **bulbus glandis** and the **pars longa glandis).**

b. The **corpus cavernosum** may be described as the cavernous tissue positioned **dorsal to the urethra.**

(1) A **tunica albuginea,** similar to but entirely separate from the one that invests the testis, invests the corpus cavernosum throughout its length.

(a) The tunica albuginea of the corpus cavernosum is well-developed and recognizable by its bright white appearance.

(b) The tunica albuginea extends inward into the substance of the corpus cavernosum, separating the relatively small cavernous spaces of this erectile tissue body.

(2) **Position**

(a) The corpus cavernosum originates as the paired **crura** of the penis. Each crus is attached by its tunica albuginea to its respective ischiatic tuberosity. The crura pass distally, cranially, and medially, converging on each other. While still separate, the crura form a part of the penile root.

(b) The crura gain the midline, fuse, and are incorporated into a single body.

(i) After the crura fuse, their corpus cavernosum forms the largest part of the penile body.

(ii) The ventral portions of the fused crura diverge slightly from each other, allowing the urethra (surrounded by the corpus spongiosum) to pass ventral to the corpus cavernosum.

(c) The corpus cavernosum continues throughout the length of the penile body. At the distal (i.e., cranial) end of the penile body, the tunica albuginea blends with the base of the os penis, a bone contained within the glans of the penis that takes the position of the corpus cavernosum through the substance of the penile glans (see Figure 52–2).

(3) **Os penis.** The os penis extends through the full length of the penile glans, and bears on its ventral surface the **urethral groove,** which accommodates the urethra. The urethral groove becomes progressively smaller moving distally, so that it disappears from the most distal end of the bone.

(a) The **base** of the os penis is attached to the end of the penile body via the tunica albuginea of the corpus cavernosum. The straight **body** of the os penis narrows as it approaches the **apex** of the os penis, which is quite pointed.

(b) The corpus spongiosum surrounding the urethra in the region of the os penis communicates with the cavernous spaces of the corpus spongiosum glandis.

Canine Clinical Correlation

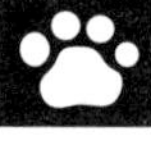

The os penis permits intromission before complete erection of the penis occurs (a characteristic of canine copulation).

3. Musculature

a. Skeletal muscles. Three sets of paired skeletal muscles assist in erection.

(1) The **ischiourethralis muscle** is a small paired muscle that originates on the dorsal surface of the ischiatic tuberosity.

(a) Each muscle passes medially to fuse with a fibrous ring that surrounds the common trunk of the major veins of the penis (i.e., the right and left dorsal veins).

(b) Contraction of the ischiourethralis muscle **obstructs venous outflow** from the penis, a necessary occurrence from the beginning of penile erection throughout copulation.

(2) The **bulbospongiosus muscle** originates from the external anal sphincter and completely covers the bulb of the penis, terminating by fusing with its fellow on the caudal midline. The muscle fibers are mainly oriented transversely to the direction of the urethra.

(3) The **ischiocavernosus muscle** originates from the ischiatic tuberosity and covers the proximal portions of the lateral and caudal surfaces of its respective crus. This muscle terminates by blending with the tunica albuginea of the crus at approximately the level of the termination of the penile bulb.

b. **Smooth muscle.** The **retractor penis muscle** is a paired muscle that **withdraws the penis into the prepuce** following erection.

(1) The retractor penis muscle originates from vertebrae Cd1 and Cd2 and courses around the lateral surfaces of the rectum to gain the caudal (i.e., ventral) surface of the penis. From the ventral surface of the penis, the retractor penis muscle continues distally along the midline to the prepuce, where it terminates by fusing with the penile body.

(2) No equivalent of the retractor penis muscle is present in females.

4. **Vascularization**

a. **Arterial supply** is provided mainly by the paired **artery of the penis,** which arises from the **internal pudendal artery.** The artery of the penis has three branches, each of which is also paired. Smaller amounts of arterial blood are provided by branches of the **external pudendal artery.** Arterial supply of the penis is described more completely in Chapter 53 I C 2 b.

b. **Venous drainage** is provided by **satellite veins.** In addition, several specializations related to venous drainage of the penis following erection, are present. Prominent among these are several communications among the arteries, venous spaces, and veins that participate in erection of the glans (see Chapter 53 II B).

c. **Lymphatic drainage** from the penis passes to the **superficial inguinal lymph nodes.**

5. **Innervation of the penis**

a. **Somatic innervation,** both **motor** and **sensory,** is provided by the **pudendal nerve.**

(1) **Motor innervation.** All three skeletal muscles and the retractor penis muscle are innervated by the **deep perineal branches** of the pudendal nerve.

(2) **Sensory innervation** passes to the penis, the preputial skin, and the skin surrounding the anus and scrotum via the paired **dorsal nerve of the penis.** This nerve, the direct continuation of the pudendal nerve after the perineal branches arise, parallels the artery and vein of the same name.

b. **Autonomic innervation** passes through the **pelvic plexus.**

(1) **Sympathetic** tone favors ejaculation and resolution of erection.

(2) **Parasympathetic** tone preserves erection.

G. The **prepuce** is the sheath of skin that houses the penile glans when the penis is not erect.

1. **Form.** The prepuce is formed from a doubled fold of integument.

a. The **external lamina** is formed of skin that is identical to that of the external body surface in the immediate area.

b. The **preputial orifice** is the ring at the cranial end of the prepuce that opens into the **preputial cavity.** At this point, the external lamina reflects inward to form the internal lamina (see Figure 52–1).

c. The **internal lamina,** a hairless, moist mucous membrane, is apposed to the surface of the glans. The internal lamina continues caudally from the preputial orifice until it reaches the blind end of the preputial cavity. Here the skin of the internal lamina reflects onto the surface of the glans penis, forming a blind "gutter," the **preputial fornix.**

2. **Musculature.** The **preputial muscle** is a paired slip of the cutaneous trunci muscle that extends between the xiphoid region and the dorsal preputial wall.
   a. When the penis is flaccid, the preputial muscle prevents the prepuce from dangling from the end of the glans.
   b. During erection, the preputial muscle relaxes and allows the glans to protrude from the prepuce; following erection, the muscle contracts and draws the prepuce back over the penile glans.

3. **Vascularization**
   a. **Arterial supply** to the prepuce arrives through the **external pudendal artery.**
   b. **Venous drainage** occurs via the **satellite vein** of the external pudendal artery.
   c. **Lymphatic drainage** passes to the **superficial inguinal lymph nodes.**

4. **Innervation** of the prepuce is sensory.
   a. The **preputial orifice** and **internal lamina** are supplied by branches of the **preputial branches of the dorsal penile nerve.**
   b. The **external lamina** is supplied by branches of the **genitofemoral nerve.**

Chapter 53

Vasculature of the Pelvic and Perineal Regions

I. ARTERIES OF THE PELVIC AND PERINEAL REGIONS. The **external** and **internal pudendal arteries,** branches of the **external** and **internal iliac arteries,** provide the main arterial supply to the pelvic region. The **caudal gluteal artery** plays a small role in arterial supply of the region. **Note that in the following description, all named vessels are paired.**

A. Caudal gluteal artery. The **dorsal perineal artery** departs from the caudal gluteal artery and supplies the skin in the region of the anus.

B. External pudendal artery. The external pudendal artery is a terminal branch of the pudendoepigastric trunk (which departs from the deep femoral artery, a branch of the external iliac artery). The external pudendal artery provides the:

1. **Ventral labial branch** (in females)
2. **Ventral scrotal branch** and branches to the **internal** and **external lamina of the prepuce** and **skin of the glans penis** (in males)

C. Internal pudendal artery. The internal pudendal artery, the more ventral of the two terminal branches of the internal iliac artery, is the **main source of blood to the pelvic region.** (The other terminal branch of the internal iliac artery is the caudal gluteal artery, which is discussed in Chapter 60 I B). The internal pudendal artery supplies essentially all of the internal pelvic viscera, the erectile organ (i.e., the clitoris or the penis), and the labia or the scrotum.

1. **Vaginal** or **prostatic artery.** After arising from the internal iliac artery, the internal pudendal artery courses caudally and slightly ventrally, giving off a large branch (the vaginal or prostatic artery, depending on the gender of the animal) that passes over the lateral surface of the rectum and supplies most of the internal pelvic viscera (Figure 53–1, Table 53–1). Despite several gender-specific branches, the **general pattern of arterial supply is similar in both sexes.**
   a. The **vaginal artery** terminates into two main branches (see Figure 53–1A).
      (1) **Cranial branch.** The more cranial of the vaginal artery's branches is essentially the ventral continuation of the vaginal artery. This branch supplies the urinary organs, as well as the uterus and vagina.
         (a) The **caudal vesical artery** supplies the caudal portion of the urinary bladder, overlapping fields with the cranial vesical artery (a branch of the umbilical artery). The caudal vesical artery provides:
            (i) A **ureteral branch** that ascends about halfway up the caudal part of the ureter
            (ii) A **urethral branch** to the part of the urethra adjacent to the urinary bladder's neck
         (b) The **urethral artery** supplies the main portion of the urethra.
         (c) The **uterine artery** passes cranially in the broad ligament of the uterus (adjacent to the lateral surface of the uterine cervix and body). This "proper" uterine artery anastomoses with the descending uterine branch of the ovarian artery.
         (d) **Proper vaginal branches** supply the cranial vaginal region.
      (2) **Caudal branch.** The more caudal of the vaginal artery's branches supplies more of the vagina, as well as the middle part of the rectum.
         (a) The **middle rectal artery** supplies the midregion of the rectum. The field of distribution of the middle rectal artery overlaps with that of the cranial rectal artery (a branch of the caudal mesenteric artery) and the caudal rectal artery (a later branch of the internal pudendal artery).

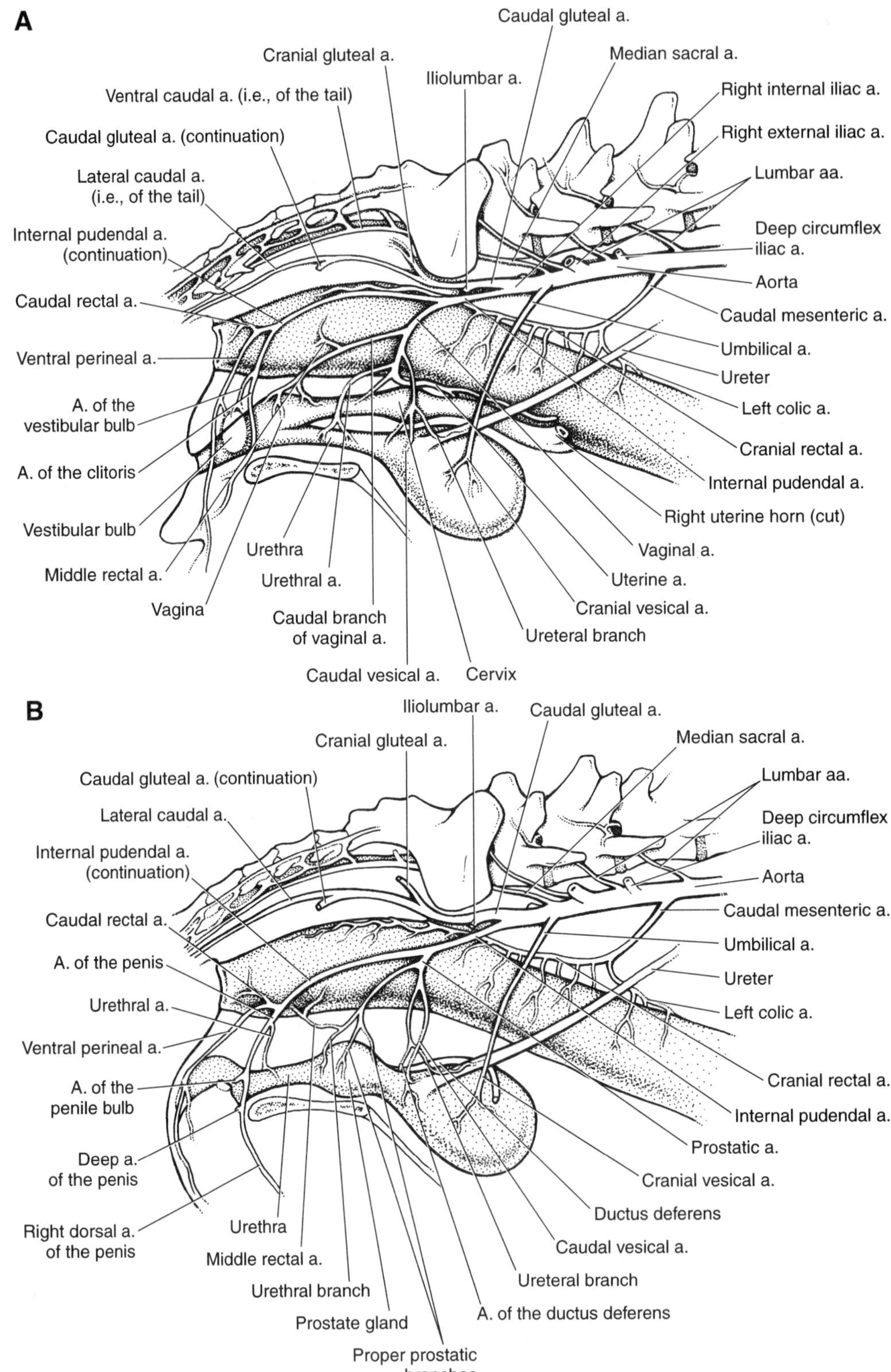

FIGURE 53–1. Arteries of the pelvic cavity. (A) Female, right lateral view. (B) Male, right lateral view. (Redrawn with permission from Evans HE, 1993, *Miller's Anatomy of the Dog,* 3e. Philadelphia, WB Saunders, p 673.)

TABLE 53–1. Structures Supplied by the Vaginal and Prostatic Arteries

Organ System	Vaginal Artery (Female)	Prostatic Artery (Male)
Urinary	Ureters, urinary bladder, urethra	Ureters, urinary bladder, urethra
Reproductive	Uterus, vagina	Prostate gland, ducti deferentia
Gastrointestinal	Rectum	Rectum

(b) The terminal **proper vaginal branches** supply the more caudal vaginal area.

(c) A few **urethral branches** supply the portion of the urethra immediately ventral to the vagina.

b. The **prostatic artery** also terminates into two main branches that supply several pelvic cavity organs (see Figure 53–1B).

(1) Cranial branch. Like the more cranial branch of the vaginal artery, the more cranial branch of the prostatic artery essentially continues the ventral course of the prostatic artery, supplying the urinary organs, the prostate gland, and the ductus deferens.

(a) The **caudal vesical artery** supplies the caudal portion of the urinary bladder and provides a:

(i) Ureteral branch, which ascends the caudal part of the ureter

(ii) Urethral branch to the portion of the urethra adjacent to the neck of the urinary bladder and the prostate gland

(b) The **artery of the ductus deferens,** which is homologous to the uterine artery, gains the ductus deferens as that organ passes into the prostate gland. The artery of the ductus deferens passes retrograde along the ductus deferens to reach the epididymis; here its final branches overlap with those of the testicular artery.

(2) Caudal branch. The more caudal of the prostatic artery's branches supplies the prostate gland, as well as the middle part of the rectum. Vessels arising from this arterial branch are the:

(a) Middle rectal artery, to the midregion of the rectum

(b) Prostatic branches, to the prostate gland

(c) Urethral branches, to the prostatic and pelvic regions of the urethra

2. Continuation of the internal pudendal artery. After giving rise to the vaginal or prostatic artery, the internal pudendal artery continues caudally and passes lateral to the levator ani muscle. Upon emerging caudal to this muscle, the artery supplies the caudal rectum, the anal canal, the external anal sphincter, and the external genitalia and perineum (see Figure 53–1).

a. Caudal rectal and **ventral perineal arteries.** As the internal pudendal artery nears the caudal border of the levator ani muscle, it gives rise to a common trunk for the caudal rectal and ventral perineal arteries.

(1) The **caudal rectal artery** passes to the lateral surface of the **caudal region of the rectum** and the **anal canal,** where it arborizes. The caudal rectal artery also provides branches to the **anal sac, external anal sphincter,** and **circumanal glands.**

(2) The **ventral perineal artery** passes caudally to provide branches to the perineal structures.

(a) Its more **dorsal branches** pass to the **skin surrounding the pelvic outlet.**

(b) Its more **ventral branch** passes through the deeper regions of the perineal area and may supply arterial branches to the anal regions. The ventral branch then passes more directly caudally to exit through the pelvic inlet and terminate as branches to gender-specific structures.

(i) In **females,** the terminal branch is the **dorsal labial branch.**

(ii) In **males,** the terminal branch is the **dorsal scrotal branch.** (The corresponding ventral scrotal branch arises from the external pudendal artery.)

b. **Artery of the penis** or **clitoris.** This artery is the continuation of the internal pudendal artery after the origin of the common trunk of the caudal rectal and ventral perineal arteries. Apart from size and with the exception of an additional urethral artery in the male, the branching of the arteries of the clitoris and penis are similar.

(1) **Artery of the penis.** The paired artery of the penis has several branches, all of which are paired.

(a) The **urethral branch** arises from the artery of the penis and is a **third source of arterial blood to the male urethra.** This artery is lacking in females.

(b) After providing the urethral branch, the artery of the penis continues distally and terminates by dividing into three branches—the artery of the penile bulb, the deep artery of the penis, and the dorsal artery of the penis (Table 53–2, Figure 53–2).

(i) The **artery of the penile bulb** is a short but relatively wide artery that plunges through the bulbospongiosus muscle into its respective half of the penile bulb. The artery of the penile bulb divides into two to three branches, each of which arborizes within the substance of the corpus spongiosum of the bulb and then anastomoses with the terminal branches of the dorsal and deep penile arteries within the pars longa glandis.

(ii) The **deep artery of the penis** enters the penile crus near the ischiatic tuberosity. **Helicine arteries,** the end-arteries of the deep artery of the penis, are groups of looped arteries that open directly into the cavernous spaces of the corpus cavernosum.

(iii) The **dorsal artery of the penis** courses dorsally along the superficial surface of the penis (deep to the skin) toward the glans. As it reaches the bulbus glandis, the artery terminates by dividing into three branches, which supply specific areas of the glans as well as other structures (see Table 53–2, Figure 53–2).

(2) **Artery of the clitoris.** This artery branches in a pattern similar to that of the artery of the penis.

(a) The **artery of the vestibular bulb** is the female homologue of the male artery of the penile bulb.

(b) Branches that correspond to the **dorsal** and **deep branches** of the artery of the penis supply the **clitoral glans** and **corpus cavernosum,** respectively.

TABLE 53–2. Structures Supplied by the Artery of the Penis

Branch	Structures Supplied
Urethral branch	Urethra
Artery of the penile bulb	Corpus spongiosum penis of the penile bulb
	Corpus spongiosum penis surrounding the penile urethra
	Penile urethra
	Corpus spongiosum glandis of the pars longa glandis
Deep artery of the penis	Corpus cavernosum
	Os penis
Dorsal artery of the penis	
Preputial branch	Dorsal region of the pars longa glandis and the preputial wall
Superficial branch	Ventral region of the pars longa glandis
Deep branch	Distal region of the pars longa glandis and the os penis

II. VEINS OF THE PELVIC AND PERINEAL REGIONS.

Most of the veins of the pelvic region are **satellites** of the named arteries; however, some specializations of venous drainage in the pelvic region require mention.

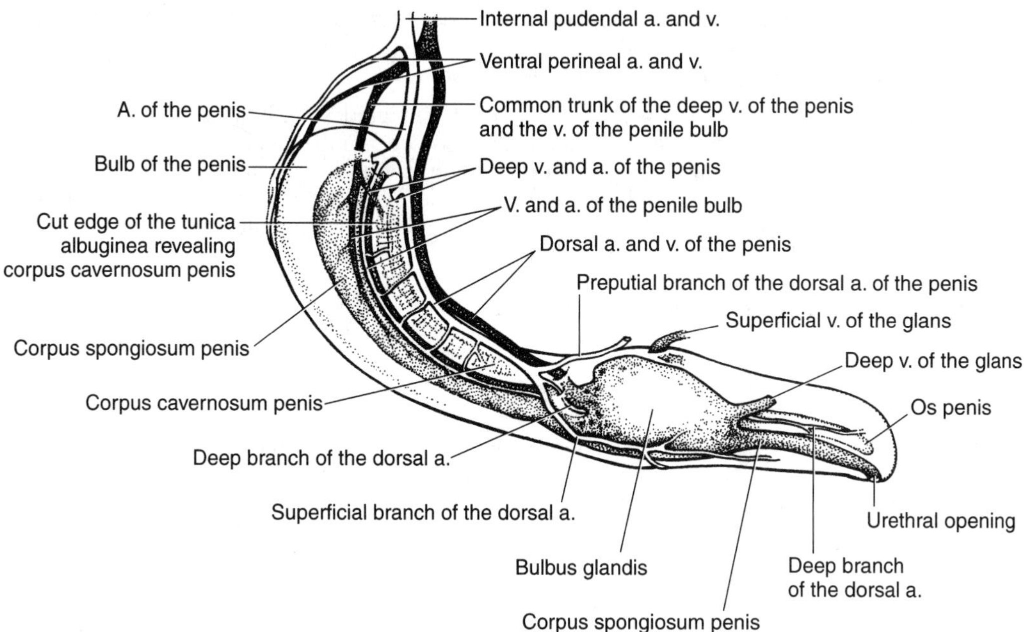

FIGURE 53–2. Arteries and veins of the penis, right lateral view. (Redrawn with permission from Evans HE, 1993, *Miller's Anatomy of the Dog,* 3e. Philadelphia, WB Saunders, p 520.)

A. Female pelvic region

1. The **vestibular plexus** is an extensive venous network that surrounds the external opening of the vulva and occupies a considerable portion of both labia. Engorgement of the vestibular plexus is associated with sexual behavior.
2. The **vein of the clitoris** originates within the vestibular bulb rather than within the clitoris. This is logical considering that the vestibular bulb is the homologue of the penile bulb.

B. Male pelvic region (see Figure 53–2)

1. The **deep vein of the penis** and the **vein of the penile bulb** form a **common trunk,** as opposed to entering the dorsal vein of the penis separately.
2. The **superficial vein of the glans** leaves the deep portion of the pars longa glandis and enters the external pudendal vein.
3. The **deep vein of the glans** provides a connection between the cavernous spaces of the pars longa glandis and the bulbus glandis, playing a role in erection of the glans. The deep vein of the glans also communicates with the dorsal vein of the penis.

III. LYMPHATIC VESSELS OF THE PELVIC AND PERINEAL REGIONS

A. Lymphocenters.

The lymphatic drainage of the pelvic region is handled by the lymphocenters of the abdominal wall (see Chapter 41 V C).

1. The **iliosacral lymphocenter** (see Chapter 41 V C 2) receives most of the efferent vessels from the pelvic region.
   a. The **medial iliac lymph nodes** are present as a pair of large single or doubled nodes positioned between the deep circumflex and external iliac arteries.

b. The **hypogastric lymph nodes** are small nodes situated in the angle between the internal iliac and median sacral arteries.
c. The **sacral lymph nodes** are small and inconstant.

2. The **lumbar lymphocenter** (see Chapter 41 V C 1) includes the **lumbar aortic lymph nodes,** which are variably present along the aorta and caudal vena cava.
3. The **superficial inguinal (inguinofemoral) lymphocenter** (see Chapter 41 V C 3) includes the **superficial inguinal lymph nodes.** These nodes usually number two on each side and are positioned in the region of the superficial inguinal ring. In males, the nodes lie on each side of the dorsolateral penile border.

B. **Lymphatic drainage of the pelvic organs** is summarized in Table 53–3.

TABLE 53–3. Major Routes of Lymphatic Drainage of the Pelvic Cavity

Structure	Lymphocenter	Nodes Receiving Drainage
Urinary bladder	Iliosacral	Hypogastric, medial iliac
	Lumbar	Lumbar aortic
Rectum and anal canal	Iliosacral	Hypogastric, sacral
Cranial uterus		
Caudal uterus	Iliosacral	Hypogastric, sacral
	Iliosacral, lumbar	Medial iliac, lumbar aortic
Vagina	Iliosacral	Hypogastric
Vestibule	Iliosacral	Hypogastric, sacral
	Superficial inguinal	Superficial inguinal
Clitoris and vulva	Superficial inguinal	Superficial inguinal
Testes and epididymis	Iliosacral	Medial iliac
	Lumbar	Lumbar aortic
Ducti deferentia	Iliosacral	Hypogastric, sacral
Prostate gland	Iliosacral	Medial iliac, hypogastric
Penis and prepuce	Superficial inguinal	Superficial inguinal

Chapter 54

Innervation of the Pelvic and Perineal Regions

I. AUTONOMIC INNERVATION

A. Overview. Autonomic innervation of the pelvic and perineal regions is **similar to that of the abdominal region:** sympathetic and parasympathetic input is delivered separately to a plexus of nerves (i.e., the **pelvic plexus)** near a main vascular trunk. After mingling within the plexus, fibers from each autonomic division leave the plexus and are distributed to target organs along the surfaces of the arteries that serve the same organs.

1. **Main departures from the abdominal pattern** include the following:
   - **a.** The **sympathetic fibers** entering the plexus are **mostly postganglionic,** having passed through and synapsed in the caudal mesenteric ganglion (in the abdomen).
   - **b.** The paired pelvic plexuses are **laterally placed** (and therefore, **relatively widely separated from one another).** This is in contrast to the plexuses in the abdominal region, which blend into a single large mass on the midline.
   - **c.** The paired plexuses are **located on the surface of an organ,** rather than on the surfaces of large arteries.

B. Pelvic plexus (Figure 54–1). The paired pelvic plexuses are located on the lateral surfaces of the **rectum.** The autonomic fibers from the plexus are delivered to target organs along the branches of the **vaginal** or **prostatic artery. Target organs** of the pelvic plexus include those of the pelvic cavity (i.e., the caudal rectum, anal canal, urinary bladder, urethra, prostate gland, uterus, cervix, and vagina), as well as the erectile organ (i.e., the penis or clitoris).

1. **Sympathetic input** to each pelvic plexus arrives through the paired **hypogastric nerves,** prominent strands that arise from the **caudal mesenteric ganglion** in the caudal abdominal region.
   - **a.** The hypogastric nerves are the only source of sympathetic fibers to the pelvic plexus (and therefore, to the pelvic organs).
   - **b.** The lateral horn of the spinal cord—the sole location of sympathetic cell bodies—terminates in the lumbar region; therefore, sympathetic fibers must reach the pelvic cavity by passing from their origin in the lumbar sympathetic trunk through the lumbar splanchnic nerves to the caudal mesenteric ganglion.
2. **Parasympathetic input** to each pelvic plexus arrives from the **pelvic nerve.** This nerve arises directly from the adjacent sacral spinal cord and takes a ventral course directly to the pelvic plexus. In addition, the pelvic nerve supplies parasympathetic fibers to the caudal mesenteric ganglion.
   - **a.** The pelvic nerve usually contains fibers from all three sacral nerves.
   - **b.** The sacral region of the spinal cord represents the "sacral" part of the craniosacral distribution of parasympathetic nerve cell bodies; therefore, the pelvic nerves are short and direct.

II. SOMATIC INNERVATION of the pelvic and perineal regions is provided by the **pudendal nerve,** which arises from the ventral branches of all three of the sacral nerves.

A. Structures supplied. The pudendal nerve supplies the gastrointestinal, urinary, and reproductive organs of the pelvic region, as well as the skin of the perineal region.

B. Course. The pudendal nerve arises from the sacral region near the internal pudendal vessels and courses caudoventrally. After passing lateral to the coccygeus muscle, the nerve be-

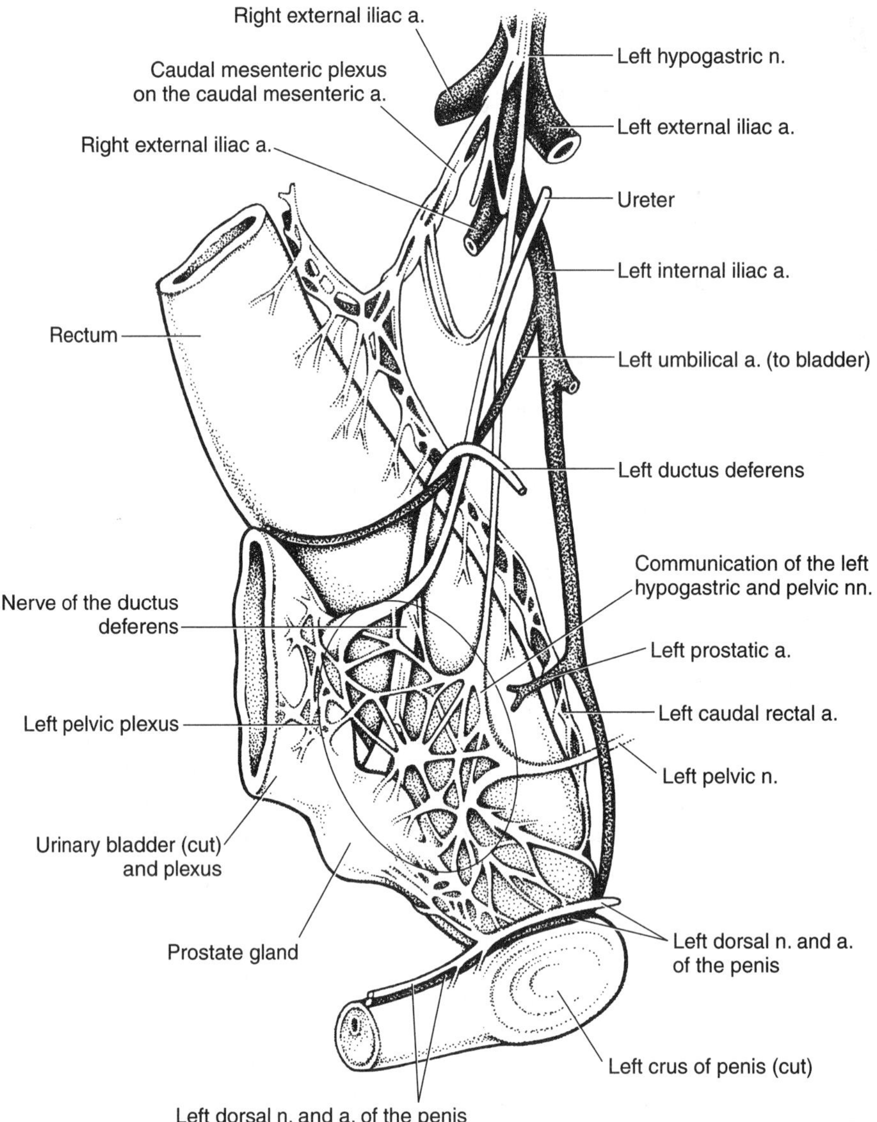

FIGURE 54–1. The autonomic nerves of the pelvic region, left lateral view. (Redrawn with permission from Anderson WD: *Atlas of Canine Anatomy.* Baltimore, Williams & Wilkins, 1994, p 729.)

comes superficial near the superficial gluteal muscle. Here, at the pelvic outlet, it divides into its terminal branches, which provide sensory innervation over a wide area.

1. The **caudal rectal nerve,** in company with the vessels of the same name, enters and supplies the **external anal sphincter.**
2. The **superficial perineal branches** supply several areas.
   a. A large branch serves the **proximal penis.**
   b. Major branches supply the **skin of the perineum** from the anal area to the vulva or scrotum, as well as the **caudomedial thigh.**
   c. The **caudal scrotal nerves,** the most distal branches of the pudendal nerve, supply part of the **scrotal skin.** No branches corresponding to the caudal scrotal nerves are present in female dogs.

Chapter 55

Prominent Palpable Features of the Pelvic and Perineal Regions

I. BONY STRUCTURES

A. In animals of normal body weight, the cranial border of the **iliac crest** can be appreciated from the cranial dorsal iliac spine almost as far as the cranial ventral iliac spine.

Canine Clinical Correlation

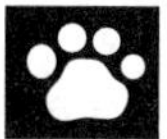

The marrow cavity of the dorsal portion of the iliac wing is often accessed for diagnostic bone marrow aspiration; therefore, palpation of the dorsal part of the iliac crest is essential for planning needle placement.

Canine Clinical Correlation

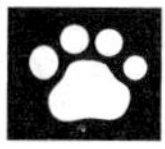

The articulation of the iliac wings with the sacrum is normally symmetrical. One is often able to see, as well as to palpate, asymmetry in patients with sacroiliac luxation.

B. The **ischiatic tuberosity** is plain, even in most obese animals, as a rounded bony prominence in the caudolateral pelvic region obliquely ventrolateral from the anus at the proximal end of the caudal thigh.

C. The **ischiatic arch** is partially palpable as the bony edge leading cranially and medially away from the ischial tuberosity.

D. The **pubic brim (pecten pubis),** which forms the ventral part of the pelvic inlet, is palpable on each side of the ventral midline.

II. SOFT TISSUE STRUCTURES

A. The **ischiorectal fossa** is a deep hollow bounded medially by the rectum and laterally by the levator ani and coccygeus muscles. Colloquially, the ischiorectal fossa may be thought of as lying lateral to the base of the tail. The ischiorectal fossa is typically filled with fat in well-nourished dogs, and largely obliterated by fat in obese animals.

Canine Clinical Correlation

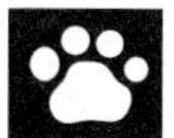

Mobilization of this fat depot during starvation is responsible for the "hollow-tailed" appearance of emaciated animals.

B. The **sacrotuberous ligament** is palpable in dogs of normal body weight as a rigid structure that extends craniomedially and slightly dorsally from the ischiatic tuberosity.

1. When the leg that is being palpated is bearing weight, the ligament feels much like a bone.
2. When the dog shifts its weight from the leg that is being palpated, the sacrotuberous ligament yields slightly.

C. Male reproductive organs

1. **Penis**
   a. The **crura of the penis** may be appreciated arising from each ischiatic tuberosity.
   b. The **penile body** is palpable through the skin along the ventral midline. The groove along its ventral surface that houses the urethra may also be detectable.
   c. The **os penis** within the glans is readily palpable through the skin of the prepuce.
2. The **spermatic cord** may be gently palpated along its full length between the scrotum and the superficial inguinal ring.
3. The **testes** and the **epididymal tail** may be gently palpated through the thin skin of the scrotum.
4. The **prostate gland** is palpable by digital palpation through the rectal wall, just ventral to the rectum.

Canine Clinical Correlation

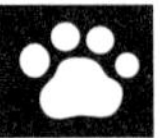

Veterinarians should digitally palpate the prostate gland of all male dogs of sufficient body size during physical examination in order to develop an appreciation for the normal dimensions of the gland, making departures from normal more immediately recognizable.

D. The **superficial inguinal lymph nodes** are occasionally faintly palpable, but they are not readily detectable unless they are enlarged.

E. **Coccygeus muscle.** Gently lifting the tail dorsally reveals the caudal end of the coccygeus muscle beneath the fold of skin that is raised when the muscle contracts.

STUDY QUESTIONS

DIRECTIONS: Each of the numbered items or incomplete statements in this section is followed by answers or by completions of the statement. Select the ONE numbered answer or completion that is BEST in each case.

1. Which one of the following is a boundary of the pelvic inlet?

(1) Dorsally, the wing of the ilium
(2) Laterally, the shaft of the ilium
(3) Ventrally, the prepubic tendon
(4) Laterally, the external abdominal oblique muscle

2. What is the tuber coxae?

(1) A convexity on the caudolateral-most area of the ischium
(2) A knob on the ventral surface of the iliac shaft just cranial to the acetabulum
(3) An elevation near the termination of the iliac shaft on its ventral surface, where the ilium fuses with the pubis
(4) The portion of the iliac wing between the cranial and caudal ventral iliac spines

3. What is the greater ischiatic notch?

(1) A concavity along the caudal part of the dorsal border of the iliac shaft cranial to the iliac spine
(2) A concavity along the dorsal edge of the ischiatic body caudal to the ischiatic spine
(3) A deep, broad, "U"-shaped concavity at the caudal-most extremity of the pelvis where the rami of the two ischia meet
(4) A concavity along the cranial border of the symphysis pelvis where the two pubes meet

4. What is the auricular surface of the pelvis?

(1) The curved surface within the acetabulum that articulates with the femoral head
(2) The curved surface of the iliac wing that articulates with the sacrum
(3) The roughened surface surrounding the obturator foramen where the obturator muscles attach
(4) The roughened surface on the ischiatic tuberosity where the sacrotuberous ligament attaches

5. Which one of the following structures is associated with the pubovesical pouch?

(1) Ilium
(2) Vagina
(3) Prostate gland
(4) Rectum

6. Which one of the following peritoneal pouches is least developed in the male?

(1) Vesicogenital
(2) Rectogenital
(3) Pubovesical
(4) Pararectal fossa

7. Which region of the anal canal is characterized by the openings of the circumanal glands?

(1) Internal region of the cutaneous anal zone
(2) External region of the cutaneous anal zone
(3) Intermediate zone of the anal canal
(4) Columnar zone of the anal canal

8. What structure marks the point of demarcation between the vagina and the vestibule?

(1) Fossa of the clitoris
(2) Urethral tubercle
(3) Vaginal fornix
(4) Clitoris

9. Which structure associated with the urinary bladder carries the round ligament of the bladder?

(1) Median ligament
(2) Trigone
(3) Lateral ligament
(4) Urachus

10. In the male reproductive tract, a tunica albuginea surrounds the:

(1) testes and penis.
(2) testes and corpus cavernosum.
(3) penile root and corpus cavernosum.
(4) penis and corpus cavernosum.

11. Which erectile body directly surrounds the urethra in male dogs?

(1) Corpus urethralis
(2) Corpus cavernosum
(3) Corpus spongiosum penis
(4) Corpus spongiosum glandis

12. The os penis represents the cranial continuation of the:

(1) penile root.
(2) corpus cavernosum.
(3) corpus spongiosum penis.
(4) corpus spongiosum glandis.

13. In order for the initial stages of erection to occur, which muscle must contract?

(1) Retractor penis muscle
(2) Ischiourethralis muscle
(3) Bulbospongiosus muscle
(4) Ischiocavernosus muscle

14. Arterial supply to the testis arrives from a branch of the:

(1) aorta.
(2) renal artery.
(3) artery of the penis.
(4) internal pudendal artery.

15. Arterial blood to the urinary bladder is provided by the:

(1) internal and external iliac arteries.
(2) internal iliac and umbilical arteries.
(3) internal and external pudendal arteries.
(4) internal pudendal and caudal mesenteric arteries.

16. Which one of the following statements concerning the pattern of blood supply of the pelvic viscera in the male and female is correct?

(1) The pattern is essentially similar, with the ductus deferens replacing the uterus.
(2) The pattern is essentially similar, with the prostate gland replacing the uterus.
(3) The pattern is widely different, owing to the large size of the penis and its cavernous spaces.
(4) The pattern differs only in the blood supply to the vulva and scrotum.

17. Which structure receives branches from the internal and the external pudendal arteries?

(1) Clitoris
(2) Rectum
(3) Scrotum
(4) Os penis

18. The erectile tissue of the penile glans is most directly supplied by the:

(1) dorsal artery of the penis.
(2) external pudendal artery.
(3) deep artery of the penis.
(4) artery of the penile bulb.

19. Sympathetic input to the pelvic organs arrives through branches of the:

(1) pelvic nerve.
(2) pudendal nerve.
(3) hypogastric nerve.
(4) iliohypogastric nerve.

20. During palpation of the caudal pelvic region, a firm structure is palpated extending dorsally and craniomedially from the ischiatic tuberosity. This structure is most likely the:

(1) iliac shaft.
(2) ischiatic arch
(3) sacrotuberous ligament.
(4) lateral border of the obturator foramen.

DIRECTIONS: Each of the numbered items or incomplete statements in this section is negatively phrased, as indicated by a capitalized word such as NOT, LEAST, or EXCEPT. Select the ONE numbered answer or completion that is BEST in each case.

21. Which one of the following organs is NOT contained within the pelvic cavity?

(1) Vagina
(2) Anal canal
(3) Uterine body
(4) Neck of the urinary bladder

22. All of the following are features of the ilium EXCEPT the:

(1) pecten.
(2) ischiatic spine.
(3) gluteal surface.
(4) tuberosity for the rectus femoris.

23. Which statement regarding the coccygeus muscle is INCORRECT?

(1) It is the more lateral of the two muscles of the pelvic diaphragm.
(2) It is covered by the superficial gluteal muscle.
(3) It depresses the tail and compresses the rectum.
(4) It attaches to the ischial spine.

24. All of the following nerves deliver innervation to the urinary bladder or its associated sphincters EXCEPT the:

(1) pudendal nerve.
(2) hypogastric nerve.
(3) pelvic nerve.
(4) internal iliac nerve.

25. Arteries providing branches to the rectum include all of the following EXCEPT the:

(1) vaginal or prostatic artery.
(2) caudal mesenteric artery.
(3) internal pudendal artery.
(4) external pudendal artery.

26. Lymph nodes receiving drainage from the pelvic viscera include all of the following EXCEPT the:

(1) sacral lymph nodes.
(2) hypogastric lymph nodes.
(3) deep inguinal lymph nodes.
(4) superficial inguinal lymph nodes.

27. The autonomic innervation of the pelvic region differs from that of the abdominal region in several ways, including all of the following EXCEPT:

(1) The sympathetic fibers entering the pelvic plexus are mostly preganglionic.
(2) The paired pelvic plexuses are laterally placed, and as a result, remain distinct.
(3) The paired pelvic plexuses are formed on the surface of a visceral organ, rather than on the surfaces of large arteries.
(4) The parasympathetic fibers entering the pelvic plexus arrive from a nearby source.

ANSWERS AND EXPLANATIONS

1. The answer is 2 [Chapter 49 I B 1 a]. The lateral border of the pelvic inlet is formed by the arcuate line along the medial surface of the iliac shaft. The dorsal border of the pelvic inlet is formed by the sacral promontory and the ventral border is formed by the pecten (i.e., the cranial border) of the pubis.

2. The answer is 4 [Chapter 50 I B 1 a (3)–(4); Figure 50–1A]. The tuber coxae is the ventral border of the iliac wing. Therefore, the tuber coxae can be described as the cranial and caudal ventral iliac spines and the space between them. The ischiatic tuberosity is a prominent convexity on the caudolateral-most area of the ischium. The tuberosity for the rectus femoris is a knob on the ventral surface of the iliac shaft just cranial to the acetabulum. The iliopubic eminence is an elevation near the termination of the iliac shaft on its ventral surface, where the ilium fuses with the pubis.

3. The answer is 1 [Chapter 50 I B 1 b (1)]. The greater ischiatic (sciatic) notch is a concavity along the caudal part of the dorsal border of the iliac shaft. The lesser ischiatic (sciatic) notch is a concavity along the dorsal edge of the ischiatic body caudal to the ischiatic spine. The ischial arch is the deep, broad, "U"-shaped concavity at the caudal-most extremity of the pelvis, formed by the junction of the rami of the ischia. The border formed by the two pubes is straight, not concave.

4. The answer is 2 [Chapter 50 I B 1 a (5)]. The auricular surface is a "C"-shaped region on the medial surface of the iliac wing that articulates with the sacrum. The lunate surface is the "C"-shaped region within the acetabulum that articulates with the femoral head. The sacrotuberous ligament does attach to the ischiatic tuberosity, but its area of attachment is not called the auricular surface. The obturator muscles attach to the area surrounding the obturator foramen, but this area does not have a specific name.

5. The answer is 3 [Chapter 51 II A 4 a]. The pubovesical pouch is positioned between the pubis (not the ilium) and the neck of the urinary bladder. Therefore, in male dogs, the pubovesical pouch is also associated with the prostate gland, which surrounds the neck of the urinary bladder.

6. The answer is 1 [Chapter 51 II A 3 b]. The vesicogenital pouch lies between the urinary bladder and the uterus (in females) or ducti deferentia (in males). Because the ducti deferentia are small in comparison with the uterus, the vesicogenital pouch is more poorly developed in males than in females. Often, the rectogenital and vesicogenital pouches blend together in male dogs to form the rectovesical pouch.

7. The answer is 2 [Chapter 51 III B 3 b (1)]. The external region of the cutaneous anal zone is the area surrounding the anus on the surface of the skin; the circumanal glands open onto the skin surface here.

8. The answer is 2 [Chapter 51 IV A 2 a (1)]. The urethral tubercle is a ridge along the vestibular floor that marks the point where the vagina and the urethra become continuous. The vestibule is the caudal region of the urogenital tract that receives both the reproductive and urinary tracts.

9. The answer is 3 [Chapter 51 II B 2 a (2) (a)]. The round ligaments of the bladder are the remnants of the umbilical arteries that entered at the umbilicus and passed centrally through the lateral ligaments of the bladder. The median ligament of the bladder holds nothing but fat. The urachus is the remnant of the allantoic stalk that originally connected the apex of the bladder to the umbilical cord, and the trigone is a triangular region on the dorsal surface of the bladder demarcated by the entrance of the ureters and the exit of the urethra.

10. The answer is 2 [Chapter 52 III B 2 a, F 2 b (1)]. Like the corpus caversosum of the penis, the testes are surrounded by a tunica albuginea ("white tunic"). Option 3, "penile root and corpus cavernosum," is incorrect because the penile root includes the penile bulb, which is not covered by a tunica albuginea.

11. The answer is 3 [Chapter 52 III F 2]. The corpus spongiosum, which encompasses the corpus spongiosum penis and the corpus spongiosum glandis, surrounds the urethra in male dogs. The corpus spongiosum penis directly surrounds the urethra, while the corpus spongiosum glandis directly surrounds the os penis (and therefore indirectly surrounds the urethra). The corpus cavernosum lies dorsal to the urethra. The term "corpus urethralis" is fanciful.

12. The answer is 2 [Chapter 52 III F 2 b (3)]. The os penis takes the position of the corpus cavernosum through the substance of the penile glans. (The corpus cavernosum extends from the penile root through the penile body.) A groove on the ventral surface of the os penis, the urethral groove, houses the urethra. Note that the urethra lies ventral to the corpus cavernosum and the os penis.

13. The answer is 2 [Chapter 52 III F 3 a (1)]. The ischiourethralis muscle passes over the dorsal surface of the major veins that drain the penis. Contraction of this muscle traps blood within the penis, which is necessary for erection to begin.

14. The answer is 1 [Chapter 52 III B 3 a]. The testicular arteries are paired branches of the abdominal aorta.

15. The answer is 2 [Chapter 53 I C 1 a (1) (a)]. The bladder is vascularized by the cranial and caudal vesical arteries. The cranial vesical arteries are the terminations of the portion of the umbilical arteries that remains patent after birth. The caudal vesical arteries are branches of the vaginal or prostatic arteries, which arise from the internal pudendal arteries. The internal pudendal artery is a branch of the internal iliac artery. The external iliac and the caudal mesenteric arteries do not play a role in vascularizing the urinary bladder.

16. The answer is 1 [Chapter 53 I C]. In both sexes, the internal pudendal artery supplies most of the pelvic structures, and the arterial pattern is largely similar, regardless of gender. Major gender-based differences in the arterial supply to the pelvic region include the "substitution" of the prostate for the vagina, and the ductus deferens for the uterus.

17. The answer is 3 [Chapter 53 I B 2, C 2 a (2) (b) (ii)]. The scrotum is one of the few structures to receive arterial supply from both the internal and the external pudendal arteries. The dorsal scrotal branch arises from the internal pudendal artery, and the ventral scrotal branch arises from the external pudendal artery.

18. The answer is 1 [Table 53–2]. The dorsal artery of the penis supplies the erectile tissue of the penile glans (i.e., the pars longa glandis and, ultimately, the bulbus glandis). The deep artery of the penis supplies the corpus cavernosum; the artery of the penile bulb supplies the penile bulb and the remainder of the corpus spongiosum penis; and the external pudendal artery supplies a portion of the prepuce and the skin of the glans, but no erectile tissue.

19. The answer is 3 [Chapter 54 I B 1]. The hypogastric nerves carry postganglionic sympathetic fibers from the caudal mesenteric ganglion to the pelvic plexus. From the pelvic plexus, the hypogastric nerves are distributed (along with the parasympathetic fibers, carried to the plexus by the pelvic nerves) to the pelvic viscera. The pudendal nerve supplies the pelvic region, but is a somatic nerve. The iliohypogastric nerves (i.e., the ventral branches of spinal nerves L1 and L2, respectively) deliver sensory innervation to the skin of the lateral abdominal wall and flank.

20. The answer is 3 [Chapter 55 II B]. The sacrotuberous ligament is palpable as a firm structure extending craniomedially and slightly dorsally away from the ischiatic tuberosity. The iliac shaft is not palpable, nor is the obturator foramen. The ischiatic arch is angled cranially, but not dorsally.

21. The answer is 3 [Chapter 49 I B 2]. The caudal part of the uterine cervix, not the uterine body, is contained within the pelvic cavity. The uterine body lies within the abdomen. The pelvic cavity also houses the vagina, the anal canal, and the neck of the urinary bladder.

22. The answer is 1 [Chapter 50 I B 1, C 2]. The ilium presents the ischiatic spine (i.e., the small elevation on the dorsal surface of the ilium where the ilium joins the ischium), the gluteal surface (i.e., the lateral surface of the ilium where the middle and deep gluteal muscles attach), and the tuberosity for the rectus femoris muscle. The pecten of the pubis, a feature of the pubis, is the cranial border of the fused pelvic girdle formed by the fused cranial rami of the right and left pubes.

23. The answer is 3 [Chapter 50 III B 1]. The coccygeus muscle acts only to depress the tail; the levator ani compresses the rectum during defecation. The coccygeus muscle, the more lateral of the two muscles, extends from the ischial spine to the transverse processes of vertebrae Cd2–Cd5. The cranial part of the coccygeus muscle is covered by the superficial gluteal muscle.

24. The answer is 4 [Chapter 51 V B 5, C 2 b, 4 b]. The urinary bladder and its associated sphincters (i.e., the external and internal urethral sphincters) receive sympathetic and parasympathetic innervation (via the pelvic plexus) and somatic innervation (via the pudendal nerve). The hypogastric nerve and pelvic nerves supply sympathetic and parasympathetic fibers to the pelvic plexus, respectively. The hypogastric nerve delivers sympathetic innervation that constricts the internal urethral sphincter and relaxes the bladder, and the pelvic nerve delivers fibers to the detrusor muscle of the bladder that contract it, leading to micturition. The external urethral sphincter, which is formed of skeletal muscle, receives somatic (voluntary) innervation from the pudendal nerve. The "internal iliac nerve" is fanciful.

25. The answer is 4 [Chapter 51 III A 3]. The cranial, middle, and caudal rectal arteries supply the rectum. The cranial rectal artery arises from the caudal mesenteric artery; the middle rectal artery arises from the vaginal or prostatic artery; and the caudal rectal artery arises from the continuation of the internal pudendal artery after the vaginal or prostatic artery arises. The external pudendal artery does not contribute to the arterial supply of the rectum.

26. The answer is 3 [Chapter 53 III; Table 53–3]. The deep inguinal lymph nodes do not receive drainage from the pelvic viscera. The sacral lymph nodes receive drainage from the rectum, anal canal, caudal uterus, vestibule, and ducti deferentia. The hypogastric lymph nodes receive drainage from the urinary bladder, rectum, anal canal, caudal uterus, vagina, vestibule, ducti deferentia, and prostate gland. The superficial inguinal lymph nodes receive drainage from the vestibule, clitoris, vulva, penis, and prepuce.

27. The answer is 1 [Chapter 54 I A 1]. The autonomic innervation of the pelvic and abdominal regions is similar in many ways; however, significant differences exist. First of all, the sympathetic fibers entering the pelvic plexus are mostly postganglionic (as opposed to preganglionic in the abdominal region). The parasympathetic fibers of the pelvic plexus originate in the sacral spinal cord, as compared with those of the abdominal plexuses, which originate in the brain as part of cranial nerve X (i.e., the vagus nerve). The paired pelvic plexuses are located on either side of the rectum, and as a result, do not blend along the midline as the plexuses in the abdominal region do.

PART VIII

PELVIC LIMB

Chapter 56

Introduction to the Pelvic Limb

I. COMPARISON WITH THORACIC LIMB

A. Similar features. Many characteristics of the thoracic limb are shared by the pelvic limb.

1. **Number of bones.** Each major region in the pelvic limb has the same number of bones as the corresponding region in the thoracic limb.
2. **Type and location of joints.** The joints in the pelvic limb correspond to those in the thoracic limb, in terms of type and location:
   - **a.** A ball-and-socket joint is found between the proximal two bones of the limb.
   - **b.** A joint with mainly hinge motion is found between the second and third limb regions.
   - **c.** Numerous gliding joints are found between the third and fourth limb regions.
   - **d.** Several hinge joints are found in the most distal limb regions.
3. **Form of the paw.** The overall form of the paw is almost identical to that of the thoracic limb, except that the hindpaw has four digits while the forepaw has five.
4. **Alternating flexor surface positions.** The flexor surface positions alternate from one surface of the limb to the other from the hip to the tarsus.
5. **Density of muscle according to region.** As in the thoracic limb, the muscles covering the proximal pelvic limb are thick, while those in the distal pelvic limb are smaller and tend to taper to tendons.
6. **Positioning of vascular and nervous structures.** As in the thoracic limb, most major vessels and nerves lie in a more protected position on the medial surface of the limb.
7. **Two sets of veins.** Both a deep set of satellite veins and a subcutaneous set of superficial veins are present.
8. **One key nerve.** The femoral nerve in the pelvic limb is similar to the radial nerve in the thoracic limb. Should the function of either of these nerves become impaired, the limb is rendered useless because it is unable to hold in extension and bear weight.

B. Unique features. The pelvic limb differs from the thoracic limb in the following ways:

1. **Bony and cartilaginous attachment to the axial skeleton.** Unlike the thoracic limb, which has an entirely muscular attachment to the body, the pelvic limb is attached to the axial skeleton by means of the sacroiliac joint.
2. **Fusion of the two most proximal bony elements of the limbs with each other across the ventral midline.** The two ossa coxarum are united across the ventral midline at the symphysis pelvis.
3. **Flexor surface positioning.** On the pelvic limb, the most proximal flexor surface faces caudally (rather than cranially, as it does in the thoracic limb). In addition, the flexor surfaces alternate from cranial to caudal (as opposed to caudal to cranial in the thoracic limb) as far as the tarsus.
   - **a.** These two features produce a rather marked difference in the action of the muscles of the shank (i.e., the cranial and caudal tibial region).
   - **b.** Because the flexor surface for the tarsal (ankle) joints is positioned opposite the flexor surface of the digits, the muscles that extend the tarsus flex the digits, a situation different from that in the forelimb, where carpal extensors are also digital extensors.
4. **Absence of the first digit.** Digit I (i.e., the dewclaw) of the hindpaw is usually absent in dogs.

II. REGIONS. Like the thoracic limb, the pelvic limb can be thought of as having five regions (Figure 56–1).

A. The **pelvic region** is the most proximal region of the pelvic limb. This portion of the limb overlaps the pelvic region of the body as a whole and assists in the formation of the pelvic inlet, the pelvic outlet, and the walls of the pelvic cavity.

1. **Bones.** The bone of the pelvic region of the pelvic limb is the **os coxae** (see Chapter 50 I A 1, B).
2. **Muscles.** The pelvic region of the pelvic limb (like the scapular region of the thoracic limb) is highly muscular. Most of the lateral surface of the os coxae is clothed in deep layers of muscles that act to extend the hip and propel the body forward during locomotion.

B. The **thigh** is the region of the pelvic limb extending between the hip and the knee.

1. **Bones.** Like the corresponding part of the thoracic limb (i.e., the brachium), the skeleton of the thigh consists of one bone, the **femur,** which is the largest and strongest single bone in the body.
2. **Muscles.** The thigh (like the brachium) is a highly muscular region. Most of the femur is thickly clothed in muscle along its full length, as well as around its full circumference.

C. The **crus (leg)** is the region of the pelvic limb extending between the knee and the tarsus (ankle).

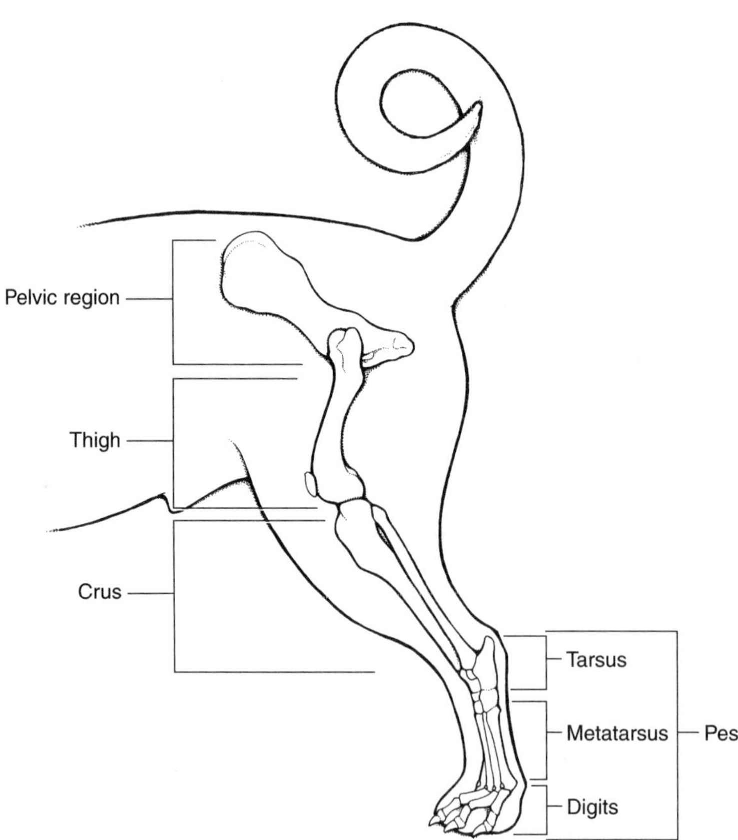

FIGURE 56–1. Regions of the pelvic limb.

Canine Clinical Correlation

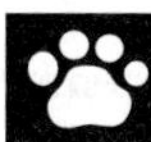

The word "leg" is frequently used colloquially to refer to the entire pelvic limb; however, anatomically, this term refers only to the portion of the limb that houses the tibia and fibula (i.e., the crus). Therefore, the term "leg" is not applicable to the other regions of the pelvic limb, or to the thoracic limb at all, and the terms "hindleg" and "front leg" are erroneous.

1. **Bones.** Like the corresponding part of the thoracic limb (i.e., the antebrachium), the crus contains two bones, the **tibia** and **fibula.** The tibia, the weight-bearing bone of the crus, is markedly stouter than the fibula.
2. **Muscles.** The crus is variably ensheathed in muscle, even more so than the antebrachium.
   a. Proximocaudally and proximolaterally, the muscle bellies are large and the bone is deeply buried.
   b. Proximomedially, little muscle is present. Much of the medial surface of the tibia is subcutaneous throughout its length, and even the proximomedial region of the tibia is covered by little more than skin.

E. The **pes (hindpaw, "foot")** is the region of the pelvic limb that extends between the distal crus and the ground. The pes comprises the **tarsus, metatarsus,** and **digits,** and associated **sesamoid bones.**

1. The **tarsus (hock, ankle)** is the region of the pelvic limb extending between the distal crus and the metatarsus.
   a. **Bones.** There are seven **tarsal bones,** arranged in two irregular rows. The rows are not as regular as those of the carpal bones; thus, thinking of the tarsal bones as comprising a relatively proximal group and a relatively distal group is somewhat more helpful. Like the bones of the carpus, the more proximal bones are named and the more distal ones numbered.
      (1) **Proximal group.** The bones of the proximal group are the **talus,** the **calcaneus,** and the **central tarsal bone.**
      (2) **Distal group.** From medial to lateral, the bones of the distal group are numbered **I–IV.**
   b. **Joints.** The numerous **intertarsal joints** are designated according to the bones between which they extend (e.g., the centroquartal joint). As in the carpus, motion at the intertarsal joints is highly restricted to a small degree of sliding motion between the various tarsal elements.

2. **Metatarsus**
   a. **Bones.** Four or five **metatarsal bones** are present in the region corresponding to the arch of the human foot. These bones are designated **I–V,** from medial to lateral.
   b. **Joints.** The **metatarsophalangeal joints** are present at the articulation of the metatarsal and proximal phalangeal bones.

3. **Digits.** Four or five **digits** are also present in the hindpaw, one articulating with each metatarsal bone. Like the metatarsal bones, these digits are **designated I–V** (or II–V), from medial to lateral.
   a. **Bones.** The digits are composed of **phalanges,** as in the manus.
      (1) **Digit I,** when present, consists of two phalanges.
      (2) **Digits II–V** are each composed of three phalanges.
   b. **Joints.** The **interphalangeal joints** lie between the bones of the digits.
      (1) **Digit I.** When digit I is present, the interphalangeal joint is located between the proximal and distal phalanges.
      (2) **Digits II–V**
         (a) The **proximal interphalangeal joints** are present between the proximal and middle phalanges of digits II–V.

(b) The **distal interphalangeal joints** are present between the middle and distal phalanges of digits II–V.

4. **Sesamoid elements.** The sesamoid elements of the pes are similar to those of the manus.
   a. One **dorsal sesamoid bone,** small and round, lies embedded in each digital extensor tendon at the metatarsophalangeal joint.
   b. Paired **proximal sesamoid bones** lie plantarly at the metatarsophalangeal joints, within the substance of the tendons of the interosseous muscles.

III. JOINTS.

As in the thoracic limb, the joints of the pelvic limb are named anatomically for the regions of the limb contributing to the joint (from proximal to distal).

A. The **sacroiliac joint** is the region where the pelvic limb articulates firmly with the vertebral column. The sacroiliac joint is formed by the articulation of the **sacrum** and the **ilium** (one of the four bones that fuse to form the **os coxae).**

B. The **coxofemoral (hip) joint** is the region where the stable, largely immobile os coxae articulates with the highly mobile proximal part of the limb.

C. The **stifle (knee) joint** is the articulation between the thigh and the crus.

1. The **femur, patella, tibia,** and **fibula** contribute to the formation of the stifle joint.
2. The anatomical terms used to refer to the stifle joint depend on the portion under consideration. The **femorotibial joint** forms the main portion of the stifle joint; the complete joint also includes the **femoropatellar** and **proximal tibiofibular joints.**

D. The **talocrural (ankle) joint** is the joint between the crus (specifically the tibia) and the tarsal region (specifically the talus). Note that this joint names the distal component before the proximal one.

E. The **tarsometatarsal joint** is the joint between the tarsus and the metatarsus. Eight bones form this joint: the four members of the **distal group of tarsal bones** and the four **metatarsal bones.**

F. The **joints of the pes** (i.e., the **metatarsophalangeal** and **interphalangeal joints)** are usually referred to colloquially as the "knuckles." As in the manus, these joints are simple saddle joints.

Chapter 57

Bones of the Pelvic Limb

I. PELVIC GIRDLE.

I. PELVIC GIRDLE. The pelvic girdle, formed from the fusion of the two **ossa coxarum** (see Chapter 50 I A 1), attaches the pelvic limb to the trunk.

II. THIGH

A. Femur. The femur (Figure 57–1) is the bone of the thigh.

1. **Proximal femur**
   a. The **head** is the hemispherical portion that faces medially and articulates with the acetabulum of the os coxae. The **fovea capitis** is a roughened, roughly circular depression in the middle of the femoral head, marking the attachment site of the **ligament of the head of the femur.** This stout ligament extends between the femoral head and the acetabular cup.
   b. The **neck** is a constriction (more distinct than the humeral neck) between the femoral head and the remainder of the bone.
   c. The **greater trochanter** is a large, almost triangular eminence positioned on the proximal lateral femur essentially opposite the femoral head. Certain muscles of the gluteal region insert here.
   d. The **lesser trochanter** is a smaller but also distinct elaboration on the medial side of the femur, positioned at the junction of the head and the shaft. The iliopsoas muscle inserts on the lesser trochanter.
   e. The **intertrochanteric crest** is a low, arching line passing between the greater and lesser trochanters.
   f. The **trochanteric fossa** is a deep depression on the caudal femoral surface between the greater and lesser trochanters and caudal to the ridge extending between the neck and greater trochanter. Several small muscles originating on the bony pelvis insert in this fossa.
   g. The **third trochanter** is a named prominence that is usually unrecognizable in the dog. When visible, this obscure elevation lies at the distal end of a faint line that extends from the highest point of the greater trochanter to a point just ventral to the level of the pelvic symphysis in the articulated skeleton. The superficial gluteal muscle inserts in this region.
2. **Femoral shaft.** The body of the femur is quite round in cross-section, and smooth on all but its caudal surface. This **aspera surface** (i.e., the roughened and slightly flattened area on the caudal surface of the femur) provides attachment for the caudal thigh muscles and extends essentially along the full length of the bone. The **medial** and **lateral linea aspera** mark the respective borders of the aspera surface, which is broad proximally and distally and narrow through the midregion.
   a. The **trochanteric surface** is the proximal part of the femur's caudal surface (near the trochanters), where the lineae aspera are widely separated.
   b. The **popliteal surface** is the distal part of the femur's caudal surface (near the condyles), where the lineae aspera diverge.
3. **Distal femur.** The distal femur is considerably modified for articulation with the tibia.
   a. The **trochlea (patellar surface)** is specialized for articulation with the patella. Located on the cranial surface of the distal femur, the trochlea presents a shallow, smooth, wide groove oriented parallel with the long axis of the femur. The medial and lateral lips of the trochlea are continuous with the femoral condyles.

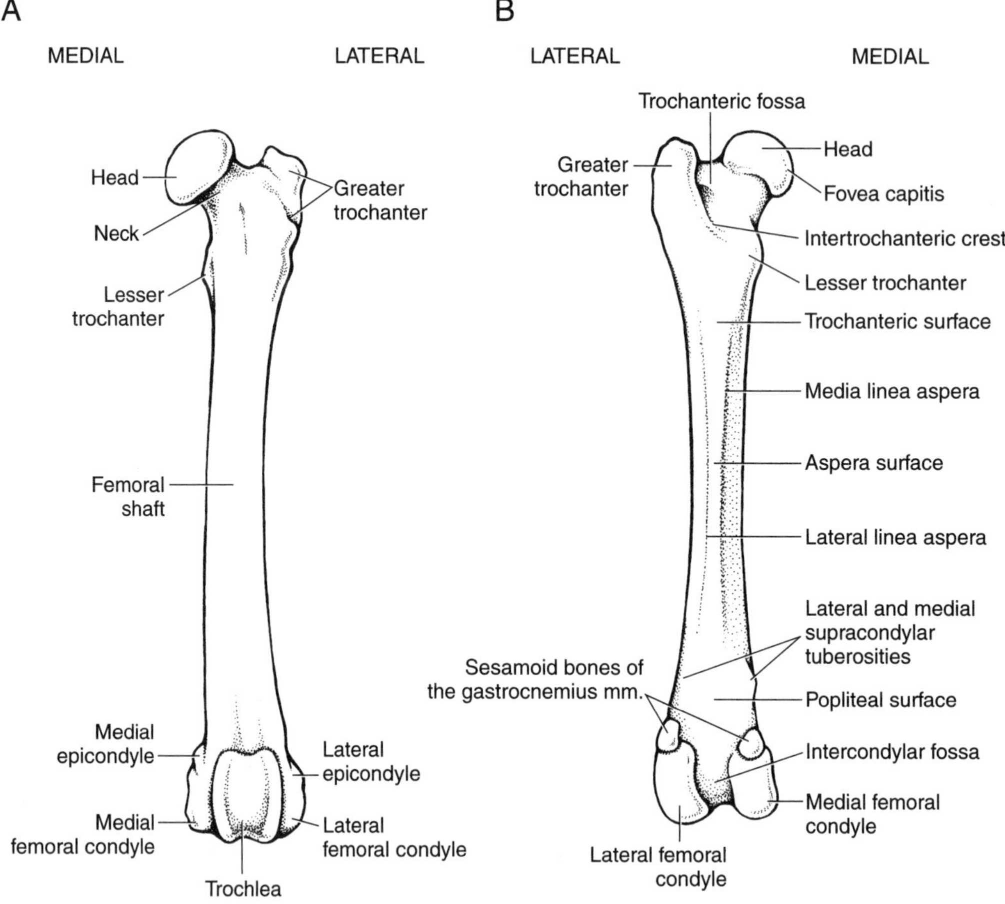

FIGURE 57–1. Left femur. (*A*) Cranial view. (*B*) Caudal view.

b. The **femoral condyles,** one **medial** and one **lateral,** articulate with the tibia. The femoral condyles are prominent, rounded projections on the caudal-most surface of the distal femur. The articular surface of each femoral condyle is very smooth.

(1) The **intercondylar fossa** is a deep depression on the caudal femoral surface separating the two femoral condyles. No structures attach here.

(2) The **extensor fossa** is a narrow, deep pit at the cranial edge of the lateral femoral condyle, where the distal edge of the lateral lip of the trochlea joins the condyle. The long digital extensor muscle originates here.

(3) The **fossa for the popliteal muscle** is a subtle dimple on the lateral surface of the lateral femoral condyle where the tendon of origin of the popliteus muscle attaches.

(4) The **articular facets for the sesamoid bones of the gastrocnemius muscles** are located on the proximal-most edges of each femoral condyle. The medial articular facet is less prominent than the lateral one, and may actually be absent.

c. The **epicondyles,** one **medial** and one **lateral,** provide the proximal attachment points for the medial and lateral collateral ligaments of the stifle (knee) joint. The epicondyles are positioned on the dorsal surface of each condyle (*epi* = "upon").

d. The **supracondylar tuberosities,** one medial and one lateral, lie proximal to the femoral condyles. The medial and lateral heads of the gastrocnemius muscle arise from these tuberosities. The lateral supracondylar tuberosity also serves as the site of origin for the superficial digital flexor muscle.

B. Sesamoid elements. Three sesamoid bones are associated with the femur.

1. The **patella,** the largest sesamoid bone in the body, is incorporated into the tendon of the quadriceps femoris muscle.
   a. **Form.** The **acorn-shaped** patella is **convex caudally** to conform to the curvature of the femoral trochlea.
   b. **Named regions**
      (1) The **base** is the blunt proximal portion (the "cap of the acorn").
      (2) The **apex** is the slightly pointed distal end.
      (3) The **articular surface,** its caudal surface, is convex and smooth.
   c. The **parapatellar fibrocartilages,** which extend from each lateral surface of the patella, conform to the ridges of the femoral trochlea.
2. The **sesamoid bones of the gastrocnemius muscle** are two small, roughly rounded bones embedded in the medial and lateral heads of the muscle. These bones articulate with the femoral condyles [see II A 3 b (4)].

III. CRUS. The **tibia** and **fibula** are the bones of the crus (Figure 57–2).

A. Tibia. The tibia is the main **weight-bearing bone** of the crus.

1. **Proximal tibia**
   a. The **tibial plateau,** the triangular **proximal articular surface** of the tibia, provides a wide, strong articular surface for the femoral condyles. Medial and lateral articular areas are separated by a central nonarticular region.
      (1) The **medial** and **lateral tibial condyles** include the articular areas, one corresponding to each femoral condyle, and also the mass of tibial substance just distal to the actual articular surfaces. The condyles of the tibia are flattened, somewhat scooped areas adapted to accommodate the more typical condyles of the femur.
      (2) The **intercondylar eminence** is a small elevation occupying the central part of the nonarticular area between the two tibial condyles. Small, distinct "knobs," the **medial** and **lateral intercondylar tubercles,** are positioned on the respective sides of the eminence.
      (3) The **cranial** and **caudal intercondylar areas** are small depressions on each respective side of the intercondylar eminence. These depressions provide attachment sites for the ligaments that hold the menisci (i.e., fibrocartilages interposed between the femur and the tibia) to the tibia.
   b. The **tibial tuberosity** is a large, stout process extending cranially from the proximal tibia that provides the insertion site for the tendon of the quadriceps femoris muscle.
   c. The **cranial border of the tibia** (formerly known as the **tibial crest)** is a prominent ridge that extends distally from the tibial tuberosity to blend with the proximal part of the tibial body.
   d. The **extensor groove,** a notch in the cranial border of the lateral tibial condyle, provides passage for the tendon of the long digital extensor. (Recall that this tendon originates from the extensor fossa of the femur.)
   e. The **proximal articular facet for the fibula** lies on the caudolateral side of the lateral tibial condyle.
   f. The **popliteal notch** is a rather deep indentation between the two tibial condyles on the caudal tibial surface.
2. **Tibial shaft**
   a. **Proximally,** where it continues distally from the triangular proximal extremity, the tibial body is three-sided.
   b. In its **midregion,** the tibial body is almost cylindrical and very smooth.

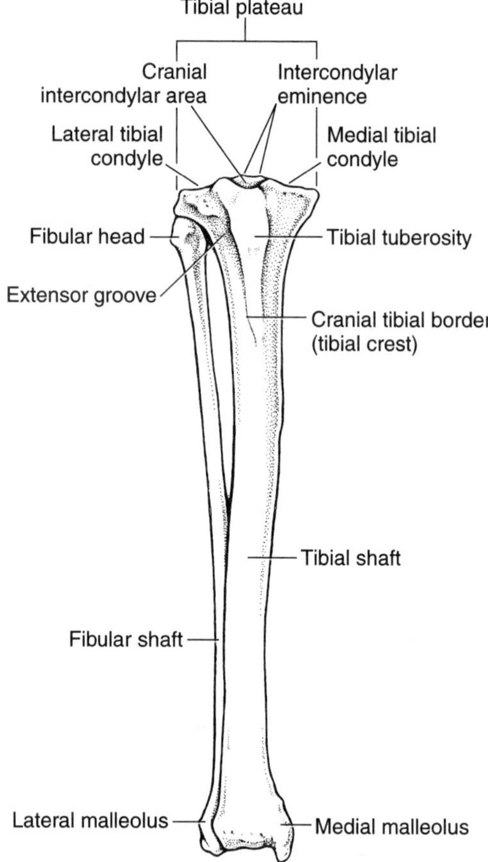

FIGURE 57–2. Right tibia and fibula, cranial view.

c. **Distally,** the tibial body becomes four-sided as it blends with the quadrangular distal extremity.

3. **Distal tibia.** The distal extremity of the tibia is rectangular and highly modified for articulation with the talus.
   a. The **distal articular surface** presents the **tibial cochlea,** two deep grooves that articulate with the trochlear ridges of the talus.
   b. The **distal articular facet for the fibula** is positioned on the lateral distal extremity of the tibia.
   c. The **medial malleolus** (i.e., the medial side of the distal tibial extremity) is the prominent bump on the medial surface of the ankle region, readily palpable in both humans and dogs.

B. Fibula. The fibula, which lies lateral to the tibia, bears little (if any) weight but provides essential attachment sites for many crural muscles.

1. **Proximal fibula.** The fibular **head** is noticeably flattened transversely, where it fits flush against the lateral tibial condyle.
2. **Fibular shaft.** The fibular **body** is rather spare and somewhat irregularly formed, being transversely flattened and slightly concave proximally, triangular in its midregions, and transversely flattened again distally.
   a. The **proximal fibular body** is separated from the tibia by a wide **interosseous space.**

The borders of the tibia and fibula that face each other across this space are referred to as the **tibial** and **fibular interosseous borders,** respectively.

b. The **distal fibular body** is markedly roughened along its medial border, a feature related to the fibula's close apposition to the tibia in this region.

3. **Distal fibula (lateral malleolus).** The lateral malleolus forms the prominent bony bulge on the lateral side of the ankle (the same bony bulge that humans tend to knock into furniture with painful regularity).
   a. The **medial surface** presents an **articular facet** for articulation with the tibia.
   b. The **lateral surface** presents a distinct groove that houses the tendons of the lateral digital extensor and peroneus brevis muscles.

C. Sesamoid elements. A small sesamoid bone lies within the tendon of origin of the popliteus muscle on the caudolateral surface of the lateral tibial condyle, about midway along its medial-to-lateral length at the level of the fibular head.

IV. PES.

The bones of the hindpaw include the bones of the tarsus, metatarsus, and digits, as well as several sesamoid bones associated with the digits (Figure 57–3).

A. Tarsus. Seven bones compose the tarsus, arranged in two groups.

1. **Proximal group**
   a. The **talus** is positioned the most medially among the proximal group of tarsal bones.
      (1) The talus articulates with the:
         (a) Tibia and fibula (proximally)
         (b) Central tarsal bone (distally)
         (c) Calcaneus (laterally)
      (2) The talus presents several readily identifiable regions:
         (a) The **trochlea** of the talus is a prominent pair of ridges that articulates with the tibial cochlea.
         (b) The **body** of the talus is the massive central part of the bone.
         (c) The **lateral process** of the talus articulates with the calcaneus.
         (d) The **neck** of the talus is a slightly restricted region distal to the body.
         (e) The slightly rounded **head** of the talus articulates distally with the central tarsal bone.
   b. The **calcaneus** is positioned most laterally in the proximal group.
      (1) The calcaneus articulates with the:
         (a) Talus (medially)
         (b) Central and fourth tarsal bones (distally)
      (2) The calcaneus presents the following features:
         (a) The **calcaneal tuber** (the proximal half of the calcaneus and what is colloquially referred to as the **"heel bone"** in the human foot) projects proximally from the remainder of the bones in the tarsus. The calcaneal tuber provides the attachment point for the tendon of the gastrocnemius muscle, and acts as a lever for extension at the hock (ankle). In form and function, the calcaneal tuber is similar to the olecranon process of the ulna.
         (b) The **sustentaculum tali** is a ledge of bone that projects from the medial side of the midportion of the calcaneus. The sustentaculum tali provides a bearing surface over which the tendon of the lateral head of the deep digital flexor passes.
   c. The **central tarsal bone** is positioned medially and distally in the proximal group.
      (1) The central tarsal bone articulates with all of the other tarsal bones.
      (2) The central tarsal bone presents a concavity (which receives the head of the talus) and a plantar process.

2. **Distal group**
   a. **Tarsal bones I–III** are relatively small (in comparison with tarsal bone IV) and restricted to the medial half of the tarsus. In some individuals, tarsal bone I is a separate

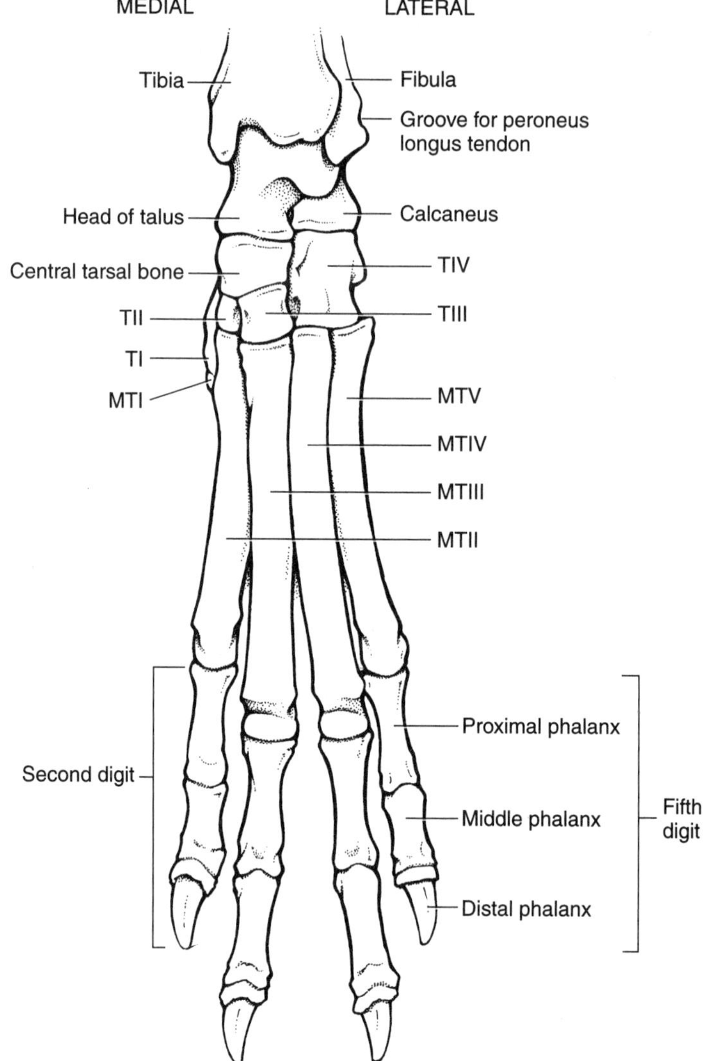

FIGURE 57–3. Bones of the left distal crus and pes, dorsal view. Note that a tiny first metatarsal bone was present in this specimen. *T1, TII, TIII, TIV*—tarsal bones I–IV; *MTI, MTII, MTIII, MTIV, MTV*—metatarsal bones I–V.

bone, while in others, it is fused to the first metatarsal bone. Tarsal bones I–III articulate with the:

(1) Central tarsal bone (proximally)
(2) Metatarsal bones I or II–III (distally)
(3) Fourth tarsal bone and each other (medially and laterally)

b. Tarsal bone IV is positioned on the lateral edge of the tarsus. This bone articulates with the:

(1) Calcaneus (proximally)
(2) Fourth and fifth metatarsal bones (distally)
(3) Central and third metatarsal bones (medially)

B. Metatarsus. Four or five metatarsal bones are present. In comparison with the metacarpal region, the metatarsal region is proportionately longer and more compressed laterally.

1. **Metatarsal bone I** may be:
   a. **Absent**
   b. **Fused with the second metatarsal bone**
   c. **Divided into two portions,** joined to each other by either fibrous tissue or a synovial joint
2. **Metatarsal bones II–IV.** Like the metacarpal bones, metatarsal bones II–IV have a base, body (shaft), and head, and are equipped with interosseous spaces (see Chapter 26 IV B).

C. **Digits.** Four or five digits are present, corresponding with the metatarsal bones. Most breeds of dogs possess only four toes on the hindpaw.

1. **Digit I** (the "dewclaw"), when present, is highly irregular. Its bony composition can range from a complete digit (i.e., two phalanges supported by a single- or double-elemented metatarsal bone), to simply a claw attached to the metatarsal region by skin and supported by the distal phalanx alone.

Canine Clinical Correlation

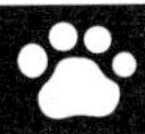

The presence or absence of digit I on the hindpaw is a matter of critical importance in some breed registries (e.g., Great Pyrenees). Some breed registries that require the presence of the dewclaw require the presence of a single toe, while others require the presence of a double toe.

2. **Digits II–V** are similar to those of the forepaw. Each consists of a proximal, middle, and distal phalanx, with the distal end of the terminal phalanx shaped like the claw it supports externally (see Chapter 26 IV C).

D. **Sesamoid elements of the pes** are essentially identical to those of the manus (see Chapter 26 IV D).

Chapter 58

Joints and Ligaments of the Pelvic Limb

I. SACROILIAC JOINT.

SACROILIAC JOINT. The sacroiliac joint, between the sacrum and the wing of the ilium, is the region where the pelvic limb articulates firmly with the vertebral column. There are two sacroiliac joints, one dorsal and one ventral, on each side, for a total of four.

A. Motion. Although the sacroiliac joint firmly attaches the limb to the axial skeleton, it is capable of a small range of motion. This flexibility allows the joint to absorb the shock transmitted when the pelvic limb contacts the ground.

B. Structure. The sacroiliac joint is largely a **synarthrosis (fibrous joint),** but it also has a small **synovial part.** The fibrous portion imparts stability to the joint, while the synovial portion allows the normal small range of motion.

II. COXOFEMORAL (HIP) JOINT

A. Motion. The hip joint is a **ball-and-socket joint,** which allows a wide range of motion (i.e., extension, flexion, abduction, adduction, and some degree of circumduction).

B. Structure

1. **Bones** contributing to the hip joint are proximally, the **os coxae** (at the **acetabulum)** and distally, the **femur** (by its **head).**
2. **Joint capsule.** The hip joint capsule is generously sized, extending from the acetabular edge to the distal area of the femoral head.
3. **Ligaments**
   a. The **ligament of the head of the femur** is a thick, well-developed ligament that extends between the fovea capitis and the acetabular fossa.
   b. No regular thickenings organized into ligaments (e.g., the collateral ligaments) are incorporated into the substance of the joint capsule of the hip. However, minor, irregularly placed thickenings are variably present.

III. STIFLE (KNEE) JOINT.

STIFLE (KNEE) JOINT. This joint is the most complex joint in the body. Its complexity is largely attributable to the poor fit of the bones that form the joint.

A. Motion. Although the stifle joint is a condylar joint, it is best thought of as a **ginglymus (hinge) joint** because its motion is largely restricted to flexion and extension.

B. Structure

1. **Bones.** Four bones—the **femur, patella, tibia,** and **fibula—** contribute to the stifle joint, although not all four are mobile. Three mobile subjoints are formed among these four bones:
   a. The **femorotibial joint** is oriented in a **proximal-to-distal** direction.
      (1) **Contributing bones.** The femorotibial joint is formed proximally by the **femoral condyles** and distally by the **tibial condyles.**
      (2) **Function.** This articulation provides both the **flexion–extension motion** and the **weight-bearing function** of the joint.
   b. The **femoropatellar joint** is oriented in a **cranial-to-caudal** direction.

(1) **Contributing bones.** The femoropatellar joint is formed cranially by the **patella,** and caudally by the **femoral trochlea.**

(2) **Function.** This articulation **protects the quadriceps femoris muscle** by providing a wider bearing surface for its tendon, thus distributing pressure over a wider area and reducing wear.

c. The **proximal tibiofibular joint** is formed by the **caudolateral surface** of the **lateral tibial condyle** and the **medial surface** of the **fibular head.** Normally, little to no motion takes place at this joint.

2. **Menisci.** The medial and lateral menisci are "C"-shaped **fibrocartilages interposed between the femur** and **tibia** to improve the fit of these two incongruous bones.

a. **Position**

(1) Each meniscus is positioned with its opening facing its fellow across the midline, and the rounded portion facing medially or laterally, respectively (Figure 58–1).

(2) The placement of the menisci over the tibial plateau reduces the area of contact between the tibia and femur to a rather small area in the center of each tibial condyle.

b. **Form.** The menisci are thinner at their open ends, and thicker on their rounded periphery.

c. **Ligaments.** Six named ligaments attach the menisci to the tibia and to each other—one pair attaches the cranial edge of each meniscus to the tibia, one pair attaches the caudal edge of each meniscus to the tibia, one individual ligament attaches the menisci to each other, and one individual ligament attaches the lateral meniscus to the femur (see Figure 58–1).

(1) **Cranial tibial ligaments.** There are two cranial tibial ligaments: the **cranial tibial ligament of the medial meniscus,** and the **cranial tibial ligament of the lateral meniscus.** These ligaments attach the cranial edge of the open part of the "C" of each meniscus to the cranial intercondylar area of the tibia.

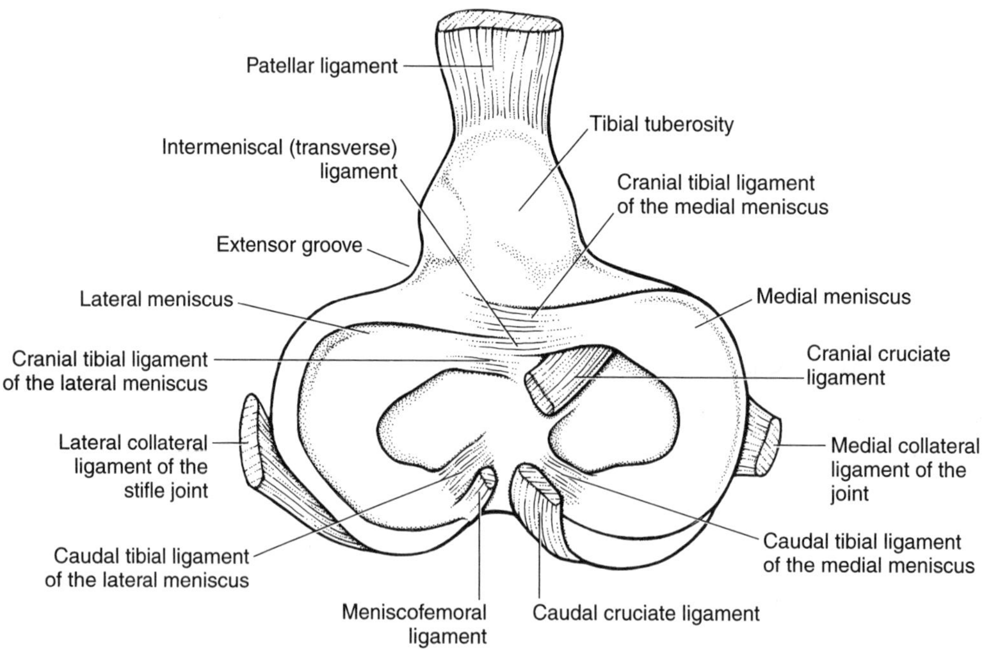

FIGURE 58–1. Menisci and ligaments of the stifle (knee) joint. The menisci are similar to each other in form, although the medial one is slightly larger and more open than the lateral one.

(2) **Caudal tibial ligaments.** There are two caudal tibial ligaments: the **caudal tibial ligament of the medial meniscus,** and the **caudal tibial ligament of the lateral meniscus.** These ligaments attach the caudal edge of the open part of the "C" of each meniscus to the caudal intercondylar area of the tibia.

(3) The **intermeniscal (transverse) ligament** extends between the free cranial ends of the two menisci.

(4) The **meniscofemoral ligament** (the **femoral ligament of the lateral meniscus)** extends dorsally from the caudal open edge of the lateral meniscus to the medial ("inner") side of the medial femoral condyle.

3. **Joint capsule.** One joint capsule composed of **three subparts** serves the stifle joint. All three subparts intercommunicate, simplifying diagnostic and therapeutic manipulations of the joint. (Note that this is not the case in large animals.)
   a. The **medial** and **lateral femorotibial joint sacs** are positioned between the respective femoral and tibial condyles. Each femorotibial sac extends caudally and proximally between the sesamoid bones of the gastrocnemius muscles and the femoral condyles.
      (1) The menisci indent each femorotibial joint sac into **femoromeniscal** and **tibiomeniscal parts.**
      (2) The **lateral femorotibial joint sac is further divided** into one portion related to the head of the fibula, and two portions related to the tendons of origin of the long digital extensor and popliteus muscles.
   b. The **femoropatellar joint sac** lies between the patella and the femoral trochlea.
      (1) The femoropatellar joint sac is very large.
      (2) A diverticulum of this sac extends a short distance proximally deep to the quadriceps femoris tendon, reducing the friction between the tendon and the femur.

4. **Ligaments.** Thirteen ligaments are associated with the stifle joint.
   a. **Collateral ligaments.** The **medial** and **lateral collateral ligaments** are distinct, stout thickenings of the joint capsule formed on each side of the joint (see Figure 58–1). These ligaments **prevent medial-to-lateral displacement of the femur and tibia relative to each other.**
      (1) The **lateral (fibular) collateral ligament** attaches proximally to the lateral femoral epicondyle, and distally to the lateral surface of the fibular head (a few fibers pass to the adjacent tibia, as well).
      (2) The **medial (tibial) collateral ligament** attaches proximally to the medial femoral epicondyle, and distally to the medial surface of the tibia, just distal to its medial condyle.
   b. **Cruciate ligaments.** The **cranial** and **caudal cruciate ligaments** are **intracapsular** (i.e., they are completely enclosed by the joint capsule) and **cross each other, forming an "X"** (*cruciate* = "cross"). These ligaments **prevent cranial-to-caudal displacement of the femur and tibia relative to each other.** The cruciate ligaments are **named for their tibial attachment.**
      (1) The **cranial cruciate ligament** originates on the **cranial intercondyloid area of the tibia** and inserts on the caudomedial part of the **lateral femoral condyle.**
      (2) The **caudal cruciate ligament** originates near the popliteal notch on the **caudal edge of the tibia** and inserts on the caudomedial part of the **medial femoral condyle.**
   c. **Ligaments associated with the patella**
      (1) **Femoropatellar ligaments.** The **medial** and **lateral femoropatellar ligaments** are relatively indistinct bands of fibers within the joint capsule that extend transversely between the respective surfaces of the patella and the femur. These ligaments **prevent medial-to-lateral displacement of the patella.**
      (2) The **patellar ligament** is the **portion of the tendon of the quadriceps femoris muscle** that lies distal to the patella (see Figure 58–1). The patellar ligament, which **maintains the position of the patella,** is simply the continuation of the parent muscle (as opposed to a specialized ligament).
   d. **Ligaments associated with the menisci.** The six ligaments associated with the menisci are detailed in III B 2 c.

Canine Clinical Correlation

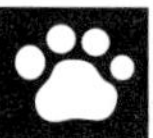

The incongruity of the bones contributing to the stifle joint results in fairly frequent injury to the ligamentous and cartilaginous structures supporting it.

- **Rupture of the cranial cruciate ligament** is a particularly common injury in dogs (as well as in humans). Physical examination of a patient with a ruptured cranial cruciate ligament reveals a positive "cranial drawer sign," in which the tibia can be pulled cranially from beneath the femur, similar to pulling a drawer out of a desk.
- **Strain or rupture of the collateral ligaments** is also rather common.
- **Trapping of the menisci** between the tibial plateau and the rolling femoral condyles results in meniscal tears familiar to veterinary and human orthopedic surgeons alike.

IV. TIBIOFIBULAR JOINTS.

Two **synovial joints** are present between the **tibia** and **fibula.** In addition, a **stiff membrane** connects much of the medial surfaces of the two bones where they are separated from each other.

A. The **proximal tibiofibular joint** is small. Minimal movement normally occurs at this joint.

1. The **ligament of the fibular head** is a small collection of fibers extending transversely between the fibular head and the proximal tibia.
2. The **synovial membrane** of the proximal tibiofibular joint is an extension of the synovial membrane associated with the lateral femorotibial joint.

B. The **distal tibiofibular joint,** like the proximal one, is small and tight.

1. The **cranial tibiofibular ligament** passes transversely between the lateral malleolus (i.e., the distal end of the fibula) and the tibia.
2. The **synovial membrane** of the distal tibiofibular joint is an extension of the synovial membrane associated with the talocrural joint.

C. The **interosseous membrane** of the crus binds the tibia and fibula together. The membrane extends along almost the full length of the tibia and fibula, but is most recognizable in the interosseous space.

V. TARSAL JOINTS

A. Overview. As in the carpus, there are three main joints of the tarsus.

1. The **talocrural (ankle) joint,** between the tibia proximally and the talus distally, provides the greatest range of motion at the tarsal region (hock).
2. The **intertarsal joints** each have two subjoints because of the positioning of the central tarsal bone between the talus and the metatarsus.
   a. The **proximal intertarsal joint** lies between the talus and central tarsal bone medially and the calcaneus and tarsal bone IV laterally. A small degree of motion is possible at the proximal intertarsal joint.
   b. The **distal intertarsal joint** lies between the central tarsal bone and tarsal bones II and III medially. (No corresponding part is present laterally because of the height of tarsal bone IV; see Chapter 57, Figure 57–3.)
3. The **tarsometatarsal joints** lie between the distal row of tarsal bones and the metatarsal bones.

B. Motion. Motion at the hock takes place primarily at the **talocrural joint,** which functions as a **ginglymus** joint and thus permits mainly extension–flexion. A limited amount of flexion–extension and gliding (i.e., lateral movement) are also possible at the proximal intertarsal joint. Motion at the many other individual joints of the hock is normally minimal.

C. Structure

1. **Bones.** The bones that form the tarsal joints are enumerated in V A.
2. **Joint capsule.** The tarsal joint capsule extends like a sheath across the entire area of the joints. The capsule has **seven subdivisions,** four positioned medially and three positioned laterally.
   a. The largest compartment surrounds the talocrural joint, which is the most mobile of the tarsal joints.
   b. Communications are variably present among the compartments, but they are not always constant or clinically significant.

Canine Clinical Correlation

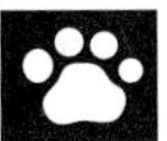

Only the talocrural joint is accessible to needle puncture.

3. **Ligaments**
   a. **Collateral ligaments**
      (1) The **medial collateral ligament** is a prominent thickening of the joint capsule that extends between the medial malleolus (i.e., the tibia) and tarsal bone I. (Much weaker attachments to metatarsal bones I and/or II are also present.)
      (2) The **lateral collateral ligament** extends between the lateral malleolus (i.e., the fibula) and the base of metatarsal bone V.
   b. **Extensor retinacula** (see Chapter 59, Figure 59–4). Three extensor retinacula are present near and on the tarsus (as opposed to one in the carpus). As in the carpus, the extensor retinacula hold the tendons of the extensor muscles of the tarsus and digits close to the adjacent bone.
      (1) The **crural (proximal) extensor retinaculum** is a rather narrow band of fibers attached to the tibia a considerable distance proximal to the hock. The crural extensor retinaculum binds the tendons of the long digital extensor and the cranial tibial muscles.
      (2) The **tarsal (distal) extensor retinaculum** is a small but distinct loop attached to the calcaneus about halfway down its length. This loop retains the tendon of the long digital extensor muscle.
      (3) The **peroneal muscle retinaculum** is a transverse band situated on the lateral tibial surface just proximal to the tarsus. This band retains the tendons of the peroneus longus and brevis muscles, as well as the tendon of the lateral digital extensor.
   c. The **flexor retinaculum** is a thickening of the tarsal fascia on the plantar and medial surfaces of the joint. The flexor retinaculum attaches plantarly to the **calcaneal tuber** and medially to the **distal tibia** and the **tarsal bones.**
   d. The **plantar tarsal fibrocartilage** ("ligament") is a thick layer of fibrocartilaginous tissue applied intimately to the plantar surface of the tarsal bones. This layer smooths the plantar surface of the tarsal bones, providing an even surface for passage of the flexor tendon over the hock.
   e. The **special ligaments of the tarsus** are individually named ligaments extending between the individual tarsal bones. The most clinically significant of these, the **long plantar ligament,** is a prominent and fairly thick band of fibers extending from the proximal end of the calcaneus directly distally to the first (when present) and second metatarsal bones. Strain of this ligament is sometimes associated with lameness.
4. **Tarsal canal.** The tarsal canal, positioned on the plantar surface of the joint, essentially lies between the sustentaculum tali of the tarsus and the flexor retinaculum.

The passageway, similar to the carpal canal of the forelimb, transmits several structures:

a. **Muscular structures** include the tendons of the lateral head of the deep digital flexor.
b. **Vascular structures** include the plantar branches of the saphenous artery and vein.
c. **Nervous structures** include the medial and lateral plantar nerves.

VI. METATARSAL AND INTERPHALANGEAL JOINTS. The metatarsal and interphalangeal joints of the pelvic limb are almost identical to those of the thoracic limb (see Chapter 27 V–VI).

Chapter 59

Muscles of the Pelvic Limb

I. EXTRINSIC MUSCLES. In the case of the pelvic limb, the extrinsic muscles are the **hypaxial (sublumbar) muscles of the back** (see Chapter 20 II C 2 b (1)–(3); Table 20–5). These muscles originate on the axial skeleton in the abdominal region (i.e., from the last three thoracic vertebrae and all of the lumbar vertebrae) and extend through the pelvic cavity to insert on the pelvic girdle. (Recall that the pelvic girdle is considered part of the pelvic limb, rather than the axial skeleton.)

A. The **quadratus lumborum** and **psoas minor** muscles insert on the iliac wing, and mainly act to flex or stabilize the vertebral column. Although they have little effect on the pelvic limb, these two muscles are included among the extrinsic pelvic limb muscles because of their attachment to the pelvic girdle, which is defined as part of the pelvic limb.

B. The **iliopsoas** (formed from the **psoas major,** an extrinsic muscle, and the **iliacus,** an intrinsic muscle) inserts on the iliac shaft and the lesser trochanter of the femur. Because the femur is more mobile than the vertebral column, the main action of this muscle is on the pelvic limb (i.e., it flexes the hip). However, when the limb is stabilized, the iliopsoas muscle acts to stabilize or flex the vertebral column.

II. INTRINSIC MUSCLES (Table 59–1) arise and insert on the pelvic limb. The intrinsic muscles essentially surround the limb on all sides in most places.

A. Muscles of the hip extend between the pelvic girdle and the femur.

1. The **iliacus** is discussed in Chapter 20 II C 2 b and Table 20–5.
2. The **muscles of the lateral pelvic surface (rump)** are powerful extensors of the hip joint.
   a. The **superficial gluteal,** a relatively thin sheet of muscle, is the most superficial of the three muscles of the rump (Figure 59–1).
      (1) The cranial region of the muscle is thinner than the caudal region.
      (2) The tendon of the superficial gluteal muscle passes over (but does not attach to) the greater trochanter of the femur; often, an opportunistic **synovial bursa** is present beneath the tendon. (A synovial bursa is a "bubble" of synovial membrane positioned between a soft structure and a hard one that serves as a cushion and lubricated "slide" to reduce wear.)
   b. The **middle gluteal** lies between the superficial and deep gluteal muscles (see Figure 59–1).
   c. The **deep gluteal muscle** is positioned most deeply among the gluteal muscles. An opportunistic synovial bursa is found between its tendon and the greater trochanter.
3. **Muscles caudal to the hip joint,** often referred to as the **"small pelvic muscles,"** are mainly associated with rotating the thigh outward at the hip.
   a. **Small pelvic association (inner pelvic group)**
      (1) The **internal obturator** (Figure 59–2) is a flaring muscle that covers the dorsal (inner) surface of the obturator foramen, and therefore lies within the pelvic cavity (hence its name).
      (2) The **gemellus** (see Figure 59–2) is formed from two muscles fused into a single mass (*gemini* = twins). Its tendon fuses with that of the internal obturator to insert on the trochanteric fossa.
      (3) The **quadratus femoris** is a short muscle positioned at the caudal edge of the small pelvic association muscles, near the ischial tuber (see Figure 59–2B). **The**

TABLE 59–1. Intrinsic Muscles of the Pelvic Limb

Muscle	Action	Innervation	Course
Hip muscles			
Iliacus	Flexes the hip (when limb is free); stabilizes or flexes the vertebral column (when limb is bearing weight)	Ventral branches of the lumbar spinal nerves	**Arises** from the ventral surface of the body of the ilium **Courses** caudodistally **Inserts** on the lesser trochanter of the femur
Superficial gluteal	Extends the hip; also abducts the thigh	Caudal gluteal nerve	**Arises** from the deep gluteal fascia, the tuber sacrale of the ilium, and the lateral sacral surface **Courses** caudodistally **Inserts** on the third trochanter of the femur
Middle gluteal	Extends the hip; also abducts the thigh and rotates the limb medially	Cranial gluteal nerve	**Arises** from the iliac crest and the gluteal (lateral) surface of the ilium **Courses** caudoventrally **Inserts** on the greater trochanter of the femur
Deep gluteal	Extends the hip; also abducts the thigh, and rotates the limb medially	Cranial gluteal nerve	**Arises** from the iliac shaft **Courses** caudoventrally **Inserts** on the greater trochanter of the femur
Internal obturator	Rotates the limb laterally at the hip	Sciatic nerve	**Arises** from the dorsal pubis and ischium surrounding the obturator foramen **Courses** laterally **Inserts** in the trochanteric fossa of the femur
Gemellus	Rotates the limb laterally at the hip	Sciatic nerve	**Arises** on the lateral ischium **Courses** laterally **Inserts** in the trochanteric fossa of the femur
Quadratus femoris	Rotates the limb laterally at the hip	Sciatic nerve	**Arises** near the ischial tuber on the ventral surface of the ischium **Courses** cranially **Inserts** just distal to the trochanteric fossa of the femur
External obturator	Rotates the limb laterally at the hip	Obturator nerve	**Arises** from the ventral pubis and ischium surrounding the obturator foramen **Courses** laterally **Inserts** in the trochanteric fossa of the femur

continued

TABLE 59–1. Intrinsic Muscles of the Pelvic Limb

Muscle	Action	Innervation	Course
Thigh muscles			
Sartorius			
Cranial belly	Flexes the hip and extends the stifle	Femoral nerve	**Arises** from the iliac crest, the cranial ventral iliac spine, and the lumbodorsal fascia **Courses** distally **Inserts** on the patella
Caudal belly	Flexes the hip and stifle	Femoral nerve	**Arises** from the cranial ventral iliac spine and the adjacent iliac shaft **Courses** distally **Inserts** on the cranial tibial border
Tensor fasciae latae	Tenses the fascia lata during locomotion; also flexes the hip and extends the stifle	Cranial gluteal nerve	**Arises** from the tuber coxae and the aponeurosis of the middle gluteal muscle **Courses** distally **Inserts** into the fascia lata
Quadriceps femoris			
Rectus femoris	Extends the stifle and flexes the hip	Femoral nerve	**Arises** from the tuberosity for the rectus femoris on the ilium **Courses** distally **Inserts** on the tibial tuberosity
Vastus lateralis	Extends the stifle	Femoral nerve	**Arises** from the proximal lateral femur **Courses** distally **Inserts** on the tibial tuberosity
Vastus medialis	Extends the stifle	Femoral nerve	**Arises** from the proximal medial femur **Courses** distally **Inserts** on the tibial tuberosity
Vastus intermedius	Extends the stifle	Femoral nerve	**Arises** from the proximal lateral femur **Courses** distally **Inserts** on the tibial tuberosity
Biceps femoris	Extends the hip, and hock; extends or flexes the stifle	Sciatic nerve	**Arises** from the sacrotuberous ligament and the ischial tuberosity **Courses** distally and cranially **Inserts** on the fascia lata, crural fascia, and tuber calcanei

continued

TABLE 59–1. Intrinsic Muscles of the Pelvic Limb

Muscle	Action	Innervation	Course
Semimembranosus	Extends the hip and flexes or extends the stifle	Sciatic nerve	**Arises** from the ischial tuber **Courses** distally and cranially **Inserts** on the distal medial aspera line of the femur and on the medial tibial condyle
Semitendinosus	Extends the hip, flexes the stifle, and extends the hock	Sciatic nerve	**Arises** from the ischial tuber **Courses** distally and cranially **Inserts** on the medial tibial body and the tuber calcanei
Gracilis	Adducts the thigh; also extends the hip, flexes the stifle, and extends the hock	Obturator nerve	**Arises** from the symphysis pelvis and the symphyseal tendon **Courses** distally and caudally **Inserts** on the cranial tibial border and the tuber calcanei
Pectineus	Adducts the thigh	Obturator nerve	**Arises** from the cranial pubis **Courses** distally **Inserts** on the distomedial femur
Adductor	Adducts the thigh; also extends the hip	Obturator nerve	**Arises** from the symphyseal tendon and the ventral ischium and pubis **Courses** distally and cranially **Inserts** along the entire lateral edge of the medial linea aspera on the femur
Crural muscles			
Cranial tibial	Flexes the tarsus; also inverts the paw (i.e., rotates the plantar surface of the paw medially)	Deep peroneal nerve	**Arises** from the cranial proximal tibia **Courses** distally **Inserts** on the plantar surfaces of metatarsal bones I and/or II
Long digital extensor	Extends the digits; also extends the stifle and flexes the tarsus	Deep peroneal nerve	**Arises** in the extensor fossa of the femur **Courses** distally through the extensor sulcus of the tibia **Inserts** on the extensor processes (on the distal phalanges) of digits II–V

continued

TABLE 59–1. Intrinsic Muscles of the Pelvic Limb

Muscle	Action	Innervation	Course
Peroneus longus	Flexes the tarsus and everts the paw (i.e., rotates the plantar surface of the paw laterally)	Deep peroneal nerve	**Arises** from the proximal fibula, the lateral tibial condyle, and the lateral collateral ligament of the stifle **Courses** distally and plantarly **Inserts** on the plantar surface of tarsal bone IV and on the bases of metatarsal bones I–IV
Lateral digital extensor	Extends and abducts digit V	Superficial peroneal nerve	**Arises** from the proximal third of the fibula **Courses** distally **Inserts** on the extensor process of digit V
Peroneus brevis	Flexes the tarsus	Superficial peroneal nerve	**Arises** from the distal two thirds of the lateral tibia and fibula **Courses** distally **Inserts** on the base of metatarsal bone V
Gastrocnemius	Extends the tarsus; also flexes the stifle	Tibial nerve	**Arises** from the lateral and medial supracondylar tuberosities of the femur **Courses** distally **Inserts** on the tuber calcanei
Superficial digital flexor	Flexes the proximal two joints of the digits; also flexes the stifle and extends the hock	Tibial nerve	**Arises** from the lateral supracondylar tuberosity of the femur **Courses** distally **Inserts** on the plantar surfaces of the proximal and middle phalanges of digits II–V
Deep digital flexor	Flexes the digits and extends the tarsus	Tibial nerve	**Arises** from the proximolateral and proximomedial caudal tibia and fibula **Courses** distally **Inserts** on the plantar surfaces of the distal phalanges of digits II–V
Popliteus	Rotates crus medially; may play a role in proprioceptive sensing of the position of the stifle	Tibial nerve	**Arises** via a long tendon from the lateral femoral condyle **Courses** caudally **Inserts** on the proximal third of the caudal tibia

continued

TABLE 59–1. Intrinsic Muscles of the Pelvic Limb

Muscle	Action	Innervation	Course
Hindpaw muscles			
Interossei	Flex the metatarso-phalangeal joints	Tibial nerve	**Arise** from the plantar basal surfaces of metatarsal bones II–V **Insert** on the plantar basal surfaces of the proximal phalanges of digits II–V

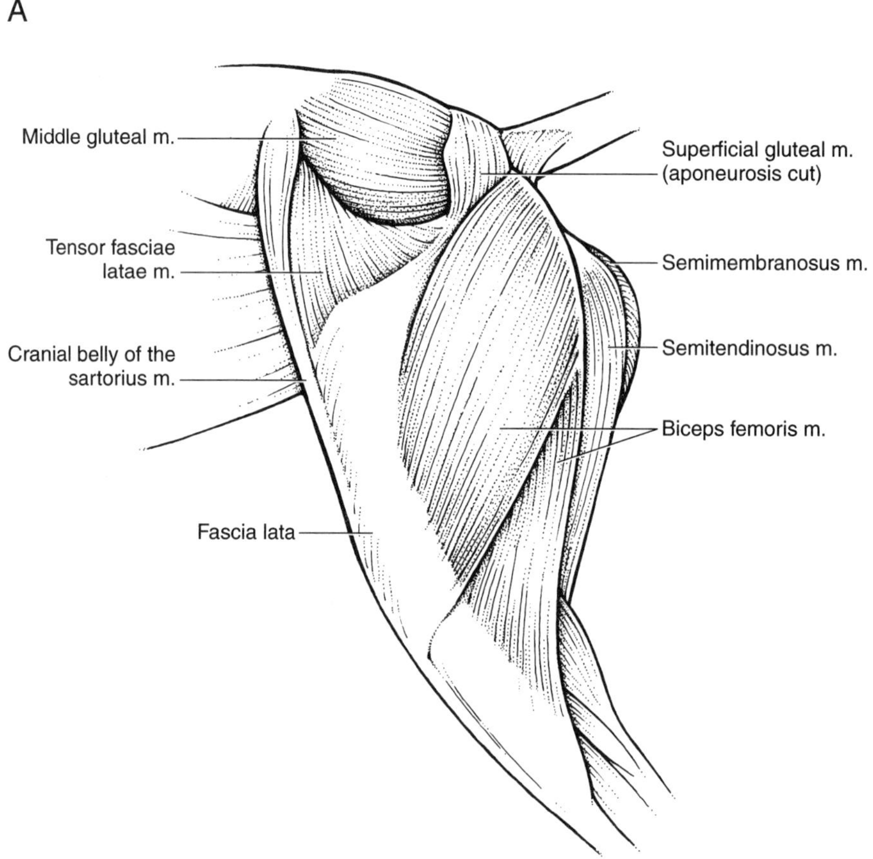

FIGURE 59–1. Muscles of the left lateral pelvic region (rump) and thigh, lateral view. (*A*) Superficial muscles. *continued*

quadratus femoris must not be confused with the quadriceps femoris, one of the cranial thigh muscles (see II B 1 c).

b. External obturator. This muscle is essentially a mirror image of its internal fellow in terms of positioning. The fibers of the external obturator form a long, strong tendon that passes ventral to the ischial ramus.

B. Muscles of the thigh. The thigh muscles can be categorized as "cranial," "caudal," or "medial," largely based on the position of the muscle bellies on the femur.

1. Cranial thigh musculature. These muscles extend distally from the pelvic girdle or proximal femur to insert on the patella. Their primary action is to **extend the stifle.**

a. The **cranial belly of the sartorius** muscle is positioned most cranially of all muscles on the thigh (see Figure 59–1B). However, a large portion of the muscle also extends to the medial thigh surface (Figure 59–3).

b. The **tensor fasciae latae** (see Figure 59–1A) is a thin sheet of muscle extending between the ilium and the lateral femoral surface, where it terminates by blending into the fascia lata.

(1) The **fascia lata** (see Figure 59–1A) is a thick portion of the deep fascia of the thigh covering approximately one third of the lateral surface of the thigh.

(a) The fascia lata covers portions of the quadriceps femoris, biceps femoris, semimembranosus, and semitendinosus muscles.

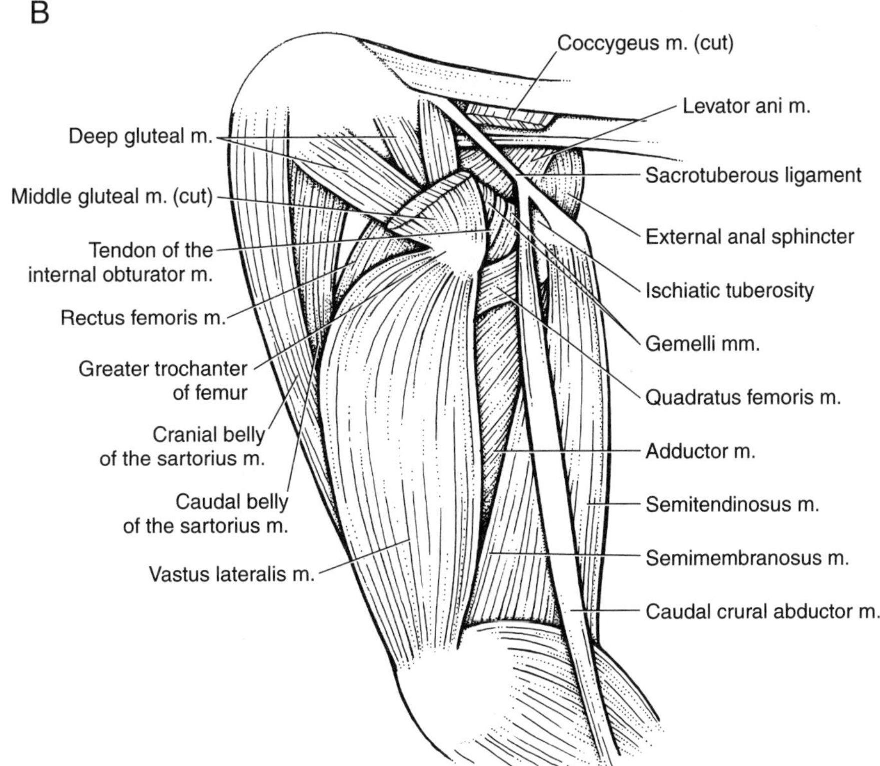

FIGURE 59–1—*continued* (*B*) Deeper muscles. The semimembranosus muscle is often confused with the adjacent semitendinosus muscle; one way to distinguish the two is to note that the semi**"m"**embranous muscle lies more **"m"**edially in the caudal thigh. (Redrawn with permission from Evans HE and deLahunta A: *Miller's Guide to Dissection of the Dog,* 4th ed. Philadelphia, WB Saunders, 1996, p 69.)

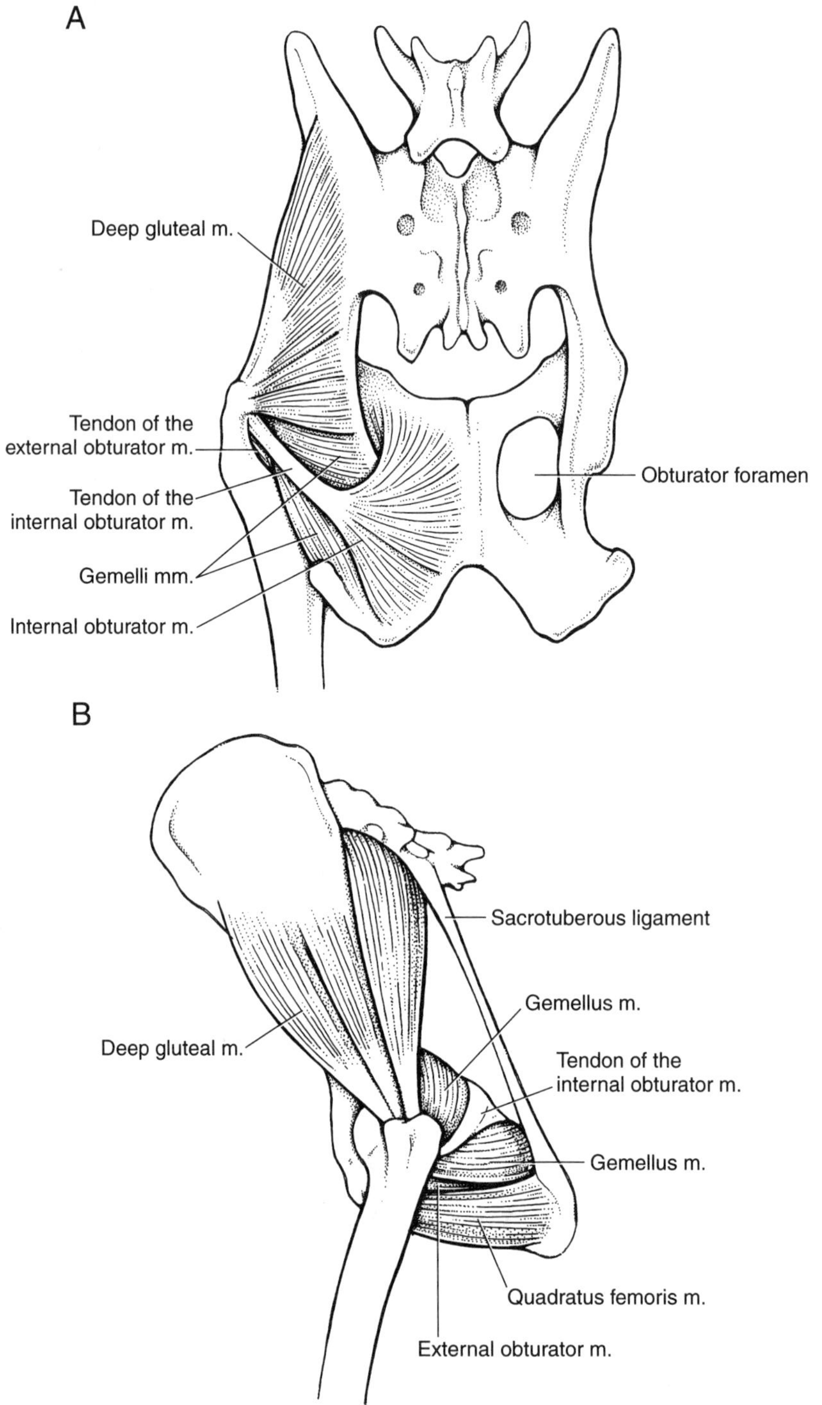

FIGURE 59–2. (*A*) The deep muscles of the dorsal pelvic girdle, dorsal view. The internal obturator originates along the entire dorsal boundary of the obturator foramen, and therefore has attachments to both the pubis and the ischium. As it courses laterally, its fibers converge on its robust and rather long tendon. The tendon passes ventral to the sacrotuberous ligament and crosses the dorsal surface of the ischial ramus by passing through the lesser sciatic notch. At this point, the tendon forms a deep groove in the dorsal surface of the gemelli muscles, over which it passes (*B*). Lateral view. As would be expected with a tendon passing tightly over an adjacent surface, various synovial bursae are usually associated with the tendon in this region. (Part *A* redrawn with permission from Evans HE, 1993, *Miller's Anatomy of the Dog,* 3e. Philadelphia, WB Saunders, p 360.)

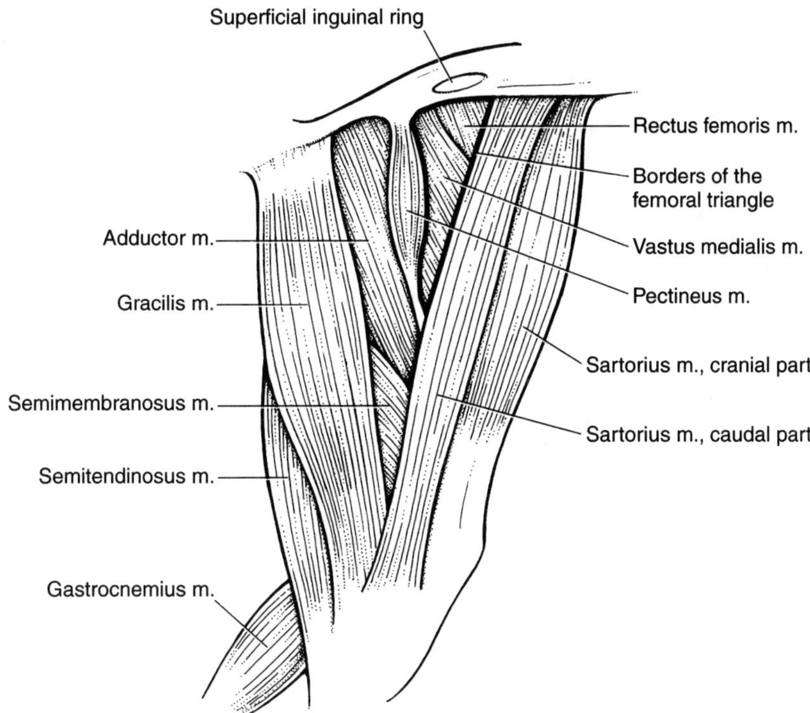

FIGURE 59–3. Musculature of the left thigh, medial view. Portions of the deeper muscles (e.g., the vastus medialis, semimembranosus, and adductor muscles) can also be seen. The medial thigh muscles are powerful adductors of the thigh. One way to remember the action of the sartorius muscle is to picture a tailor with his legs crossed (i.e., flexed at the hip and stifle and outwardly rotated) and his sewing in his lap—the sartorius muscle (*sartor,* Latin, "tailor") enables the tailor to obtain this position. (Redrawn with permission from Evans HE and deLahunta A: *Miller's Guide to Dissection of the Dog,* 4th ed. Philadelphia, WB Saunders, 1996, p 68.)

(b) Portions of the tensor fasciae latae and the biceps femoris muscles terminate by blending with the fascia lata, which itself terminates by blending with the tibial crest, patella, and femoral condyles.

(2) The tensor fasciae latae muscle is sometimes considered a muscle of the rump, owing to its innervation by the cranial gluteal nerve. However, topographically, the tensor fasciae latae is positioned on the cranial thigh, and shares an insertion site with the muscles of this region.

c. The **quadriceps femoris,** the major muscle of the cranial thigh surface, is composed of **four bellies** that closely cover the femur on its medial, lateral, and cranial surfaces. The four portions blend to **form a single tendon that incorporates the patella in its substance** prior to inserting on the tibial tuberosity.

(1) The **rectus femoris,** the most cranial belly of the quadriceps femoris, is roughly cylindrical in form (see Figure 59–1B and Figure 59–3).

(a) Arising from the ilium just cranial to the acetabulum, the rectus femoris is the only portion of the quadriceps femoris that arises from a bone other than the femur.

(b) The rectus femoris is embraced closely on each side by the vastus lateralis and the vastus medialis.

(2) The **vastus lateralis,** the largest of the four heads of the quadriceps femoris, covers the cranial half of the lateral femoral surface (see Figure 59–1B). Through part of its course, the fibers of the vastus lateralis blend intimately with those of the rectus femoris, so that the two are inseparable without sharp dissection.

(3) The **vastus medialis** is considerably smaller than its lateral counterpart (see Figure 59–3). Unlike the vastus lateralis, the vastus medialis blends with the rectus femoris only in its more distal regions.

(4) The **vastus intermedius,** the smallest of the four heads of the quadriceps femoris, directly covers the cranial surface of the femur over most of the femoral shaft, and thus lies directly deep to the rectus femoris.

d. The **articularis coxae** is a tiny spindle-shaped muscle that lies on the surface of the articular capsule of the hip joint. The articularis coxae arises from the iliopubic eminence, together with the rectus femoris, and dissipates over the craniolateral joint capsule. This muscle is incised during surgery of the hip joint to gain access to the joint cavity and presumably heals spontaneously.

2. Caudal thigh musculature. These muscles, colloquially termed the **"hamstring" muscles,** originate on the ischiatic tuberosity and extend distally to terminate on the distal femur or the proximal crus. Some of the muscles in this group pass to the lateral surface of the thigh, while others pass to its medial surface. The caudal thigh muscles **extend the hip and flex the stifle.**

a. The **biceps femoris** is a large, powerful muscle positioned in the caudolateral region of the thigh (see Figure 59–1). Although the origins of the biceps femoris are distinct, the fibers of the muscle fan out and terminate in a wide aponeurotic band associated with both the fascia lata and the crural fascia.

(1) The biceps femoris comprises **two heads,** a larger **superficial** head and a smaller **deep** one.

(2) The muscle fibers from the two heads regroup topographically to form **cranial, middle,** and **caudal parts** that are generally recognizable grossly, and have remarkably different actions.

(a) The **cranial part** blends with the **fascia lata** to terminate on the patella, patellar ligament, and cranial tibial border.

(i) Although mainly innervated by the **sciatic nerve,** the cranial portion receives some fibers from the **caudal gluteal nerve.**

(ii) This portion of the biceps femoris **extends the hip** and **stifle.**

(b) The **middle part** blends with the **crural fascia** to terminate on the lateral tibial body. This portion of the biceps femoris acts only to **extend the hip.**

(c) The **caudal part** terminates on the **tuber calcanei** by means of its contribution to the common calcanean tendon. This portion of the biceps femoris **extends the hip and the tarsus** and **flexes the stifle.**

b. The **caudal crural abductor** (see Figure 59–1B) is a narrow, long muscle that parallels the caudal border of the biceps femoris. This muscle is not clinically significant but is often encountered during dissection.

c. The **semimembranosus** is a robust muscle comprising two bellies of approximately equal size (see Figure 59–1B). The muscle is entirely fleshy, forming no pronounced tendons. The semimembranosus inserts by way of its two bellies at sites proximal and distal to the stifle joint.

(1) The **cranial belly** inserts onto the distal end of the medial lip of the aspera surface of the femur. The cranial belly extends the hip and stifle.

(2) The **caudal belly** inserts on the medial tibial condyle. The caudal belly extends the hip and flexes or extends the stifle, depending on the position and weight-bearing status of the limb.

d. The **semitendinosus** (see Figures 59–1B and 59–3) forms a large part of the caudal contour of the thigh. Shortly before its termination, the muscle becomes largely aponeurotic and inserts in two regions.

(1) The **cranial part** inserts on the **medial tibial body.** This attachment allows the muscle to flex the stifle.

(2) The **caudal part** attaches to the **tuber calcanei.** This attachment allows the muscle to extend the tarsus.

3. **Medial thigh musculature.** The medial thigh muscles are **powerful adductors of the thigh.** Care must be taken to distinguish between the "adductor muscles" as a group and the specific adductor muscle, one particular muscle in the group.
   a. **Superficially placed adductor muscles**
      (1) The **caudal belly of the sartorius** muscle is positioned fully on the medial surface of the thigh and inserts on the cranial tibial border by blending with the aponeurotic insertion of the gracilis muscle (see Figure 59–3).
      (2) The **gracilis** covers the caudal half of the thigh's medial surface (see Figure 59–3). The gracilis is rather thin, although it thickens appreciably along its caudal border. Interestingly, the muscle is aponeurotic at both its origin and insertion.
   b. **Deeply placed adductor muscles**
      (1) The **pectineus** is a short, fusiform muscle with a long, thin tendon. The muscle belly is considerable in size, but rapidly tapers to form the tendon in the proximal third of the thigh (see Figure 59–3).

Canine Clinical Correlation

Transection of the tendon of the pectineus is sometimes performed in patients with hip dysplasia. Although this procedure does nothing to treat the underlying disease, it is often associated with notable (but temporary) lessening of pain.

      (2) The **adductor muscle** occupies the proximal part of the thigh on the caudal femoral surface, between the semimembranosus and the pectineus muscles (see Figure 59–3).

Canine Clinical Correlation

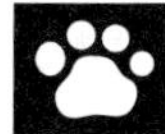

The **femoral triangle** (Fig. 59–3) is a significant landmark on the medial surface of the thigh. The borders are formed by the caudal belly of the sartorius muscle (cranially), the pectineus muscle (caudally), and the vastus medialis muscle (laterally). Several large nervous and vascular structures pass through the femoral triangle, including the femoral artery and vein and the saphenous nerve.

C. **Muscles of the crus.** The lateral half of the cranial surface, the lateral surface, and the caudal surface of the tibia are deeply covered by muscles. However, the medial tibial surface is mainly subcutaneous along nearly all of its length.

1. **Craniolateral crural muscles.** These muscles generally **flex the tarsus** and **extend the digits.**
   a. The **cranial tibial muscle,** the most superficial muscle on the cranial crural surface, is fleshy throughout most of its length. Medially, it lies in direct contact with the tibial shaft, and laterally, it overlies the other craniolateral muscles of the crus (Figure 59–4). At the tarsus, the muscle tapers to a flattened tendon, which passes under the crural extensor retinaculum.
   b. The **long digital extensor** lies immediately lateral to the cranial tibial muscle (see Figure 59–4).
      (1) The long digital extensor derives its name ("long") from the fact that it is the only one of the craniolateral crural muscles to arise from the femur.
      (2) This spindle-shaped, fleshy muscle narrows to a long, strong tendon about midway distally along the tibia. The tendon of the long digital extensor is flanked medially by the tendon of the cranial tibial muscle.
         (a) The long digital extensor's tendon passes deep to the crural and tarsal extensor retinacula.

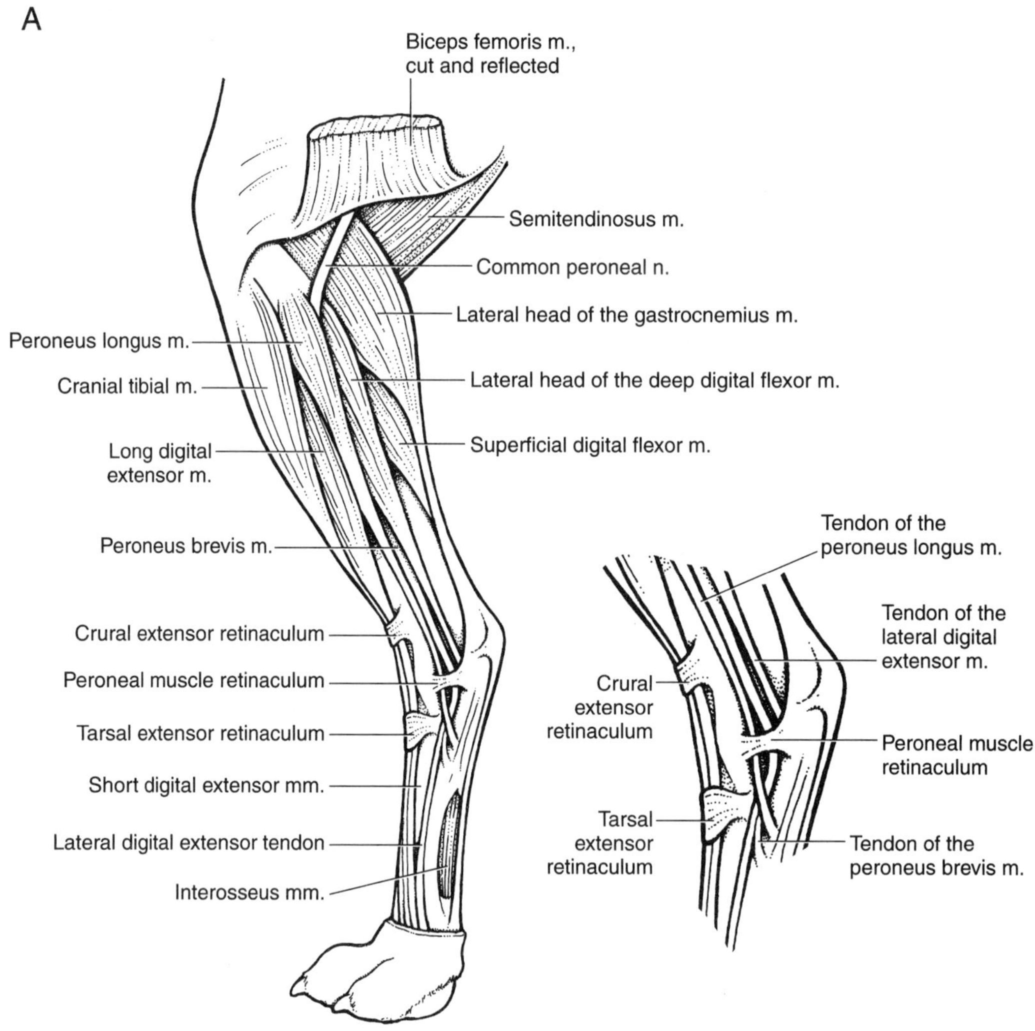

FIGURE 59–4. Superficial muscles of the left crus and pes. (*A*) Lateral view. *continued*

(b) On gaining the dorsal surface of the tarsus, the extensor tendon divides into four tendons, one for each digit. These tendons continue distally, receiving branches from the interosseus muscles, and insert separately on the distal phalanges of digits II–V.

c. The **peroneus longus** is located just cranial to the fibula.
   (1) The belly of this muscle ends about one third of the way distally along the crus, and continues via a long tendon onto the tarsus (see Figure 59–4).
   (2) The tendon takes a sharp turn plantarly at the distal end of tarsal bone IV to gain the plantar tarsal surface preparatory to insertion.

d. The **lateral digital extensor** has a short, fusiform belly positioned deep to the peroneus longus and the lateral head of the deep digital flexor. The belly is not visible on superficial view, although the tendon is (see Figure 59–4). The tendon joins with the lateral-most slip of the long digital extensor tendon midway down the proximal phalanx.

e. The **peroneus brevis** has short fibers that remain closely applied to the lateral tibial and fibular surfaces. The tendon of the peroneus brevis passes deep to the tendons of

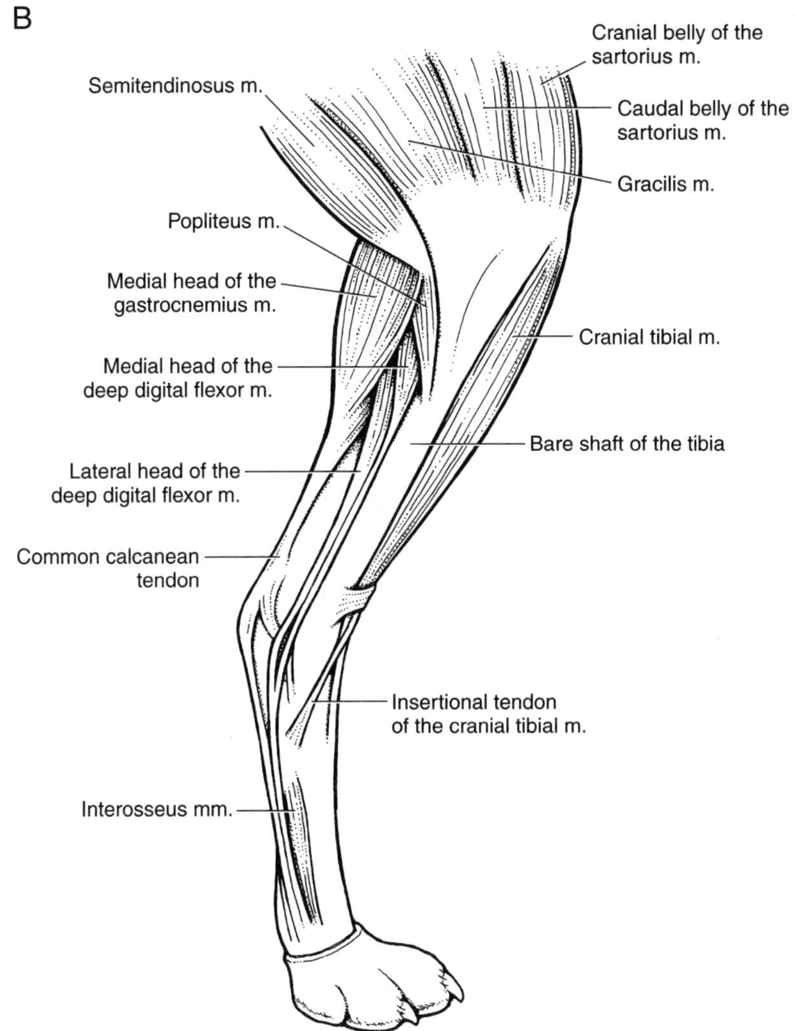

FIGURE 59–4—*continued* (*B*) Medial view. (Redrawn with permission from Dyce KM, Sack WO, Wensing CJG: *Textbook of Veterinary Anatomy,* 2nd ed. Philadelphia, WB Saunders, 1996, p 97.)

both the peroneus longus and the lateral digital extensor, and then through the groove on the lateral malleolus together with the tendon of the lateral digital extensor.

2. **Caudal crural muscles.** These muscles generally **extend the tarsus** and **flex the digits.**
   a. The **gastrocnemius** forms the largest bulge of the caudal crus in the intact state (*gastr* = "belly," *cnem* = "crus"). This muscle is the most superficial of the muscles in the caudal crus, and comprises a medial and a lateral head (see Figure 59–4).
      (1) The large **sesamoid bones of the gastrocnemius** reside within the tendon of origin of each head.
      (2) The two heads surround the substance of the superficial digital flexor muscle.
   b. The **superficial digital flexor** is a spindle-shaped muscle sandwiched between the two heads of the gastrocnemius muscle superficially and the popliteus and deep digital flexor muscles deeply (see Figure 59–4). Owing to a shared point of origin, much of the proximal part of the superficial digital flexor is fused with the lateral head of the gastrocnemius.

(1) The superficial digital flexor forms a strong tendon shortly after emerging from beneath the gastrocnemius. Initially, this tendon lies deep to the tendon of the gastrocnemius, but at the tuber calcanei, the tendon of the superficial digital flexor becomes superficial to that of the gastrocnemius. This change in position allows the tendon of the gastrocnemius tendon to insert on the tuber calcanei, while the flexor tendon continues distally to attain the digits.
(2) Like the tendon of the long digital extensor on the dorsal surface of the tarsus, the tendon of the superficial digital flexor splits into four tendons (one for each digit) as it approaches the metatarsal region.
(3) The tendons of the superficial digital flexor split just proximal to their insertion to allow the tendons of the deep digital flexor to pass through and continue to their insertion site on the distal phalanges.

Canine Clinical Correlation

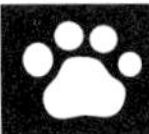

The **common calcanean tendon ("Achilles" tendon)** is the tendinous structure that attaches to the point of the tuber calcanei. The biceps femoris, semitendinosus, gracilis, gastrocnemius, and superficial digital flexor muscles contribute to the formation of this tendon.

c. The **deep digital flexor** lies against the caudal tibial surface. The deep digital flexor has **two heads,** one lateral and one medial (see Figure 59–4).
(1) After passing through the **tarsal canal,** the tendons of the two heads fuse.
(2) The combined tendon divides into four tendons (one for each weight-bearing digit), which (as in the forepaw) pass through perforations in the tendons of the superficial digital flexor muscle, and insert on the plantar surface of the distal phalanges of digits II–V.

d. The **popliteus** muscle is positioned deeply on the proximal part of the caudal crus, adjacent to the joint capsule.
(1) Despite its small size, the popliteus is a powerful medial rotator of the crus.
(2) Unusual among limb muscles, the popliteus arises by an elongate tendon and inserts by blending directly with the bony surface.

Canine Clinical Correlation

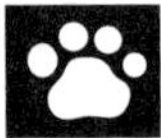

A **sesamoid bone** is incorporated into the tendon of origin at its junction with the muscle fibers; this sesamoid bone is visible radiographically and should not be mistaken for a bone fragment.

(3) As the tendon gains the caudal tibial surface, it fans into a wide triangular belly that covers much of the proximal caudal tibia.

D. Muscles of the pes (hindpaw). Like the forepaw, the hindpaw has numerous specialized muscles, most of which are of academic interest only. The four **interosseous muscles** of the hindpaw are similar to those of the forepaw (see Chapter 28 II D).

III. MUSCLE ACTION

A. General principles

1. The **flexor surfaces** of the pelvic limb joints **alternate** from the **cranial** to the **caudal surface** of the limb from the hip through the tarsus and then remain on the plantar surface of the limb from the tarsus distally (Figure 59–5).

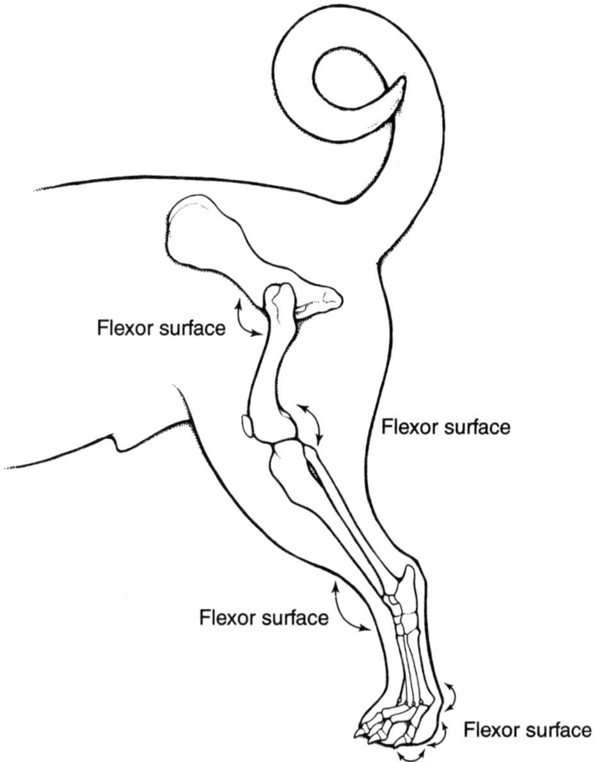

FIGURE 59–5. Flexor surfaces of the joints of the pelvic limb.

2. The **same muscle can act on multiple joints.**
   a. Either the muscle belly or the tendon may pass more than one joint in the pelvic limb. Because muscles act on any joint they cross, many muscles serve multiple functions in the pelvic limb.
   b. Because the flexor surfaces of the tarsus and digital joints are positioned on opposite sides of the limb, muscles passing on the caudal surface of the tarsus and digits have inverse actions at these two sets of joints (i.e., digital flexors also act as tarsal extensors). This arrangement differs from that seen in the thoracic limb, where the flexor surfaces of the carpus and digits are both positioned on the same surface (see Chapter 28, Figure 28–4).

B. **Coxofemoral (hip) joint.** The flexor surface faces cranially.

1. Muscles with tendons passing on or to the **cranial side** of the hip are **hip flexors.** These muscles include the:
   a. **Iliopsoas** (major flexor)
   b. **Rectus femoris** (on the cranial thigh; major flexor)
   c. **Sartorius** and **tensor fasciae latae** (on the medial thigh; minor flexors)

2. Muscles with tendons passing on or to the **caudal side** of the hip are **hip extensors.** These muscles include the:
   a. Superficial, middle, and deep **gluteals** (on the pelvic girdle; major extensors)
   b. **Semimembranosus, semitendinosus,** and **biceps femoris** (on the caudal thigh; moderate extensors)
   c. **Adductor** and **gracilis** (on the medial thigh; moderate extensors)

C. Stifle joint. The flexor surface lies caudally.

1. Muscles with tendons passing on or to the **caudal side** of the stifle are **stifle flexors.** These muscles include the:
   a. **Semitendinosus** and **caudal part of the biceps femoris** (on the caudal thigh; major flexors)
   b. **Caudal part of the sartorius** and the **gracilis** (on the medial thigh; minor flexors)
   c. **Gastrocnemius** and **superficial digital flexor** (on the caudal crus; moderate flexors)
2. Muscles with tendons passing on or to the **cranial side** of the stifle are **stifle extensors.** These muscles include the:
   a. **Quadriceps femoris** (on the cranial thigh; major extensor)
   b. **Cranial part of the biceps femoris** (on the caudal thigh; moderate extensor)
   c. **Cranial part of the sartorius** and the **tensor fasciae latae** (on the medial thigh; minor extensors)

D. Talocrural joint. The flexor surface lies cranially.

1. Muscles with tendons passing on or to the **cranial** and **lateral sides** of the tarsus are **tarsal flexors.** The following muscles of the crus are tarsal flexors:
   a. **Cranial tibial** (major flexor)
   b. **Long digital extensor** (major flexor)
   c. **Peroneus longus** (moderate flexor)
   d. **Peroneus brevis** (minor flexor)
2. Muscles with tendons passing on or to the **caudal side** of the tarsus are **tarsal extensors.** The numerous muscles in this group are the:
   a. **Biceps femoris** and **semitendinosus** (on the caudal thigh; moderate extensors)
   b. **Gracilis** (on the medial thigh; minor extensor)
   c. **Gastrocnemius** and the **superficial and deep digital flexors** (on the crus; major extensors)

E. Metatarsophalangeal joints. The flexor surface lies caudally.

1. Muscles with tendons passing on or to the **cranial side** of the metatarsus are **metatarsophalangeal extensors.** Muscles in this group include the **long digital extensor.**
2. Muscles with tendons passing on or to the **caudal side** of the metatarsus are **metatarsophalangeal flexors.** Muscles in this group include the **superficial** and **deep digital flexors.**

F. Interdigital joints. The flexor surface lies caudally.

1. Muscles on the **cranial side** of the digits are **digital extensors.** Muscles in this group include the **long** and **lateral digital extensors.**
2. Muscles on the **caudal side** of the digits are **digital flexors.** Muscles in this group include the **superficial** and **deep digital flexors.**

Chapter 60

Vasculature of the Pelvic Limb

I. ARTERIES OF THE PELVIC LIMB (Figure 60–1, Table 60–1). The typical branching pattern is described in this section. The reader must keep in mind that variations are relatively common, and that **arteries are named for the structures they supply, rather than for the source from which they branch.**

A. Introduction

1. **Position.** As in the thoracic limb, most arteries of the pelvic limb are positioned on the medial side of the limb, deeply among the muscles (which protects against surface trauma) and on the flexor surface of joints (which minimizes stretching of the artery during limb motion).
2. **Flow of arterial blood to the pelvic limb.** Arterial supply to the pelvic limb arrives from two sources: one supplies the **lateral pelvic (gluteal) region,** and one supplies the **limb from the thigh distally.** A central continuous channel, from which smaller branches arise to deliver blood to regional structures, can be identified for each of these major areas. As in the thoracic limb, these corridors change name from area to area, although the main vessel really continues uninterrupted through much of its course.
   a. The main channel that supplies the **lateral pelvic structures** is oriented **cranial** to **caudal** and takes the following sequence:
      (1) **Internal iliac artery**
      (2) **Caudal gluteal artery**
   b. The main channel that supplies the **free portion of the pelvic limb** is oriented **proximal** to **distal** and takes the following sequence:
      (1) **External iliac artery**
      (2) **Femoral artery**
      (3) **Popliteal artery**
      (4) **Cranial tibial artery**
      (5) **Dorsal pedal artery**
      (6) **Perforating metatarsal artery**
      (7) **Plantar common digital arteries**
      (8) **Plantar proper digital arteries**

B. Arteries of the lateral pelvic region.

The **caudal gluteal artery** is the main artery to the lateral pelvic region.

1. **Origin.** The caudal gluteal artery is the larger, more dorsal **terminal branch** of the **internal iliac artery.**
2. **Course.** The caudal gluteal artery extends from the sacroiliac joint to the caudal thigh ("hamstring") muscles.
   a. From its origin inside the pelvic cavity, the caudal gluteal artery travels along the ventral sacral surface, and then across the iliac shaft toward the lesser ischiatic notch.
   b. The artery provides regional branches between its origin and the level of the sacrotuberous ligament (dorsal to the lesser ischiatic notch).
   c. After sending off its last branch, the caudal gluteal artery continues along the sacrotuberous ligament, toward the ischial tuberosity, and terminates by ramifying in the substance of the caudal thigh muscles.
3. **Branches**
   a. The **iliolumbar artery** is a small branch that usually arises from the caudal gluteal artery, although it may arise directly from the internal iliac artery.
      (1) **Course.** Typically, the iliolumbar artery arises from the caudal gluteal artery, close to the latter artery's origin (about midway along the ventral border of the

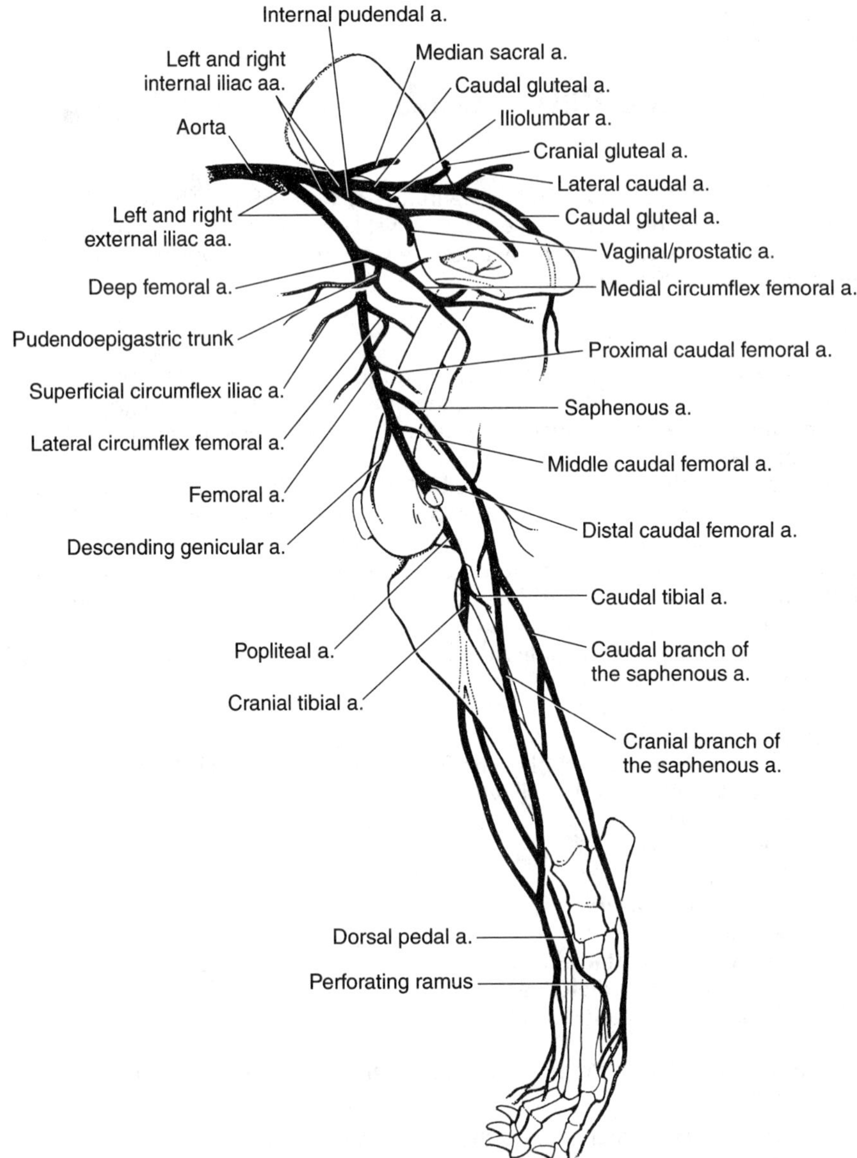

FIGURE 60–1. Arteries of the right pelvic limb, medial view. (Redrawn with permission from Evans HE and deLahunta A: *Miller's Guide to Dissection of the Dog,* 4th ed. Philadelphia, WB Saunders, 1996, p 228.)

iliac shaft) and courses ventral to the ilium and out of the pelvic cavity to approach its target muscles.

(2) **Structures supplied** include the **ilium** and the **middle gluteal** and **abdominal wall muscles.**

b. The **cranial gluteal artery** arises from the caudal gluteal artery on the medial surface of the iliac shaft.

(1) **Course.** The cranial gluteal artery passes out of the pelvic cavity via the greater ischiatic notch and approaches the deep surface of the middle gluteal muscle, sending a superficial branch toward the skin. The artery then continues between the middle and deep gluteal muscles, supplying both.

TABLE 60–1. Main Arterial Supply of the Major Pelvic Limb Muscles

Muscle	Main Arterial Supply	Parent Artery
Gluteal muscles		
Superficial gluteal	Caudal gluteal Lateral circumflex femoral	Internal iliac Femoral
Middle gluteal	Cranial gluteal Lateral circumflex femoral	Caudal gluteal Femoral
Deep gluteal	Cranial gluteal	Caudal gluteal
Small pelvic association muscles	Caudal gluteal Obturator branch	 Medial circumflex femoral
Internal obturator		
Gemelli		
Quadratus femoris		
External obturator		
Caudal hip muscles		
External obturator	Obturator branch	Medial circumflex femoral (deep femoral)
Cranial thigh muscles		
Cranial belly of the sartorius	Superficial circumflex iliac	Femoral
Tensor fasciae latae	Superficial circumflex iliac Lateral circumflex femoral	Femoral Femoral
Quadriceps femoris	Lateral circumflex femoral Medial circumflex femoral	Femoral Deep femoral
Caudal thigh muscles		
Biceps femoris	Distal caudal femoral Caudal gluteal	Femoral Internal iliac
Semimembranosus	Medial circumflex femoral Distal caudal femoral Middle caudal femoral Caudal gluteal	Deep femoral Femoral Femoral Internal iliac
Semitendinosus	Distal caudal femoral Caudal gluteal	Femoral Internal iliac
Medial thigh muscles		
Caudal belly of the sartorius	Superficial circumflex iliac Saphenous	Femoral Femoral
Gracilis	Proximal caudal femoral Saphenous	Femoral Femoral
Pectineus	Proximal caudal femoral	Femoral
Adductor	Proximal caudal femoral Middle caudal femoral Distal caudal femoral Medial circumflex femoral	Femoral Femoral Femoral Deep femoral
Craniolateral crural muscles	Cranial tibial	Popliteal
Cranial tibial		
Long digital extensor		
Peroneus longus		
Lateral digital extensor		
Peroneus brevis		

continued

TABLE 60–1. Main Arterial Supply of the Major Pelvic Limb Muscles

Muscle	Main Arterial Supply	Parent Artery
Caudal crural muscles		
Popliteus	Popliteal	Femoral
Gastrocnemius	Popliteal Distal caudal femoral	Femoral Femoral
Superficial digital flexor	Distal caudal femoral	Femoral
Deep digital flexor	Popliteal Caudal tibial	Femoral Popliteal
Interosseous muscles	Medial plantar Lateral plantar	Saphenous (femoral) Saphenous (femoral)

(2) **Structures supplied** by the cranial gluteal artery include the **middle** and **deep gluteal muscles,** as well as the **skin and fat** over the **dorsal rump** and **caudal thigh.**

c. The **lateral caudal artery** (i.e., the laterally positioned artery directed toward the **tail)** departs from the caudal gluteal artery just as this artery passes caudal to the dorsal border of the iliac shaft.

(1) **Course.** The lateral caudal artery passes out of the pelvic cavity between the tail and the superficial gluteal muscle. Providing numerous cutaneous branches on its way, the caudal gluteal artery courses to the tip of the tail, dorsal to the transverse processes of the caudal vertebrae.

(2) **Structures supplied** include the **skin** over the **dorsal** and **lateral rump,** and the **skin** and **muscles of the tail.**

d. The **dorsal perineal artery** leaves the caudal gluteal artery just before the caudal gluteal reaches the caudal thigh muscles.

(1) **Course.** The dorsal perineal artery courses medially (toward the anal region) and ventrally (toward the perineum).

(2) **Structures supplied** include the **external anal sphincter muscle** and the **perineal skin.**

e. The **continuation of the caudal gluteal artery** is the major supplier of arterial blood to the **biceps femoris, semimembranosus,** and **semitendinosus muscles,** and may also provide branches to the small pelvic association muscles (i.e., the **internal obturator, gemelli,** and **quadratus femoris muscles).** This part of the caudal gluteal also provides a named branch, the **satellite artery of the sciatic nerve,** which accompanies the large sciatic nerve throughout most of its length.

C. Arteries of the thigh

1. The **external iliac artery,** which extends from the aorta to the deep femoral artery, is the main source of blood for the mobile part of the pelvic limb.

a. **Origin.** The external iliac artery arises from the **lateral aortic surface** at the level of vertebra L5 or L6.

b. **Course.** The external iliac artery courses obliquely caudoventrally toward the medial surface of the thigh.

c. **Branches**

(1) The **deep femoral artery** is the only constant branch of the internal iliac. Blood from this artery eventually reaches many structures, including the caudal thigh muscles, the ventral abdominal wall muscles, the external genitalia, and the mammary gland.

(a) **Course.** The deep femoral artery courses away from the external iliac artery at a 45-degree angle, leaving the abdomen through the caudal angle of the vascular lacuna (i.e., an oblique opening between the thigh musculature and the abdomen that conducts the femoral artery and vein).

(b) **Branches.** The branch of the deep femoral artery is the **pudendoepigastric trunk.** This trunk branches to supply the ventral abdominal wall and mammary gland (via the **caudal epigastric artery),** as well as the inguinal structures and scrotum or labia (via the **external pudendal artery).**

(2) The **medial circumflex femoral artery** is the **continuation of the deep femoral artery,** following the origin of the pudendoepigastric trunk.

(a) **Course.** The medial circumflex femoral artery courses caudoventrally in the original direction of the deep femoral artery, passing between the vastus medialis and pectineus muscles to plunge into the substance of the adductor muscle.

(b) **Branches**

(i) The **transverse branch** arises from the medial circumflex femoral artery to supply the adductor muscle *en route* to the semimembranosus muscle.

(ii) The **deep branch** passes between and supplies the vastus medialis and adductor muscles.

(iii) The **obturator branch** passes through the obturator foramen and supplies the adductor muscle, the obturator muscles, and the small pelvic association muscles.

(c) **Structures supplied** include the small pelvic association muscles, the quadratus lumborum, the psoas minor, the iliopsoas, the internal and external obturators, the coccygeus, the levator ani, the adductor, the vastus medialis adductor, and the semimembranosus.

2. The **femoral artery,** the **direct continuation of the external iliac artery,** extends from the vascular lacuna to the stifle and supplies numerous branches to most of the muscles surrounding the femur.

a. **Course.** The femoral artery originates distal to the vascular lacuna and courses distally through the medial thigh, at first superficially and then deeply among the medial and caudal thigh musculature.

Canine Clinical Correlation

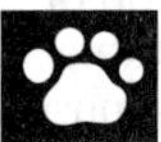

The superficial portion of the femoral artery lies in the femoral triangle and is the **preferred site for taking the pulse** in the dog.

b. **Branches.** The femoral artery does not follow the pattern of its thoracic counterpart, the brachial artery, which typically has branches that alternate regularly from its cranial and caudal surface (see Chapter 29 I C 4).

(1) The **superficial circumflex iliac artery** is a small artery that leaves the lateral surface of the femoral artery just distal to the vascular lacuna. The artery arises close to the origin site of the lateral circumflex femoral artery; in fact, the two may arise from a common trunk.

(a) **Course.** The superficial circumflex iliac artery courses between the caudal belly of the sartorius muscle and the tensor fasciae latae.

(b) **Structures supplied** include the two muscles that surround the artery (i.e., both sartorius bellies and the tensor fasciae latae), as well as a cutaneous region over the craniolateral thigh.

(2) The **lateral circumflex femoral artery** is a rather large artery that arises from the caudolateral surface of the femoral artery.

(a) **Course.** The lateral circumflex femoral artery courses caudally, immediately plunging deep between the rectus femoris and the vastus medialis muscles.

(b) **Branches.** The vessel has two named branches, in addition to numerous unnamed ones.
(c) **Structures supplied** include the quadriceps femoris, iliopsoas, tensor fasciae latae, and deep and middle gluteal muscles, and the hip joint capsule. The lateral circumflex femoral artery provides the **main arterial supply to all four heads of the quadriceps femoris.**

(3) The **proximal caudal femoral artery** arises from the caudal surface of the femoral artery at the level of the distal end of the pectineus muscle, and passes to the caudal femoral region.
(a) **Course.** The proximal caudal femoral artery courses caudally over the adductor muscle at a level even with the site where the pectineus changes from muscle to tendon, and then dips deep to the gracilis muscle. Its terminal branches ramify within the gracilis muscle.
(b) **Structures supplied** include the pectineus, adductor, and gracilis muscles.

(4) The **saphenous artery** leaves the caudal surface of the femoral artery shortly before the femoral artery descends into the caudal femoral musculature, just proximal to the stifle. Despite its small size, the saphenous artery is important to the arterial supply to both surfaces of the paw.
(a) **Course.** The saphenous artery courses distally across the medial side of the semimembranosus muscle before dividing into two branches.
(i) The **cranial branch of the saphenous artery** arises at the proximal end of the tibia and courses over the bare portion of the medial tibial shaft, past the tarsus, and into the paw, where it contributes to the three dorsal metatarsal arteries (see I F).

Canine Clinical Correlation

The **pulse** may be obtained from the saphenous artery as it crosses the medial side of the tibia, about two-thirds of the way distally along its shaft.

(ii) The **caudal branch of the saphenous artery** is the main continuation of the saphenous artery. This vessel arises at the proximal end of the tibia and courses along the tibial shaft just cranial to the gastrocnemius muscle. The caudal branch continues into the tarsus and pes, where it divides to form the medial and lateral plantar arteries (see I E 3 f).
(b) **Structures supplied.** In the thigh, the caudal belly of the sartorius muscle lies cranial to the artery, and the gracilis muscle lies caudal to it. The saphenous artery supplies small twigs to these muscles, but the major role of the saphenous artery is in supplying **structures of the distal-most limb.**

(5) The **descending genicular artery** is a small artery that usually arises from the cranial surface of the femoral artery not far distal to the origin of the saphenous artery.
(a) **Course.** The descending genicular artery courses craniodistally over the medial surface of the stifle.
(b) **Structures supplied** include mainly the **stifle joint capsule.** The descending genicular artery also sends tiny twigs into the vastus medialis muscle.

(6) The **middle caudal femoral artery** is a rather small artery arising from the caudal surface of the femoral artery immediately before the femoral artery plunges into the thigh muscles.
(a) **Course.** The middle caudal femoral artery courses directly caudally over the adductor muscle.
(b) **Structures supplied** include the adductor and the semimembranosus muscles.

(7) The **distal caudal femoral artery** is a large vessel that leaves the caudal surface of the terminal part of the femoral artery. The distal caudal femoral artery is buried deeply in the caudal musculature of the distal thigh.

(a) **Course.** The distal caudal femoral artery courses caudally, and then both proximally and distally after dividing into its two main branches.

(b) **Structures supplied.** Ascending and descending branches of the distal caudal femoral artery supply the distal thigh muscles, both heads of the gastrocnemius muscle, and the skin over the distal femoral and proximal crural regions.

3. The **popliteal artery,** the **direct continuation of the femoral artery,** extends from the popliteal surface of the femur to the level of the interosseous space between the tibia and fibula, where it terminates as the cranial and caudal tibial arteries.

a. **Origin.** When the femoral artery gains the popliteal surface of the femur (i.e., the caudal surface between the femoral condyles), it becomes the popliteal artery.

b. **Course.** The popliteal artery courses directly distally over the popliteal surface of the femur and through the popliteal notch of the tibia, passing between the two heads of the gastrocnemius muscle and over the surface of the superficial digital flexor muscle.

c. **Branches** of the popliteal artery include the small caudal genicular arteries to the stifle joint capsule, as well as branches to the popliteus, deep digital flexor, and gastrocnemius muscles.

D. Arteries of the crus. The **cranial** and **caudal tibial arteries** are the sole arteries of the crus.

1. The **caudal tibial artery** is the smaller of the two terminal branches of the popliteal artery. This vessel plunges into and supplies the lateral head of the deep digital flexor muscle. In addition, it supplies the nutrient artery of the tibia.

2. The **cranial tibial artery** represents the main source of arterial blood to the cranial crural region.

a. **Origin.** The cranial tibial artery originates at the terminal bifurcation of the popliteal artery into the cranial and caudal tibial arteries.

b. **Course.** The cranial tibial artery courses cranially through the interosseous space between the tibia and fibula. On gaining the cranial crural surface, the cranial tibial artery inclines laterally and passes distally to the dorsal surface of the tarsus, where it continues as the dorsal pedal artery.

c. **Branches.** The cranial tibial artery has several branches. One of the more significant is the **superficial branch,** which supplies the skin and fascia on the dorsal surface of the distal crus and the pes, and then passes to the plantar side of the paw to contribute to the arterial supply there.

d. **Structures supplied** include the **cranial tibial, long digital extensor, lateral digital extensor, peroneus longus,** and **peroneus brevis muscles.**

E. Arteries of the pes

1. The **dorsal pedal artery** is the **main continuation of the cranial tibial artery** into the pes.

a. **Origin.** The dorsal pedal artery originates over the talocrural joint as the cranial tibial artery gains the dorsal surface of the pes.

b. **Course.** The dorsal pedal artery courses directly distally over the dorsum of the tarsus and terminates in the interosseous space between metatarsal bones II and III (see Figure 60–1 and Chapter 61, Figure 61–3).

c. **Branches.** The dorsal pedal artery supplies small twigs to nearby structures.

(1) Relatively large and constant branches passing to each of the collateral ligaments are named the **medial** and **lateral tarsal arteries** (a departure from the usual naming convention).

(2) The **arcuate artery** (see Chapter 61, Figure 61–3) leaves the lateral surface of the dorsal pedal artery and courses transversely across the tarsus, adjacent to the tarsometatarsal joints. The arcuate artery provides the dorsal metatarsal arteries II or III–V.

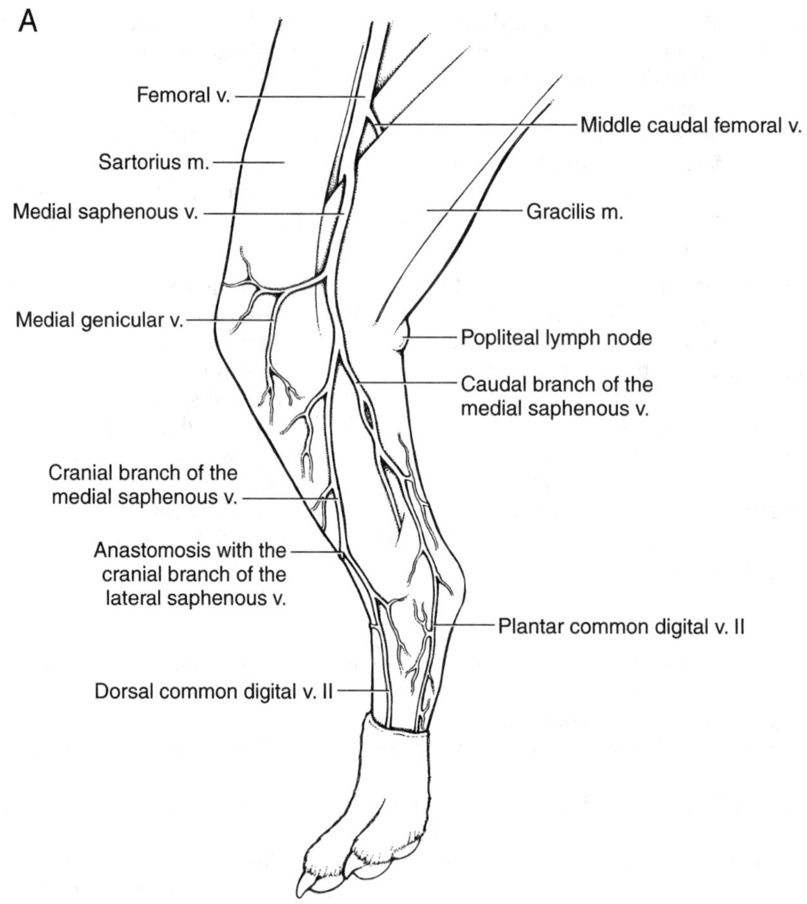

FIGURE 60–2. (*A*) Medial saphenous vein of the right pelvic limb (medial view). *continued*

Canine Clinical Correlation

The **pulse** can be readily palpated where the dorsal pedal artery crosses the dorsal surface of the tarsus, between the tendons of the cranial tibial and long digital extensor muscles.

2. The **perforating metatarsal artery** is the **direct continuation of the dorsal pedal artery.** This vessel courses from the dorsal to the plantar surface of the pes by passing between the proximal ends of metatarsal bones II and III. On gaining the plantar surface, it joins with the caudal branch of the saphenous artery, and is instrumental in forming the arteries of the plantar region which, like those of the thoracic region, provide the major arterial supply to the pes.
3. **Arteries of the pes.** In the pelvic limb, the general pattern of arterial supply for the dorsal and plantar surfaces of the hindpaw is essentially the same as that of the dorsal and palmar surfaces of the forepaw (see Chapter 29 I E 1).
   a. The **dorsal common digital arteries** (see Chapter 61, Figure 61–3) arise from a common trunk formed from anastomosis of the **cranial branch of the saphenous artery** and the **superficial branch of the cranial tibial artery.** (The contribution from the latter artery is very small.)

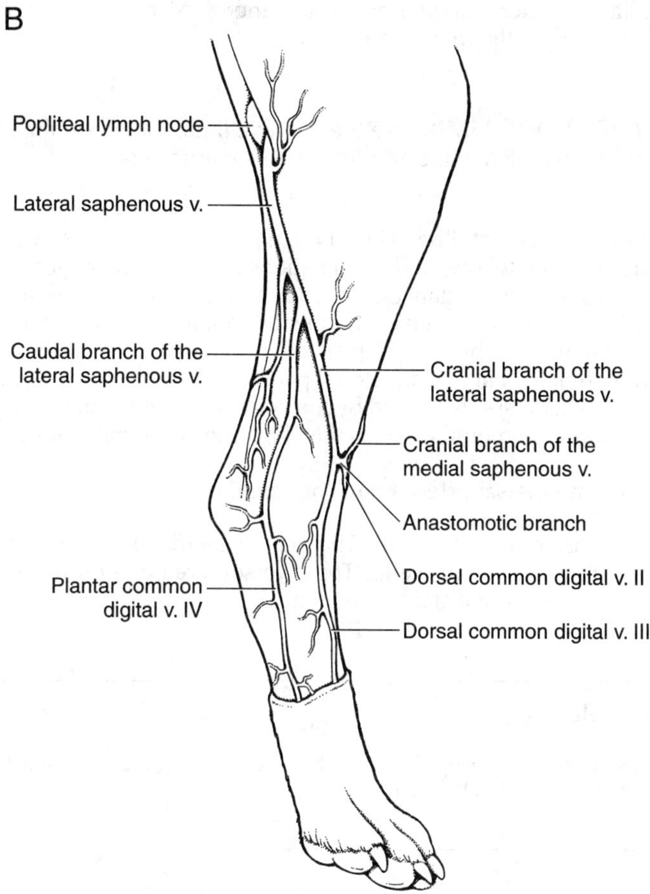

FIGURE 60–2—*continued* (*B*) Lateral saphenous vein of the right pelvic limb (lateral view). (Redrawn with permission from Evans HE, 1993, *Miller's Anatomy of the Dog,* 3e. Philadelphia, WB Saunders, pp 701–702.)

b. The **dorsal metatarsal arteries** (see Chapter 61, Figure 61–3), like all metatarsal arteries in both limbs, are small and of little significance. These arteries arise somewhat variably, but usually in the following pattern:
   (1) **Dorsal metatarsal artery II** usually arises directly from the **dorsal pedal artery,** but may arise as a branch of the arcuate artery.
   (2) **Dorsal metatarsal arteries III** and **IV** arise from the **arcuate artery.**
c. The **plantar common digital arteries** (see Chapter 61, Figure 61–4) arise from the **medial plantar artery,** a branch of the **caudal branch of the saphenous artery.** The plantar common digital arteries, which are the major suppliers of arterial blood to the hindpaw, represent the continuation of the main channel of arterial supply. Thus, the main channel flow passes from the dorsal surface to the plantar surface of the hindpaw.
d. The **plantar metatarsal arteries** (see Chapter 61, Figure 61–4) arise from the **deep plantar arch.** The deep plantar arch is formed from the **perforating metatarsal artery** and the **lateral plantar artery,** a branch of the caudal branch of the saphenous artery. (The contribution from the latter is small.)
e. The **axial** and **abaxial dorsal and plantar proper digital arteries** (see Chapter 61, Figure 61–4) arise by contributions from the respective dorsal and plantar common digital and metatarsal arteries, just as in the forepaw.

f. The **medial** and **lateral plantar arteries,** branches of the caudal branch of the saphenous artery, supply the **interosseous muscles.**

II. VEINS OF THE PELVIC LIMB.

Like the thoracic limb, the pelvic limb has **two sets of veins,** a deeper set paralleling the arteries, and a superficial set that has no relation to the arteries.

A. The **deep veins** are largely **satellite veins** of the named arteries. These veins take the same name as the arteries they follow, and drain regions similar to the regions supplied by their companion arteries. In some instances, the satellite veins are doubled, in which case the two veins simply share a name with each other as well as with the companion artery. Departures from the pattern within the deep set of veins include the following:

a. The **common iliac vein** has no arterial parallel, although it is a member of the deep set of veins. This vessel is formed by the confluence of the **internal** and **external iliac veins.** The two common iliac veins then become confluent to form the **caudal vena cava.**

b. The **plantar metatarsal arteries** have no satellite veins.

B. The **superficial veins** are subcutaneous. The major superficial veins of the pelvic limb are the **medial** and **lateral saphenous veins.** These vessels are best considered in the direction of their blood flow (i.e., from distal to proximal).

Canine Clinical Correlation

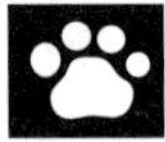

The large, subcutaneous medial and lateral saphenous veins are accessible to venipuncture, although they often "roll" abysmally.

1. The **medial saphenous vein,** located on the medial surface of the crus and distal thigh, is essentially the satellite of the saphenous artery. (This represents a departure from the pattern established in the thoracic limb, where the superficial veins are not associated with any arteries.) The medial saphenous vein is prominent from its origin in the proximal crus to its termination in the femoral vein in the distal third of the thigh (Figure 60–2A).

   a. **Origin.** The medial saphenous vein is formed by the confluence of its two tributaries. (Note that these vessels are referred to as "branches," although technically, they are tributaries.) The formation of the tributaries is often variable.

      (1) The **cranial branch of the medial saphenous vein,** the smaller tributary, commonly forms as the continuation of **dorsal common digital vein II.**

         (a) Dorsal common digital vein II ascends the dorsal pedal surface, becoming the cranial branch of the medial saphenous vein as it reaches the tarsus.

         (b) At the distal tibia, the cranial branch of the medial saphenous vein inclines caudally to course across the cranial tibial muscle and the bare part of the tibial shaft toward the caudal surface of the stifle. Near the stifle, the cranial branch of the medial saphenous vein becomes confluent with its caudal fellow to form the medial saphenous vein, proper.

         (c) The cranial branch of the medial saphenous vein becomes confluent with the cranial branch of its lateral fellow in the distal fourth of the crus.

      (2) The **caudal branch of the medial saphenous vein** is quite small.

         (a) This vessel forms relatively proximally, continuing proximally from the medial tarsal vein.

         (b) On reaching the distal tibia, the caudal branch of the medial saphenous vein inclines centrally to course toward the central region of the proximal medial tibia. The caudal branch becomes confluent with its cranial fellow on or near the caudal surface of the stifle to form the medial saphenous vein, proper.

b. **Course.** From the stifle, the medial saphenous vein continues proximally across the surface of the gracilis muscle. About halfway between its origin and termination, the medial saphenous vein usually receives another large tributary, the **medial genicular vein.**

2. The **lateral saphenous vein,** located on the lateral surface of the crus, extends from the mid-tibial region to the popliteal region of the crus. Like its medial fellow, the lateral saphenous vein has two main tributaries.
   a. The **cranial branch of the lateral saphenous vein,** the larger of the two tributaries, forms from the confluence of all three dorsal common digital veins.
      (1) The vessel formed from this confluence ascends the dorsal pedal surface, becoming the cranial branch of the lateral saphenous vein as it reaches the tarsus.
      (2) At the hock, the cranial branch of the lateral saphenous vein inclines caudally to pass over the tarsal flexor and digital extensor muscles. The vessel gains the caudolateral tibial surface midway up the tibia, where it receives the caudal branch of the lateral saphenous vein to form the lateral saphenous vein, proper.
      (3) The cranial branch of the lateral saphenous vein anastomoses with the cranial branch of its medial fellow in the distal fourth of the crus.
   b. The **caudal branch of the lateral saphenous vein** is the continuation from the **superficial plantar arch,** which receives blood from all three plantar common digital arteries.
      (1) The caudal branch of the lateral saphenous vein takes its definitive name as it gains the crus.
      (2) On reaching the distal tibia, the caudal branch of the lateral saphenous vein inclines toward the central region of the proximal lateral tibia. The caudal branch becomes confluent with the cranial branch about midway proximally along the tibia, forming the lateral saphenous vein, proper. The lateral saphenous vein plunges between the biceps femoris and semitendinosus muscles to terminate in the femoral vein (Figure 60–2B).

III. LYMPHATIC VESSELS OF THE PELVIC LIMB.

Three systems of lymphatic vessels and potentially three named regions of lymph nodes serve the pelvic limb. Because the vessels network in such a way that vessels from one system may enter multiple nodes, the vessels and nodes are best considered separately.

A. Vessels

1. The **superficial lateral system** of vessels originates on the dorsum of the paw and passes proximally, largely paralleling the lateral saphenous vein. These lymphatic vessels terminate in the **popliteal lymph node.**
2. The **superficial medial system** originates just proximal to the tarsus, and drains mainly skin. These vessels pass proximally over the gracilis muscle and terminate in the **superficial inguinal lymph node.**
3. The **deep medial system** also originates just proximal to the tarsus. These vessels pass toward the gastrocnemius muscle, skirt the popliteal node, and continue proximally to terminate in the **iliac lymph node.**

B. Lymphocenters

1. **Popliteal lymphocenter.** The popliteal lymphocenter is constant.
   a. **Lymph nodes.** The **popliteal lymph node,** usually single, is a relatively large, constant node. The ovoid node is positioned at the caudal surface of the stifle, tucked between the distal portions of the biceps femoris and the semitendinosus muscles.

Canine Clinical Correlation

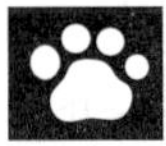

The popliteal lymph node, the most readily palpable lymph node of the pelvic limb, can be fairly easily stabilized with the fingers during palpation. Thus, this node is well-suited for lymph node biopsy by needle aspiration.

b. **Lymphatics**
   (1) **Afferent lymphatics** arrive from all parts of the limb distal to the node.
   (2) **Efferent lymphatics** pass along the medial saphenous vein and terminate in the **superficial inguinal lymph node.**

2. **Superficial inguinal (inguinofemoral) lymphocenter.** This lymphocenter is also constant.
   a. **Lymph nodes.** The **superficial inguinal (inguinofemoral) lymph nodes,** usually double, are constant nodes that lie in the groove between the abdominal wall and the medial surface of the thigh. These nodes are often palpable in healthy dogs, although not as readily as the popliteal node.
   b. **Lymphatics**
      (1) **Afferent vessels.** The inguinofemoral lymphocenter drains the inguinal and femoral regions (see also Chapter 41 V C 3).
         (a) Afferent vessels related to the pelvic limb arrive from the ventral pelvic surface and the medial surfaces of the thigh, stifle, and crus. In addition, the superficial inguinal lymph nodes receive the efferent vessels from the popliteal lymph node, thus forming an important staging site for the lymphatic drainage of much of the pelvic limb.
         (b) The superficial inguinal nodes also receive the efferent vessels from the mammary gland in the bitch; the penis, prepuce, and scrotum in the dog; and the ventral half of the abdominal wall in both sexes.
      (2) **Efferent lymphatics** from the superficial inguinal lymph node pass to the **medial iliac lymph nodes** (see Chapter 41 V C 2 a).

3. **Deep inguinal (iliofemoral) lymphocenter.** This lymphocenter is inconstant.
   a. **Lymph nodes**
      (1) The **femoral lymph node** is small and inconstant in occurrence. When present, the tiny node is positioned deep to the femoral vessels in the femoral triangle.
      (2) The **iliofemoral lymph node** is also inconstant. This node lies near the insertion of the tendon of the psoas minor, between the internal and external iliac veins.
   b. **Lymphatics**
      (1) **Afferent vessels.** The breadth of the drainage field served by the femoral lymph node belies the small size and inconstant nature of the node. The drainage field includes the skin over much of the medial surface of the pelvic limb from the stifle on distally, the stifle and hock joints, the patella and bones of the crus and pes, the tendons over the crus and pes, and the popliteal lymph node.
      (2) **Efferent vessels** pass to the **iliofemoral** or **medial iliac lymph nodes** (see Chapter 41 V C 2 a, 4 a) and to the **sacral lymph nodes** (see Chapter 41 V C 2 c).

Chapter 61

Innervation of the Pelvic Limb

I. LUMBOSACRAL PLEXUS

A. Definition. The lumbosacral plexus is the network of nerves that supplies most structures of the pelvic limb with both sensory and motor innervation. (Note that "sensory" includes cutaneous information, as well as sensory information from the muscle spindle fibers, periosteum, and joint capsule.)

B. Formation (Figure 61–1)

1. **Roots.** Like the brachial plexus of the thoracic limb (see Chapter 30 I), the lumbosacral plexus of the pelvic limb is formed from the **ventral branches of spinal nerves,** specifically, **lumbar nerves 3, 4, 5, 6,** and **7 (L3, L4, L5, L6, L7)** and **sacral nerves 1, 2,** and **3 (S1, S2, S3).** These nerves are referred to as the roots of the lumbosacral plexus.
   a. The ventral branches of the contributing spinal nerves cross the adjacent muscles and intercommunicate extensively to form the plexus.
   b. In some individuals, the lumbosacral plexus may be clearly divided into lumbar and sacral plexuses; however, in such instances, numerous communications are present between the two.

2. **Derivatives.** From the network that is the lumbosacral plexus, fibers from multiple nerve roots (i.e., **branches)** coalesce to form the **named nerves** of the plexus. These named nerves pass into the pelvic limb along constant routes.
   a. Formation of the named nerves from the branches of the lumbosacral plexus is fairly constant.
   b. When multiple branches within the plexus contribute to a named nerve, not all contributions are necessarily equal.

II. NERVES OF THE LUMBOSACRAL PLEXUS IN THE PELVIC LIMB AND ADJACENT AREAS.

Only the nerves of the lumbosacral plexus that serve the pelvic limb are discussed here. The pelvic and pudendal nerves are discussed in Chapter 54 I B 2 and II.

A. The **ilioinguinal nerve** is formed from the ventral branches of **L3.**

1. From its origin at the intervertebral foramen, the ilioinguinal nerve **courses** caudodistally over the caudolateral abdominal and cranial thigh regions.
2. The ilioinguinal nerve provides **motor branches** to the **psoas minor, psoas major,** and **iliacus muscles,** and **sensory branches** to the **skin of the craniolateral thigh.**

B. The **lateral cutaneous femoral nerve** is formed mainly from the ventral branches of **L4,** but also receives branches from L3 and L5.

1. The lateral cutaneous femoral nerve **courses** caudolaterally through the psoas minor muscle.
2. In spite of its name, the lateral cutaneous femoral nerve provides motor innervation as well as cutaneous innervation.
   a. The lateral cutaneous femoral nerve supplies **motor fibers** to the **psoas minor** and **adjacent hypaxial muscles.**
   b. The nerve supplies **sensory fibers** to a **wide swathe of skin** extending from the dorsal midline, over the iliac wing, and distally over the lateral thigh as far as the stifle.

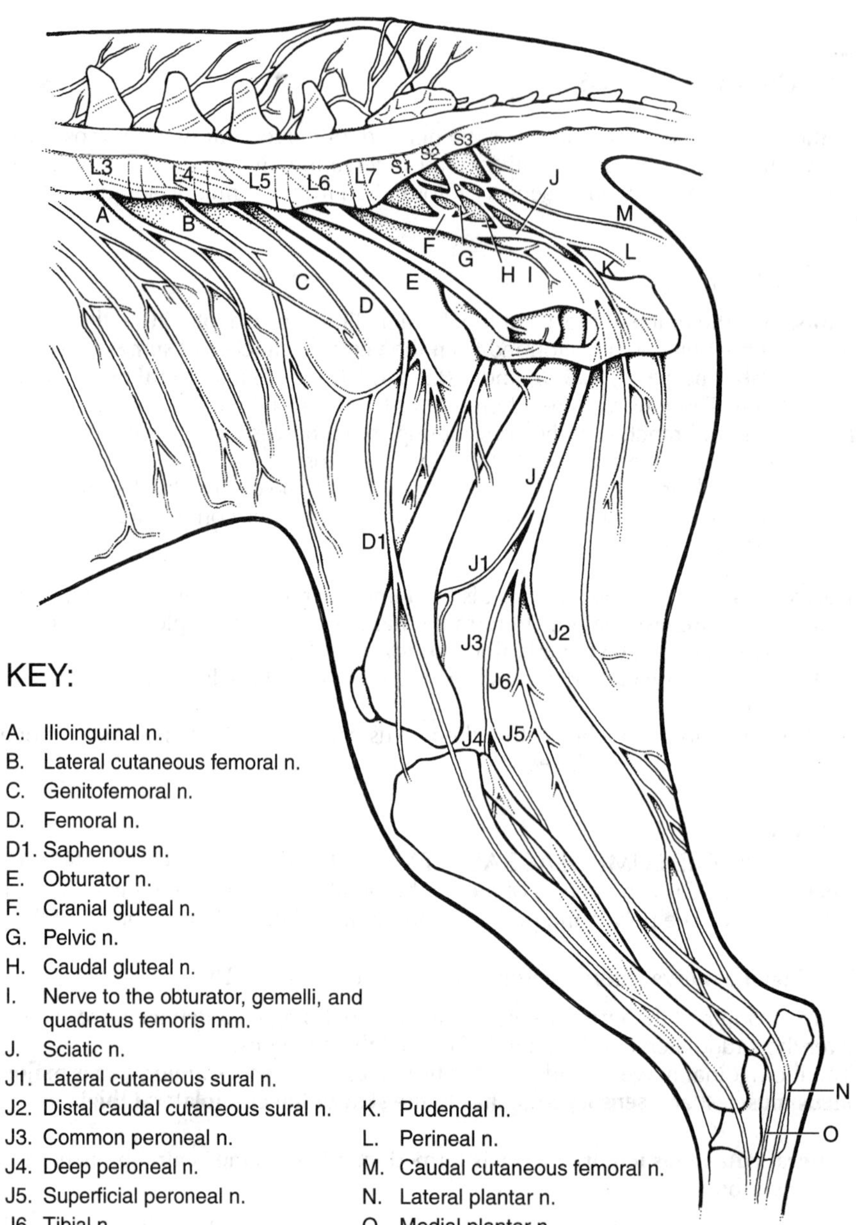

FIGURE 61–1. Schematic medial view of the sacrolumbar plexus and its named branches. (Modified with permission from Evans HE, 1993, *Miller's Anatomy of the Dog,* 3e. Philadelphia, WB Saunders, p 866.)

C. The **genitofemoral nerve** is formed from the ventral branches of **L3** and **L4.**

1. The genitofemoral nerve **courses** caudodistally through the inguinal canal to gain the inguinal region.
2. **Structures supplied**
   a. The genitofemoral nerve provides **motor fibers** to the **cremaster muscle of the dog,** but has no motor branch in the bitch.
   b. The nerve provides **sensory fibers** to a wide triangular region of skin extending from the tip of the prepuce (or the equivalent point on the skin of the ventral abdomen in the bitch) to almost the stifle, and back almost as far as the ischiatic tuberosity. Included in this field are the **prepuce** in the dog or the **mammary gland** in the bitch, as well as a large region of **skin over the medial thigh.**

D. The **femoral nerve** is formed from the ventral roots of **L4, L5,** and **L6.** Like the radial nerve of the thoracic limb, the femoral nerve is often described as the **key nerve of the pelvic limb.** The femoral nerve innervates the muscles that function to extend the stifle joint, which must remain fixed in order for the limb to bear weight. Fortunately, the deep positioning of the femoral nerve renders it less susceptible to injury than its more vulnerable counterpart in the thoracic limb.

1. **Course.** The femoral nerve courses caudally and longitudinally through the iliopsoas muscle, giving off its single superficial branch (i.e., the saphenous nerve) and leaving the abdominal cavity while still enclosed within the muscle. After leaving the abdominal cavity, the femoral nerve plunges into the substance of the quadriceps femoris muscle. Note that the femoral nerve remains buried among muscles throughout most of its course, and therefore is concealed. However, splitting the iliopsoas muscle longitudinally reveals the femoral nerve as a white cord within its depths.
2. **Branches.** The **saphenous nerve** courses with femoral nerve longitudinally through the iliopsoas muscle. On leaving the abdominal cavity, the saphenous nerve parts company with its parent, and courses laterally toward the sartorius muscle. The saphenous nerve travels adjacent to the femoral artery through the femoral triangle and proximal thigh, and then becomes intimately associated with the saphenous artery in its distal course to the paw.
3. **Structures supplied**
   a. **Femoral nerve**
      (1) Motor fibers. The femoral nerve provides motor innervation to the **iliopsoas, quadriceps femoris,** and **articularis coxae muscles.** The **sartorius muscle** is also supplied by the femoral nerve, either by direct motor branches, or more indirectly by branches of the saphenous nerve.
      (2) Sensory fibers originating from the femoral nerve pass through its superficial branch (i.e., the saphenous nerve).
   b. **Saphenous nerve.** The saphenous nerve may divide into separate motor and sensory branches.
      (1) Motor fibers. The saphenous nerve supplies motor innervation to both bellies of the **sartorius muscle, when the femoral nerve does not.**
      (2) Sensory fibers. The saphenous nerve supplies sensory innervation to a wide area, including the:
         (a) Skin of the **medial thigh, cranial** and **lateral regions of the crus,** and **medial stifle**
         (b) Deep structures of the medial surface of the stifle (e.g., ligaments, joint capsule)
         (c) Skin of the **dorsomedial tarsus** and **metatarsus**
         (d) Skin of the **medial-most surface of the medial-most digit**

E. The **obturator nerve** is formed from the ventral branches of **L4, L5,** and **L6** within the substance of the iliopsoas muscle.

1. After quickly exiting the iliopsoas muscle, the obturator nerve **courses** caudoventrally along the iliac shaft. The nerve passes out of the pelvic cavity through the cranial part of

the obturator foramen (along with the small obturator branch of the medial circumflex femoral artery) and then passes through the internal obturator muscle to ramify in the adductor muscles of the thigh.

2. The obturator nerve provides **motor fibers** to the **external obturator, pectineus, gracilis,** and **adductor muscles.**

F. The **cranial gluteal nerve** is formed from the ventral branches of **L6, L7,** and **S1.**

1. **Course.** The cranial gluteal nerve leaves the pelvic cavity via the greater ischiatic (sciatic) notch, and immediately enters the middle and deep gluteal muscles. The terminal branch of the cranial gluteal nerve usually pierces the cranial edge of the deep gluteal muscle (or simply passes over it) to end in the tensor fasciae latae muscle.
2. The cranial gluteal nerve provides **motor fibers** to the **middle gluteal, deep gluteal,** and **tensor fasciae latae muscles.**

G. The **caudal gluteal nerve** is formed from the ventral branch of **L7.**

1. The caudal gluteal nerve **courses** along the medial surface of the iliac shaft and exits the greater sciatic foramen to enter the superficial gluteal muscle.
2. The caudal gluteal nerve provides **motor fibers** to the **superficial gluteal muscle,** as well as tiny twigs to the **piriformis muscle,** which it crosses. The nerve may also send a branch into the **middle gluteal muscle.**

H. The **sciatic nerve,** the **largest nerve** of the lumbosacral plexus (and of the pelvic limb), is formed from the ventral branches of **L6, L7,** and **S1.** The sciatic nerve innervates an immense amount of muscle mass, including the small pelvic association muscles, the caudal muscles of the thigh, and all of the muscles distal to the stifle. The branches of the sciatic nerve also provide significant cutaneous innervation to the crus.

1. **Sciatic nerve proper**
   a. **Course.** The sciatic nerve courses caudally along the ilium and exits the pelvic cavity over the greater ischiatic (sciatic) notch. The nerve continues caudally a bit further, and then turns distally to pass between the greater trochanter of the femur cranially and the ischiatic tuberosity caudally. From here, the nerve passes distally along the lateral surface of the thigh deep to the biceps femoris. The sciatic nerve terminates by dividing into the **common peroneal** and **tibial nerves.**

Canine Clinical Correlation

The sciatic nerve is vulnerable to iatrogenic injury at the point where it turns sharply distally and passes between the greater trochanter and the caudal part of the ischium, as well as in the more distal part of the lateral thigh region, where it lies deep to the thinning caudal edge of the biceps femoris muscle. Intramuscular injections should be placed in about the middle third of the caudal thigh to avoid the sciatic nerve in these two vulnerable sites. Alternately, the injections may be placed in the cranial muscle mass of the thigh, which does not house any large nerves.

   b. **Structures supplied.** The sciatic nerve proper provides various motor and sensory branches as it courses distally along the lateral surface of the thigh.
      (1) The sciatic nerve proper provides **motor innervation** to the **small pelvic association muscles** (i.e., the internal obturator, gemelli, and quadratus femoris) and the **caudal thigh ("hamstring") muscles** (i.e., the biceps femoris, semimembranosus, semitendinosus, and caudal crural abductor muscles).
      (2) The sciatic nerve proper provides **sensory fibers** to the **lateral and caudal regions of the crus.**

2. **Branches**
   a. **Unnamed muscular branches** arise directly from the sciatic nerve as the nerve crosses the caudal thigh muscles (i.e., the semimembranosus, semitendinosus, and biceps femoris).
   b. The **muscular branch** of the sciatic nerve leaves the main trunk far proximally, and courses adjacent to the sacrotuberous ligament with the caudal gluteal artery and vein.
      (1) Several **motor branches** arise from the muscular branch to supply the **hamstring muscles.**
      (2) A **sensory branch** (i.e., the **proximal caudal cutaneous sural nerve)** leaves the muscular branch near the intertrochanteric fossa, and passes distally to the crus to supply the **skin over the proximal caudal crus.**
   c. The **lateral cutaneous sural nerve** ("sural" refers to the crus) leaves the sciatic nerve about two-thirds of the way down the thigh. This nerve passes between the two heads of the biceps femoris, becomes subcutaneous in the proximolateral crus, and supplies only the **skin of the central part of the lateral crural region.**
   d. The **distal caudal cutaneous sural nerve** arises approximately 1 centimeter distal to the lateral cutaneous sural nerve and passes caudally toward the popliteal region. The nerve then passes distally along the surface of the gastrocnemius muscle, where it is closely associated with the lateral saphenous vein, and then continues to the tarsus.
      (1) At the tarsus, the distal caudal cutaneous sural nerve provides a **sensory branch** to the **joint capsule skin over the calcaneal tuber.**
      (2) A **motor branch** of the distal caudal cutaneous sural nerve joins the tibial nerve, follows that nerve distally, and is distributed to the **plantar muscles of the pes.**
   e. The **common peroneal nerve** is the smaller of the two terminal divisions of the sciatic nerve. (Note that the peroneal nerve is not the same as the perineal nerve.)
      (1) **Course.** The common peroneal nerve courses distally from the sciatic nerve, usually at a level just proximal to the stifle. The nerve crosses the lateral head of the gastrocnemius muscle and passes deeply between the lateral digital extensor and the peroneus longus muscles to terminate by dividing into the superficial and deep peroneal nerves.
         (a) The **superficial peroneal nerve,** the more caudal of the two terminal branches, leaves the common peroneal nerve a short distance distal to the stifle joint, deep to the muscle belly of the peroneus longus muscle. The nerve then passes distally along the lateral digital extensor (deep to the peroneus longus muscle), becoming subcutaneous about two-thirds of the way distally along the crus, and continuing into the pes alongside the dorsal branch of the saphenous artery. The superficial peroneal nerve provides **motor** fibers to the **peroneus brevis** and **lateral digital extensor muscles,** and **sensory fibers** (via a cutaneous branch) to the **craniolateral crus.**
         (b) The **deep peroneal nerve,** the more cranial of the two terminal branches of the common peroneal nerve, passes distally deep to the crural muscles (specifically, the deep digital flexor and the lateral digital extensor) and adjacent to the bone. On reaching the hock, the deep peroneal nerve continues into the pes. In the early part of its course, the deep peroneal nerve provides several **motor branches** to the **cranial tibial, long digital extensor,** and **peroneus brevis muscles.**
      (2) **Structures supplied.** Including both of its terminal divisions, the common peroneal nerve supplies the **muscles of the craniolateral crus** and the **dorsum of the paw,** as well as the **skin covering its main field of muscular distribution.**
   f. The **tibial nerve** is the larger, more caudal terminal branch of the sciatic nerve.
      (1) **Course.** The tibial nerve usually leaves the sciatic nerve in the distal two thirds of the thigh, and passes caudodistally over the surface and between the medial and lateral heads of the gastrocnemius muscle. The nerve then continues distally through the crus on the surface of the lateral head of the deep digital flexor.
         (a) Just proximal to the tarsus, the tibial nerve **receives the communicating**

branch from the distal caudal cutaneous sural nerve, which carries motor fibers to be distributed along with those of the tibial nerve to the muscles of the plantar paw.

(b) At the level of the tarsus, the tibial nerve provides a small cutaneous branch, and then divides into the **medial** and **lateral plantar nerves,** which continue into the pes.

(2) **Structures supplied.** In general, the tibial nerve supplies:

(a) **Motor fibers** to all of the muscles on the **caudal surface of the crus** and **plantar surface of the pes**

(b) **Sensory fibers** to the **stifle, tarsal,** and **digital joints,** as well as to the **skin of the plantar surface of the paw** and the **foot pads**

I. The **caudal cutaneous femoral nerve** is formed mainly from the ventral branches of **S1** and **S2,** although the exact source of the fibers varies widely among individuals.

1. The caudal cutaneous femoral nerve **courses** caudally through the pelvic cavity together with the pudendal nerve, leaving the cavity by crossing the ischiatic arch.
2. As it leaves the pelvic cavity, the caudal cutaneous femoral nerve detaches the **caudal cluneal nerves,** which are **sensory** to a patch of **skin over the greater trochanter of the femur.** The caudal cutaneous femoral nerve terminates by supplying a broad area of **skin over the caudolateral surfaces of the thigh** as far distally as the stifle.

III. NERVES OF THE LUMBOSACRAL PLEXUS IN THE PES.

The saphenous, superficial peroneal, deep peroneal, and tibial nerves provide motor and sensory innervation of the pes (Table 61–1, Figure 61–2).

A. General pattern of innervation. The nerves of the pes are identified by position and number, as in the manus (see Chapter 30 III A).

1. **Metatarsal region.** As in the metacarpal region of the manus, the nerves of the metatarsal region of the pes are divided into **dorsal** and **plantar sets.**
2. **Digital region.** The **proper digital nerves** are formed essentially like those of the forelimb.

B. Sensory innervation

1. **Metatarsal region**

a. **Dorsal metatarsal region**

(1) **Dorsal common digital nerves II–V** are formed mainly from the **superficial per-**

TABLE 61–1. Summary of the Contributions of the Saphenous, Superficial Peroneal, Deep Peroneal, and Tibial Nerves to the Innervation of the Pes

Nerve	Sensory Innervation	Motor Innervation
Saphenous nerve	Medial border of the most medial digit	None
Superficial peroneal nerve	Skin over most of the dorsum of the paw	None
Deep peroneal nerve	Skin over a small portion of the dorsum of the paw	Muscles on the dorsal surface of the paw
Tibial nerve	Skin over the entire plantar surface of the paw (via the medial and lateral plantar nerves)	Muscles on the plantar surface of the paw

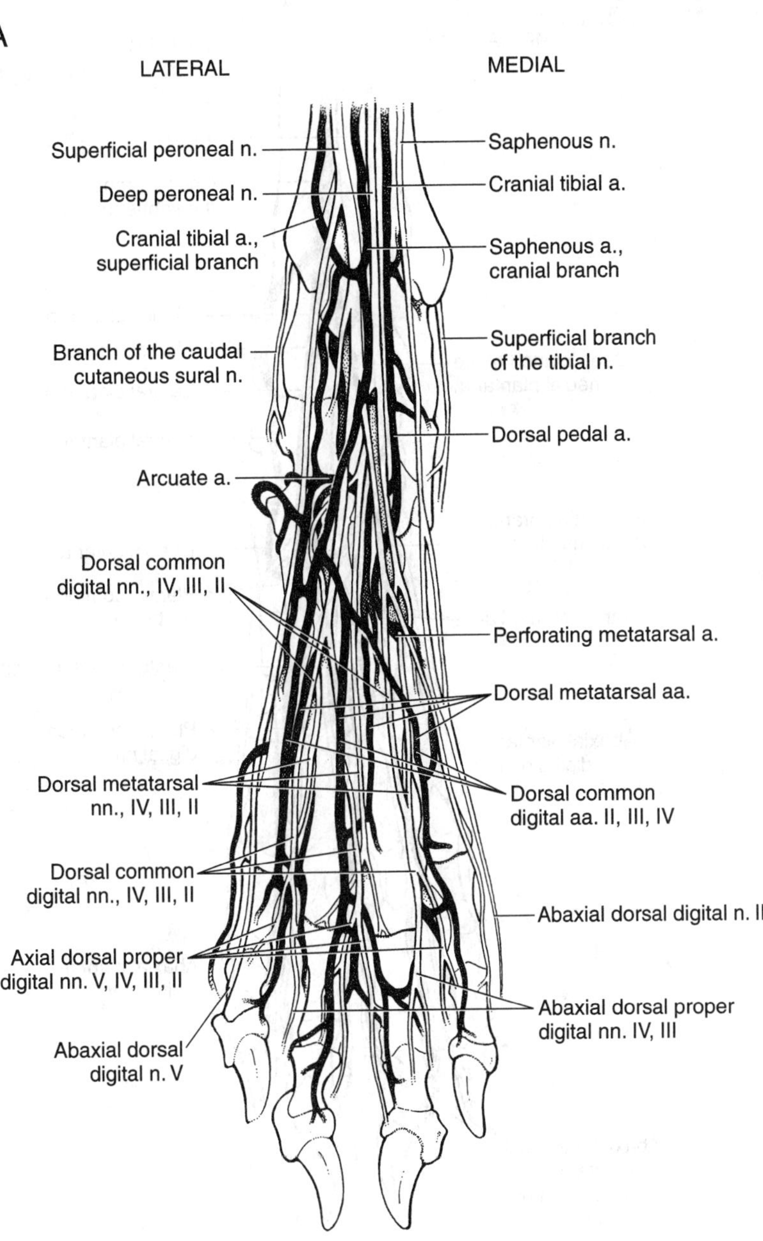

FIGURE 61–2. Nerves and arteries of the right pes. (*A*) Dorsal view. *continued*

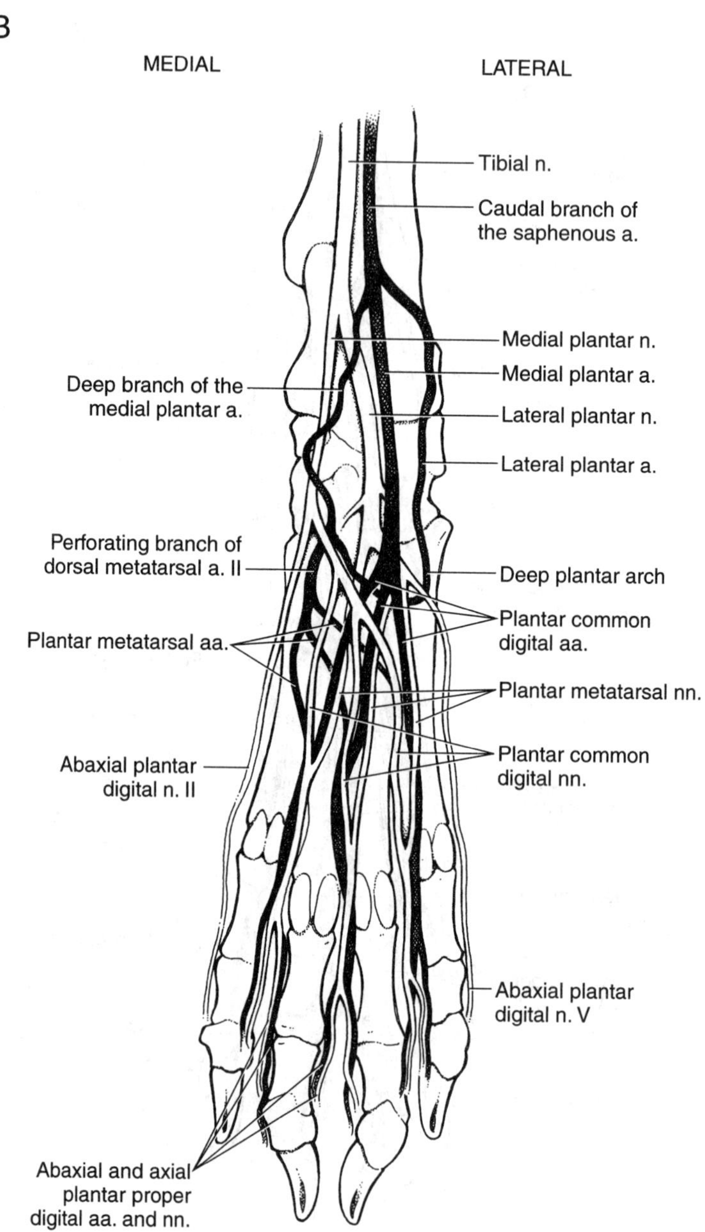

FIGURE 61–2—*continued* (*B*) Plantar view. (Redrawn with permission from Evans HE, 1993, *Miller's Anatomy of the Dog,* 3e. Philadelphia, WB Saunders, pp 890 and 887.)

oneal nerve. Thus, cutaneous supply to most of the dorsum of the paw is provided by the superficial peroneal nerve, with the following exceptions:
- **(a)** A small cutaneous area between digits II and III
- **(b)** The medial surface of the metatarsus and medial-most digit, which receives fibers from the saphenous nerve

(2) Dorsal metatarsal nerves II–IV are formed by the branchings of the **deep peroneal nerve.** The area supplied by these branches overlaps that supplied by the superficial peroneal nerve, and also covers the most medial part of the paw (which is not served by the superficial peroneal nerve).

b. Plantar metatarsal region

(1) Plantar common digital nerves II–IV are provided by the branchings of the **medial plantar nerve** from the **tibial nerve.** These nerves supply the skin over most of the plantar surface of the metatarsus.

(2) Plantar metatarsal nerves II–IV are provided by the branchings of the **lateral plantar nerve** from the **tibial nerve.**

2. Digital region. The **axial** and **abaxial dorsal** and **plantar proper digital nerves** arise mainly from the dorsal common digital nerves in a pattern essentially like that seen in the manus.

a. Dorsal digital region. The dorsal common digital nerves receive the dorsal metatarsal nerves, and the combined trunk bifurcates to provide an axial and abaxial dorsal proper digital nerve to two adjacent digits. Fairly constant exceptions arise for the supply to the most medial surface of the most medial digit and the most lateral surface of the most lateral digit:

(1) Abaxial dorsal proper digital nerve II arises from a continuation of the saphenous nerve.

(2) Abaxial dorsal proper digital nerve V arises from a continuation of the superficial peroneal nerve.

b. Plantar digital region. The nerves of the plantar surface of the digits are similarly formed from their respective common digital and metatarsal nerves.

(1) Abaxial plantar proper digital nerve II arises from a more direct continuation of the medial plantar nerve.

(2) Abaxial plantar proper digital nerve V arises from a more continuation of the lateral plantar nerve.

C. Motor innervation

1. Dorsal surface. Motor innervation to the **short digital extensor** (a muscle of little clincial significance) is provided by fibers originating in the **deep peroneal nerve.**

2. Plantar surface. Motor innervation to the plantar surface of the pes is provided by fibers originating in the **lateral plantar nerve,** a branch of the **tibial nerve.**

Chapter 62

Prominent Palpable Features of the Pelvic Limb

I. BONY STRUCTURES

A. Lateral pelvic region. The readily palpable features of the pelvic girdle (i.e., the **iliac crest, ischiatic tuberosity, ischiatic arch,** and **pubic brim**) are described in Chapter 55 I.

B. Thigh region. The **femur,** which is ensheathed in muscle, presents only a few palpable features:

1. The **greater trochanter** is prominent on the proximal lateral thigh.
2. The **lateral surfaces of both condyles** are palpable on each side of the proximal stifle.

C. Stifle joint region

1. The **joint** itself is palpable between the femur and the tibia.
2. The **patella** is readily palpable within the substance of the tendon of the quadriceps femoris muscle, proximal to the actual stifle joint. Placing the dog in lateral recumbency so that the limb is not weight-bearing and the muscles are relaxed allows appreciation of the patella as a bony density within the tendon that can be displaced slightly medially and laterally.

D. Crural region

1. **Tibia**
   a. The **tibial tuberosity** and **tibial crest** are subcutaneous on the cranial tibia, just distal to the femur.
   b. The **bare shaft of the tibial body** is subcutaneous on the medial side of the crus. The tibial body can be palpated over almost its full length from the stifle to the hock.
   c. The **medial malleolus** is a prominent, jutting mound of bone on the medial side of the tibia's distal extremity, just proximal to the hock.
2. **Fibula**
   a. The **head** of the fibula can be felt as a rather large, rounded bump on the lateral surface of the crus just distal to the stifle joint.
   b. The **body** of the fibula is largely obscured by the mass of muscle that encloses it; however, the hardness of the underlying bone becomes detectable through the muscles and the tendons in the distal third or quarter of the crus on its lateral side.
   c. The **lateral malleolus** is as prominent as the medial malleolus, but on the lateral side of the distal end of the crus, just proximal to the tarsus.

E. Tarsal region

1. The **tarsal bones as a group** can be appreciated distal to the distal ends of the medial and lateral malleoli.
2. Only the **calcaneus** can be individually identified. Its proximally projecting **calcanean tuber** is visible as well as palpable.

F. Tarsal joint region. The **talocrural joint** is the only joint that can be appreciated in the tarsal region. Recall that this is the only joint in the region with a wide range of motion.

G. Metatarsal region. The **metatarsal bones** are palpable both as a group (more proximally) and individually (more distally, where they diverge to meet the proximal phalanges of the digits). The bony substance of the metatarsal bones is best appreciated from the dorsal surface, because on the plantar surface, they are largely covered by the substantive interosseous muscles.

H. **Digital region.** The only structures that can be appreciated by palpation in this region are the **proximal interdigital joints.** The distal interdigital joints are largely obscured by the digital pads.

II. SOFT TISSUE STRUCTURES

A. Lateral pelvic region

1. The **superficial** and **middle gluteal muscles,** although not individually distinguishable, are subcutaneous and palpable over most of the lateral rump region.
2. The **sacrotuberous ligament** is also palpable (see Chapter 55 II B).

B. Thigh region

1. **Muscles**
   a. The **stifle extensors** are readily palpable as the large muscle mass in the **cranial thigh region.**
   b. The **stifle flexors** are readily appreciated as the very large mass of muscle in the **caudal thigh region.**
   c. The **thigh adductors** are appreciable in the **medial thigh region.**
      (1) This group of muscles is thinner than those of the cranial and caudal thigh.
      (2) Among this muscle group, the **pectineus muscle** is prominent as a firm, cord-like structure just under the skin at the proximal part of the medial thigh surface, just cranial to the femur. The muscle belly is readily palpable, but the tendon not so much so.
2. The **femoral triangle** is easily identified on the medial surface of the limb where the thigh joins the body, at the midpoint of the cranial-to-caudal extent of the proximal thigh. The triangle is appreciated as a soft, yielding area between the muscles that form its borders.
   a. The **pectineus muscle** is easily felt at its caudal border.
   b. The **caudal belly of the sartorius muscle** is a bit more difficult to appreciate at its cranial border.
   c. The **femoral artery** is readily palpable as a firm, cylindrical structure within the femoral triangle. The **pulse** is easily obtained here.
3. The **popliteal lymph node** is normally palpable as a small, firm, oval structure between the diverging heads of the biceps femoris and the semitendinosus muscles at the caudal surface of the stifle.

C. Stifle joint region

1. The **patellar ligament** can be identified subcutaneously distal to the patella and at its attachment site, the tibial tuberosity.
2. The **tendon of the biceps femoris** is easily palpable in the standing dog at the lateral border of the caudal surface of the stifle region.
3. The **tendons of the semimembranosus and semitendinosus muscles** can be easily distinguished on the medial—caudal border of the stifle region.

D. Crural region

1. **Tendons.** The **common calcanean tendon** is plain as a thick, cord-like structure on the caudal crural surface. The tendon is separated from the remaining structures of the caudal crus by a wide gap that is covered only by skin. This plain area is "visually palpable" as the indentation between the tendon and the caudal surface of the crus.

2. **Muscles**
   a. The **flexors of the hock** and **extensors of the digits** can be identified as the large, soft tissue mass on the proximal medial tibia. This mass extends distally through most of the cranial crural region.
   b. The **extensors of the hock** and **flexors of the digits** form a large, almost hemispherical mass of muscle on the caudal proximal tibia.
      (1) Most of this palpable mass is formed by the **gastrocnemius muscle.**
      (2) The narrowing of the mass as it blends with the common calcanean tendon can also be readily appreciated.
   c. The **lateral head of the deep digital flexor** muscle is palpable as the soft tissue on the distal caudal tibia.
3. The **pulse in the saphenous artery** is sometimes detectable where the saphenous artery passes across the medial side of the distal third of the tibia.
4. The **common peroneal nerve** can be detected subcutaneously as a fine, cord-like structure against the head of the fibula. If the skin over the fibular head is gently stroked in a proximal to distal direction, the nerve will roll under the fingertip.

E. Metatarsal region

1. **Tendons**
   a. The **digital extensor tendons** are palpable as they cross the dorsal surface of the metatarsal bones. The tendons can be rolled transversely against the metatarsal bones beneath them, and in this manner tendons passing to individual digits can sometimes be appreciated.
   b. The **digital flexor tendons** are palpable as part of the soft mass on the palmar surface of the metatarsal bones. However, they cannot be distinguished from the interosseous muscle mass.
2. **Muscles.** The **interosseous muscles** can be appreciated as a yielding soft tissue mass on the plantar surface of the metatarsus.
3. The **pulse in the dorsal pedal artery** can be obtained as the artery passes across the tarsal region and into the proximal metatarsal region.

STUDY QUESTIONS

DIRECTIONS: Each of the numbered items or incomplete statements in this section is followed by answers or by completions of the statement. Select the ONE numbered answer or completion that is BEST in each case.

1. Which one of the following is a unique feature of the pelvic limb (as compared with the thoracic limb)?

(1) Manner of attachment of the limb to the trunk
(2) Presence of a single "key" nerve
(3) Tapering of the muscle bellies to tendons in the more distal regions of the limb
(4) Number of bones in the most proximal limb region

2. The condyles of the femur articulate with the:

(1) patella.
(2) head of the tibia.
(3) condyles of the tibia.
(4) heads of the tibia and fibula.

3. Which tarsal bone provides a lever for the muscles that extend the hock?

(1) Talus
(2) Tarsal bone IV
(3) Central tarsal bone
(4) Calcaneus

4. Which ligament attaches to the fovea capitis on the head of the femur?

(1) Acetabular ligament
(2) Cotyloid ligament
(3) Articular ligament of the femur
(4) Ligament of the head of the femur

5. Which ligaments attach to the intercondylar areas of the tibia?

(1) Intermeniscal ligaments
(2) Cruciate ligaments
(3) Collateral ligaments of the stifle
(4) Cranial and caudal tibial ligaments

6. Rupture of which one of the following stifle ligaments would most likely result in excessive lateral motion of the tibia?

(1) Medial collateral ligament
(2) Lateral collateral ligament
(3) Cranial cruciate ligament
(4) Caudal cruciate ligament

7. Which tarsal joint is correctly paired with the bones that form it?

(1) Talocrural joint: talus distally and fibula proximally
(2) Proximal intertarsal joint: talus and central tarsal bone medially and the calcaneus and tarsal bone IV laterally
(3) Distal intertarsal joint: Central tarsal bone and tarsal bones II and III laterally, no medial component
(4) Intratarsal joints: the distal row of tarsal bones proximally and the metatarsal bones distally

8. Which statement regarding the flexor surfaces of the pelvic limb joints is correct?

(1) They are consistently located on the cranial surface of the limb from proximal to distal.
(2) They alternate from cranial to caudal from the hip through the tarsus.
(3) They remain on the plantar surface from the stifle distally.
(4) They alternate from cranial to caudal from the metatarsus distally.

9. What is the action of muscles on the caudal surface of the thigh?

(1) Flex the hip
(2) Adduct the thigh
(3) Circumduct the thigh
(4) Flex the stifle

10. Which one of the following statements correctly describes the action of the crural muscles?

(1) The major extensors of the tarsus are also extensors of the digits.
(2) The major extensors of the tarsus are also extensors of the stifle.
(3) The major extensors of the digits are also extensors of the tarsus.
(4) The major extensors of the digits are also flexors of the tarsus.

11. Which muscle is positioned laterally on the crus and attaches at the plantar surface along the full width of the metatarsus?

(1) Peroneus brevis
(2) Peroneus longus
(3) Lateral digital extensor
(4) Lateral head of the deep digital flexor

12. Which muscle positioned deeply on the proximocaudal surface of the crus extends between the lateral femoral condyle and the proximal medial tibia, possesses a sesamoid bone in its long tendon of origin, and acts to rotate the crus?

(1) Popliteus
(2) Short head of the deep digital flexor
(3) Medial head of the deep digital flexor
(4) Accessory head of the gastrocnemius

13. Which of the following parts of the quadriceps femoris differs the most from the others on the basis of attachments?

(1) Rectus femoris
(2) Vastus lateralis
(3) Vastus medialis
(4) Vastus intermedius

14. Which pelvic limb muscle extends the hip, stifle, and hock and flexes the stifle?

(1) Semitendinosus muscle
(2) Semimembranosus muscle
(3) Biceps femoris muscle
(4) Caudal crural abductor muscle

15. Which artery arises from the femoral artery and passes distally along the medial surface of the thigh, terminating by dividing into cranial and caudal branches that contribute to the arterial supply of the paw?

(1) Saphenous artery
(2) Medial pedal trunk
(3) Medial saphenous artery
(4) Proximal accessory pedal artery

16. What is the sequence of the main channel arterial flow to the lateral pelvic (gluteal) region?

(1) External iliac artery, caudal gluteal artery
(2) Internal iliac artery, cranial gluteal artery, caudal gluteal artery
(3) Internal iliac artery, caudal gluteal artery, iliolumbar artery
(4) Internal iliac artery, caudal gluteal artery

17. What artery arises from the main arterial channel to the pelvic limb while the main channel is still inside the abdominal cavity and provides blood that will ultimately supply the adductor, vastus medialis, and semimembranosus muscles?

(1) Iliolumbar
(2) Deep femoral
(3) Deep circumflex iliac
(4) Lateral circumflex femoral

18. If blood flow to the semimembranosus muscle via the caudal gluteal artery were compromised, which one of the following vessels could potentially supply collateral flow to this muscle and the other members of its group?

(1) Femoral artery
(2) Popliteal artery
(3) Cranial gluteal artery
(4) Distal caudal femoral artery

19. Arterial flow to the pes would be most compromised by interruption of blood flow through which of the following arteries?

(1) Cranial and caudal tibial arteries
(2) Dorsal pedal and saphenous arteries
(3) Saphenous and dorsal metatarsal arteries
(4) Caudal tibial and plantar pedal arteries

20. While performing surgery on a black Labrador retriever, a veterinarian accidentally lacerates the lateral circumflex femoral artery in the proximal thigh. Which one of the following muscles would be most compromised?

(1) Tensor fasciae latae muscle
(2) Quadriceps femoris muscle
(3) Middle gluteal muscle
(4) Biceps femoris muscle

21. The efferent vessels of the popliteal lymph node pass to the:

(1) femoral lymph node.
(2) lumbar lymphatic trunk.
(3) deep inguinal lymph node.
(4) superficial inguinal lymph node.

22. The lumbosacral plexus is formed from:

(1) the dorsal roots of lumbar nerves 3–7 (L3–L7) and sacral nerves 1–3 (S1–S3).
(2) the dorsal roots of L5–L7 and S1–S3.
(3) the ventral roots of L3–L7 and S1–S3.
(4) the ventral roots of L1–L7 and S1–S2.

23. Which one of the following nerves includes both motor and sensory fibers in its composition?

(1) Cranial gluteal nerve
(2) Caudal gluteal nerve
(3) Lateral cutaneous sural nerve
(4) Lateral cutaneous femoral nerve

24. Trauma to the greater trochanter of the femur would affect muscles innervated by the:

(1) cranial gluteal nerve.
(2) cranial and caudal gluteal nerves.
(3) femoral nerve.
(4) sciatic nerve.

25. Injury to the sciatic nerve at a level just proximal to its division into the tibial and common peroneal nerves would most likely impair the dog's ability to:

(1) bear weight.
(2) bear weight, flex the hock, and extend the digits.
(3) extend the digits, flex the hock, and detect cutaneous sensation over the medial crus and tarsus.
(4) extend the digits and flex the hock.

26. Which one of the following nerves has a motor component in the dog but not in the bitch?

(1) Caudal gluteal nerve
(2) Genitofemoral nerve
(3) Ilioinguinal nerve
(4) Femoral nerve

27. Which nerve innervates the outward rotators of the hip?

(1) Sciatic nerve
(2) Femoral nerve
(3) Caudal gluteal nerve
(4) Cranial gluteal nerve

28. Which one of the following nerves is located in the femoral triangle alongside the femoral artery and femoral vein?

(1) Femoral nerve
(2) Saphenous nerve
(3) Common peroneal nerve
(4) Medial branch of the femoral nerve

29. Compromise of the obturator nerve would most directly affect the ability of the pelvic limb to:

(1) bear weight.
(2) be pulled medially.
(3) be pulled laterally.
(4) be rotated outwardly.

30. According to position, what nerve would be most susceptible to blunt trauma to the lateral crural surface in the area of the fibular head?

(1) Superficial peroneal nerve
(2) Common peroneal nerve
(3) Sciatic nerve
(4) Tibial nerve

31. Which nerve passes on the dorsal surface of the paw in the space between the second and third metatarsal bones?

(1) Dorsal common digital nerve II
(2) Dorsal metatarsal nerve II
(3) Dorsal common digital nerve III
(4) Dorsal metatarsal nerve III

32. The plantar common digital nerves carry fibers from the:

(1) sciatic nerve.
(2) femoral nerve.
(3) dorsal cutaneous sural nerve.
(4) lateral cutaneous femoral nerve.

33. What is the large bony protuberance that is palpable at the proximal lateral end of the femur, just caudal to the hip joint?

(1) Third trochanter
(2) Lesser trochanter
(3) Greater trochanter
(4) Crest of the femoral head

34. What nerve is palpable subcutaneously against the head of the fibula?

(1) Sciatic nerve (distal-most portion)
(2) Common peroneal nerve
(3) Superficial peroneal nerve
(4) Lateral branch of the tibial nerve

35. Which tarsal bone can be individually palpated?

(1) Talus
(2) Central tarsal bone
(3) Fourth tarsal bone
(4) Calcaneus

36. Which one of the following muscles would be palpable on the lateral side of the caudal surface of the proximal tibia?

(1) Popliteus
(2) Lateral digital extensor
(3) Lateral head of the gastrocnemius
(4) Lateral head of the deep digital flexor

DIRECTIONS: Each of the numbered items or incomplete statements in this section is negatively phrased, as indicated by a capitalized word such as NOT, LEAST, or EXCEPT. Select the ONE numbered answer or completion that is BEST in each case.

37. Which of the following major nerves of the pelvic limb is NOT readily visualized through most of its course?

(1) Tibial nerve
(2) Sciatic nerve
(3) Femoral nerve
(4) Saphenous nerve

38. Sesamoid bones are associated with all of the following muscles of the pelvic limb EXCEPT the:

(1) popliteus muscle.
(2) gastrocnemius muscle.
(3) semitendinosus muscle.
(4) quadriceps femoris muscle.

39. Which of the following structures is NOT a feature of the femur?

(1) Trochlea
(2) Greater tubercle
(3) Greater trochanter
(4) Condyle

40. All of the following statements regarding the tibia are true EXCEPT:

(1) The tibial tuberosity forms the medial malleolus.
(2) The extensor groove is a notch in the cranial border of the lateral tibial condyle that provides passage for the tendon of the long digital extensor.
(3) The popliteal notch is an indentation on the caudal tibial surface between the two tibial condyles.
(4) The tibial body is almost cylindrical in its midregion, but becomes four-sided as it blends with the distal extremity.

41. All of the following statements regarding the femur are true EXCEPT:

(1) The aspera surface is a roughened area covering most of the cranial femoral surface.
(2) The extensor fossa is a prominent, deep pit at the cranial edge of the lateral condyle where the long digital extensor muscle originates.
(3) Articular facets for the sesamoid bones of the gastrocnemius muscles are present on the proximal-most edges of each femoral condyle.
(4) The popliteal fossa is a small pit on the distal end of the lateral femoral condyle.

42. The talus articulates with all of the following bones EXCEPT the:

(1) fibula.
(2) calcaneus.
(3) central tarsal bone.
(4) metatarsal bone II.

43. All of the following muscles act on the tarsus EXCEPT the:

(1) Cranial tibial
(2) Peroneus longus
(3) Long digital extensor
(4) Lateral digital extensor

44. Which of the following muscles does NOT include stifle extension among its actions?

(1) Rectus femoris
(2) Biceps femoris
(3) Long digital extensor
(4) Caudal belly of the sartorius

45. Which among the following is NOT characteristic of the three gluteal muscles as a group?

(1) General placement
(2) General insertion area
(3) Major action
(4) Innervation

46. Traumatic interruption of flow in the distal caudal femoral artery would compromise flow to all of the following structures EXCEPT the:

(1) peroneus longus muscle.
(2) adductor muscle.
(3) biceps femoris muscle.
(4) gastrocnemius muscle.
(5) skin over the proximal region of the crus.

47. Which statement regarding the saphenous veins is INCORRECT?

(1) Both are accessible to venipuncture.
(2) Both possess a cranial and a caudal branch.
(3) Both pass deeply and terminate just as they reach the stifle.
(4) They communicate with each other across the tibia.

48. Which of the following structures is NOT a palpable feature at the caudal surface of the stifle?

(1) Popliteal lymph node
(2) Pulse in the popliteal artery
(3) Tendon of the biceps femoris muscle
(4) Tendon of the semitendinosus muscle

ANSWERS AND EXPLANATIONS

1. The answer is 1 [Chapter 56 I B 1]. The attachment of the pelvic limb to the trunk is bony and cartilaginous, and takes place directly between the proximal limb and the axial skeleton. In contrast, the attachment of the thoracic limb to the trunk is entirely muscular. Both the pelvic and thoracic limbs have a single "key" nerve (the femoral nerve and the radial nerve, respectively)—compromise of these nerves renders the limb incapable of bearing weight. In both the pelvic and thoracic limbs, the muscle bellies taper to form tendons in the distal regions of the limb. Each major region in the pelvic limb has the same number of bones as the corresponding region in the thoracic limb.

2. The answer is 3 [Chapter 57 II A 3 b]. The femoral condyles articulate with the tibial condyles. The patella articulates with the femoral trochlea. The tibia does not have a "head," only a proximal extremity, and the head of the fibula articulates with the tibial condyle.

3. The answer is 4 [Chapter 57 IV A 1 b]. The calcaneal tuber provides the attachment site for the tendon of the gastrocnemius muscle and acts as a lever for extension at the hock.

4. The answer is 4 [Chapter 58 II B 3 a]. The ligament of the head of the femur extends between the fovea capitis (a roughened depression in the middle of the femoral head) and the acetabular fossa. This ligament is associated with the coxofemoral (hip) joint.

5. The answer is 4 [Chapter 58 III B 2 c (1)–(2)]. The cranial and caudal tibial ligaments, which attach to the intercondylar areas of the tibia, anchor the menisci to the tibia. The cranial tibial ligaments extend between the cranial edge of each meniscus and the cranial intercondylar area of the tibia, and the caudal tibial ligaments extend between the caudal edge of each meniscus and the caudal intercondylar area of tibia. The single intermeniscal ligament extends between the free cranial ends of the two menisci; the collateral ligaments of the stifle extend between the femoral condyles and the tibia or fibula; and the cruciate ligaments of the stifle extend between the tibia and the femur.

6. The answer is 1 [Chapter 58 III B 4 a (2)]. Rupture of the medial (tibial) collateral ligament of the stifle joint would most likely result in excessive lateral motion of the tibia, while rupture of the lateral (fibular) collateral ligament of the stifle joint would result in excessive medial motion. Rupture of the cranial cruciate ligament would result in excessive cranial displacement of the tibia (the "cranial drawer sign"), while rupture of the caudal cruciate ligament would result in excessive caudal displacement of the tibia (the "caudal drawer sign").

7. The answer is 2 [Chapter 57, Figure 57–3; Chapter 58 V A]. The proximal intertarsal joint lies between the talus and central tarsal bone medially, and the calcaneus and tarsal bone IV laterally. The talocrural joint is between the talus and the tibia, not the fibula. The distal intertarsal joint lies between the central tarsal bone and tarsal bones II and III, but is positioned medially, not laterally. The intratarsal joints are those formed among the individual bones of the tarsus.

8. The answer is 2 [Chapter 59 III A 1]. The flexor surfaces of the pelvic limb alternate from the cranial to the caudal surface from the hip through the tarsus and then remain on the plantar surface of the limb from the tarsus distally. This is in distinct contrast to the flexor surfaces of the thoracic limb, which alternate from caudal to cranial from the shoulder to the carpus, and then remain on the palmar surface of the limb.

9. The answer is 4 [Chapter 59 II B 2]. The "hamstring" muscles on the caudal surface of the thigh (i.e., the biceps femoris, semitendinosus, semimembranosus, and caudal crural abductor muscles) flex the stifle and extend the hip. Muscles that adduct the thigh are positioned on its medial surface; circumduction requires cooperation of all muscle groups of the thigh.

10. The answer is 4 [Chapter 59 III A 2 b; Figure 59–5]. The flexor angle of the tarsus faces cranially, while the flexor angles of the digits face caudally. Thus, muscles passing over the cranial surface of the crus and the dorsal surface of the pes and crossing both joints (e.g., the long digital extensor) will flex the tarsus and extend the digits. The major extensors of the tarsus have only a minor effect on the stifle, and that effect is flexion. Because of the reversed positioning of the flexor angles of the tarsus and digits, those that act to extend the digits will flex the tarsus.

11. The answer is 2 [Chapter 59 II C 1 c (2)]. The peroneus longus, one of the craniolateral thigh muscles, originates from the proximal fibula and lateral tibial condyle, courses down the lateral surface of the crus, and turns deeply and medially to insert on the plantar surface of the tarsal bone and the bases of all of the metatarsal bones. The peroneus brevis inserts on the dorsal side of only metatarsal bone V. Neither digital extensor has any plantar attachment to the metatarsal bones.

12. The answer is 1 [Chapter 59 II C 2 d]. The popliteus muscle, which acts to rotate the crus medially, is positioned deeply on the proximal part of the caudal crus, adjacent to the joint capsule and the tibial surface. Its tendon of origin contains a sesamoid bone. The medial head of the deep digital flexor muscle extends all the way to the distal phalanges. The deep digital flexor does not have a "short head," and the gastrocnemius muscle does not have an "accessory head."

13. The answer is 1 [Chapter 59 II B 1 c (1) (a)]. The rectus femoris is the only head of the quadriceps femoris that originates from the pelvic girdle (i.e., from the ilium). The vastus lateralis, vastus medialis, and vastus intermedius originate from the femur.

14. The answer is 3 [Chapter 59 II B 2 a; Table 59–1]. The biceps femoris originates on the ischiatic tuberosity and, by means of three different aponeurotic extensions, attaches to the patella and patellar ligament, the proximal lateral tibia, and the tuber calcanei. The diversity of these attachments allows the biceps femoris to extend the hip, flex and extend the stifle, and extend the tarsus (hock). The cranial part of the biceps femoris, which attaches to the patella and patellar ligament, extends the hip and stifle. The middle part of the biceps femoris, which attaches to the proximal lateral tibial body, extends the hip. The caudal part of the biceps femoris, which attaches to the tuber calcanei, extends the hip and the hock and flexes the stifle.

15. The answer is 1 [Chapter 60 I C 2 b (4)]. The saphenous artery leaves the caudal surface of the femoral artery and courses distally across the medial side of the semimembranosus muscle. The saphenous artery terminates by dividing into a cranial branch and a caudal branch and is important to the arterial supply of both surfaces of the paw.

16. The answer is 4 [Chapter 60 I A 2 a]. The caudal gluteal artery, which is a branch of the internal iliac artery, delivers the main arterial supply to the lateral pelvic (gluteal) region in a cranial to caudal direction. The cranial gluteal and iliolumbar arteries are both branches of this main channel.

17. The answer is 2 [Chapter 60 I C 1 c (1); Table 60–1]. The deep femoral artery arises from the external iliac artery just before the external iliac passes out of the abdominal cavity via the vascular lacuna to become the femoral artery. The deep femoral artery gives off the pudendoepigastric trunk, and then continues as the medial circumflex femoral artery, which supplies the caudal thigh muscles (i.e., the biceps femoris, semimembranosus, and semitendinosus muscles), the ventral abdominal wall muscles, the external genitalia, and the mammary gland.

18. The answer is 4 [Chapter 60, Table 60–1]. The semimembranosus muscle, a caudal thigh ("hamstring") muscle, is supplied by the caudal gluteal, medial circumflex femoral, middle caudal femoral, and distal caudal femoral arteries. Therefore, if blood flow via the caudal gluteal artery were compromised (e.g., owing to trauma to the internal iliac artery), the semimembranosus could still receive arterial flow from the distal or middle caudal femoral arteries (branches of the femoral artery). The femoral artery is a main channel vessel, and does not directly supply any muscles. The popliteal and cranial gluteal arteries are not involved with the arterial supply of the caudal thigh musculature.

19. The answer is 2 [Chapter 60 I E 1]. The dorsal pedal and saphenous arteries share in supplying both the dorsal and plantar surfaces of the hindpaw. The dorsal pedal artery is a part of the main channel of arterial flow to the pes; therefore, compromise of this artery would drastically affect blood supply to the distal limb. The caudal tibial artery is not significant in arterial supply to the pes. The dorsal metatarsal arteries are small and of minor importance. "Plantar pedal artery" is a spurious term.

20. The answer is 2 [Chapter 60 I C 2 b (2)]. The lateral circumflex femoral artery provides the primary flow to the quadriceps femoris muscle. The tensor fasciae latae and middle gluteal muscles receive their supply mainly from the cranial gluteal artery, and the biceps femoris muscle is supplied by the caudal gluteal and distal caudal femoral arteries.

21. The answer is 4 [Chapter 60 III B 1 b (2)]. The efferent lymphatics of the popliteal lymph node terminate in the superficial inguinal lymph node.

22. The answer is 3 [Chapter 61 I B 1]. The lumbosacral plexus is formed from the ventral branches of lumbar nerves 3–7 (L3–L7) and sacral nerves 1–3 (S1–S3).

23. The answer is 4 [Chapter 61 II B 2]. The lateral cutaneous femoral nerve, despite its name, provides motor fibers to the psoas minor and adjacent hypaxial muscles, in addition to providing sensory fibers to the lateral femoral region. The cranial and caudal gluteal nerves are only motor. The lateral cutaneous sural nerve is only sensory, supplying the skin of the central part of the lateral crural region.

24. The answer is 1 [Chapter 59 II A 2; Chapter 61 II F–G]. Trauma to the greater trochanter of the femur would affect the middle and deep gluteal muscles, which insert there. The superficial gluteal muscle inserts on the third trochanter. The middle and deep gluteal muscles are innervated by the cranial gluteal nerve.

25. The answer is 4 [Chapter 61 II H]. Injury to the sciatic nerve at a level just proximal to its division into the tibial and common peroneal nerves would most likely impair the dog's ability to extend the digits and flex the hock. The sciatic nerve is not involved to a significant degree in extending the stifle, and therefore does not play an essential role in weight-bearing. The skin over much of the medial surface of the pelvic limb from the thigh to the pes is supplied by the saphenous nerve, a branch of the femoral nerve. Thus, this area of cutaneous sensation would be preserved.

26. The answer is 2 [Chapter 61 II C 2]. The genitofemoral nerve has a motor component in the male dog (i.e., to the cremaster muscle), but not in the bitch. It provides sensory fibers in both sexes to a triangular region of skin on the ventral abdomen and medial thighs.

27. The answer is 1 [Chapter 61 II H]. The sciatic nerve innervates the small pelvic association muscles (i.e., the internal obturator, gemelli, and quadratus femoris muscles), which are the major outward rotators of the hip. The femoral nerve innervates the major stifle extensor. The cranial gluteal nerve innervates the middle and deep gluteal muscles as well as the tensor fasciae latae. The caudal gluteal nerve innervates the superficial gluteal muscle and, in some individuals, part of the middle gluteal muscle.

28. The answer is 2 [Chapter 61 II D 2]. The saphenous nerve, a branch of the femoral nerve, travels with the femoral artery through the femoral triangle and proximal thigh before becoming associated with the saphenous artery in its distal course to the paw. The femoral nerve dissipates immediately and deeply within the quadriceps femoris muscle and is never seen superficially. The common peroneal nerve arises just proximal to the stifle, and is not seen superficially until the mid-level of the crus. The femoral nerve does not have a "medial" branch.

29. The answer is 2 [Chapter 61 II E]. The obturator nerve innervates the adductor muscle group (i.e., those muscles that adduct or draw the limb medially). The muscles innervated by the femoral nerve allow the dog to bear weight on the pelvic limb. The muscles innervated by the gluteal nerve allow the pelvic limb to be pulled laterally. The muscles innervated by the sciatic nerve allow the pelvic limb to be rotated outwardly.

30. The answer is 2 [Chapter 61 II H 2 e]. The common peroneal nerve would be most susceptible following blunt trauma to the lateral crural surface in the area of the fibular head. The nerve passes relatively superficially in this area before sinking between the muscle bellies and dividing into its two terminal branches, the superficial and deep peroneal nerves. The superficial peroneal nerve, named for the more superficial position it gains in the more distal crus, actually branches from the parent nerve deep to the lateral muscle bellies on the crus. The tibial nerve has a deep course and is thus more protected. The sciatic nerve has already divided into its two terminal branches, the common peroneal and the tibial nerves, proximal to the fibular head.

31. The answer is 2 [Chapter 61 III A 1, B 1 a (2)]. Dorsal metatarsal nerve II passes on the dorsal surface of the paw in the space between the second and third metatarsal bones. Nerves passing on the surface of the metatarsal bones are named metatarsal nerves. By convention, these nerves take the name of the lower-numbered metatarsal bone with which they are associated.

32. The answer is 1 [Chapter 61 III B 1 b (1)]. The plantar common digital nerves arise from the medial plantar nerve, which arises as a terminal branch of the tibial nerve, itself one of the two terminal branches of the sciatic nerve.

33. The answer is 3 [Chapter 57 II A 1 c; Chapter 62 I B 1]. The greater trochanter is the large bony protuberance that is palpable at the proximal lateral end of the femur, just caudal to the hip joint. The third trochanter and the lesser trochanter are too small to palpate. In addition, the lesser trochanter is positioned medially, rather than laterally. There is no "crest of the femoral head."

34. The answer is 2 [Chapter 62 II D 4]. The common peroneal nerve is palpable against the head of the fibula, where it has departed from the sciatic nerve and is coursing cranially prior to dividing into the superficial and deep peroneal nerves. The superficial peroneal nerve is named for the superficial position it takes much further distally in the crus.

35. The answer is 4 [Chapter 62 I E 2]. The calcaneus, which provides a lever for the action of the common calcanean tendon, projects far proximally and caudally from the remaining tarsal bones, and is the only tarsal bone that can be individually identified by palpation.

36. The answer is 3 [Chapter 62 II D 2 b]. The two heads of the gastrocnemius form the major palpable mass on the caudal side of the proximal tibia. The popliteus and lateral digital extensor muscles are buried too deeply to be appreciated. The lateral head of the deep digital flexor muscle is palpable on the distal caudal tibia, but is too deep proximally to be accessible.

37. The answer is 3 [Chapter 61 II D]. The femoral nerve forms in, and remains buried within, the iliopsoas muscle throughout most of its course. On reaching the quadriceps femoris muscle, the femoral nerve enters the muscle and ramifies immediately and deeply within it, so that little to none of the nerve is visible without directly invading muscle masses.

38. The answer is 3 [Chapter 57 II B 1–2; III C]. The semitendinosus muscle is not associated with a sesamoid bone. A small sesamoid bone within the tendon of origin of the popliteus muscle lies on the caudolateral surface of the tibial condyle. The sesamoid bones of the gastrocnemius muscle are embedded in the muscle's medial and lateral heads. These bones articulate with the femoral condyles. The sesamoid bone of the quadriceps femoris muscle is the patella.

39. The answer is 2 [Chapter 57 II A 1 c, 3]. The greater tubercle is a feature of the proximal humerus, not the femur. The trochlea of the femur, on its distal cranial surface, is the groove with which the patella articulates. The greater trochanter is the most prominent feature on the proximolateral surface of the femur. The femoral condyles, at the distal end of the femur, articulate with the tibial condyles.

40. The answer is 1 [Chapter 57 III A 1 b, 3 c]. The medial malleolus, a bony bump on the distal medial tibial surface, is not related to the tibial tuberosity. The tibial tuberosity is a feature of the proximal, cranial tibia where the tendon of the quadriceps femoris muscle attaches. The remaining statements are true: The extensor groove is a notch in the cranial border of the lateral tibial condyle that provides passage for the tendon of the long digital extensor. The popliteal notch is an indentation on the caudal tibial surface between the two tibial condyles. The tibial body is almost cylindrical in its midregion, but becomes four-sided as it blends with the distal extremity.

41. The answer is 1 [Chapter 57 II A 2]. The aspera surface is the roughened area on the caudal, not the cranial, femoral surface. The caudal thigh musculature attaches to the aspera surface of the femur. Articular surfaces for the sesamoid bones of the gastrocnemius muscles are present on the proximal-most edges of each femoral condyle. The extensor fossa is a pit on the distal end of the lateral femoral condyle. The long digital extensor muscle originates from the extensor fossa. The popliteal fossa is a subtle dimple on the surface of the lateral femoral condyle, where the tendon of origin of the popliteus muscle attaches.

42. The answer is 4 [Chapter 57 IV A 1 (a) (1); Figure 57–3]. The talus articulates with the fibula (proximally), the calcaneus (laterally), and the central tarsal bone (distally), but not metatarsal bone II (the central tarsal bone is interposed between the talus and the metatarsus).

43. The answer is 4 [Chapter 59, Table 59–1]. Most of the craniolateral crural muscles act on the tarsus, with the exception of the lateral digital extensor. This muscle passes so closely along the lateral side of the tarsus that it has essentially no action on it, either to flex or extend it. The cranial tibial, long digital extensor, and peroneus longus muscle all flex the hock.

44. The answer is 4 [Chapter 59 II B 3 a (1); Table 59–1]. The caudal belly of the sartorius inserts too far caudally to extend the stifle. The rectus femoris is a head of the quadriceps femoris muscle, the most powerful of stifle extensors. The biceps femoris extends the stifle via its fascial attachment to the patella and patellar ligament. The long digital extensor extends the stifle by originating from the extensor fossa of the femur and passing across the cranial joint surface.

45. The answer is 4 [Chapter 59, Table 59–1]. The superficial gluteal muscle is innervated by the caudal gluteal nerve, while the others are innervated by the cranial gluteal nerve. Together, the gluteal muscles lie over the lateral pelvic region, insert on the proximal lateral surface of the femur, and act to extend the hip.

46. The answer is 1 [Chapter 60 I C 2 b (7); Table 60–1]. The peroneus longus muscle, a craniolateral crural muscle, is supplied by the cranial tibial artery. The distal caudal femoral artery supplies the distal thigh muscles (e.g., biceps femoris, adductor), both heads of the gastrocnemius muscle, and the skin over the distal femoral and proximal crural regions.

47. The answer is 3 [Chapter 60 II B]. The lateral saphenous vein terminates in the popliteal vein, but the medial saphenous vein remains superficial and passes all the way proximally to the femoral triangle before terminating in the femoral vein. Both the lateral and the medial saphenous veins are superficial and therefore accessible to venipuncture. Both possess a cranial and a caudal branch. The cranial branch of the medial saphenous vein anastomoses with the cranial branch of the lateral saphenous vein in the distal fourth of the crus.

48. The answer is 2 [Chapter 60 I C 3; Chapter 62 II B 3, C 2–3]. The popliteal artery is buried too deeply among the thigh muscles to be accessible. The popliteal lymph node, and the tendons of the biceps femoris and semitendinosus muscles are palpable at the caudal surface of the stifle.

QUESTIONS

DIRECTIONS: Each of the numbered items or incomplete statements in this section is followed by answers or by completions of the statement. Select the ONE numbered answer or completion that is BEST in each case.

1. A veterinarian must access the heart through the chest wall. Which site is associated with the least chance of puncturing the lung?

(1) The area between the cranial and caudal lobes of the left lung at the level of the sternum
(2) The area between the cranial and caudal parts of the cranial lobe of the right lung at the level of the costochondral junction
(3) The area between the cranial and middle lobes of the right lung at the distal quarter of the fourth rib
(4) The area between the cranial and caudal lobes of either the right or left lungs at the distal quarter of the fourth rib.

2. During nephrectomy (surgical removal of the kidney), which one of the following is most likely to present possible complications?

(1) The retroperitoneal positioning of the kidney
(2) The possible presence of multiple renal arteries
(3) The tight adherence of the renal capsule to the kidney
(4) The complexity of the renal nervous plexus in the perihilar region

3. Which one of the following intraarticular structures of the elbow joint develops from a separate ossification center and may remain separate from the final bone, causing lameness requiring surgical correction?

(1) Radial head
(2) Articular circumference of the radius
(3) Anconeal process
(4) Olecranon tuber

4. Select the correct pairing of foramen and structures passing through it.

(1) Orbital fissure: cranial nerves III, IV, V_1, and VI and the external ophthalmic vein
(2) Hypoglossal canal: cranial nerve XII and the basilar artery
(3) Round foramen: mandibular nerve
(4) Caudal alar foramen: maxillary nerve
(5) Tympanooccipital fissure: facial nerve

5. Where is cystocentesis performed?

(1) On the ventral midline, a short distance caudal to the pelvic brim
(2) On the ventral midline, a short distance cranial to the pelvic brim
(3) One centimeter to the left of the ventral midline, at the level of the pelvic inlet
(4) One centimeter to the right or the left of the ventral midline, at the level of the pelvic inlet

6. The space accessed during thoracocentesis lies between:

(1) two layers of parietal pleura.
(2) one parietal layer and one visceral layer of pleura.
(3) the two serous layers of the pericardium.
(4) the fibrous and parietal serous layer of the pericardium.

7. Features of the cervical vertebrae that are normally clearly palpable in healthy dogs include the:

(1) spinous processes.
(2) transverse processes.
(3) ventral borders of the vertebral bodies.
(4) transverse foramina.

8. A female golden retriever is hit by a car, causing a fracture in the midshaft of her femur. In what direction would the distal fragment be displaced following pull of the "hamstring" muscles?

(1) Laterally
(2) Medially
(3) Caudally and proximally
(4) Cranially and proximally

9. Which one of the following covers the caudal wall of the thoracic cavity?

(1) Costal pleura
(2) Visceral pleura
(3) Pulmonary pleura
(4) Diaphragmatic pleura

10. A dog sustains an injury to the radial nerve at the level just proximal to the nerve's division into superficial and deep branches. What would be the most likely result?

(1) The dog's ability to bear weight is impaired, but extension of the carpus and digits is preserved.
(2) The dog's ability to extend the carpus and digits is impaired, and cutaneous sensory function is lost.
(3) The dog's ability to bear weight and flex the carpus and digits is impaired.
(4) The dog's ability to extend the carpus and digits is impaired, but cutaneous sensory function is preserved.

11. Which one of the following statements regarding the middle tunic of the eye is true?

(1) It is highly vascular in nature and supplies nutrition to the innermost layer by diffusion.
(2) It is sensitive to light over its caudal-most regions but not over the cranial-most ones.
(3) It possesses thick bundles of connective tissue that impart considerable strength to the tunic.
(4) It possesses a light-reflecting layer from the equator posteriorly.

12. What does the term "common integument" refer to?

(1) The skin over the entire surface of the body
(2) Unspecialized regions of the skin
(3) The skin and its associated hair, glands, pads, and claws
(4) Structures visible only on the external surface of the body
(5) Haired regions of the skin

13. Which one of the following nerves provides both motor and sensory innervation to the region it supplies?

(1) Trochlear nerve (cranial nerve IV)
(2) Maxillary nerve (cranial nerve V_2)
(3) Facial nerve (cranial nerve VII)
(4) Vestibulocochlear nerve (cranial nerve VIII)
(5) Hypoglossal nerve (cranial nerve XII)

14. Which of the following organs are normally palpable within the abdomen?

(1) The transverse colon and ileum
(2) The right and left kidneys
(3) The ovaries and adrenal glands
(4) The jejunum and descending colon

15. In dogs, the attachment of the thoracic limb to the axial skeleton is typically:

(1) a conventional bony attachment.
(2) a greatly reduced bony attachment.
(3) ligamentous.
(4) muscular.

16. What is the correct adult dental formula?

(1) 2(I 4/4, C 1/1, P 4/4, M 2/3)
(2) 2(I 3/4, C 1/1, P 4/4, M 2/3)
(3) 2(I 3/3, C 1/1, P 4/4, M 2/3)
(4) 2(I 3/3, C 1/1, P 3/4, M 2/3)
(5) 2(I 3/3, C 1/1, P 3/4, M 3/2)

17. A client brings her 4-year-old beagle to the veterinarian and complains that the dog has been "scooting." The veterinarian diagnoses impaction of the:

(1) circumanal glands.
(2) anal sinuses.
(3) anal glands.
(4) anal sacs.

18. Select the list that represents the body regions with musculature that overlies or attaches to the thoracic wall.

(1) Neck, abdomen
(2) Abdomen, pelvic limb
(3) Abdomen, pelvic limb, thoracic limb
(4) Neck, abdomen, thoracic limb

19. A dog has sustained a nerve injury that results in an impaired gait—he has difficulty flexing the elbow as part of bringing the limb forward, and as a result, his toes drag on the ground. Which nerve is most likely injured?

(1) Axillary nerve
(2) Radial nerve
(3) Median nerve
(4) Musculocutaneous nerve

20. Select the correct sequence of arteries in the main channel of blood flow to the head.

(1) Common carotid, external carotid, infraorbital, maxillary
(2) Common carotid, external carotid, maxillary, infraorbital
(3) External carotid, common carotid, maxillary, infraorbital
(4) Maxillary, infraorbital, common carotid, external carotid
(5) External carotid, common carotid, maxillary, infraorbital

21. Which one of the following statements regarding the linea alba is true?

(1) The linea alba is a white line formed on the deep surface of the abdominal wall along the ventral midline where the parietal peritoneum fuses with the underlying musculature.
(2) The linea alba presents a poor site for placement of a ventral midline incision because it is densely populated with afferent (sensory) nerves.
(3) The linea alba is the termination site of the various muscles contributing to the formation of the rectus sheath.
(4) The linea alba is a paired white line (one on each side of the midline) that represents the lateral border of the rectus abdominis muscle.

22. Identify the correct combination of fetal circulatory feature, organ the feature is designed to bypass, and remnant of the fetal structure in the adult.

(1) Ductus venosus/ pulmonary circulation/ round ligaments of the lungs
(2) Ductus arteriosus/ pulmonary circulation/ ligamentum arteriosum
(3) Foramen ovale/ hepatic circulation/ fossa ovalis
(4) Ductus venosus/ hepatic circulation/ falciform ligament
(5) Ductus arteriosus/ hepatic circulation/ round ligament of the liver

23. How many regions are found in the vertebral column?

(1) Three
(2) Four
(3) Five
(4) Six
(5) Seven

24. Which sequence represents the main channel arterial flow through the pelvic limb?

(1) External iliac, popliteal, femoral, dorsal pedal, cranial tibial
(2) External iliac, femoral, popliteal, cranial tibial, dorsal pedal
(3) Femoral, external iliac, cranial tibial, popliteal, dorsal pedal
(4) Popliteal, external iliac, femoral, cranial tibial, dorsal pedal

25. What is the vestibular plexus?

(1) A plexus of autonomic nerves on the lateral vestibular walls that functions in engorgement of the vulva
(2) A plexus of sensory nerves on the lateral vestibular walls that functions during copulation
(3) A plexus of arteries within the medial vestibular wall that engorges the vestibular bulb during copulation
(4) a plexus of veins around the vulvar opening that functions in sexual behavior

26. What is the "dewclaw"?

(1) Digit V
(2) Digit I
(3) The proximal sesamoid bone of digit I
(4) A supernumerary digit resulting from embryonic digital duplication

27. A 6-year-old dalmatian must be intubated using a nasogastric tube. Through what meatus should the veterinarian seek access to the nasal cavity?

(1) Dorsal nasal meatus
(2) Middle nasal meatus
(3) Ventral nasal meatus
(4) Common nasal meatus

28. Which muscle is palpable at the caudal border of the axilla?

(1) Superficial pectoral muscle
(2) Deep pectoral muscle
(3) Teres major muscle
(4) Teres minor muscle

29. How many spinal cord segments are in each region of the vertebral column?

(1) Cervical (7), thoracic (13), lumbar (7), sacral (3), caudal (20–23)
(2) Cervical (8), thoracic (13), lumbar (7), sacral (3), caudal (20–23)
(3) Cervical (8), thoracic (13), lumbar (7), sacral (3), caudal (5)
(4) Cervical (8), thoracic (12), lumbar (7), caudal (20–23)
(5) Cervical (7), thoracic (13), lumbar (7), caudal (4–5)

30. The tapering of the spinal cord in its caudal-most extent is the:

(1) cauda equina.
(2) conus medullaris.
(3) conus sacralis.
(4) filum terminale.

31. Which one of the following structures forms the palpable part of the pelvic inlet?

(1) Pecten pubis
(2) Ischium
(3) Iliac crest
(4) Iliac shaft

32. Which cranial nerve develops as an outgrowth of the diencephalon and hence retains meningeal coverings and histologically resembles brain tissue?

(1) Olfactory nerve (cranial nerve I)
(2) Optic nerve (cranial nerve II)
(3) Oculomotor nerve (cranial nerve III)
(4) Trochlear nerve (cranial nerve IV)

33. Which one of the following structures is located in the cranial mediastinum?

(1) Aortic arch
(2) Tracheal bifurcation
(3) Brachiocephalic trunk
(4) Tracheobronchial lymph nodes

34. Traumatic injury to which of the following nerves would render the pelvic limb incapable of bearing weight?

(1) Sciatic nerve
(2) Femoral nerve
(3) Cranial gluteal nerve
(4) Common peroneal nerve

35. Which one of the following statements regarding dorsal intercostal arteries 1–12 is true?

(1) They are branches of the thoracic aorta.
(2) They course along the cranial border of the associated rib.
(3) They supply the muscle, but not the skin, of the lateral thoracic wall.
(4) They provide a spinal branch to the spinal cord within the vertebral canal.

36. A dog has a fractured humerus. The fracture is located in the midshaft of the humerus, and the proximal fragment is displaced. Pull of which muscle is most likely responsible for the displacement?

(1) Biceps brachii
(2) Triceps brachii
(3) Deltoideus
(4) Pronator teres

37. Which one of the following statements regarding the mammary glands of the dog is true?

(1) They are modified sweat glands; the progenitors develop in both sexes but regress in males.
(2) They share glandular interconnections of secretory tissue throughout their length.
(3) They each receive exclusive arterial supply solely from the adjacent intercostal artery.
(4) They receive autonomic, but no sensory, innervation.
(5) They lack lymphatic drainage, which increases the efficiency of milk production.

38. All serous membranes adhere to the wall of the cavity that contains them. In the abdomen, which one of the following structures is the equivalent of the endothoracic fascia in the thorax?

(1) Enteric abdominal fascia
(2) Deep abdominal fascia
(3) Intermuscular fascia
(4) Transversalis fascia

39. Which statement regarding the diaphragm is correct?

(1) The central tendinous portion of the diaphragm securely attaches it to the subcostal musculature.
(2) The muscular periphery is perforated in three places to provide passageway for structures passing between the thorax and abdomen.
(3) The lumbar part includes the right and left diaphragmatic crura, from which strong muscular bundles radiate.
(4) The costal part is separated from the lumbar part by prominent aponeuroses on both the right and the left.

40. A dog suffering from a cerebellar disorder would most likely demonstrate signs related to:

(1) visual deficit.
(2) impaired memory.
(3) miscoordination of heart rhythm.
(4) coordination deficit.

41. Which of the following ventilatory muscles differs from the others on the basis of innervation?

(1) Diaphragm
(2) Rectus thoracis
(3) Serratus dorsalis caudalis
(4) Internal intercostal muscles

42. The greatest structural modifications of the ulna:

(1) are present distally.
(2) involve articulation with the carpus.
(3) contribute to the formation of the elbow.
(4) are related to the tremendous pull of the insertion of the triceps brachii muscle.

43. What is the correct sequence of the flow of semen through the male reproductive tract?

(1) Ductus deferens, epididymis, pelvic urethra, prostatic urethra
(2) Epididymis, ductus deferens, prostatic urethra, pelvic urethra
(3) Epididymis, prostatic urethra, ductus deferens, penile urethra
(4) Prostatic urethra, epididymis, ductus deferens, pelvic urethra

44. A veterinarian sees a dog with a pelvic limb nerve injury that is manifested as lameness. The dog is unable to extend the hock or flex the digits, but other limb functions have been preserved. Which nerve is most likely to have sustained damage?

(1) Tibial nerve
(2) Sciatic nerve
(3) Common peroneal nerve
(4) Tibial and common peroneal nerves

45. Which two tissues are most similar in terms of ability to heal?

(1) Hyaline cartilage and diaphyseal bone
(2) Hyaline cartilage and ligament
(3) Elastic cartilage and irregular bone
(4) Ligament and diaphyseal bone
(5) Fibrocartilage and flat bone

46. Which one of the following statements regarding palpable head features is correct?

(1) Normal lymph nodes are too small to detect.
(2) The laryngeal cartilages are placed too deeply for palpation.
(3) The opening of the parotid duct may be visualized in the oral vestibule lateral to the lower carnassial tooth.
(4) The infraorbital foramen is readily palpable on the maxilla at approximately halfway the distance between the eye and external nose.

47. Which statement describing the pharyngeal musculature is correct?

(1) It serves to hold the pharyngeal opening (aditus) securely closed during nasal breathing
(2) It receives motor innervation from the glossopharyngeal nerve (cranial nerve IX) and the accessory nerve (cranial nerve XI).
(3) It consists of one dilator and several constrictors.
(4) It blends imperceptibly with the laryngeal musculature.

48. The numerous ligamentous and cartilaginous specializations of the stifle joint are necessary to:

(1) support the joint through its normal diverse range of motion.
(2) compensate for the lack of well-developed collateral ligaments.
(3) compensate for the lack of a good fit between the apposing bony surfaces.
(4) support the stifle joint as the part of the pelvic limb that bears most of the individual's weight.

49. A first-year veterinary student auscultates a 4-month-old puppy over the bony thorax in the area of the eleventh intercostal space midway down the thorax and is alarmed to hear gut sounds rather than air sounds. On examining the puppy, the student's instructor confirms her observations. Which one of the following is the correct conclusion?

(1) The puppy should have thoracic and abdominal survey radiographs to rule out the possibility of a congenital diaphragmatic hernia.
(2) The presence of digestive viscera within the caudal thorax is normal at this developmental stage, and the gut will regress to the abdomen once the diaphragm closes.
(3) The caval foramen of the diaphragm periodically admits some gut loops into the caudal thorax; these loops of intestine usually return to their proper position spontaneously.
(4) The presence of digestive viscera within the caudal thorax is normal.

50. Which statement regarding the peritoneal ligaments is true?

(1) They are bands of peritoneum that connect one organ to another.
(2) They are doubled folds of peritoneum that connect organs to the dorsal body wall.
(3) They are stout bands of collagenous fibers that anchor the stomach, liver, and descending colon to the dorsal body wall.
(4) They are narrow bands of peritoneum that conduct vessels and nerves to the intestinal wall.

51. What is the sequence of peritoneal pouches in the pelvic region, from dorsal to ventral?

(1) Pubovesical, pararectal fossae, vesicogenital, rectogenital
(2) Vesicogenital, rectogenital, pubovesical, pararectal fossae
(3) Pararectal fossae, rectogenital, vesicogenital, pubovesical
(4) Rectogenital, pararectal fossae, pubovesical, vesicogenital

52. Which one of the following statements regarding the arterial supply to the brain is true?

(1) It arrives to the arterial circle of the brain from the internal carotid and rostral cerebral arteries.
(2) It is distributed by two paired arteries arising from each side of the circle.
(3) It is distributed from the arterial circle to essentially the entire cerebrum and the rostral part of the cerebellum.
(4) The caudal cerebellar arteries are the largest arteries supplying the brain.

53. Which fascial layer possesses characteristics that facilitate the subcutaneous injection of fluids in the caudal cervical region?

(1) Superficial cervical fascia
(2) Superficial layer of the deep cervical fascia
(3) Deep layer of the deep cervical fascia
(4) Dorsolateral cervical fascia

54. A client wishes to have her Siberian husky artificially inseminated. The clinician must first pass the artificial insemination rod directly:

(1) dorsally, in order to bypass the ischiatic arch.
(2) cranially, in order to access the vestibular canal.
(3) ventrally, in order to avoid the clitoral fossa.
(4) ventrally, in order to circumvent the urethral tubercle.

55. What is the omental bursa?

(1) A cavity that is continuous with the peritoneal cavity.
(2) A layer of peritoneum that enfolds the omentum.
(3) A specialization of peritoneum that is associated with the inguinal canal.
(4) A synonym for the ovarian bursa, which is formed from an omental diverticulum.

56. Rupture of which one of the following elbow ligaments would most likely result in excessive lateral motion of the proximal radius and ulna?

(1) Medial collateral ligament
(2) Lateral collateral ligament
(3) Annular ligament
(4) Oblique ligament

57. Select the correct pairing of muscle and action.

(1) Platysma—draws the external ear caudally and ventrally
(2) Buccinator—draws the angle of the mouth caudally
(3) Orbicularis oculi—closes the lips
(4) Caninus—raises the upper lip
(5) Mentalis—raises the upper lid

58. Which joint of the pelvic limb has a single joint capsule, five contributing bones, and no collateral ligaments?

(1) Coxofemoral (hip) joint
(2) Stifle (knee) joint
(3) Talocrural (hock, ankle) joint
(4) Metatarsophalangeal joint

59. Which one of the following statements regarding the lateral funiculus is true?

(1) It contains neuronal cell bodies of the parasympathetic nervous system.
(2) It is positioned between the dorsal and ventral horns of the spinal cord.
(3) It conducts impulses to the intermediate horn.
(4) It is positioned superficial to the pia mater along the ventrolateral cord surface.

60. Which carpal joint is most difficult to access by needle puncture?

(1) Antebrachiocarpal joint
(2) Radiocarpal joint
(3) Middle carpal joint
(4) Carpometacarpal joint

61. What is the proper cranial-to-caudal sequence of the gut regions?

(1) Descending duodenum, ascending duodenum, jejunum, ileum, ascending colon, transverse colon, descending colon
(2) Descending duodenum, ascending duodenum, ileum, jejunum, ascending colon, transverse colon, descending colon
(3) Ascending duodenum, ileum, descending duodenum, jejunum, descending colon, transverse colon, ascending colon
(4) Ascending duodenum, descending duodenum, jejunum, ileum, ascending colon, descending colon, transverse colon

62. Hemal arches are characteristic of:

(1) cervical vertebrae, for transmission of the vertebral artery.
(2) thoracic vertebrae, for transmission of the thoracic aorta.
(3) lumbar vertebrae, for transmission of the otherwise unprotected abdominal aorta.
(4) caudal vertebrae, for transmission of the median caudal artery.

63. During intestinal surgery, temporary occlusion of which one of the following arteries would reduce blood flow to the cecum?

(1) Celiac artery
(2) Ileocolic artery
(3) Middle colic artery
(4) Caudal mesenteric artery

64. Select the sequence that reflects the main channel arterial flow through the thoracic limb.

(1) Axillary, subclavian, brachial, median, palmar proper digital, palmar common digital
(2) Axillary, subclavian, median, brachial, palmar proper digital, palmar common digital
(3) Subclavian, axillary, brachial, median, palmar common digital, palmar proper digital
(4) Subclavian, axillary, median, brachial, palmar common digital, palmar proper digital

65. Which statement concerning the ligaments of the stifle is true?

(1) The cranial cruciate ligament attaches to the femur cranially and the tibia caudally.
(2) The intermeniscal ligament extends from the free cranial edge of one meniscus to the free caudal edge of the other meniscus.
(3) The meniscofemoral ligament extends between the femur and the lateral meniscus.
(4) The medial and lateral femoropatellar ligaments are subdivisions of the medial and lateral collateral ligaments.

66. Which one of the following salivary glands is sometimes accompanied by accessory salivary glands of the same name?

(1) Parotid salivary gland
(2) Zygomatic salivary gland
(3) Mandibular salivary gland
(4) Monostomatic portion of the sublingual salivary gland

67. The venous drainage of the spinal cord takes place:

(1) mainly by satellite veins that directly parallel the named arteries of the cord.
(2) by a set of enlarged veins within the dorsal lamina of the dura mater.
(3) by a large venous plexus that entirely surrounds the cord within the vertebral canal.
(4) by three variably developed venous plexuses, some within and some outside of the vertebral canal.

68. The biceps brachii and the long head of the triceps brachii are similar in that they both:

(1) have similar insertion sites.
(2) have multiple heads.
(3) are innervated by the same nerve.
(4) completely bridge the brachium with no attachment to it.

69. Of the three potential lymphocenters of the thoracic region, which is the most constant?

(1) Ventral thoracic lymphocenter
(2) Dorsal thoracic lymphocenter
(3) Mediastinal lymphocenter
(4) Cranial mediastinal lymph nodes

70. Parasympathetic innervation to the liver would be most affected by transection of the:

(1) right vagus nerve.
(2) dorsal vagal trunk.
(3) ventral vagal trunk.
(4) left dorsal vagal branch.

71. Which statement regarding the internal substance of the spinal cord is correct?

(1) The peripherally located grey matter is composed largely of neuronal cell bodies.
(2) The white matter is composed of myelinated axonal processes together with neuronal cell bodies.
(3) The grey matter of the dorsal horn has sensory function.
(4) The intermediate horn of the cervical region is composed of sympathetic neuronal bodies.

72. In the pelvic limb, which artery is located on the medial side of digit II on the ground-facing surface of the paw?

(1) Palmar common digital artery II
(2) Plantar proper digital artery II
(3) Axial plantar proper digital artery II
(4) Axial palmar proper digital artery II

73. The internal pudendal artery supplies both the scrotum and the vulva, a fact that is most causally related to:

(1) the similar location of the two organs.
(2) the similar layered structure of the two organs.
(3) the similar developmental origin of the two organs.
(4) the common internal mesenteric support of the two organs.

74. Select the correct statement regarding the lymph nodes of the head.

(1) They lie adjacent to and take the same names as the deep salivary glands because they send efferent lymphatics through the salivary glands.
(2) They send their efferent vessels to the more superficial nodes.
(3) They are not always constant in occurrence and number.
(4) They drain soft tissues but not bone.

75. During ovariohysterectomy, which supporting structure of the ovary offers the most resistance to sectioning?

(1) Suspensory ligament
(2) Proper ligament
(3) Broad ligament
(4) Mesovarium

76. Blood flow to the triceps brachii muscle through the deep brachial artery is compromised. Which one of the following arteries can provide alternate blood flow, preventing the muscle from becoming completely ischemic?

(1) Caudal circumflex humeral artery
(2) Cranial circumflex humeral artery
(3) Bicipital artery
(4) Suprascapular artery

77. Which thoracic vertebra is described as follows: small body, costal foveae, short spinous process that is not inclined cranially or caudally.

(1) T1
(2) T7
(3) T11
(4) T13

78. Which one of the following statements regarding endolymph is true?

(1) It fills the semicircular canals.
(2) It fills the cochlear and semicircular ducts.
(3) Its primary function is to provide nutrition to the bony labyrinth.
(4) It drains from the inner ear through the vestibular window.

79. The most prominently palpable lymph node of the pelvic limb in the healthy dog is the:

(1) femoral lymph node.
(2) popliteal lymph node.
(3) medial iliac lymph node.
(4) superficial inguinal lymph node.

80. Which large, ventrally directed first branch of the internal pudendal artery supplies the greatest number of pelvic structures in the male?

(1) Dorsal artery of the penis
(2) Internal pelvic artery
(3) Great perineal artery
(4) Prostatic artery

81. What are the arterial plexuses in relation to the thoracic autonomic nerves?

(1) They are specialized nervous networks controlling blood flow through the coronary arteries.
(2) They are sympathetic networks placed at strategic points to coordinate closure of the heart valves.
(3) They are supplementary parasympathetic networks that form to mimic the placement of the cervicothoracic and middle cervical ganglia, for which there are no parasympathetic correlates.
(4) They are networks of autonomic fibers that surround the major arteries.

82. Which portion of the uterus is specialized for the gestation of fetuses?

(1) Uterine body
(2) Uterine horn
(3) Uterine tube
(4) Uterine cervix

83. An artery arising from the brachial artery and passing to the latissimus dorsi muscle as its sole supply will be named the:

(1) collateral dorsal artery.
(2) collateral thoracodorsal artery.
(3) brachial thoracodorsal artery.
(4) thoracodorsal artery.

84. Which one of the following statements regarding the sacrum is true?

(1) Fusion of the four sacral vertebrae forms the sacrum.
(2) A single, partially mobile joint lies at the original junction of the first and second sacral vertebrae.
(3) It articulates with the ischial wing.
(4) The dorsal sacral foramina transmit the dorsal sacral nerves and vessels.

85. The bulbar conjunctiva is most easily distinguished from the palpebral conjunctiva by its:

(1) location.
(2) vascularity.
(3) lack of innervation by a sensory nerve.
(4) possession of goblet cells.

86. Where should the thoracic wall be percussed to access the hollow sound of an air-filled lung?

(1) Ribs 6–9
(2) Ribs 5–10
(3) Intercostal spaces 6–9
(4) Intercostal spaces 5–10

87. Which artery is located on the medial surface of the dorsal side of digit II?

(1) Dorsal common digital artery II
(2) Dorsal proper digital artery II
(3) Axial dorsal proper digital artery II
(4) Abaxial dorsal common digital artery II

88. Select the correct statement from those below concerning the relations among the various cavities of the thoracic region.

(1) The thoracic cavity contains the pleural and pericardial cavities and the mediastinal space.
(2) The thoracic cavity contains the pleural cavity but not the pericardial cavity and mediastinal space.
(3) The pleural cavity contains the pericardial cavity, and both are contained by the thoracic cavity.
(4) The pleural cavity lies within the mediastinal space, and both are contained by the thoracic cavity.

89. What is the cervical intumescence?

(1) An enlargement in the vertebral canal that accommodates the larger-than-normal spinal ganglia of the thoracic regions of the spinal cord
(2) An enlargement of the spinal cord caused by the increased number of neurons associated with innervation of the thoracic limb
(3) An area particularly prone to intervertebral disc rupture
(4) Intermittent swelling of the cervical region of the spinal cord

90. Which one of the following statements regarding the facial vein is true?

(1) It closely follows the artery of the same name.
(2) It forms from the confluence of the deep and superficial facial veins.
(3) It forms part of the linguofacial trunk.
(4) It enters the common carotid vein.

91. The brachial plexus is formed from:

(1) the dorsal branches of C5, C6, C7, T1, and T2.
(2) the ventral branches of C5, C6, C7, T1, and T2.
(3) the dorsal branches of C6, C7, C8, T1, and T2.
(4) the ventral branches of C6, C7, C8, T1, and T2.

DIRECTIONS: Each of the numbered items or incomplete statements in this section is negatively phrased, as indicated by a capitalized word such as NOT, LEAST, or EXCEPT. Select the ONE numbered answer or completion that is BEST in each case.

92. All of the following bones contribute to the formation of the viscerocranium EXCEPT the:

(1) frontal bone.
(2) maxilla.
(3) incisive bone.
(4) palatine bone.
(5) temporal bone.

93. The adrenal glands and the kidneys share certain basic structural features. Which one of the following is NOT among these general features?

(1) Retroperitoneal positioning
(2) A cortex and a medulla
(3) A hilus to allow ingress and egress of arteries and veins
(4) A thick covering of fat

94. Portions of which one of the following muscles would NOT be readily palpable on the caudal surface of the thigh?

(1) Biceps femoris muscle
(2) Semitendinosus muscle
(3) Semimembranosus muscle
(4) Caudal crural abductor muscle

95. Which one of the following statements concerning the mobility of the vertebral column is NOT true?

(1) Extension and flexion in the cervical region is the vertebral column's most significant contribution to the running gait.
(2) The caudal cervical region is the region of the vertebral column associated with the most mobility.
(3) Rotation is mainly accomplished in the thoracic region of the vertebral column.
(4) The ability of the dog to curl up when sleeping is mainly afforded by the relatively great lateral mobility of the thoracolumbar area.

96. All of the following portions of the abdominal wall are largely or entirely muscular EXCEPT the:

(1) cranial abdominal wall.
(2) caudal abdominal wall.
(3) lateral abdominal wall.
(4) ventral abdominal wall.

97. All of the following statements describing the dural venous sinuses of the brain are true EXCEPT:

(1) They drain the deeper structures of the brain.
(2) They drain the diploe of the skull.
(3) They are located between the arachnoid and the dura mater.
(4) Some sinuses are paired and some are not.

98. Which of the following spaces is NOT accessible to diagnostic needle puncture for obtaining a sample of cerebrospinal fluid?

(1) Cerebellomedullary cistern
(2) Lumbar cistern
(3) Central canal
(4) Subarachnoid space

99. Which one of the following is NOT a member of the thoracolumbar hypaxial muscle group?

(1) Quadratus lumborum muscle
(2) Quadratus femoris muscle
(3) Iliacus muscle
(4) Psoas major muscle
(5) Psoas minor muscle

100. Arteries of the pelvic limb from which the pulse can be readily palpated include all of the following EXCEPT the:

(1) femoral artery.
(2) saphenous artery.
(3) dorsal pedal artery.
(4) cranial gluteal artery.

101. All of the following bones contribute to the bony pelvis EXCEPT the:

(1) ilium.
(2) sacrum.
(3) acetabulum.
(4) Vertebra Cd1.

102. Nerves sensory to the superficial thoracic wall and shoulder region near the thorax include branches of all of the following EXCEPT the:

(1) dorsal branches of the thoracic spinal nerves.
(2) ventral branches of the thoracic spinal nerves.
(3) axillary nerve.
(4) lateral thoracic nerve.

103. Which one of the following lymphoid structures does NOT contribute to the ring of lymphoid tissue surrounding the entrance to the deeper regions of the respiratory and digestive tracts?

(1) Palatine tonsil
(2) Medial retropharyngeal lymph node
(3) Lingual tonsil
(4) Pharyngeal tonsil

104. Which one of the following structures is NOT located within the femoral triangle?

(1) femoral vein
(2) femoral nerve
(3) femoral artery
(4) saphenous nerve

105. Which one of the following statements regarding the tracheal trunk is NOT true?

(1) It is the major lymphatic channel of the neck.
(2) It is positioned deeply along the trachea.
(3) It originates as efferents of the deep cervical lymph nodes.
(4) It terminates in either the thoracic duct or the great veins of the heart.

106. Which one of the following statements regarding the peritoneum is INCORRECT?

(1) The parietal and visceral peritoneum are directly continuous.
(2) The peritoneal cavity extends into the pelvic cavity.
(3) Intraperitoneal organs are located within the peritoneal cavity.
(4) The peritoneum produces a small amount of serous fluid that contributes to the mobility of the abdominal organs.

107. All of the following are a source of autonomic innervation to the urinary bladder EXCEPT the:

(1) pelvic nerve.
(2) lumbar sympathetic trunk.
(3) hypogastric nerves.
(4) pudendal nerve.

108. Which one of the following structures is NOT common to both cardiac ventricles?

(1) Chordae tendineae
(2) Papillary muscles
(3) Trabeculae carneae
(4) Trabecula septomarginalis

109. Arterial supply to the back arrives through all of the following vessels EXCEPT the:

(1) 12 dorsal intercostal arteries in the thoracic region.
(2) 7 lumbar arteries in the lumbar region.
(3) costoabdominal artery.
(4) direct branches of the aorta.
(5) collateral branches of the renal, gonadal, and external iliac arteries.

110. All of the following muscles contribute to the common calcanean tendon EXCEPT the:

(1) medial head of the gastrocnemius muscle.
(2) superficial digital flexor muscle.
(3) semitendinosus muscle.
(4) peroneus longus muscle.

111. Which one of the following statements regarding the cervical spinal nerves is INCORRECT?

(1) They have an exit from the vertebral canal relative to the vertebral body of the same number.
(2) The medial division of the dorsal branch is cutaneous in nature.
(3) The dorsal branches of nerves C6–C8 contribute to the brachial plexus.
(4) The cervical spinal nerves supply both the hypaxial and epaxial musculature.
(5) The dorsal branches of nerves C1 and C2 form large named nerves with specialized function.

112. All of the following organs are supplied by the pelvic plexus EXCEPT the:

(1) uterus.
(2) penis.
(3) rectum.
(4) ovary.

113. Components of the carotid sheath include all of the following EXCEPT the:

(1) vagosympathetic trunk.
(2) external carotid artery.
(3) tracheal lymphatic duct.
(4) internal jugular vein.

114. The cranial mesenteric artery supplies all of the following organs EXCEPT the:

(1) cecum.
(2) spleen.
(3) pancreas.
(4) descending colon.

115. Intercostal arteries can arise from all of the following arteries EXCEPT:

(1) the descending aorta.
(2) the internal thoracic artery.
(3) the vertebral artery.
(4) the thoracic vertebral artery.

116. Which statement regarding the veins of the heart is INCORRECT?

(1) The veins of the heart are largely satellite veins of arteries and share the arterial name.
(2) Some veins of the heart open directly into the right and left ventricles.
(3) Most cardiac veins are paired.
(4) Most blood from the heart wall reaches the right atrium via the coronary sinus.

117. The pulse can be readily obtained in the pelvic limb in all of the following sites EXCEPT the:

(1) femoral artery, where it passes through the femoral triangle.
(2) dorsal pedal artery, where it crosses the tarsus into the metatarsus.
(3) saphenous artery, as it departs from the femoral artery on the medial thigh.
(4) saphenous artery, as it crosses the medial side of the tibial shaft.

ANSWERS AND EXPLANATIONS

1. The answer is 3 [Chapter 37 II D 3 a (4)]. The pericardium and heart are accessible to needle puncture through the cardiac notch, a triangular space between the cranial and middle lobes of the right lung. The cardiac notch is formed where the borders of the associated lobes diverge from each other, leaving a significant portion of the pericardial wall uncovered by lung tissue. The apex of the cardiac notch is positioned at the distal quarter of the fourth rib.

2. The answer is 2 [Chapter 47 I G 1]. During development, the kidney "ascends" from its original, more caudal, position to its definitive position, which is located more cranially in the abdomen. As the kidney ascends, it is vascularized by progressively more cranial branches of the aorta. Not uncommonly, two or three of these branches are retained into the definitive form. Therefore, during nephrectomy, care must be taken to identify and ligate all of the renal arteries. Neither the retroperitoneal position nor the adherence of the capsule to the renal surface present an obstacle to nephrectomy. There is no renal nervous plexus in the perihilar region.

3. The answer is 3 [Chapter 26 III B 2 a (2) (a)]. The anconeal process is a sharp, beak-like process on the proximal end of the trochlear notch of the ulna that, in full extension, is seated within the olecranon fossa of the humerus. The anconeal process develops from a separate ossification center than the rest of the ulna. In many large breeds, faulty fusion of this process with the olecranon occurs, resulting in ununited anconeal process, a condition characterized by painful lameness that must be treated surgically.

4. The answer is 1 [Chapter 8 II A 2 b (3) (b) (ii); Table 9–1]. The orbital fissure transmits the oculomotor nerve (cranial nerve III), the trochlear nerve (cranial nerve IV), the opthalmic component of the trigeminal nerve (cranial nerve V_1), the abducent nerve (cranial nerve VI), and the external opthalmic vein. Only cranial nerve XII passes through the hypoglossal canal. The mandibular nerve passes through the oval foramen, not the round foramen. The maxillary nerve passes through only the rostral alar foramen. The facial nerve passes through the stylomastoid foramen, not the tympanooccipital fissure.

5. The answer is 2 [Chapter 40 III B 2]. Cystocentesis, a procedure that allows the clinician to obtain a sterile urine sample with minimal discomfort to the animal, takes advantage of the fact that the full (distended) urinary bladder can extend across the pelvic brim, gaining access to the floor of the abdominal region. A needle is inserted through the ventral midline a short distance cranial to the pubic brim to obtain the urine sample.

6. The answer is 1 [Chapter 37 III B 2 a]. The target during thoracocentesis is the pleural cavity between the costal and diaphragmatic layers of parietal pleura.

7. The answer is 1 [Chapter 24 I B]. The spinous processes of the vertebrae are palpable from vertebra C3 through L7. Although a general firmness can be appreciated at the level of the transverse processes in healthy animals, these structures become distinctly palpable only in emaciated animals. The ventral borders of the vertebral bodies and the transverse foramina are not palpable, even in emaciated dogs.

8. The answer is 3 [Chapter 59 II B 2]. In a dog with a broken femur, pulling of the caudal thigh muscles (i.e., the "hamstring" muscles), which extend between the ischiatic tuberosity and the distal femur, would tend to draw the distal fragment caudally and proximally.

9. The answer is 4 [Chapter 37 I A 3 b (2)]. The diaphragmatic pleura covers the diaphragm, which forms the caudal wall of the thoracic cavity. The costal pleura, which lies over the internal surfaces of the ribs, covers the lateral as well as most of the dorsal and ventral walls of the thoracic cavity. The visceral (pulmonary) pleura directly covers the lungs.

10. The answer is 2 [Chapter 30 II K 2 a (1), b]. At the level where the radial nerve divides into superficial and deep branches, the triceps brachii has already received its motor innervation, so the limb could still be fixed in extension and thus bear weight. Injury to the nerve proximal to its division impairs function of both branches: the superficial branch is involved with cutaneous sensory function, and the deep branch is involved with motor function of the extensors of the carpus and digits—therefore, both of these functions would be lost.

11. The answer is 1 [Chapter 15 II B 2]. The middle tunic of the eye, the vascular tunic, is (as the name would suggest) highly vascular and it supplies nutrition to the innermost tunic, the retina (nervous) tunic by diffusion. The retina, not the vascular tunic, is sensitive to light over its caudal-most regions. The fibrous tunic, consisting of the sclera and cornea, possesses thick bundles of connective tissue that help the eyeball maintain its shape. The tapetum lucidum, a light-reflecting layer, is present in the choroid (part of the vascular layer), but it is positioned in the dorsal region of the fundus.

12. The answer is 3 [Chapter 2 I A 1]. The term "common integument" refers to the skin, along with its associated hair, glands, pads, and claws.

13. The answer is 3 [Chapter 10 II D, E 2 b, G, H, L]. The facial nerve (cranial nerve VII) is motor to the muscles of facial expression, and sensory to part of the ear canal. The vestibulocochlear nerve (cranial nerve VIII) and maxillary nerve (cranial nerve V_2) are sensory only, while the trochlear nerve (cranial nerve IV) and hypoglossal nerve (cranial nerve XII) are motor only.

14. The answer is 4 [Chapter 48 II]. The jejunum and the descending colon are normally palpable within the abdomen. The ileum and transverse colon are too cranial and have too short a mesentery to be detected. Only the left kidney is palpable over its full length. The ovaries are too small and located too far cranially to be palpable, and the adrenal glands are too small and too deeply situated in fat at the cranial pole of each kidney to be accessible.

15. The answer is 4 [Chapter 25 I; Chapter 26 I A]. Although most dogs possess an ossified clavicle, the bone is very small and embedded entirely within the substance of the brachiocephalicus muscle. The attachment of the thoracic limb in dogs, as in most domestic quadrupeds, is entirely muscular.

16. The answer is 3 [Chapter 8 IV B 3]. The adult dog has 42 permanent teeth, written as follows: 2 (I 3/3, C 1/1, P 4/4, M 2/3). There are 12 incisors (6 on the upper arcade and 6 on the lower arcade), 4 canines (2 on the upper arcade and 2 on the lower arcade), 16 premolars (8 on the upper arcade and 8 on the lower arcade), and 10 molars (4 on the upper arcade and 6 on the lower arcade).

17. The answer is 4 [Chapter 51 III C 4 b]. The contents of this beagle's anal sacs need to be expressed. The paired anal sacs receive the numerous openings of the tiny glands of the anal sacs, but it is the single duct from each anal sac that may become obstructed. These ducts open onto the internal region of the cutaneous zone of the anal canal. "Anal glands" is an incomplete term that is not specific enough to identify which glands associated with the anal region are under discussion. The circumanal glands are microscopic glands that open onto the skin surrounding the anal opening; although they can become enlarged or even tumorous, they cannot be manually expressed. The anal sinuses are simply the depressions between the anal columns in the columnar region of the anal canal.

18. The answer is 4 [Chapter 34 I A–D]. Muscles of the neck (i.e., the longus colli, scalenus), the abdomen (i.e., the external and internal obliques and the rectus abdominis), and the thoracic limb (i.e., much of the musculature of the shoulder) are associated with the thoracic wall.

19. The answer is 4 [Table 28–2; Chapter 30 II G 2]. Inability to flex the elbow indicates loss of function of the cranial brachial muscle group (including the biceps brachii and brachialis). These muscles are primarily innervated by the musculocutaneous nerve.

20. The answer is 2 [Chapter 9 I A 2 a]. The correct sequence of arteries representing the central channel of arterial blood flow to the head is the common carotid artery, the external carotid artery, the maxillary artery, and the infraorbital artery.

21. The answer is 3 [Chapter 41 III B 1]. The linea alba is a single, poorly vascularized and poorly innervated collagenous structure along the ventral midline. It extends from the superficial to the deep surface of the abdominal wall. The terminal aponeuroses of all of the muscles that contribute to the rectus sheath attach to it, either superficially or deeply.

22. The answer is 2 [Chapter 5 I C 2; Figure 5–2]. The ductus arteriosus bypasses the pulmonary circulation in the fetus and persists in adults as the ligamentum arteriosum. The foramen ovale also bypasses the pulmonary circulation; the remnant in the adult is the fossa ovalis. The ductus venosus bypasses the hepatic circulation. The round ligament of the liver is the adult remnant of the umbilical vein.

23. The answer is 3 [Chapter 18 I B 1]. There are five regions in the vertebral column: the cervical, thoracic, lumbar, sacral, and caudal and regions.

24. The answer is 2 [Chapter 60 I A 2 b]. In the pelvic limb, from proximal to distal, the main channel of arterial flow passes from the external iliac artery to the femoral artery, then to the popliteal artery, the cranial tibial artery, and the dorsal pedal artery.

25. The answer is 4 [Chapter 53 II A 1]. The vestibular plexus is an extensive venous network that surrounds the vulvar opening. Engorgement of the plexus and the associated vulvar enlargement are early steps in sexual behavior.

26. The answer is 2 [Chapter 25 II E 1 b]. By definition, the dewclaw is digit I.

27. The answer is 3 [Chapter 8 II G 1 b]. The ventral nasal meatus is the only passage that leads to the nasopharynx and thence to the esophagus. The dorsal and middle meati end blindly in the nasal cavity and attempts to pass a nasogastric tube through these meati will result in epistaxis. The common nasal meatus is not related to the nasopharynx throughout its dimension, and, because of its small diameter, will not accept a nasogastric tube.

28. The answer is 3 [Chapter 31 II A 1 b]. The teres major muscle is palpable along the caudal border of the axilla. The pectoral muscles are more related to the cranial edge of the axilla. The teres minor has nothing to do with defining the axillary space.

29. The answer is 3 [Chapter 19 II A]. There are 8 cervical spinal cord segments, 13 thoracic spinal cord segments, 7 lumbar spinal cord segments, 3 sacral spinal cord segments, and 5 caudal spinal cord segments. The spinal cord segments correlate with the vertebrae in the thoracic, lumbar, and sacral regions, but deviate in the cervical and caudal regions. (There are 7 cervical vertebrae and 20–23 caudal vertebrae, as opposed to 8 and 5 segments, respectively.)

30. The answer is 2 [Chapter 4 II A 2 b (3)]. The conus medullaris is the gradually narrowing region of the spinal cord caudal to the lumbar intumescence. Spinal cord segments S2 through Cd5 compose the conus medullaris, which terminates at approximately the level of vertebrae L6–L7. The cauda equina is the collection of elongated nerve roots in the caudal part of the vertebral canal, and the filum terminale is the termination of the dura mater. "Conus sacralis" is a fanciful term.

31. The answer is 1 [Chapter 55 I D]. The pecten pubis (pubic brim) forms the ventral part of the pelvic inlet and is palpable. The dorsal part, or sacral promontory, is not palpable, nor are the lateral parts, which are formed by the arcuate line along the medial surface of the iliac shafts. Although the iliac crest is palpable, this structure is not related to the pelvic inlet. The ischium is positioned too far caudally to contribute to the pelvic inlet.

32. The answer is 2 [Chapter 15 VI B 1]. The optic nerve (cranial nerve II) develops as an outgrowth of the optic cup of the diencephalon. Like brain tissue, the optic nerve is surrounded by neuroglia (as opposed to Schwann cells, which surround most peripheral nerves). The optic nerve also has meninges, complete with a subarachnoid space that is continuous with that of the brain.

33. The answer is 3 [Chapter 37 VI A 1]. The brachiocephalic trunk is located in the dorsal portion of the cranial mediastinum. The aortic arch, tracheal bifurcation, and tracheobronchial lymph nodes are located in the dorsal portion of the middle mediastinum.

34. The answer is 2 [Chapter 61 II D]. The femoral nerve, the "key" nerve of the pelvic limb, innervates the quadriceps femoris muscle—the major extensor of the stifle. Without normal functioning of this nerve, the dog cannot bear weight on the limb because the stifle cannot be held in extension.

35. The answer is 4 [Chapter 21 II A 1 b (1) (b); Chapter 35 I B 1 a]. Dorsal intercostal arteries 1–12 each give off a spinal branch, which enters the vertebral canal to contribute to the arterial supply of the spinal cord. Only dorsal intercostal arteries 4 or 5–12 arise from the thoracic aorta; the first several are branches of the thoracic vertebral artery. The dorsal intercostal arteries course distally along the caudal border of the associated rib, not the cranial border. They supply both the skin and the muscle of the lateral thoracic wall.

36. The answer is 3 [Chapter 28 II A 3 a]. Of the muscles listed (i.e., the biceps brachii, triceps brachii, pronator teres, and deltoideus), the deltoideus is the only muscle that has its distal attachment to the upper humerus, and thus would displace the humerus as described.

37. The answer is 1 [Chapter 2 II B]. The mammary glands are modified sweat glands. The progenitors develop in both sexes, but regress in males. The glandular tissue of each gland is separate from the others. Arterial supply is shared among several glands and arrives from numerous arteries, including the intercostals. The glands have an extensive and partially interconnecting meshwork of lymphatic drainage, a fact that becomes important when one considers the treatment of mammary adenocarcinoma. Sensory innervation is supplied to the mammary glands.

38. The answer is 4 [Chapter 42 I A]. The transversalis fascia anchors the parietal peritoneum to the internal abdominal wall, just as the endothoracic fascia anchors the parietal pleura to the internal thoracic wall. The intermuscular fascia of the abdomen are external to the transversalis fascia.

39. The answer is 3 [Chapter 34 I E; Figure 34–2]. The lumbar part of the diaphragm includes the right and left diaphragmatic crura, from which strong muscular bundles radiate. The central tendinous portion of the diaphragm is completely surrounded by the muscular part on all sides, and does not directly attach to the body wall at any point. The caval foramen lies in the central tendon—the esophageal hiatus has at least partly muscular borders, and the aortic hiatus is simply the passageway between the crura. The costal and lumbar portions of the muscular part of the diaphragm are smoothly continuous.

40. The answer is 4 [Chapter 13 IV A 1 a]. The cerebellum is the seat of control of coordination and posture.

41. The answer is 1 [Chapter 34 I E 2; Table 34–1]. The diaphragm is innervated by the phrenic nerve, which is derived from the ventral roots of cervical spinal nerves 5, 6, and 7. The rectus thoracis, serratus dorsalis caudalis, and internal intercostal muscles are innervated by branches of adjacent intercostal nerves.

42. The answer is 3 [Chapter 26 III B 1 a, 2 a]. The modifications of the ulna into the trochlear notch, radial notch, and medial and lateral coronoid processes all deal with articulations at the elbow. Distal to the marked specializations for articulation with the humerus, the ulna narrows to an unspecialized shaft of bone that generally tapers to a nondescript termination at the carpus.

43. The answer is 2 [Chapter 52 III]. The correct sequence of the flow of semen through the male reproductive tract is epididymis, ductus deferens, prostatic urethra, pelvic urethra. The epididymis is the convoluted tubular structure that stores maturing spermatozoa following their production by the testis. The tail of the epididymis is continuous with the ductus deferens. The ductus deferens passes through the inguinal canal (as part of the spermatic cord) to reach the prostatic urethra. From the prostatic urethra, the semen flows to the pelvic urethra, and then to the penile urethra, which leads to the exterior of the body.

44. The answer is 1 [Chapter 61 II H 2 f]. This dog has most likely sustained injury to the tibial nerve, which innervates the hock extensors and digital flexors. The common peroneal nerve innervates the hock flexors and digital extensors, and hence is not involved in this lameness. Both the tibial and common peroneal nerves are branches of the sciatic nerve; therefore, injury to the sciatic nerve would be reflected as compromise of the functions of both the tibial and common peroneal nerves.

45. The answer is 2 [Chapter 3 II A, B, D]. Hyaline cartilage and ligaments are both avascular; therefore, these tissues heal poorly. All forms of bone are well vascularized and therefore heal well. Therefore, any pairing of bone with either ligament or cartilage is incorrect, and only the pairing of ligament and cartilage is correct.

46. The answer is 4 [Chapter 16 I A 4]. The infraorbital foramen is readily palpable on the maxilla a little less than halfway along the distance between the eye and the external nose. The mandibular lymph nodes are palpable in normal dogs, as are two of the laryngeal cartilages. The parotid duct does open into the oral vestibule, but opposite the upper carnassial tooth.

47. The answer is 3 [Chapter 12 III A 2]. The pharyngeal musculature consists of one dilator (the stylopharyngeus muscle) and several constrictors (the pterygopharyngeus, palatopharyngeus, hyopharyngeus, and thyropharyngeus cricopharyngeus muscles). These muscles aid in swallowing and are all innervated by the glossopharyngeal and vagus nerves (cranial nerves IX and X, respectively). The musculature receives no innervation from the accessory nerve (cranial nerve XI) and is distinct from the laryngeal musculature.

48. The answer is 3 [Chapter 58 III]. The articulation between the rounded femoral condyles and the flattened tibial condyles is notably poor. The menisci and their associated ligaments, including the cruciate ligaments, all assist in improving the fit between the femur and the tibia. The range of motion of the normal stifle is quite narrow, restricted mainly to extension and flexion. The thoracic limbs, not the pelvic limbs, bear 60% of the body's weight.

49. The answer is 4 [Chapter 32 I B 1 b]. The diaphragm forms a convex arc that extends into the bony thorax. The cranial placement of some of the digestive viscera (caudal to the diaphragm) results in the ability to hear digestive sounds over a considerable portion of the caudoventral bony thorax during auscultation in dogs of all ages. It would be erroneous to order radiographs or rush to perform surgery on this puppy!

50. The answer is 1 [Chapter 42 III C 2]. Peritoneal ligaments are bands of peritoneum that connect one organ to another. They contain few (if any) vascular or nervous structures. Mesenteries connect abdominal organs to the abdominal wall and transmit nervous and vascular structures.

51. The answer is 3 [Chapter 51 II A; Figure 51–1A]. The peritoneum forms five pouches within the pelvic region, two of which are paired. From dorsal to ventral, these pouches are the paired pararectal fossae, the rectogenital pouch, the vesicogenital pouch, and the pubovesical pouch. Remembering the dorsal to ventral order of the three organ systems that are represented in the pelvic region—the gastrointestinal system, the reproductive system, and the urinary system—can help one to remember the order of the peritoneal pouches: the paired pararectal fossae extend laterally along each side of the rectum, the rectogenital pouch lies between the rectum and the uterus or prostate gland, the vesicogenital pouch lies between the uterus or ducti deferentia and the urinary bladder (*vesico* = hollow organ), and the pubovesical pouch lies between the neck of the urinary bladder and the pubis.

52. The answer is 3 [Chapter 13 VI A]. Arterial blood arrives to the arterial circle of the brain from the basilar and internal carotid arteries and is distributed a total of eight arteries (i.e., four sets of paired arteries), supplying the cerebrum and rostral cerebellum. The middle cerebral artery is the largest artery supplying the brain.

53. The answer is 1 [Chapter 20 III A 1]. The superficial cervical fascia is very loose in its attachments, while all parts of the deep cervical fascia are very tight. The looseness of the superficial fascial attachment in the cervical region allows the skin to be readily grasped and elevated, providing a convenient site for the administration of subcutaneous injections. There is no "dorsolateral cervical fascia."

54. The answer is 1 [Figure 51–2A; Chapter 52 II]. The vulva depends considerably ventrally to the ischiatic arch, and thus the rod must be directed dorsally until the bony pelvis is passed; only then can the rod be successfully directed cranially into the vagina and then into the uterus. Direct cranial passage of an instrument through the vulvar lips will lodge the instrument in the clitoral fossa.

55. The answer is 1 [Chapter 42 III D 2 c]. The omental bursa (i.e., the space between the superficial and deep walls of the greater omentum) is continuous with the peritoneal cavity through the epiploic foramen. The ovarian bursa is formed from two parts of the broad ligament of the uterus (i.e., the mesovarium and mesosalpinx).

56. The answer is 1 [Chapter 27 II B 3 a (1)]. Rupture of the medial collateral ligament of the brachioantebrachial (elbow) joint would result in excessive lateral motion of the proximal radius and ulna. Rupture of the lateral collateral ligament would result in excessive medial motion. Rupture of the annular ligament would result in separation of the radial head from the ulnar notch (i.e., cranial movement of the radius). Rupture of the oblique ligament would lead to hyperextension.

57. The answer is 4 [Table 11–1]. The caninus draws the upper lip up and back, exposing the teeth. The platysma draws the angle of the lips caudally, the buccinator draws the cheek against the teeth, the orbicularis oculi closes the eyelids, and the mentalis stiffens the apical regions of the lower lip.

58. The answer is 1 [Chapter 50 I C 1; Chapter 58 II B 1]. Among the joints of the pelvic limb listed in the question, only the coxofemoral (hip) joint has five bones contributing to it: four in the os coxae (i.e., the ilium, ischium, pubis, and acetabular bone) and the femur. The four bones of the os coxae form the acetabulum, a deep cup on the lateral surface of the pelvis that houses the femoral head.

59. The answer is 2 [Chapter 4, Figure 4–4]. The lateral funiculus has nothing to do with the parasympathetic nervous system or the intermediate horn. Like all other components of the spinal cord, the lateral funiculus is covered by (rather than being superficial to) the pia mater.

60. The answer is 4 [Chapter 27 IV B 2]. The carpometacarpal joint is capable of very limited movement, making it difficult to access this joint via needle puncture. The antebrachiocarpal joint (of which the radiocarpal joint is a part) and the middle carpal joint open widely on full flexion of the carpus, facilitating needle puncture access.

61. The answer is 1 [Chapter 43 I C–D]. From cranial to caudal, the sequence of the intestinal regions is: descending duodenum, ascending duodenum, jejunum, ileum, ascending colon, transverse colon, descending colon.

62. The answer is 4 [Chapter 18 III E 2 b]. The hemal arches are associated with the caudal vertebrae and transmit the median caudal artery. The transverse canal transmits the vertebral artery. Options 2 and 3 are fanciful.

63. The answer is 2 [Chapter 44 I B 3 a; Table 44–1]. The ileocolic artery, a branch of the cranial mesenteric artery, supplies the cecum by way of the cecal branch (ileocecal artery). The middle colic artery supplies most of the transverse colon. Neither the celiac artery nor the caudal mesenteric artery supplies blood to the cecum.

64. The answer is 3 [Chapter 29 I A 2]. Arterial flow to and through the thoracic limb is proximal to distal via a central continuous channel that takes the following sequence: subclavian artery, axillary artery, brachial artery, median artery, palmar common digital artery, palmar proper digital artery.

65. The answer is 3 [Chapter 58 III B 2 c (4)]. The meniscofemoral ligament (also called the femoral ligament of the lateral meniscus) extends between the lateral meniscus and the medial condyle of the femur. The cruciate ligaments are named for their attachments to the tibia, not the femur; therefore, the caudal cruciate ligament (not the cranial cruciate ligament) attaches to the femur cranially and the tibia caudally. The intermeniscal ligament extends between the free cranial edges of the two menisci. The femoropatellar ligaments are entirely separate from the collateral ligaments.

66. The answer is 1 [Chapter 11 I B 1 a]. The parotid salivary gland is sometimes accompanied by accessory parotid glands, which lie along the course of, and empty into, the parotid duct.

67. The answer is 4 [Chapter 19 IV B]. Venous drainage of the spinal cord takes place through the variably developed internal, dorsal external, and ventral external venous plexuses. The three main arterial channels of the spinal cord do not have well developed satellite veins. Options 2 and 3 are fanciful.

68. The answer is 4 [Chapter 28 II B 1 b (1), 2 a (1)]. The biceps brachii inserts on the radial and ulnar tuberosities, has a single head (despite its name), and is innervated by the musculocutaneous nerve. The triceps brachii inserts on the olecranon tuber, and is innervated by the radial nerve. Both the biceps brachii and the long head of the triceps brachii originate on the scapula and insert on the antebrachium, and thus have no humeral attachment.

69. The answer is 3 [Chapter 35 III B 1]. The mediastinal lymphocenter is the most constant of the three potential lymphocenters of the thoracic region. The dorsal and ventral thoracic lymphocenters are highly variable. The cranial mediastinal lymph nodes are simply those of the ventral thoracic lymphocenter.

70. The answer is 3 [Chapter 45 II E 2]. The liver receives parasympathetic innervation directly from two large branches of the ventral vagal trunk, and one branch of the dorsal vagal trunk. Therefore, transection of the ventral vagal trunk would affect the parasympathetic innervation of the liver most severely. The dorsal branches from the right and left vagus nerves combine to form the dorsal vagal trunk, and the ventral branches from the right and left vagus nerves combine to form the ventral vagal trunk. Therefore, sectioning of the left dorsal vagal branch would remove only half of the input to the dorsal vagal trunk, and would have only half of the effect of sectioning the dorsal vagal trunk.

71. The answer is 3 [Chapter 4 II A 2 c, B 1 a]. The grey mater of the dorsal horn has sensory function. Grey matter is centrally, not superficially, located within the cord, and white matter does not contain neuronal cell bodies. The intermediate horn does house sympathetic neurons, but it is located in the thoracolumbar, not the cervical, region of the spinal cord.

72. The answer is 3 [Chapter 29 I E 1, 3 a; Chapter 60 I E 3 c]. In the pelvic limb, axial plantar common digital artery II is located on the medial side of digit II on the ground-facing surface of the paw. The axis of the digits passes between digits III and IV; the medial surface of digit II faces toward this axis and thus is termed "axial." The artery carries blood to only one digit, and therefore is termed "proper" (rather than "common"). Because the paw in question is that of the hindlimb, the modifier "plantar" must be used, rather than "palmar."

73. The answer is 3 [Chapter 52 I]. The scrotum and the vulva share the same developmental origin; as the primordium is vascularized, it retains its arterial supply into the definitive form. The positions of the scrotum in males and the vulva in females are not completely similar, and although the scrotum is a layered structure, the vulva is not.

74. The answer is 3 [Chapter 11 I B 2; II B 3]. Many lymph nodes of the head are variable in either occurrence (such as the lateral retropharyngeal nodes), number (such as the parotid and mandibular nodes), or both. Although the parotid and mandibular salivary glands do have "namesake" lymph nodes, the zygomatic and sublingual salivary glands do not; moreover, lymph nodes receive afferent lymphatics from, rather than sending efferent lymphatics to, the salivary glands. Lymphatic flow runs from superficial to deep, rather than the other way around. Bones of the head (as well as other regions of the body) do have efferent lymphatics.

75. The answer is 1 [Chapter 44 II C 1]. The suspensory ligament of the ovary resembles a ligament of the limb in form more than it resembles the other "ligaments" of the body cavities. This ligament is so stout that it requires separate sectioning during ovariohysterectomy. The proper ligament of the ovary and the mesovarium are not sectioned during ovariohysterectomy. Even if the mesovarium were sectioned, it is merely a peritoneal fold and would mount little resistance. The broad ligament is a thin peritoneal fold that, even when laden with fat, offers little resistance to tearing or cutting.

76. The answer is 1 [Table 29–1]. The caudal circumflex humeral artery, which arises from the subscapular artery (a branch of the axillary artery) actually supplies the greatest amount of blood to the triceps brachii muscle. In addition, the triceps brachii receives blood from the deep brachial and collateral ulnar arteries.

77. The answer is 3 [Chapter 18 III B 5 a (2) (c)]. Small bodies and costal foveae are characteristics of thoracic vertebrae in general, but only T11, the anticlinal vertebra, is characterized by a short spinous process that inclines neither cranially nor caudally.

78. The answer is 2 [Chapter 14 IV B 1 a–b]. Endolymph fills the membranous labyrinth, of which the cochlear and semicircular ducts are a part. The semicircular canals are part of the bony labyrinth, which is filled with perilymph. Endolymph is removed from the inner ear via the endolymphatic duct and sac.

79. The answer is 2 [Chapter 60 III B 1 a]. The superficial inguinal lymph nodes may be palpable in healthy dogs, but not as readily as the popliteal lymph node. This node is normally palpable at the caudal surface of the stifle, between the heads of the semimembranosus and biceps femoris muscles. The femoral nodes are inconstant, and even when present, are too small and too deep to be detected. The medial iliac lymph nodes are large and constant, but they are positioned adjacent to the abdominal aorta between the deep circumflex iliac and external iliac arteries and are not palpable.

80. The answer is 4 [Chapter 53 I C 1]. The prostatic artery is the large, ventrally directed first branch of the internal pudendal artery that supplies most of the pelvic structures in male dogs. The dorsal artery of the penis is the terminal continuation of the internal pudendal artery. The "internal pelvic artery" and the "great perineal artery" are spurious.

81. The answer is 4 [Chapter 36 III E 1]. The arterial plexuses are networks of autonomic fibers, both sympathetic and parasympathetic, that surround the major arteries as they travel into the thoracic limb. The plexuses branch with the arteries and are distributed to essentially the same area as the vessels.

82. The answer is 2 [Chapter 46 IV C 1]. The uterine horns are the elongate paired portions of the uterus where the litter is gestated. The uterine tube is the small-bore tube that serves to conduct the oocyte (before fertilization) and the ovum (after fertilization) to the uterine horn. The uterine body is a short region at the juncture of the horns that serves simply to conduct the fetuses to the cervix, which is the muscular sphincter between the uterus and the vagina.

83. The answer is 4 [Chapter 29 I]. Arteries are named by what they supply; therefore, the main artery supplying the latissimus dorsi is the thoracodorsal artery, regardless of the artery's source. (The latissimus dorsi covers a large part of the lateral thoracic wall.)

84. The answer is 4 [Chapter 18 III D]. The dorsal sacral foramina transmit the dorsal branches of the sacral nerves and vessels. The sacrum is formed from the fusion of the three sacral vertebrae, and articulates with the iliac wing (not the ischial wing). The bone is completely fused, with no mobile parts.

85. The answer is 1 [Chapter 15 IV A]. The bulbar and palpebral conjunctiva are essentially identical in structure and are distinguishable only by position. The bulbar conjunctiva covers the sclera and becomes continuous with the epithelium at the level of the limbus. The palpebral conjunctiva lines the inner surface of the upper, lower, and third eyelids.

86. The answer is 3 [Chapter 39 I]. Percussion of the thoracic wall over intercostal spaces 6–9 should reveal the hollow sound of an air-filled lung. Percussion is performed over the intercostal spaces rather than the ribs. The spaces cranial to space 6 are covered by the shoulder musculature, and those caudal to space 9 overlie the diaphragm or digestive viscera rather than the lungs.

87. The answer is 3 [Chapter 29 I E 3 a (2); Figure 29–2]. The artery located on the medial surface of the dorsal side of digit II is the axial dorsal proper digital artery II. The axis of the digits passes between digits III and IV; the medwial surface of digit II faces toward this axis and thus is termed "axial." The artery carries blood to only one digit, and hence is termed "proper" (as opposed to "common").

88. The answer is 1 [Chapter 32 I B 2 a]. The thoracic cavity encloses and thus contains the pleural and pericardial cavities and the mediastinal space. The pleural cavity lies external to the mediastinal space. Neither the pleural nor pericardial cavities contain anything other than serous fluid.

89. The answer is 2 [Chapter 4 II A 2 b (1)]. The cervical intumescence is an enlargement of the spinal cord between spinal cord segments C6 and T1. This enlargement is caused by the increased number of neurons associated innervating the thoracic limb.

90. The answer is 3 [Chapter 9 II B 2 a (2)]. The facial vein, formed from the confluence of the dorsal nasal vein and the angular vein of the eye, significantly departs from the course of the facial artery. The facial vein terminates by entering the linguofacial trunk. There is no common carotid vein in the body.

91. The answer is 4 [Chapter 30 I B 1]. The brachial plexus is formed from the ventral branches of cervical nerves 6, 7, and 8 (C6, C7, C8) and thoracic nerves 1 and 2 (T1, T2).

92. The answer is 5 [Chapter 8 I A 2 a (1)]. Among the bones listed (the frontal bone, maxilla, incisive bone, palatine bone, and temporal bone), only the temporal bone does not contribute to the viscerocranium (i.e., the facial region). Though the frontal bone also contributes to the formation of the neurocranium, its rostral regions form part of the face.

93. The answer is 4 [Chapter 6 II E; Chapter 47 III B]. Although both the adrenal glands and the kidneys possess a hilus, only the adrenal vein exits the adrenal gland at the adrenal hilus. The arterial supply to the adrenal gland arrives via arterioles that penetrate the fibrous capsule of the gland on all surfaces. Both the kidneys and the adrenal glands are positioned retroperitoneally and covered in a thick layer of retroperitoneal fat. Both organs also possess a cortex and a medulla.

94. The answer is 4 [Chapter 59 II B 2; Chapter 62 II B 2]. The caudal crural abductor is both too small and too deep to be palpable. The other caudal thigh muscles (i.e., the biceps femoris, the semitendinosus, and the semimembranosus) are readily palpable.

95. The answer is 1 [Chapter 17 I A 1; Chapter 18 III B 4]. The great extension–flexion ability of the thoracolumbar area, not the cervical region, represents the vertebral column's largest contribution to the running gait. The caudal cervical region is the region of the vertebral column associated with the most mobility. Rotation is mainly accomplished in the thoracic region of the vertebral column. The ability of the dog to curl up when sleeping is mainly afforded by the relatively great lateral mobility of the thoracolumbar area.

96. The answer is 2 [Chapter 40 III A 2]. The abdomen essentially lacks a caudal wall, because the caudal region of the abdominal cavity is continuous with the pelvic cavity. The diaphragm forms the cranial boundary of the abdominal cavity, and the abdominal oblique muscles (internal and external) and the transversus abdominis muscle form the lateral and ventral walls of the abdomen.

97. The answer is 3 [Chapter 13 VI B 1 b]. The dural venous sinuses are located between the two layers of the dura mater. They drain the deeper structures of the brain and the diploe of the skull. Some of the sinuses are paired, and some are not.

98. The answer is 3 [Chapter 4 II A 2 d (2)]. Although the central canal contains cerebrospinal fluid, it is located at the center of the spinal cord. Attempts to access the central canal would result in spinal cord injury. The subarachnoid space contains cerebrospinal fluid and is accessible at the lumbosacral junction (i.e., the lumbar cistern, a dilatation of the subarachnoid space between the spinal cord and the dorsal region of the vertebral column). The cerebellomedullary cistern is also a dilatation of the subarachnoid space and is sometimes accessed to obtain cerebrospinal fluid for analysis.

99. The answer is 2 [Table 20–5]. The quadratus femoris is an intrinsic muscle of the pelvic limb, extending between the pelvis and femur. The quadratus lumborum, iliacus, and psoas major and minor muscles are all members of the thoracolumbar hypaxial muscle group.

100. The answer is 4 [Chapter 60 I B 3 b]. The cranial gluteal artery lies buried deeply below major muscle masses throughout its course and is inaccessible to palpation. The pulse can be detected in the femoral artery (at the femoral triangle), in the dorsal pedal artery (at the dorsal surface of the tarsus), and in the saphenous artery (approximately two thirds of the way along the tibial shaft).

101. The answer is 3 [Chapter 50 I A 1, C 1]. The acetabulum is not a bone; it is the deep cup on the lateral surface of the articulated bony pelvis, contributed to by the ilium, the ischium, the pubis, and the acetabular bone. The bony pelvis is the bony ring formed by the four bones of the pelvic girdle (i.e., the ilium, the ischium, the pubis, and the acetabular bone), the sacrum, and the first two caudal vertebrae.

102. The answer is 4 [Chapter 30 II J; Table 36–1]. The lateral thoracic nerve is not sensory; rather, it is motor to the cutaneous trunci and deep pectoral muscles. Branches of the dorsal branches of the thoracic spinal nerves, ventral branches of the thoracic spinal nerves, and axillary nerve are sensory to the superficial thoracic wall and shoulder region.

103. The answer is 2 [Chapter 11 II B 3 a; Chapter 12 III B 1 b (3), 2 b (1)–(2)]. The medial retropharyngeal lymph node is positioned dorsal to the wall of the pharynx, ventral to the wing of the atlas, and is too deep and too caudal to contribute to the ring of lymphoid tissue that surrounds the entrance to the deeper regions of the respiratory and digestive tracts. The palatine and pharyngeal tonsils are distinct aggregations of lymphoid tissue located on the lateral oropharyngeal wall and in the nasopharynx, respectively. The lingual tonsil is a diffuse collection of lymphoid tissue that is located in the oropharyngeal mucosa and contributes to the ring of lymphoid tissue guarding the deeper regions of the respiratory and digestive tracts.

104. The answer is 2 [Chapter 59 II B 3 b (2)]. The femoral triangle is a landmark on the medial surface of the thigh formed by the caudal belly of the sartorius muscle, the pectineus muscle, and the vastus medialis muscle. Several large nervous and vascular structures, including the femoral artery and vein and the saphenous nerve, pass through this triangle. The femoral nerve dissipates so quickly in the substance of the quadriceps femoris muscle that it never reaches the femoral triangle, although its sensory branch, the saphenous nerve, does.

105. The answer is 3 [Chapter 21 I C 2]. The tracheal trunk, the largest lymphatic vessel in the neck, receives efferents from the medial retropharyngeal lymph node (not the deep cervical lymph nodes). The left tracheal duct enters the thoracic duct, and the right tracheal duct enters the great vessels cranial to the heart.

106. The answer is 3 [Chapter 42 III B 1 a]. No organs are contained within the peritoneal cavity. The "intraperitoneal" organs (e.g., the liver, gonads, uterus) are organs that are covered on almost all surfaces by visceral peritoneum, as opposed to the "retroperitoneal" organs, which are applied to the body wall, and therefore have only one surface that is covered with visceral peritoneum.

107. The answer is 4 [Chapter 51 V B 5]. The pudendal nerve is a somatic nerve, and therefore, is not involved with autonomic innervation. The lumbar sympathetic trunk provides the fibers that travel to the caudal mesenteric plexus and thus ultimately give rise to the hypogastric nerves, which deliver sympathetic fibers to the pelvic plexus. The pelvic nerve delivers parasympathetic fibers to the same plexus.

108. The answer is 4 [Chapter 38 II D 3 e, 4 d]. The trabecula septomarginalis is a band of muscle that crosses the lumen of the right ventricle, carrying conduction fibers to the free right ventricular wall. The trabecula septomarginalis is found only in the right ventricle. Both ventricles have chordae tendineae, papillary muscles, and trabeculae carneae.

109. The answer is 5 [Chapter 21 III A]. The back receives its blood supply from the dorsal intercostal arteries and the costoabdominal artery (i.e., the segmental artery following the last rib) in the thoracic region, and from the lumbar arteries in the lumbar region. The intercostal, costoabdominal, and lumbar arteries are all direct branches of the aorta. No collateral branches are supplied by the renal, gonadal, or external iliac arteries.

110. The answer is 4 [Chapter 59 II B 2 a (2) (c), d (2), 3 a (2), C 2 a, b (1); Table 59–1]. The peroneus longus muscle does not contribute to the common calcanean tendon. This tendon attaches to the tuber calcanei and is formed from the tendons of the biceps femoris, semitendinosus, gracilis, gastrocnemius, and superficial digital flexor muscles.

111. The answer is 3 [Chapter 22 II]. The ventral branches, not the dorsal branches, of nerves C6–C8 contribute to the brachial plexus. The cutaneous nature of the medial division of the dorsal branch of the cervical nerves is characteristic of cervical nerves. Cervical nerves supply the epaxial musculature by their dorsal branches and the hypaxial musculature by their ventral branches. The dorsal branches of nerves C1 and C2 form the suboccipital nerve (nerve C1) and the greater occipital, great auricular, and transverse cervical nerves (nerve C2).

112. The answer is 4 [Chapter 54 I B]. The gonads (i.e., the ovaries or the testes) originate in the abdominal cavity and are innervated by the lumbar splanchnic nerves, as opposed to the pelvic plexus. The pelvic plexus supplies autonomic innervation to the rectum and anal canal, as well as to the uterus, vagina, and clitoris in females and the penis in males.

113. The answer is 2 [Chapter 23 IV B]. The common carotid artery, not the external carotid artery, is located within the carotid sheath. Other structures housed by the carotid sheath include the vagosympathetic trunk, the tracheal lymphatic duct, the internal jugular vein, and the recurrent laryngeal nerve.

114. The answer is 2 [Chapter 44 I B 1]. The spleen is supplied by the splenic artery, a branch of the celiac artery. The cranial mesenteric artery supplies the cecum by means of the ileocolic artery, the pancreas by means of the caudal pancreaticoduodenal artery, and the descending colon by means of the middle colic arteries.

115. The answer is 3 [Chapter 21 A 2; Chapter 35 I C 2 c (2) (b)]. Intercostal arteries can arise from the descending aorta, the internal thoracic artery, and the thoracic vertebral artery. The vertebral artery ascends the neck to supply its bony and soft tissue structures, as well as structures of the cranial cavity. The thoracic vertebral artery, however, is contained within the thorax and typically contributes to the arterial supply of the first three or four intercostal spaces.

116. The answer is 1 [Chapter 38 III B]. Although many of the cardiac veins are parallel to the arteries, relatively few veins share a name with the arteries they accompany. Most cardiac veins are paired. The small cardiac (Thebesian) veins are microscopic vessels in the myocardium that open directly into the associated heart chamber, including the ventricles. Most blood from the ventricular walls reaches the right atrium via the coronary sinus.

117. The answer is 3 [Chapter 62 II B 2 c, D 3, E 3]. The pulse is not accessible where the saphenous artery departs from the femoral artery on the medial thigh. However, a pulse can be detected as the saphenous artery crosses the medial side of the distal third of the tibia, as the femoral artery passes through the femoral triangle, and the dorsal pedal artery crosses the tarsus to course into the metatarsus.

Index

Page numbers in *italics* denote figures; those followed by a t denote tables; those followed by a Q denote study questions